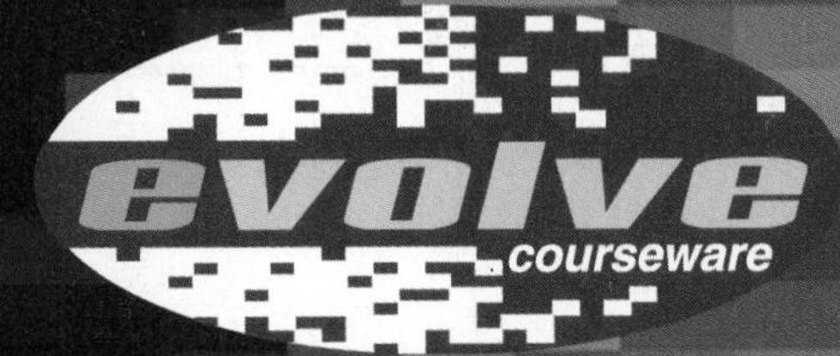

The Latest Evolution in Learning.

Evolve provides online access to free learning resources and activities designed specifically for the textbook you are using in your class. The resources will provide you with information that enhances the material covered in the book and much more.

Visit the Web address listed below to start your learning evolution today!

LOGIN: *http://evolve.elsevier.com/Shiland*

Evolve Online Courseware for *Shiland's Mastering Healthcare Terminology* offers the following features:

- **Weblinks**
  This exciting resource lets you link to hundreds of active websites keyed specifically to the content of this book. The weblinks are updated regularly, with new links added as they develop.

- **Links to Related Products**
  See what else Elsevier Science has to offer in a specific field of interest.

Think outside the book...evolve.

Mastering Healthcare Terminology

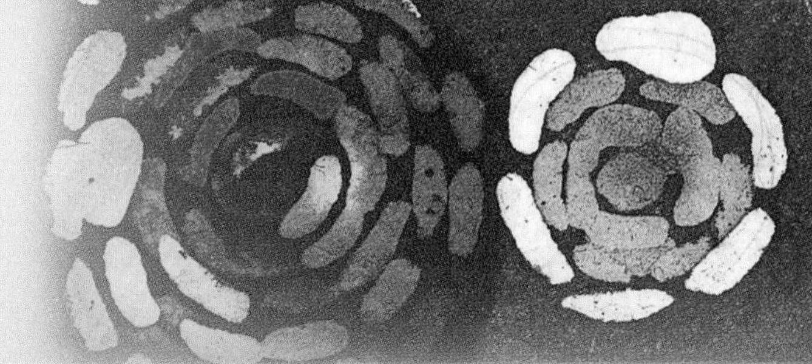

Mastering Healthcare Terminology

Betsy J. Shiland, MS, RHIA, CPHQ, CTR

Assistant Professor
Health Information Technology
Community College of Philadelphia
Philadelphia, Pennsylvania

with 376 illustrations

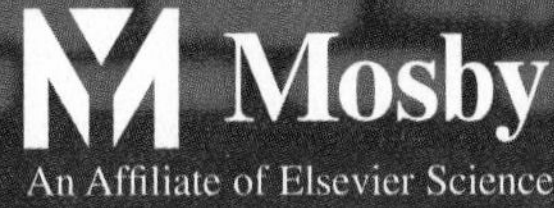

Mosby
An Affiliate of Elsevier Science

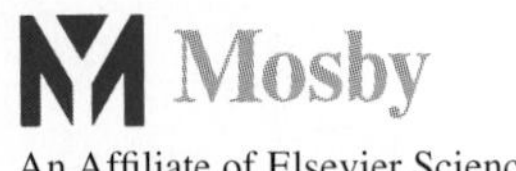

An Affiliate of Elsevier Science

11830 Westline Industrial Drive
St. Louis, Missouri 63146

MASTERING HEALTHCARE TERMINOLOGY 0-323-01615-4

NOTICE

Medical Terminology is an ever-changing field. Standard safety precautions must be followed, but as new research and clinical experience broaden our knowledge, changes in treatment and drug therapy may become necessary or appropriate. Readers are advised to check the most current product information provided by the manufacturer of each drug to be administered to verify the recommended dose, the method and duration of administration, and contraindications. It is the responsibility of the licensed prescriber, relying on experience and knowledge of the patient, to determine dosages and the best treatment for each individual patient. Neither the publisher nor the author assumes any liability for any injury and/or damage to persons or property arising from this publication.

Library of Congress Cataloging-in-Publication Data

Shiland, Betsy J.
Mastering healthcare terminology / Betsy J. Shiland.
p. ; cm.
Includes bibliographical references and index.
ISBN 0-323-01615-4 (alk. paper)
1. Medicine—Terminology. I. Title.
[DNLM: 1. Terminology. W 15 S556m 2003]
R123 .S454 2003
610'.14—dc21 2002037999

Publishing Director: Andrew Allen
Executive Editor: Jeanne Wilke
Senior Developmental Editor: Linda Woodard
Publishing Services Manager: Pat Joiner
Senior Project Manager: Rachel E. Dowell
Designer: Julia Dummitt
Medical Illustrator: Jeanne Robertson
Cover Design: Paul Fry

Printed in the United States of America

Last digit is the print number: 9 8 7 6 5 4 3 2 1

To my son, Thomas R. O'Hanlon,
who is my inspiration for all I do,
and my brother, Thomas W. Shiland,
who is my most constant supporter and mentor.

Reviewers

Gina Augustine, MLS, RT(R)
Coordinator, Advanced Level Radiographic Externship Program
St. Francis Hospital
New Castle, Pennsylvania

Marilyn Duran, RNP, MSN
Assistant Professor of Nursing
Arkansas State University
Jonesboro, Arizona

Ann Ehrlich, RT(R)
Senior Instructor, Radiology
Western States Chiropractic College;
Continuing Education Instructor, Radiography
Portland Community College
Portland, Oregon

Patricia Fergus, RN, RRT
Department of Endoscopy
Saint Louis University Hospital
St. Louis, Missouri

Sandra Hertkorn, LVN
Director Medical Office Programs
Nexus Speech Recognition,
Medical Office Careers
Sacramento, California

Kathleen Murphy, MS, CNMT, RT(N)
Associate Professor/Program Director
Gateway Community College
North Haven, Connecticut

Roxianne Snodgrass, MHSA, MT(ASCP)
Instructor, Medical Laboratory Technology
Orangeburg-Calhoun Technical College
Orangeburg, South Carolina

Sue Treitz, BSN, MA
Director, Nurse Assistant Program
Arapahoe Community College
Littleton, Colorado

Mary Weis, DVM
Professor of Biology
Collin County Community College
Plano, Texas

Brandy Ziesemer, MA, RHIA
Health Information Program Manager
Lake Sumter Community College
Leesburg, Florida

Preface

Beginning a healthcare career is like visiting a foreign country. If you want to converse with the inhabitants, you need to speak their language. If you are interested in a career in healthcare, fluency in its terminology is required. The goal of *Mastering Healthcare Terminology* is to help you learn the large number of terms that describe very specific healthcare conditions or procedures in the easiest, most effective manner possible.

We do not often think about what makes up our language, perhaps because we are so familiar with it. Prefixes, suffixes, and word roots make up both the English language and healthcare language. A student of terminology can develop a sizable vocabulary by learning these decodable word parts and the rules necessary to join them together. Memorizing eponyms, abbreviations, symbols, and nondecodable terms completes a healthcare professional's vocabulary.

ORGANIZATION OF THE BOOK

Mastering Healthcare Terminology has been designed for your success. Each feature has been chosen to help you learn this new language quickly and effectively. A variety of exercises appear at logical breaks in the text and are intended to reinforce the concepts covered.

Chapters 1 and 2 help orient you to the basic concepts necessary to learn healthcare terminology, which will be reinforced throughout the rest of the text.

Chapters 3 through 15 are body system chapters, each organized in the same way. The function of each system is introduced first, then its anatomy and physiology. Once the terms for normal function are covered, pathologic terms, diagnostic techniques, therapeutic interventions, pharmacologic terms, and common abbreviations are presented. Chapter 16 covers cancer terminology for all the body systems.

SPECIAL FEATURES

In each chapter, *Be Careful!* boxes cover the most common terminology errors and *Did You Know?* boxes relate interesting terminology factoids. Included in each body system chapter are a career box and an Internet project that is relevant to the system being studied. Each chapter ends with review exercises to test knowledge gained and a sample healthcare report that integrates that knowledge with a real-life scenario based on the case study that is threaded throughout the chapter.

APPENDIXES

The appendixes in this text should be bookmarked as your primary reference for an alphabetic listing of word components, including combining forms, prefixes, suffixes, and abbreviations. Answers to exercises and review questions follow the appendixes.

LEARNING AIDS

Included with *Mastering Healthcare Terminology* are a variety of learning aids intended to make your study of healthcare terminology as efficient and enjoyable as possible.

Mosby's Medical Terminology Online

Mosby's Medical Terminology Online to Accompany Mastering Healthcare Terminology is a great resource to supplement your textbook. This Web-delivered course supplement, available as a separate purchase, provides a range of visual, auditory, and interactive elements to reinforce your learning and synthesize concepts presented in the text. Interactive lesson reviews at the end of each module provide you with testing tools that are actually fun. Clicking on a bolded term provides you with the pronunciation. Related Internet resources can be accessed by clicking on the hypertext links provided throughout the text.

This online course supplement is accessible only if you have purchased the PIN code packaged with your book. If you did not purchase the book/PIN code package, ask your instructor for information or visit http://evolve.elsevier.com/Shiland to purchase.

CD-ROM with Extra Exercises

Your copy of *Mastering Healthcare Terminology* includes a complimentary program on CD that provides additional opportunities for word building and definition and application of language skills. This interactive program presents terminology in various healthcare documents to help you get used to seeing healthcare terms as they are presented in actual healthcare settings. A variety of exercises will help you memorize the word parts and their definitions, then combine the parts to form healthcare terms.

TO THE INSTRUCTOR

Instructor's Electronic Resource

The Instructor's Electronic Resource to accompany *Mastering Healthcare Terminology* consists of an Instructor's Manual, a Computerized Test Bank, and an Electronic Image Collection on CD. The Instructor's Manual and Computerized Test Bank are also available as a print product. Included in the Instructor's Manual is a course outline, chapter objectives, activities for the classroom, and many, many extra questions for students, including crosswords and word scrambles. The Computerized Test Bank offers over 1200 multiple-choice questions that can be sorted by subject matter and level of difficulty. The Electronic Image Collection includes all the images from the text that can be printed out.

Mosby's Medical Terminology Online

Connecting you and your students, *Mosby's Medical Terminology Online to Accompany Mastering Healthcare Terminology* was developed with a creative approach to education in mind. The more resources available to facilitate learning and the more varied your presentation, the greater the likelihood your students will comprehend and retain the material you want them to learn. Rather than replacing the textbook, this unique course supplement, delivered in a Web environment, provides a range of visual, auditory, and interactive elements to amplify text content, reinforce learning, synthesize concepts presented in the textbook, and demonstrate the practical application of medical language. Over 100 animations and slide shows convey difficult concepts that are impossible to demonstrate with static illustrations. A variety of communication options and administrative tools allow you to hold virtual office hours! See for yourself at http://evolve.elsevier.com/Shiland. Then contact your sales representative for more information about how to adapt the online companion to supplement your course.

Betsy J. Shiland

How to Use This Text

Mastering Healthcare Terminology has been designed for your success. Each feature has been chosen to help you learn healthcare language quickly and effectively. Healthcare terms are presented in logical order, beginning with each body system's anatomy and physiology, and progressing through pathology, diagnostic procedures, therapeutic interventions, and finally pharmacology. Along the way, colorful boxes, tables, and illustrations visually spark your interest, add to your knowledge, and aid in retention. Concepts, terms, and abbreviations for a topic are covered and then immediately followed by exercises that reinforce and assess your understanding and retention of the material. Each chapter ends with a review examination that asks you to apply the terms you have learned.

BEGIN AT THE BEGINNING

Chapter 1 covers the basics of word components, types of healthcare terms, pronunciation rules, singular/plural spelling, categories of healthcare terms, and study tips that you need to master before you move on to the remainder of the book. These are concepts that you will use repeatedly, and an understanding of these basics will help you successfully complete the course. If you find you are struggling in the later chapters, go back to Chapter 1 and review.

USE ALL THE FEATURES IN THE CHAPTER

Objectives

Each objective is a goal for you. An objective that asks you to "recognize, recall, and apply" terms is asking you to learn at three increasingly difficult levels. Recognition means "I know it when I see it," recall means "I can remember that term when asked what the definition is," and application means "I can use the term in context with an understanding of its definition." You should refer to these objectives before you study the chapter to see what your goals are and then again at the end of the chapter to see if you have accomplished them.

Case Study Boxes

Have you ever read an article in a newspaper that used an individual to illustrate the point of the story and find yourself skimming the rest of the article to see what happened to him or her? Would you like to have a peek into a career to see how a particular healthcare professional relates to patients? Our threaded case study boxes are designed to introduce you to a patient who is followed throughout the diagnostic and treatment process and to give you a glimpse of the responsibilities of a healthcare professional.

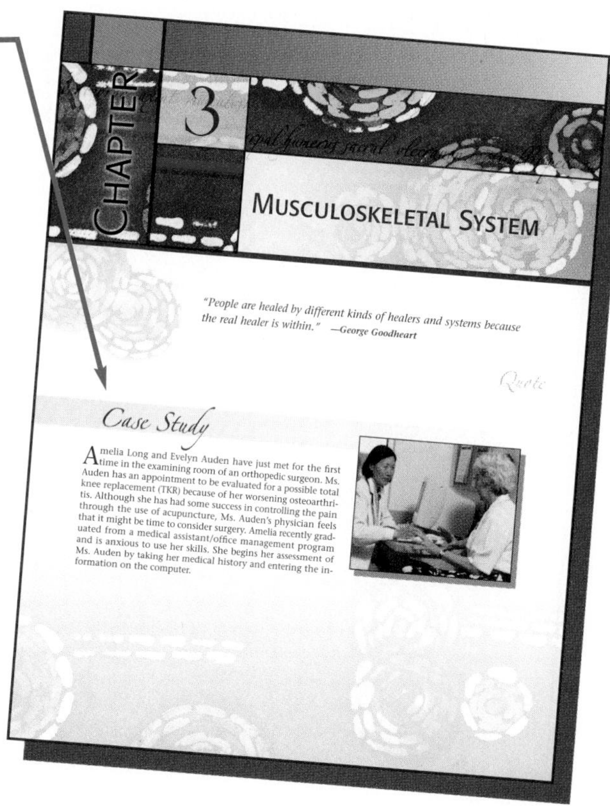

CHAPTER 3

MUSCULOSKELETAL SYSTEM

"People are healed by different kinds of healers and systems because the real healer is within." —**George Goodheart**

Case Study

Amelia Long and Evelyn Auden have just met for the first time in the examining room of an orthopedic surgeon. Ms. Auden has an appointment to be evaluated for a possible total knee replacement (TKR) because of her worsening osteoarthritis. Although she has had some success in controlling the pain through the use of acupuncture, Ms. Auden's physician feels that it might be time to consider surgery. Amelia recently graduated from a medical assistant/office management program and is anxious to use her skills. She begins her assessment of Ms. Auden by taking her medical history and entering the information on the computer.

Anatomy and Physiology

It is impossible to understand healthcare terminology without understanding the basic anatomy and physiology (A&P) of the human body. Each body system chapter describes and illustrates the relevant anatomy and physiology and explains how the system normally functions. Make sure you do the exercises after each A&P section to help you retain your new knowledge. Answers are provided in the back of the book.

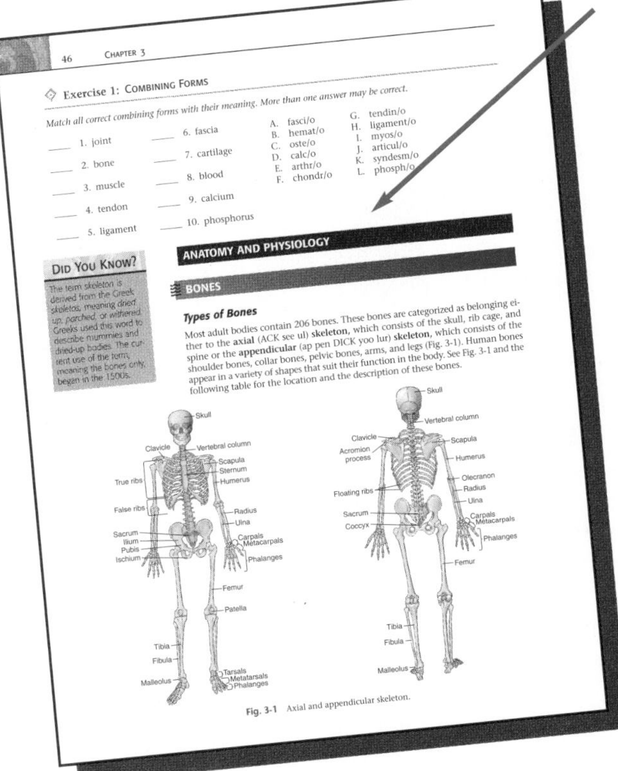

46 CHAPTER 3

Exercise 1: COMBINING FORMS

Match all correct combining forms with their meaning. More than one answer may be correct.

___ 1. joint
___ 2. bone
___ 3. muscle
___ 4. tendon
___ 5. ligament
___ 6. fascia
___ 7. cartilage
___ 8. blood
___ 9. calcium
___ 10. phosphorus

A. fasci/o
B. hemat/o
C. oste/o
D. calc/o
E. arthr/o
F. chondr/o
G. tendin/o
H. ligament/o
I. myos/o
J. articul/o
K. syndesm/o
L. phosph/o

DID YOU KNOW?

The term *skeleton* is derived from the Greek *skeletos,* meaning *dried up, parched,* or *withered.* Greeks used this word to describe mummies and dried-up bodies. The current use of the term, meaning the bones only, began in the 1500s.

ANATOMY AND PHYSIOLOGY

BONES

Types of Bones

Most adult bodies contain 206 bones. These bones are categorized as belonging either to the **axial** (ACK see ul) **skeleton,** which consists of the skull, rib cage, and spine or the **appendicular** (ap pen DICK yoo lur) **skeleton,** which consists of the shoulder bones, collar bones, pelvic bones, arms, and legs (Fig. 3-1). Human bones appear in a variety of shapes that suit their function in the body. See Fig. 3-1 and the following table for the location and the description of these bones.

Fig. 3-1 Axial and appendicular skeleton.

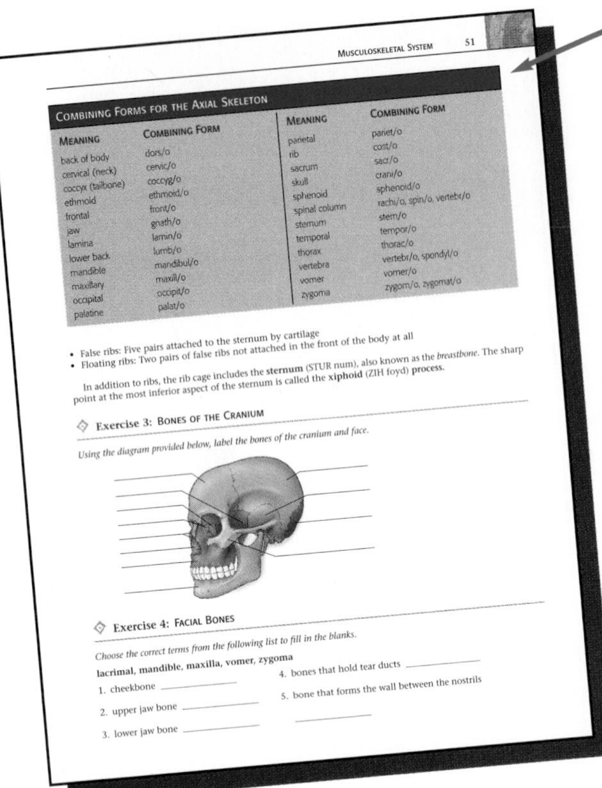

MUSCULOSKELETAL SYSTEM 51

COMBINING FORMS FOR THE AXIAL SKELETON

Meaning	Combining Form	Meaning	Combining Form
back of body	dors/o	parietal	pariet/o
cervical (neck)	cervic/o	rib	cost/o
coccyx (tailbone)	coccyg/o	sacrum	sacr/o
ethmoid	ethmoid/o	skull	crani/o
frontal	front/o	sphenoid	sphenoid/o
jaw	gnath/o	spinal column	rachi/o, spin/o, vertebr/o
lamina	lamin/o	sternum	stern/o
lower back	lumb/o	temporal	tempor/o
mandible	mandibul/o	thorax	thorac/o
maxillary	maxill/o	vertebra	vertebr/o, spondyl/o
occipital	occipit/o	vomer	vomer/o
palatine	palat/o	zygoma	zygom/o, zygomat/o

- False ribs: Five pairs attached to the sternum by cartilage
- Floating ribs: Two pairs of false ribs not attached in the front of the body at all

In addition to ribs, the rib cage includes the **sternum** (STUR num), also known as the *breastbone*. The sharp point at the most inferior aspect of the sternum is called the **xiphoid** (ZIH foyd) **process**.

Exercise 3: BONES OF THE CRANIUM

Using the diagram provided below, label the bones of the cranium and face.

Exercise 4: FACIAL BONES

Choose the correct terms from the following list to fill in the blanks.

lacrimal, mandible, maxilla, vomer, zygoma

1. cheekbone ________
2. upper jaw bone ________
3. lower jaw bone ________
4. bones that hold tear ducts ________
5. bone that forms the wall between the nostrils ________

Word Components

The majority of the terminology you learn is made of decodable word components—combining forms, prefixes, and suffixes. A sizable vocabulary can be built by learning the meanings of word components and how they go together to form healthcare terms. This text presents word components in separate tables in the anatomy and physiology section and in a separate column in the pathology, diagnostic procedures, and therapeutic interventions terms tables. Many exercises are provided to help you memorize these important terminology tools.

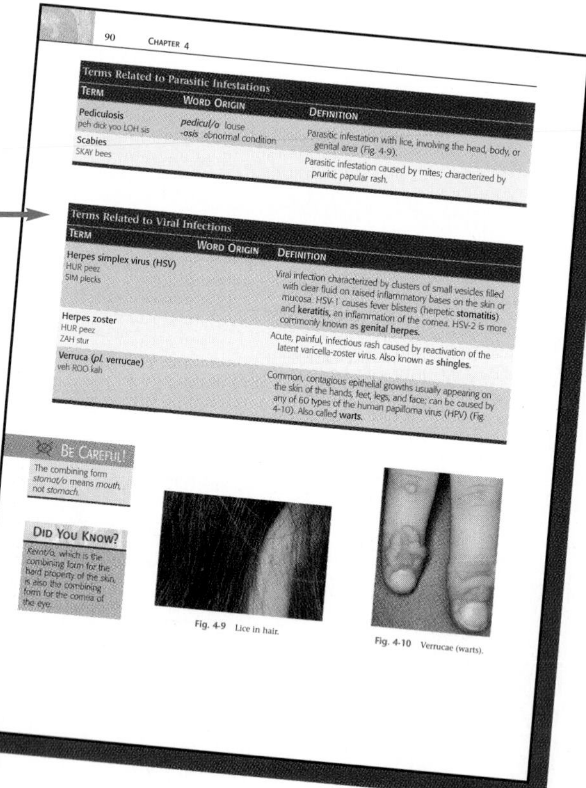

90 CHAPTER 4

Terms Related to Parasitic Infestations

Term	Word Origin	Definition
Pediculosis peh dick yoo LOH sis	*pedicul/o* louse *-osis* abnormal condition	Parasitic infestation with lice, involving the head, body, or genital area (Fig. 4-9).
Scabies SKAY bees		Parasitic infestation caused by mites; characterized by pruritic papular rash.

Terms Related to Viral Infections

Term	Word Origin	Definition
Herpes simplex virus (HSV) HUR peez SIM plecks		Viral infection characterized by clusters of small vesicles filled with clear fluid on raised inflammatory bases on the skin or mucosa. HSV-1 causes fever blisters (herpetic **stomatitis**) and **keratitis**, an inflammation of the cornea. HSV-2 is more commonly known as **genital herpes**.
Herpes zoster HUR peez ZAH stur		Acute, painful, infectious rash caused by reactivation of the latent varicella-zoster virus. Also known as **shingles**.
Verruca (*pl.* **verrucae**) veh ROO kah		Common, contagious epithelial growths usually appearing on the skin of the hands, feet, legs, and face; can be caused by any of 60 types of the human papilloma virus (HPV) (Fig. 4-10). Also called **warts**.

BE CAREFUL! The combining form *stomat/o* means *mouth*, not *stomach*.

DID YOU KNOW? *Kerat/o*, which is the combining form for the hard property of the skin, is also the combining form for the cornea of the eye.

Fig. 4-9 Lice in hair.

Fig. 4-10 Verrucae (warts).

Healthcare Terms

All pathology, diagnostic procedures, and interventions are organized in tables. Included in these tables are the pronunciation, origin, and meaning of the most frequently occurring disease and disorders and their treatment. This organization gives you a quick yet complete reference to the terminology you are most likely to encounter in a healthcare setting.

Pronunciations for the terms have been spelled out phonetically, so no knowledge of pronunciation symbols is necessary. All you have to do is read each syllable as you would if they were separate words, and make sure to put the stress on the syllable that is capitalized. It does help to read the word out loud. Once you have sounded out the syllables, try to say the word more quickly and fluidly. Audio pronunciations are available on the CD that accompanies the book.

Word origins are provided for those terms that can be "decoded." Understanding a term's origins—what its prefix, combining form, and suffix means—is immensely helpful in learning not only a single term, but a whole class of terms. Knowing that the suffix *-itis* means *inflammation* will help you recognize that any term that ends with *-itis* will be an inflammation of some part of the body, whether it be arthritis (inflammation of a joint), phlebitis (inflammation of a vein,) or gastritis (inflammation of the stomach).

Definitions of the terms are also given, along with any synonym or variation of the term.

Exercises follow these tables and the pharmacology and abbreviation sections to provide the practice needed to master the terms.

Special Information Boxes

Special information boxes are scattered throughout each chapter that offer interesting facts or cautions. *Did You Know?* boxes highlight the fascinating, sometimes strange history that underlies the origins of healthcare terms. *Be Careful!* boxes point out common pitfalls that students experience when healthcare terms and word parts are spelled similarly but have different meanings.

The Internet projects included in each chapter are intended to reinforce newly learned concepts and to help you find more information that could not be covered in the text. The interesting Websites that follow can be very educational and fun.

The career boxes are intended to give you a little more information about the job outlook, tasks, and educational requirements for the healthcare occupation featured in each chapter's case study. By following the Websites provided, you can access information on these careers. The Website in the career box in Chapter 1 provides information on all healthcare careers.

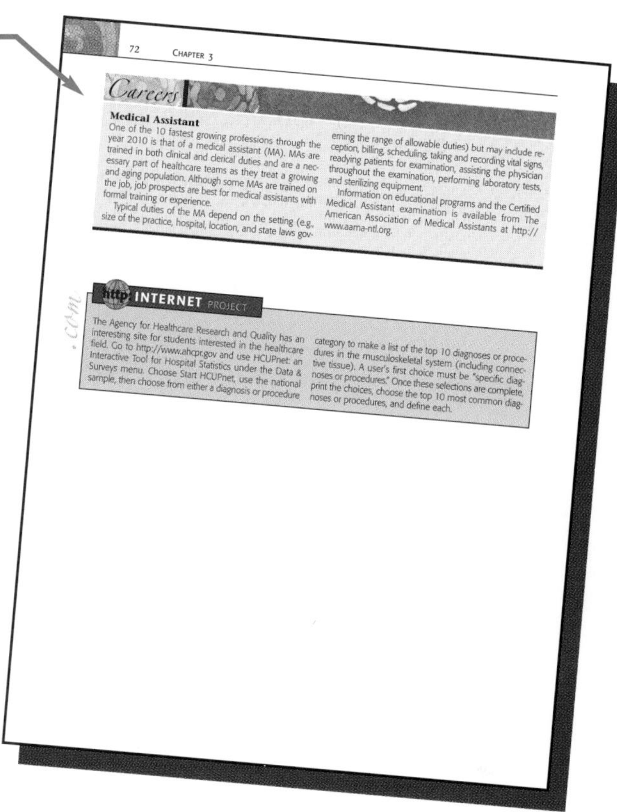

72 Chapter 3

Careers

Medical Assistant

One of the 10 fastest growing professions through the year 2010 is that of a medical assistant (MA). MAs are trained in both clinical and clerical duties and are a necessary part of healthcare teams as they treat a growing and aging population. Although some MAs are trained on the job, job prospects are best for medical assistants with formal training or experience.

Typical duties of the MA depend on the setting (e.g., size of the practice, hospital, location, and state laws governing the range of allowable duties) but may include reception, billing, scheduling, taking and recording vital signs, readying patients for examination, assisting the physician throughout the examination, performing laboratory tests, and sterilizing equipment.

Information on educational programs and the Certified Medical Assistant examination is available from The American Association of Medical Assistants at http://www.aama-ntl.org.

http: INTERNET PROJECT

The Agency for Healthcare Research and Quality has an interesting site for students interested in the healthcare field. Go to http://www.ahcpr.gov and use HCUPnet: an Interactive Tool for Hospital Statistics under the Data & Surveys menu. Choose Start HCUPnet, use the national sample, then choose from either a diagnosis or procedure category to make a list of the top 10 diagnoses or procedures in the musculoskeletal system (including connective tissue). A user's first choice must be "specific diagnoses or procedures." Once these selections are complete, print the choices, choose the top 10 most common diagnoses or procedures, and define each.

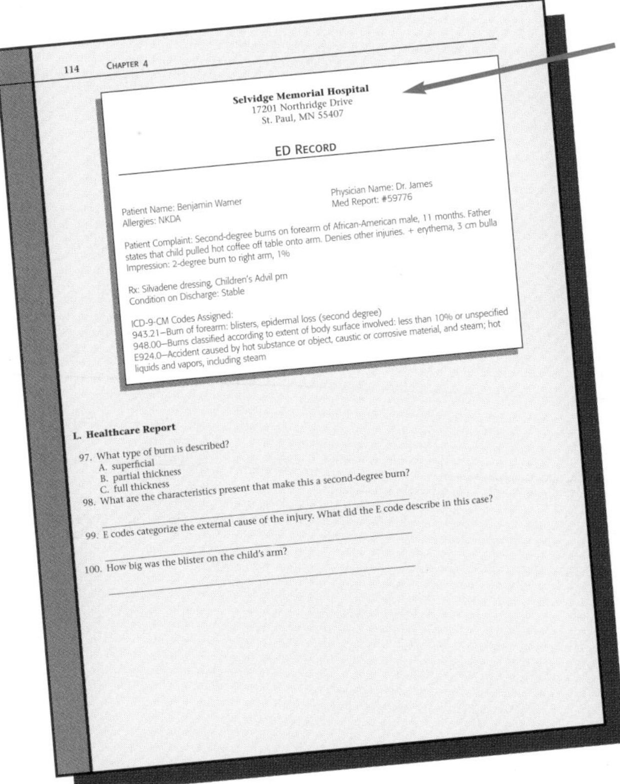

114 Chapter 4

Selvidge Memorial Hospital
17201 Northridge Drive
St. Paul, MN 55407

ED Record

Patient Name: Benjamin Warner
Allergies: NKDA

Physician Name: Dr. James
Med Report: #59776

Patient Complaint: Second-degree burns on forearm of African-American male, 11 months. Father states that child pulled hot coffee off table onto arm. Denies other injuries. + erythema, 3 cm bulla
Impression: 2-degree burn to right arm, 1%

Rx: Silvadene dressing, Children's Advil prn
Condition on Discharge: Stable

ICD-9-CM Codes Assigned:
943.21–Burn of forearm: blisters, epidermal loss (second degree)
948.00–Burns classified according to extent of body surface involved: less than 10% or unspecified
E924.0–Accident caused by hot substance or object, caustic or corrosive material, and steam; hot liquids and vapors, including steam

L. Healthcare Report

97. What type of burn is described?
    A. superficial
    B. partial thickness
    C. full thickness
98. What are the characteristics present that make this a second-degree burn?
99. E codes categorize the external cause of the injury. What did the E code describe in this case?
100. How big was the blister on the child's arm?

Healthcare Report

The healthcare reports in Chapters 2 through 16 are real-life scenarios that reflect the diagnosis and treatment of the patient followed in the case study. Included in each report are select healthcare terms that have been introduced in the chapter. These reports are representative of the different forms and medical charts that you will encounter in a healthcare setting. They give you the opportunity to apply your recently gained knowledge to real-life situations.

Chapter Review

A variety of exercises, including reviews of chapter terminology, terminology from previous chapters, boxed material, singulars and plurals, and abbreviations are included at the end of each chapter to help you test your knowledge. Answers are provided at the end of the book.

Appendixes

Appendixes include alphabetically listed combining forms, prefixes, suffixes, and abbreviations, as well as their meanings. Use them as a easy-to-access review tool or to find a term from a previous chapter.

FROM THE AUTHOR

Buying the text and showing up for class is not enough! This text will meet you halfway, but you must participate in the learning process. The more senses you can involve, the better your chance for success. Make flashcards, use color to code your notes, draw and label diagrams, and find a place where you can spend time to study without constant interruption. You need to find what study aids work for you. Knowing yourself and getting involved with your learning will help you complete all your healthcare courses successfully.

Acknowledgments

Without the talent, experience, and hard work of the *Mastering Healthcare Terminology* team, not one page of this text could have been possible. I would like to express my sincere appreciation to the executive editor, Jeanne Wilke, for having the patience and confidence to shepherd me through the proposal process and continue to oversee the entire project with humor and grace. Thanks also to Billi Sharp, my initial developmental editor, who nudged me through the first several seemingly impossible chapters. Because the visual component of the book is so important to me, I am grateful to have had Jeanne Robertson, our medical illustrator, and Julia Dummitt, our designer, as team members. Jeanne took my verbal descriptions of visual ideas and did a beautiful job of interpreting them. Julia came up with the attractive interior design that makes our book so accessible. Finally, although it seems impossible to express adequate gratitude, kudos to Linda Woodard, my developmental editor, who has been a relentless advocate for excellence, tirelessly reviewing and making the manuscript better.

I am also extremely grateful to our reviewers, who offered their years of experience by reading and commenting on well over 1000 pages of text. Again, no one person could ever succeed in an effort of this magnitude without help. The reviewers were equally valuable team members.

And thanks are also due to my students—for all of you who were willing to ask questions when it would have been easier to remain quiet and confused. I will continue to listen and look for ways to improve.

Betsy J. Shiland

Contents

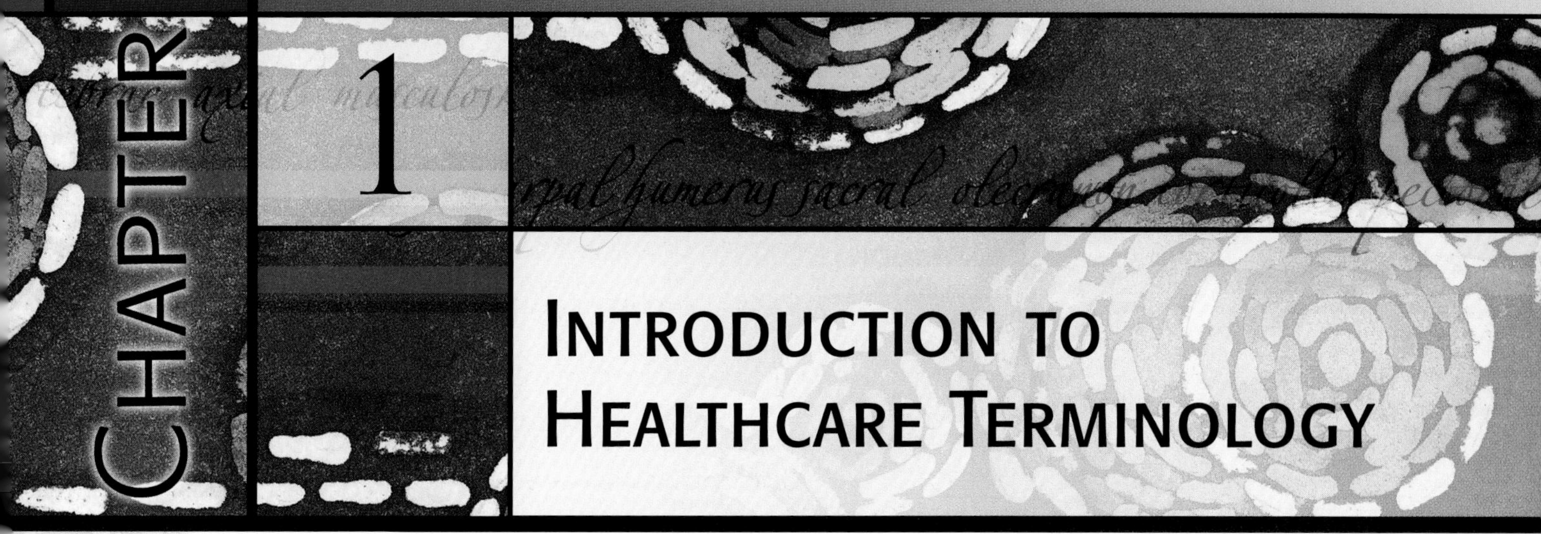

CHAPTER 1 INTRODUCTION TO HEALTHCARE TERMINOLOGY

"They do certainly give very strange, and newfangled, names to diseases." ***—Plato***

Quote

Case Study

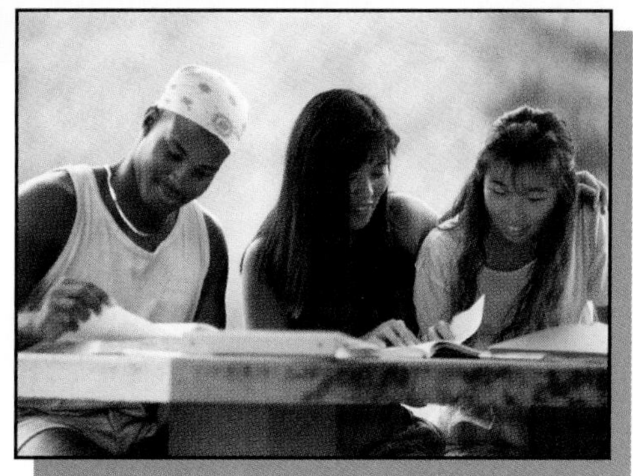

Students taking a healthcare terminology class may be right out of high school, returning to college to explore a new career, or starting college after life experience in other fields. These students are ready to learn, to apply what they know, and to absorb the material as efficiently as possible. Maya has come straight from being senior class president in a Kansas high school, whereas Izaak is returning to college after a stint in the Peace Corps in central Africa during which he realized he wanted to become a nurse. Lan worked for several years for the Chicago Transit Authority as a ticketing agent. With her children all school-age now, she is interested in trying out a new career. Working together, these three students can bring new insights and learning strategies to a study group.

OBJECTIVES

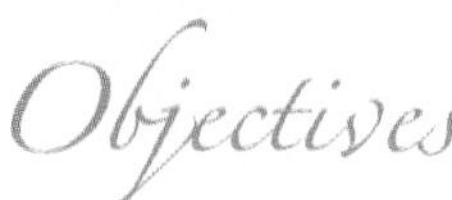

- Explain the importance of learning healthcare terminology.
- State the derivation of most healthcare terms.
- List and give an example of the different types of healthcare terms.
- List the parts of decodable healthcare terms and give an example of each.
- Explain the spelling rules for component parts and give an example of each rule.
- List the singular/plural rules and give an example of each.
- Explain the different categories of healthcare terms used in the diagnostic/treatment process.
- Name some of the common healthcare disciplines and relate them appropriately to the areas that they cover.
- List some healthcare terminology resources and explain the type of information found in each.

THE IMPORTANCE OF LEARNING HEALTHCARE TERMINOLOGY

Healthcare professionals require a vocabulary of words that describe very specific concepts unique to their discipline. Students who aspire to becoming members of a healthcare team must learn to read, speak, spell, and understand a new language. This language, healthcare terminology, has been spoken for thousands of years, with many of its roots in ancient Greek and Latin. It was during the time of the ancient Greeks and Romans that the terms we currently use were written and preserved. Like most languages, the language of healthcare continually changes to reflect current knowledge. New words are periodically added, and older terms are constantly being redefined to more accurately reflect contemporary wisdom. In addition to technologic advances in mainstream medicine, patients are using more complementary and alternative medicine (CAM) approaches, which have not been a part of contemporary healthcare practice. These varied approaches may include spiritual, herbal, physical, and other remedies. Certain CAM remedies are becoming so widely accepted that they are now included in some types of insurance coverage and have certainly entered the healthcare language.

DID YOU KNOW?

The term *hysteria* is an example whose meaning has changed since its origin. Its current definition is a condition of emotional instability that may be diagnosed in either males or females. The derivation of the term is from *hyster-*, meaning *uterus,* and the suffix *-ia,* meaning *condition.* Ancient Greeks believed that this condition was a result of an empty, discontent uterus and thus was suffered only by females who were not pregnant.

TYPES OF HEALTHCARE TERMS

Most healthcare terms fit into the following categories: decodable, nondecodable, eponyms, abbreviations, and symbols.

Decodable

Decodable terms are healthcare terms with usually Greek or Latin component parts, which can be analyzed and defined. Once the code is mastered, volumes of complex-looking terms suddenly become easier to decipher, or conversely, to build. For example, the term *cardiology* is the process of the study of the heart. But if one understands the meaning of its parts, a whole world of terms opens up. In the first place, *cardi/o* is the combining form for *heart; -logy* is the suffix for *the process of the study of.** Armed with this knowledge, it quickly becomes apparent that other

*The suffix *-logy* is actually built from the combining form *log/o,* which means *a study of,* and the suffix *-y,* meaning *the process of.* For the purpose of simplicity, this text will refer to *-logy* as meaning *the study of.*

words ending in *-logy* will be fields of study, such as *psychology* and *biology*. By the same token, the learner will also know from now on that words with *cardi/o* in them pertain in some way to the heart, such as *cardiopulmonary* or *electrocardiogram*. Many of the terms presented in the text have been decoded in this manner and are included under the "Word Origin" column of the terminology tables.

Nondecodable

Nondecodable terms cannot be broken into component parts; for these terms, the entire definition must be memorized. For example the term *cataract,* which is a progressive opacification of the lens, is derived from the Greek term meaning *waterfall*—not an especially helpful derivation. Another example is *angina,* cardiac pain caused by a lack of oxygen to the heart muscle. It comes from a Latin term meaning *strangling.*

Eponyms

Eponyms are terms that are named after the person who first identified the condition or devised the object bearing the name. Students may recognize the terms *Alzheimer's* disease, the progressive mental deterioration named by Alois Alzheimer, the German neurologist, or *cesarean* section, the removal of the infant from the uterus by incising the abdominal wall, named after the manner in which Julius Caesar was supposedly born. Sometimes eponyms have a decodable term as an alternative. For example, *Bright's disease* is the eponym for *glomerulonephritis,* an inflammation of the glomeruli in the kidneys.

Another example of an eponym is the term *Doppler,* a technique that uses ultrasound imaging to measure the behavior of a moving substance, such as blood moving through a beating heart. Doppler is used to detect areas of blockage and/or narrowing and is named after Christian Doppler, an Austrian scientist noted for his research in the variations of sound waves.

Abbreviations

Abbreviations are terms that have been shortened to a number of letters for the sake of convenience. For example, CAD stands for *c*oronary *a*rtery *d*isease. Some abbreviations are actually acronyms, pronounceable words formed from the initial letters of other words. For example, CABG (pronounced like the vegetable) is an acronym for a *c*oronary *a*rtery *b*ypass *g*raft.

Abbreviations can certainly save time, but they can be confusing because some can have more than one meaning. For example, the abbreviation OD can mean *once daily, overdose, Doctor of Optometry,* and *right eye,* among others. A further complication is that although most abbreviations are capitalized, some uppercase abbreviations have different meanings than their lowercase equivalents. An example is the abbreviation NG, meaning *nasogastric* or *nitroglycerin,* and ng, meaning *nanogram.* Every healthcare facility should have a master list of approved abbreviations, with only one meaning allowed for each abbreviation stated.

Symbols

Graphic representations called *symbols* are also used in healthcare terminology. For example, the symbol for female is ♀ and the symbol for male is ♂. Other symbols that a healthcare professional will encounter are the positive (+) sign and the negative (−) sign. Arrows are also used to indicate an increase (↑) or decrease (↓) in a value, especially in diagnostic laboratory tests.

Exercise 1: Types of Healthcare Terms

Match the following types of healthcare terms with their examples.

_____ 1. symbol

_____ 2. decodable term

_____ 3. abbreviation

_____ 4. nondecodable term

_____ 5. eponym

A. CAD
B. angina
C. cardiology
D. Doppler
E. ♀

Case Study Continued

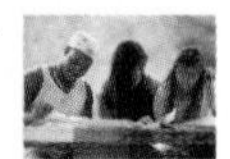

A regular time to study should be a priority for a student. For every hour of class, a student should budget 2 hours study time outside of class. For example, Maya uses the time between her classes at school and after dinner to study. Lan schedules her study time during part of her lunch break and after her children go to bed. Izaak studies while riding the bus to work and on weekends.

BUILDING HEALTHCARE TERMS

Students are always relieved to know that a large part of healthcare language can be decoded by learning the Greek and Latin counterparts of a number of **word roots, suffixes**, and **prefixes.** Mastering the few rules that determine how these component parts are joined, one can quickly learn to build and analyze thousands of healthcare terms. As with any rules, there will be exceptions. Wherever possible, these exceptions will be noted.

Word Roots

Word roots are the subject or foundation of the healthcare term. They describe what the term is about; therefore almost every term has at least one. For example, the root *oste* means *bone,* and the root *arthr* means *joint.* Word roots are seldom used alone, however. They are usually paired with a suffix and sometimes with a prefix. They often need a vowel, called a *combining vowel,* to link them to a suffix, for ease of pronunciation.

Combining Vowels

Combining vowels (usually the letter *o*) appear between certain word roots and suffixes and act to join the two by making the term easier to pronounce. For example, the *o* in the word *thermometer* serves as a combining vowel. It combines the word root *therm* (meaning *heat*) and the suffix *-meter* (meaning *an instrument that measures*) to form a word that means *an instrument that measures temperature.*

Combining Forms

Combining forms are word roots plus their appropriate combining vowel, usually an *o.* When listing and discussing word roots, it is easier to pronounce the combining form than the word root because of the ending vowel.

SOME COMBINING FORMS AND THEIR MEANINGS

COMBINING FORM	MEANING	COMBINING FORM	MEANING
arthr/o	joint	hepat/o	liver
bi/o	life	lith/o	stone
cardi/o	heart	log/o	study, knowledge
col/o, colon/o	colon (large intestine)	nat/o	birth
dent/i, odont/o	teeth	ophthalm/o	eye
derm/o, dermat/o	skin	oste/o	bone
electr/o	electrical activity	path/o	disease
enter/o	small intestine	therm/o	heat, temperature
fet/o	fetus	troph/o	nourishment, development
gastr/o	stomach	tympan/o	eardrum

Suffixes

Suffixes always come after the word root and usually qualify the term as a condition, a procedure, or a symptom. For example, adding the suffix *-logy* (the study of) to the combining form *path/o* (disease) creates the term *pathology,* which means *the study of disease.* Nearly every healthcare term will have at least one suffix. When defining a term, it is sometimes easier to start with the definition of the suffix and then move on to the word root, as demonstrated with the term *pathology.*

By using the wheel in Fig. 1-1, many terms using the combining form *arthr/o,* which means *joint,* can be made by combining it with different suffixes:

Arthritis:	Inflammation of a joint	Arthrotomy:	Incision of a joint
Arthroscopy:	Visual examination of a joint	Arthroplasty:	Surgical repair of a joint
Arthropathy:	Disease of a joint	Arthralgia:	Pain in a joint

Fig. 1-1 Combining form wheel. (Courtesy Mirele Steinig.)

SOME SUFFIXES AND THEIR MEANINGS

SUFFIX	MEANING	SUFFIX	MEANING
-al	pertaining to	-pathy	disease process
-algia	pain	-plasty	surgical repair
-dynia	pain	-rrhage	bursting forth
-ectomy	excision, removal	-rrhaphy	suture
-gram	a record	-rrhea	discharge, flow
-ia	condition	-rrhexis	rupture
-ic	pertaining to	-scopy	visual examination
-ist	one who specializes	-stomy	new opening
-itis	inflammation	-tomy	an incision
-logy	the study of	-um	noun ending usually meaning a structure
-megaly	an enlargement	-y	noun ending usually meaning the process of
-opsy	a viewing		
-osis	abnormal condition		

Case Study Continued

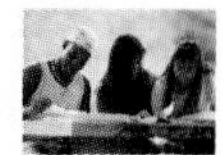

Izaak was having trouble defining the term *gastritis* on an exam one day. After deciding that panic wouldn't help anything, he looked more carefully at the word and realized that he recognized that the suffix, *-itis* means *inflammation*. Then, as he took two Tums to calm his stomach, he remembered that the word root *gastr* meant *stomach*. Voila! Izaak realized that gastritis was an inflammation of the stomach.

BE CAREFUL!

Don't confuse *ante-*, which means *before*, and *anti-*, which means *against*.

Prefixes

Prefixes come before a word root and give more information about the term described by the word root and suffix. For example, adding the prefix *hypo-* to the word root *therm* and the suffix *-ia* creates the word *hypothermia*, which means *an abnormally low body temperature*. On the other hand, exchanging the prefix *hyper-* for *hypo-* creates the word *hyperthermia*, which means *an abnormally high body temperature*, the opposite of hypothermia.

SOME PREFIXES AND THEIR MEANINGS

PREFIX	MEANING	PREFIX	MEANING
a-	not, without	hypo-	deficient, below
an-	no, not, without	in-	not, in
ante-	before, in front of	infra-	below
anti-	against	inter-	between
dys-	painful, abnormal, difficult	intra-	within
endo-	within	neo-	new
epi-	above, on top of	per-	through
ex-	outside, out	peri-	surrounding
hemi-	half, partial	pre-	before
hyper-	excessive, above	sub-	under, below

Building a Healthcare Term

By using these word parts, a healthcare term can be created. The following figure represents how the word *osteoarthritis* is formed.

Two root words—*oste*, meaning *bone*, and *arthr*, meaning *joint*—are joined by a combining vowel, *o*. The suffix *-itis*, meaning *inflammation*, is added to create a term that means *inflammation of a bone of a joint*.

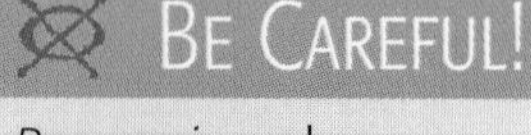

Per-, *peri-*, and *pre-* are prefixes that are very close in spelling but that have very different meanings.

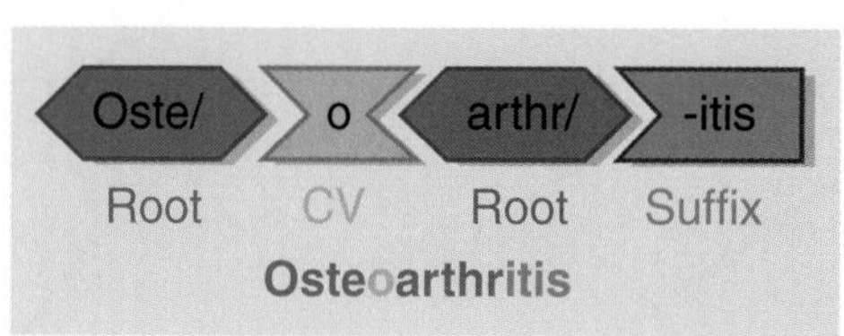

Pronunciation of Unusual Letter Combinations

Terminology is not only written, it is also spoken. One of the more difficult parts of a healthcare terminology course is to learn how to speak this new language with all of its unusual pronunciations. Below are a few letter combinations that may seem a little unusual because they occur more frequently in healthcare terminology than in everyday English.

Unusual Letter Combinations

SPELLING	PRONUNCIATION	EXAMPLE
eu	you	**euthyroid** (yoo THIGH royd): Good, healthy thyroid function
gn	n (*no*)	**gnathalgia** (nuh THAL jah): Pain in the jaw
ph	f (*fill*)	**phalanx** (FAY lanks): One of the bones of the fingers or toes
pn	n (*no*)	**pneumonitis** (noo moh NYE tis): Inflammation of the lungs
ps	s (*sort*)	**psychology** (sye KALL uh jee): Study of the mind
pt	t (*top*)	**ptosis** (TOH sis): Drooping, prolapse
x	z (*zoo*)	**xeroderma** (zeer oh DUR mah): Dry skin

Exercise 2: BUILDING HEALTHCARE TERMS

Match the following combining forms with their meanings.

____ 1. odont/o
____ 2. cardi/o
____ 3. ophthalm/o
____ 4. col/o, colon/o
____ 5. gastr/o
____ 6. path/o
____ 7. arthr/o
____ 8. derm/o, dermat/o
____ 9. bi/o
____ 10. oste/o

A. stomach
B. large intestine
C. disease
D. skin
E. bone
F. teeth
G. joint
H. eye
I. life
J. heart

Match the following suffixes with their meanings.

____ 11. -itis
____ 12. -ectomy
____ 13. -tomy
____ 14. -scopy
____ 15. -ic
____ 16. -gram
____ 17. -pathy
____ 18. -ist
____ 19. -opsy
____ 20. -logy

A. incision
B. visual examination
C. a record
D. specialist
E. study of
F. disease process
G. excision, resection
H. a viewing
I. pertaining to
J. inflammation

Match the following prefixes with their definitions.

____ 21. hemi-
____ 22. endo-
____ 23. neo-
____ 24. hyper-
____ 25. an-
____ 26. epi-
____ 27. peri-
____ 28. ex-
____ 29. anti-
____ 30. pre-

A. no, not, without
B. excessive
C. new
D. half, partial
E. against
F. surrounding
G. above, on top of
H. within
I. before
J. out, outside

Fill in the blank.

31. Most decodable healthcare terms have a ____________ and a ____________.
32. Suffixes appear at the ____________ of a healthcare term, whereas prefixes appear at the ____________ of healthcare terms.
33. Combining forms are often used because they are easier to ____________ than word roots.
34. Using some of the component parts given, how would you define dermatitis? (Hint: start with the suffix first, then use the word root.) ____________ of the ____________
35. In the term "prenatal," identify and state the meaning of the:

    A. word root ____________

    B. suffix ____________

    C. prefix ____________

    D. The definition of prenatal would be ____________

Match the word part with an example.

____ 36. prefix
____ 37. combining form
____ 38. suffix
____ 39. word root
____ 40. combining vowel

A. o
B. arthr/
C. neo-
D. dermat/o
E. -itis

Fill in the blank.

41. If the term starts with an "s" sound, try looking under s, c, or ____________. For example, you hear the term "sore EYE ah sis" to describe a patient's skin disorder. You can't find it under soriasis, so you try ____________.
42. You hear an "f" sound when the physician says the patient has an extreme "FOE bee ah" of cats. You can't find it under fobia. You should try ____________.
43. A patient calls in to have her prescription for "ZERO derm ah" (dry skin) renewed. When you check under zeroderma, it's not there, so you check ____________.
44. One of the nurses tells you that the patient who just left had "YOOP nee ah." When you try to check the spelling, you can't find it under upnea or youpnia so you try ____________.

45. The last patient of the day is diagnosed with an "abnormal condition of dust in his lungs." You thought the term was "noo moh koh nee OH sis" and spelled neumoconiosis, but it needed one more letter to be correctly spelled ______________.

SPELLING RULES

With minor exceptions, decodable healthcare terms follow a few very short spelling rules.

1. If the suffix starts with a vowel, a combining vowel is not needed to join the parts. For example, it is simple to combine *arthr* and *-itis* to make *arthritis,* an inflammation of the joint.
2. If the suffix starts with a consonant, a combining vowel is needed to join the two word parts. For example, to combine the word root *cardi* and the suffix *-logy* to make *cardiology* (a study of the heart), the combining vowel *o* is inserted.
3. If two or more word roots are used in a term, a combining vowel is used regardless of whether the word roots start with vowels or consonants. For example, in combining word roots *oste* and *arthr* with the suffix *-itis* to make *osteoarthritis,* an *o* is needed between the two roots.
4. In body systems in which there is a directionality to the anatomy, word roots that are joined should be sequenced in a logical order. Combining the word roots *esophag* (esophagus or "food tube"), *gastr* (stomach), *duoden* (for the duodenum or first part of the small intestine), and the suffix *-scopy* (visual examination) creates the word *esophagogastroduodenoscopy* (EGD)—the visual examination of the upper digestive system. An EGD begins in the esophagus, goes through the stomach, and ends in the duodenum. Fig. 1-2 shows the route of an EGD, with each of the body parts labeled.

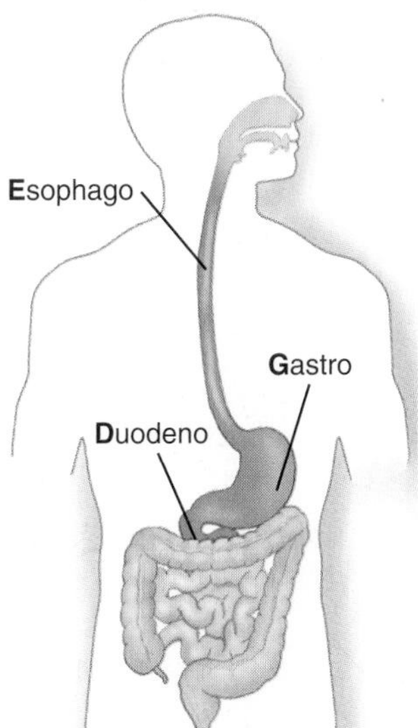

Fig. 1-2 Esophagogastroduodenoscopy (EGD).

Singular/Plural Rules

Because most healthcare terms end with Greek or Latin suffixes, making a healthcare term singular or plural is not always done the same way as it is in English. The following table gives the most common singular/plural endings and the rules for using them. Examples of unusual singular/plural endings and singular/plural exercises will be included throughout the text.

Case Study Continued

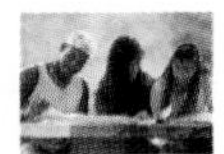

Quizzing one another on term building and definitions, Maya, Izaak, and Lan find that the act of making and using flashcards to memorize word components is extremely helpful. It is Izaak who gets the others into this great habit when he buys a pack of 3 × 5 cards, cutting them in half and using two rubber bands to hold them together. He writes the combining form (e.g., *cardi/o*) on the front and the definition *(heart)* on the back. When he has a set made for one chapter, he bands them together and puts them in his right pocket. During the day (in any 5-minute opportunity), he quizzes himself. If he knows the card, he puts it in his left-hand pocket. If he doesn't, he puts it back on the bottom of the pile for another try.

Rules for Using Singular and Plural Endings

Rule	Example
1. If a term ends in *-a,* drop the *-a* and add an *-ae* (pronounced as a long *a, e,* or *i,* depending on the term).	Singular: **vertebra** (VUR tuh brah) Plural: **vertebrae** (VUR tuh bray)
2. If a term ends in *-is,* drop the *-is* and add *-es* (pronounced *eez*)	Singular: **diagnosis** (dye agg NOH sis) Plural: **diagnoses** (dye agg NOH seez)
3. If a term ends in *-nx,* drop the *-nx* and add *-nges* (pronounced as *ng* [like in sing] + *jeez*)	Singular: **phalanx** (FAY lanks) Plural: **phalanges** (fuh LAN jeez)
4. If a term ends in *-um,* drop the *-um* and add an *-a* (pronounced *ah*)	Singular: **bacterium** (back TEER ree um) Plural: **bacteria** (back TEER ree ah)
5. If a term ends in *-us,* drop the *-us* and add an *-i* (pronounced *eye*)	Singular: **digitus** (DIJ ih tus) Plural: **digiti** (DIJ ih tye)
6. If a term ends in *-y,* drop the *-y* and add *-ies* (pronounced as *eez*)	Singular: **therapy** (THAIR ah pee) Plural: **therapies** (THAIR ah peez)

Exercise 3: Spelling Healthcare Terms

Using the component parts given from the tables so far and the appropriate spelling rules, try building terms for the following.

1. Mr. Ryan's doctor advised a/an ______________ (removal of the large intestine) because of cancer-related problems.
2. Kathleen had her wisdom teeth surgically removed; the procedure was termed a/an ______________.
3. At his biannual eye examination, Mario had a/an ______________ (visual examination of his eyes).
4. Chronic knee problems caused the football player to seek advice from his physician. He was advised to have a/an ______________ (surgical repair of his [knee] joint).
5. Paloma has always wanted to work with newborns. Her area of specialty will be ______________ (the study of newborns).
6. Sarah visited her physician after experiencing stomach pain for several days. This symptom would be termed ______________.
7. Tanisha's mother was sent for tests to determine which type of "disease involving the bones and the joints" she might have. The term would be ______________.
8. Van was diagnosed with ______________, "an inflammation of the stomach and small intestines" after she experienced diarrhea and vomiting from what she thought might be food poisoning.
9. Jeremy developed an inflammation of the skin. He had a type of ______________.
10. Mr. Ruiz' young neighbor was diagnosed with a middle ear disorder that required surgical repair of his eardrum. The term for this would be ______________

Change the following terms from singular to plural.

11. thrombus (a blood clot) ______________
12. biopsy (a viewing of living tissue) ______________

13. septum (a partition or wall) ______

14. prognosis (a prediction of disease outcome) ______

15. bulla (a large blister) ______

16. larynx (the voice box) ______

CATEGORIES OF HEALTHCARE TERMS

As a patient progresses through a healthcare intervention, from initial contact with a practitioner's office, through the diagnostic process, to the resulting treatment, his or her health record soon fills with a variety of healthcare terms that fall under the categories of signs and symptoms, diagnostic procedures, and therapeutic interventions.

Signs and Symptoms

Signs and symptoms are information that comes from the patient before any testing or imaging is done. **Symptoms** are subjective indications of disease experienced by the patient. The patient may complain of pain or itching, which are symptoms of many different diseases or conditions. When the patient is seen by the healthcare professional, he or she evaluates the patient's physical **signs**, objective findings that can be seen or measured, such as fever or rash. Frequently a diagnosis can be made on signs and symptoms alone.

Diagnostic Procedures

Aside from collecting information about the manifestations of the disease that are reported by the patient and observed and measured by the practitioner, the healthcare professional will sometimes further investigate the disorder by ordering or performing a number of laboratory tests or diagnostic imaging procedures. The most common laboratory tests are blood and urine analyses. Diagnostic imaging procedures include x-rays, ultrasounds, magnetic resonance imaging (MRIs), positron emission tomography (PET scans), or computed tomography (CT scans) (Fig. 1-3). The results from such a myriad of tests lend more information or clues to help determine the diagnosis.

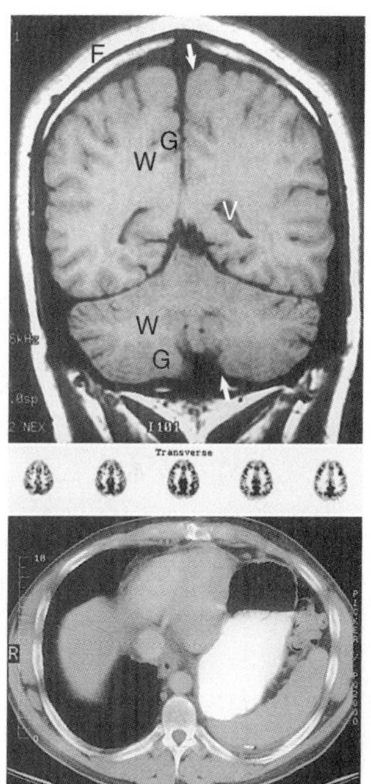

Fig. 1-3 *Top,* MRI of the brain. *Middle,* PET scan of the brain. *Bottom,* CT scan of the abdomen.

Diagnoses and Prognoses

Although similar in sound, diagnoses and prognoses are different. A **diagnosis** (dye agg NOH sis) is the disease or condition named after evaluating the patient's signs, symptoms, and history, along with possible laboratory test results and imaging procedures. A **prognosis** (prahg NOH sis) is a prediction of the probable outcome of the disease. A prognosis is based not only on the condition of the person, but on the usual course of the disease as others with the same condition or disease have experienced it. Suppose that in the course of one day, a physician records, among others, the following diagnosis: "gastritis with an excellent prognosis" and "cardiomyopathy with a poor prognosis." Both of these are conclusions about what the patient's healthcare problem is (diagnosis) and what the future holds for him or her (prognosis).

Diagnoses can be described as being **acute** (ah KYOOT) or **chronic** (KRAH nick). An acute diagnosis is one that begins abruptly and severely and ends after a short period of time. A chronic condition is one that develops slowly and lasts for a long time.

SUFFIXES USED TO DESCRIBE THERAPEUTIC INTERVENTIONS

SUFFIX	MEANING	SUFFIX	MEANING
-ectomy	excision	-stomy	a new opening
-graphy	process of recording	-therapy	treatment
-metry	process of measurement	-tomy	incision
-scopy	a visual examination	-tripsy	process of crushing

BE CAREFUL!

The procedural suffixes *-tomy, -stomy,* and *-ectomy* are spelled similarly but have different meanings.

Therapeutic Interventions

Finally, once a diagnosis has been reached, the healthcare professional will assign treatment to correct the disorder. Treatment may be traditional (surgical intervention and/or the prescribing of medicine), or may consist of a variety of complementary and alternative medical therapies. Increasingly, a combination of different treatment options are being prescribed.

Instruments

When discussing diagnostic or treatment procedures, it is inevitable that terms that describe medical instruments will be encountered. No matter their function, most instrument terms share common suffixes. For example, a fetoscope is used to listen to a fetus's heartbeat, and a tympanometer is used to measure the function of the tympanic membrane (Fig. 1-4). Some of the more common suffixes for instruments are as follows:

SUFFIXES USED TO DESCRIBE INSTRUMENTS

SUFFIX	MEANING	SUFFIX	MEANING
-graph	an instrument/machine to record	-tome	an instrument to cut
-meter	an instrument to measure	-tripter	an instrument to crush
-scope	an instrument to visually or aurally examine		

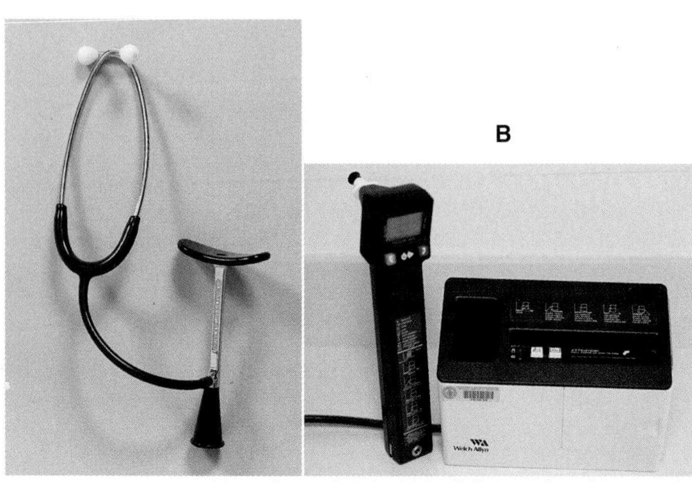

Fig. 1-4 **A,** Fetoscope. **B,** Tympanometer.

Exercise 4: CATEGORIES OF HEALTHCARE TERMS

1. A patient mentions that she has been experiencing headaches and dizziness. Her physician finds that she has a slight fever and elevated blood pressure. Which of the following are signs and which are symptoms?

   A. headache ____________ C. dizziness ____________

   B. fever ____________ D. elevated blood pressure ____________

2. Identify each of the following diagnostics procedures as being a laboratory test (L) or an imaging procedure (I).

   A. ____ urinalysis C. ____ red blood cell count

   B. ____ PET scan D. ____ ultrasound

Match the following terms and definitions.

3. ____ acute
4. ____ diagnosis
5. ____ chronic
6. ____ prognosis

A. condition that develops slowly and lasts a long time
B. condition identified after analysis of signs, symptoms, history, and lab tests or imaging
C. condition that begins abruptly and severely
D. prediction made about the outcome of a disease

Match the following suffixes with their meanings.

7. ____ -tomy
8. ____ -ectomy
9. ____ -tripsy
10. ____ -metry
11. ____ -graphy
12. ____ -therapy
13. ____ -plasty

A. process of recording
B. process of crushing
C. process of measurement
D. surgical repair
E. process of treatment
F. process of cutting
G. excision

14. Decode the following terms by using a slash (/) to separate the components and then using their meanings to define the term (Example: gastro/scopy; the process of visually examining the stomach).

    A. arthrotome ____________________

    B. electrocardiograph ____________________

    C. ophthalmoscope ____________________

    D. thermometer ____________________

    E. lithotripter ____________________

HEALTHCARE DISCIPLINES

The last category of general healthcare terms is the various healthcare disciplines. Many of the disciplines relate directly to one of the body systems, although several concern the entire body at a period in the aging process (neonatology, pediatrics, geriatrics) or a part of a system (anesthesiology) or the entire organism (pathology, oncology).

Although most of the healthcare disciplines have *-logy,* meaning *the study of,* as their suffix, a few end with the suffixes *-iatry* and *-iatrics,* which come from the combining form *iatr/o,* meaning *treatment.* Although by no means exhaustive, the following healthcare specialties cover most of the major disciplines and include a few complementary and alternative medicine (CAM) therapies.

Healthcare Disciplines

DISCIPLINE	WORD ORIGIN	DEFINITION
Acupuncture ACK yoo punk chur	*acu-* sharp	Traditional Chinese method of producing analgesia, or altering the function of a body system, by inserting fine, wire-thin needles into the skin at specific sites on the body along a series of lines called **meridians** (Fig. 1-5).
Anesthesiology an es thee see ALL uh jee	*an-* without *esthesi/o* feeling *-logy* study of	Branch of medicine concerned with the relief of pain and the administration of medication to relieve pain during surgery.
Cardiology kar dee ALL uh jee	*cardi/o* heart *-logy* study of	Branch of medicine focusing on the functions of the heart and the diagnosis and treatment of disorders that affect its function.
Chiropractic kye roh PRACK tick	*chir/o* hand *pract/o* manipulation *-ic* pertaining to	Study of methods of spinal column manipulation to ease disorders by relieving pressure on the nerves.
Dermatology dur mah TALL uh jee	*dermat/o* skin *-logy* study of	Branch of medicine that includes the study of the skin with its anatomic, physiologic, and pathologic characteristics and the diagnosis and treatment of skin disorders.
Geriatrics jair ee AT tricks	*ger/o* aging *iatr/o* treatment *-ics* pertaining to	Branch of medicine that deals with the physiologic characteristics of aging and the diagnosis and treatment of diseases affecting the aged.
Gynecology gye nuh KALL uh jee	*gynec/o* female *-logy* study of	Branch of medicine that studies and treats diseases of the female reproductive organs, including the breasts.
Hematology he mah TALL uh jee	*hemat/o* blood *-logy* study of	Branch of medicine that deals with the study and treatment of the blood and the blood-forming tissues (Fig. 1-6).

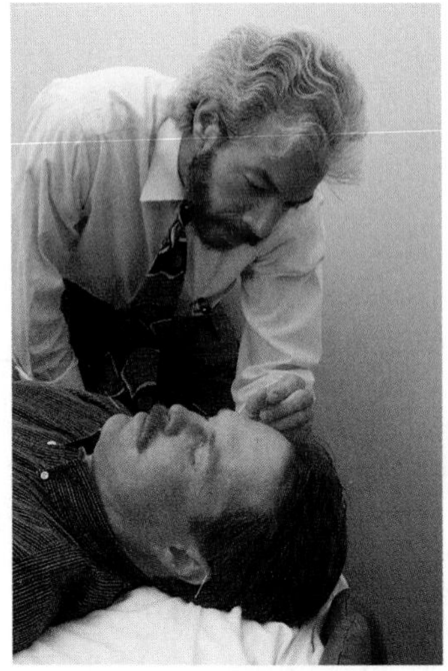

Fig. 1-5 Acupuncture.

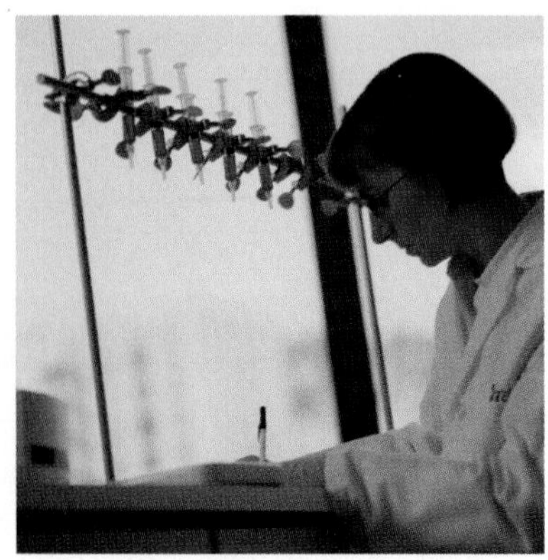

Fig. 1-6 Hematology.

Healthcare Disciplines—cont'd		
DISCIPLINE	**WORD ORIGIN**	**DEFINITION**
Homeopathy hoh mee AH puh thee	*home/o* same *-pathy* disease	System of therapeutics based on the theory of "like cures like"; medications are diluted in ratios of 1 to 10 to achieve the smallest dose of a drug that seems necessary to control the symptoms in a patient.
Immunology im myoo NALL uh jee	*immun/o* safety, protection *-logy* study of	Branch of medicine that deals with the study of the reaction of tissues of the immune system of the body to antigenic stimulation.
Neonatology nee oh nay TALL uh jee	*neo-* new *nat/o* birth *-logy* study of	Branch of medicine that concentrates on the care, diagnosis, and treatment of the newborn (Fig. 1-7).
Neurology nyoo RALL uh jee	*neur/o* nerves *-logy* study of	Branch of medicine that deals with the nervous system and its disorders.
Obstetrics ob STEH tricks	*obstetr/o* midwife *-ics* pertaining to	Branch of medicine concerned with pregnancy and childbirth and the immediate postpartum period. Currently, childbirth is the province of both nurse midwives and physicians.
Odontology oh don TALL uh jee	*odont/o* teeth *-logy* study of	Study and treatment of the teeth and surrounding structures in the oral cavity.
Oncology on KALL uh jee	*onc/o* tumor *-logy* study of	Branch of medicine concerned with the study and treatment of tumors, especially cancers.
Ophthalmology off tholl MALL uh jee	*ophthalm/o* eye *-logy* study of	Branch of medicine concerned with the study of the physiology, anatomy, pathology, diagnosis, and treatment of disorders of the eye.
Orthopedics or thoh PEE dicks	*orth/o* straight *ped/o* children *-ics* pertaining to	Branch of medicine concerned with the prevention and correction of disorders of the skeleton, muscles, joints, and related tissues (Fig. 1-8).

Continued

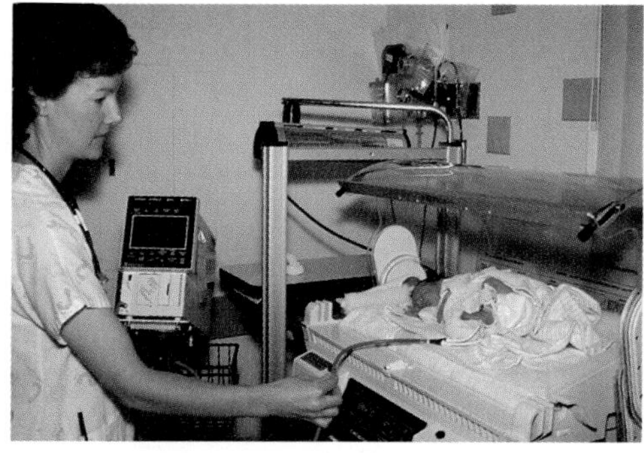

Fig. 1-7 Neonatology.

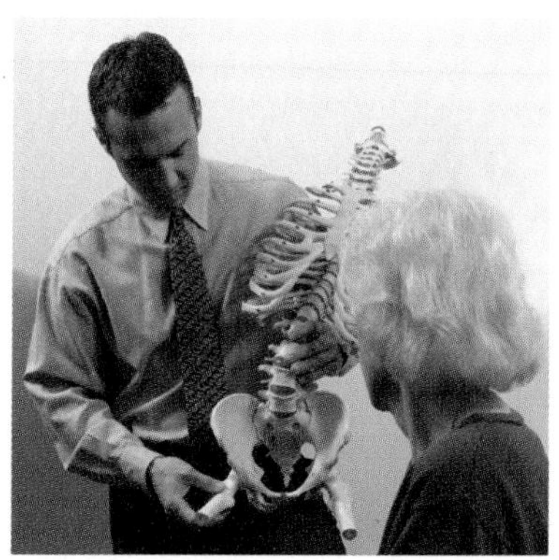

Fig. 1-8 Orthopedics.

Healthcare Disciplines—cont'd		
DISCIPLINE	**WORD ORIGIN**	**DEFINITION**
Otorhinolaryngology oh toh rye noh lair ing GALL uh jee	*ot/o* ear *rhin/o* nose *laryng/o* voice box *-logy* study of	Branch of medicine that is concerned with diseases and disorders of the ear, nose, and throat; often shortened to ENT (ear, nose, and throat). The term is a bit of a misnomer because the larynx is the voicebox and the pharynx is the throat.
Pathology puh THALL uh jee	*path/o* disease *-logy* study of	Study of the characteristics, causes, and effects of disease, as observed in the structure and function of the body.
Pediatrics pee dee AT tricks	*ped/o* children *iatr/o* treatment *-ics* pertaining to	Branch of medicine concerned with the development and care of infants and children.
Psychiatry sye KYE ah tree	*psych/o* mind *iatr/o* treatment *-y* process	Branch of medicine that deals with the causes, treatment, and prevention of mental, emotional, and behavioral disorders.
Rheumatology roo mah TALL uh jee	*rheumat/o* watery flow *-logy* study of	Branch of medicine concerned with the study of disorders characterized by inflammation, degeneration, or metabolic derangement of connective tissue and related structures of the body.
Urology yoo RALL uh jee	*ur/o* urinary system *-logy* study of	Branch of medicine concerned with the anatomy, physiology, disorders, and care of the urinary tract in both sexes and the male genital tract.

Exercise 5: Healthcare Disciplines

Match the following disciplines with their areas of concern.

__H__ 1. gynecology
__I__ 2. geriatrics
__F__ 3. hematology
__A__ 4. urology
__D__ 5. anesthesiology
__E__ 6. ophthalmology
__J__ 7. pediatrics
__G__ 8. oncology
__C__ 9. psychiatry
__B__ 10. pathology

A. The branch of medicine concerned with the anatomy, physiology, disorders and care of the urinary tract in both sexes and the male genital tract.
B. The study of the characteristics, causes, and effects of disease, as observed in the structure and function of the body.
C. The branch of medicine that deals with the causes, treatment, and prevention of mental, emotional, and behavioral disorders.
D. The branch of medicine that is concerned with the relief of pain and with the administration of medication to relieve pain during surgery.
E. The branch of medicine concerned with the study of the physiology, anatomy, pathology, diagnosis, and treatment of disorders of the eye.
F. The branch of medicine that deals with the study of the blood and the blood-forming tissues.
G. The branch of medicine concerned with the study of tumors, especially cancers.
H. The branch of medicine that studies the disease of the female reproductive organs, including the breasts.
I. The branch of medicine that deals with the physiologic characteristics of aging and the diagnosis and treatment of diseases affecting the aged.
J. The branch of medicine concerned with the development and care of infants and children.

HEALTHCARE REFERENCES AND RESOURCES

Just as it is impossible to learn every word in the English language, the same is true of healthcare terminology. The goal of a healthcare terminology course is not to attempt to teach every possible term encountered, but to give a good grounding in the majority of the terms likely to be seen and heard in today's healthcare environment. The following references are available to assist in defining, coding, or understanding healthcare terminology.

DID YOU KNOW?

Given its name from the 1600s when certain types of arthritis were noted to be marked by an effusion of fluid into the joint spaces, rheumatology evolved into a discipline that deals with musculoskeletal diseases and disorders.

Healthcare Resources and References

SOURCE	INFORMATION PROVIDED
Printed Medical References	
Mosby's Medical Dictionary	Definitions, derivations, pronunciations, and illustrations of terms.
The Merck Manual of Diagnosis and Therapy	Etiology (cause), epidemiology (spread), pathology, signs and symptoms, laboratory findings, diagnosis, prognosis, prophylaxis, and treatment of diseases.
The International Classification of Diseases (ICD-9 and ICD-10)	Morbidity classification produced by the World Health Organization; uses the standard terminology for classifying diseases throughout the world for purposes of billing in the U.S.
Current Procedural Terminology (CPT)	American Medical Association coding for physician offices; provides listing of acceptable terminology for classifying services rendered by healthcare providers.
Appendices in this textbook	Alphabetical listing (healthcare terminology to English and English to healthcare terminology) of combining forms, suffixes and prefixes, and healthcare abbreviations.
Pharmacologic References	
United States Pharmacopeia National Formulary	Complete government listing of all drugs which may be legally dispensed within the United States.
Mosby's Drug Consult	Compendium of information on pharmaceuticals currently on the market in the United States; provides the chemical, generic (common), brand name, and photographs of the drugs listed by manufacturers who choose to list their products in this reference.
Agencies and Websites	
The American Medical Association	http://www.ama-assn.org/about/guidelines.htm This site is only one of many but is a good example because it offers guidelines on the usefulness of a variety of *other* sites.
United States Pharmacopeia	Organization providing information on virtually all of the drugs available in the United States. Agency for processing reports of difficulties with medicines, such as improperly labeled drugs, medication errors, or confusing instructions. Publishes *USPDI, Advice for the Health Care Professional (Volume I)*, and *USPDI, Advice for the Patient (Volume II)*. http://www.usp.org

Continued

Healthcare Resources and References—cont'd

SOURCE	INFORMATION PROVIDED
Agencies and Websites—cont'd	
World Health Organization	http://www.who.int/health-topics
Centers for Disease Control (CDC), National Center for Infectious Diseases	http://www.cdc.gov/ncidod/diseases
National Library of Medicine MEDLINEplus Health Information Website	http://www.nlm.nih.gov/medlineplus/
CDC's National Center for Health Statistics	http://www.cdc.gov/nchs/fastats
Modern Language Association of America	http://www.mla.org (For citation information using a Website)
The United States Bureau of Labor Statistics	http://www.bls.gov/ocohome.htm

Case Study Continued

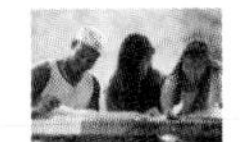

Lan, Maya, and Izaak know that the course textbook is just an introduction to healthcare terminology. As professionals in the healthcare field, they will need to learn to use reference materials to help further understand terminology. For this reason, they team up to try out one of the types of references just discussed, as well as some of the Websites recommended. Each photocopies or prints out a sample page for each of the others. As a result, when these are exchanged, they each have a sample that illustrates that source. This familiarizes each of them with the references they may very well use some day—either in research or on the job.

Abbreviations

Abbreviation	*Definition*	*Abbreviation*	*Definition*
CABG	Coronary artery bypass graft	ICD	International Classification of Diseases
CAM	Complementary and alternative medicine	MRI	Magnetic resonance imaging
CPT	Current Procedural Terminology	PET scan	Positron emission tomography scan
CT	Computed tomography	USP	United States Pharmacopeia (National Formulary)
EGD	Esophagogastroduodenoscopy		
ENT	Ear, nose, and throat		

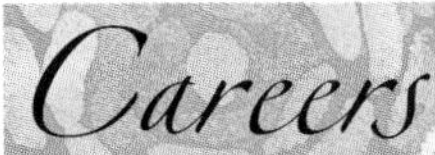

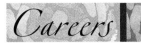

Careers

The United States Bureau of Labor Statistics publishes a constellation of career information. Anyone interested in finding information about a career—what it entails, what training is required, salary ranges, what the projected demand is for its employees—can find that information at http://www.bls.gov/ocohome.htm.

Those without access to the Internet can obtain the same information through their library. Throughout this text, the careers with the greatest potential for growth will be highlighted.

http: INTERNET PROJECT

Now that you have an introduction to healthcare terminology and realize that this is a language that is continually evolving, visit the Websites below and choose one of the diseases listed. Write a 2-page summary (double-spaced) of one of the communicable/infectious diseases that is emerging somewhere currently in the world. Be sure to identify any component word parts and explain the disease's signs and symptoms, means of diagnosis, treatment, and prognosis.

Suggested Websites:

World Health Organization: http://www.who.int/health-topics
Centers for Disease Control (CDC), National Center for Infectious Diseases: http://www.cdc.gov/ncidod/diseases
National Library of Medicine MEDLINEplus Health Information Website: http://www.nlm.nih.gov/medlineplus/
CDC's National Center for Health Statistics: http://www.cdc.gov/nchs/fastats

For citation information for using a Website, visit the Modern Language Association of America at http://www.mla.org.

Chapter Review

A. Types of Healthcare Terms

1. Most healthcare terms are from the ______________ and ______________ languages.
2. A healthcare term that is named after a person who discovered it is a/an ______________.
3. The foundation of a healthcare term is the ______________.
4. If a suffix begins with a vowel, you do/do not (circle one) need a combining vowel.
5. The term that comes before a word root is a/an ______________.
6. If two word roots are joined and the second word root begins with a vowel, you do/do not (circle one) need a combining vowel.

B. Word Roots

Match the following word roots with their definitions.

_____ 7. cardi
_____ 8. gastr
_____ 9. hepat
_____ 10. hemat
_____ 11. arthr
_____ 12. oste
_____ 13. nat
_____ 14. iatr
_____ 15. gynec
_____ 16. ur
_____ 17. radi
_____ 18. psych
_____ 19. ophthalm
_____ 20. ped
_____ 21. dent, odont
_____ 22. electr
_____ 23. onc
_____ 24. derm, dermat
_____ 25. esthesi
_____ 26. ger

A. birth
B. bone
C. urine, urinary system
D. treatment
E. blood
F. stomach
G. joint
H. liver
I. heart
J. female
K. feeling, sensation
L. teeth
M. skin
N. mind
O. old age
P. tumor
Q. rays
R. children
S. electricity
T. eye

C. Prefixes

Match the following prefixes with their definitions.

_____ 27. neo-
_____ 28. endo-
_____ 29. pre-
_____ 30. anti-
_____ 31. hemi-
_____ 32. an-
_____ 33. sub-
_____ 34. epi-
_____ 35. post-
_____ 36. ex-

A. no, not, without
B. half, partial
C. out, out of
D. before
E. after
F. above, on top of
G. inside, within
H. new
I. under
J. against

D. Suffixes

Match the following suffixes with their definitions.

______ 37. -ectomy

______ 38. -itis

______ 39. -tomy

______ 40. -logy

______ 41. -ist

______ 42. -scopy

______ 43. -meter

______ 44. -gram

______ 45. -ic, -al

______ 46. -algia

A. pain
B. a record, recording
C. one who specializes
D. an instrument to measure
E. an incision
F. a removal, a resection
G. the study of
H. a visual examination
I. inflammation
J. pertaining to

E. Word Building

Choose the appropriate prefixes, suffixes, and/or word roots and build terms that take the place of the phrase in parentheses.

47. Janice's father was on medical leave from his job as an emergency medical technician because of a/an ______________ (inflammation of the liver), type C.
48. A ______________ (resection of half of the stomach) was advised for the treatment of Mrs. Smith's stomach cancer.
49. The basketball player was sidelined for several games because the team physician sent him for a ______________ (visual examination of his knee joint).
50. A/an ______________ (incision of a bone) was done as one step of an operation within the chest cavity.
51. The term for the discipline that examines the blood and blood-forming tissues is ______________ (study of the blood).
52. Mr. Connor took his son to a pediatric ______________ (one who specializes in the study of the heart).
53. A baby is described as a newborn during the ______________ period.
54. Lower right quadrant pain, nausea, and a high fever led to a diagnosis of ______________ (inflammation of the appendix).
55. The ophthalmologist used a/an ______________ (instrument to visually examine the interior of the eye) to check Mrs. Johnson's vision.
56. Before her surgery, Ms. Owens was visited by the ______________ (one who specializes in the study of the "lack of feeling or relief of pain").

F. Word Analysis

Define the underlined healthcare term in the following sentences.

57. Wanda experienced ophthalmodynia when a bug flew in her eye.

____

58. The 77-year-old man was considered a geriatric patient.

____

59. Years of long-distance running may have been the cause of Sam's cardiomegaly.

____

60. Mrs. Spacht complained of arthralgia throughout her body.

pain in Joint.

61. A patient who fell through the ice was treated for hypothermia.

G. Procedure and Instrument Terms

Define the following terms.

62. arthroscope

63. thermometer

64. electrocardiograph

65. lithotripter

66. stethoscope

67. endoscopy

68. ophthalmoscope

69. otoscopy ear exame

70. arthrogram

71. osteotome Instrument to cut bone

H. Singulars and Plurals

Change the following from singular to plural or vice versa.

72. pleura

73. prognoses

74. pharynx

75. arthroscopies

76. septa

I. Be Careful

Define and give an example of the following.

77. pre-, per-, and peri- Before - Through - surrounding

78. ante- and anti- before - against

79. -ectomy, -tomy, and -stomy removal - incision - new opening

CHAPTER 2

Body Structure and Directional Terminology

"What a piece of work is a man! How noble in reason! How infinite in faculties! In form and moving, how express and admirable! In action how like an angel! In apprehension, how like a god! the beauty of the world! the paragon of animals!" —**William Shakespeare**

Quote

Case Study

John Greco did not break his wrist playing tennis. No, he tripped and fell *leaving* the court while trying to answer his cell phone. He broke his fall with his free hand and then landed heavily on his left shoulder. John wanted to keep playing, but his partner insisted on taking him to the emergency department at Community Memorial Hospital.

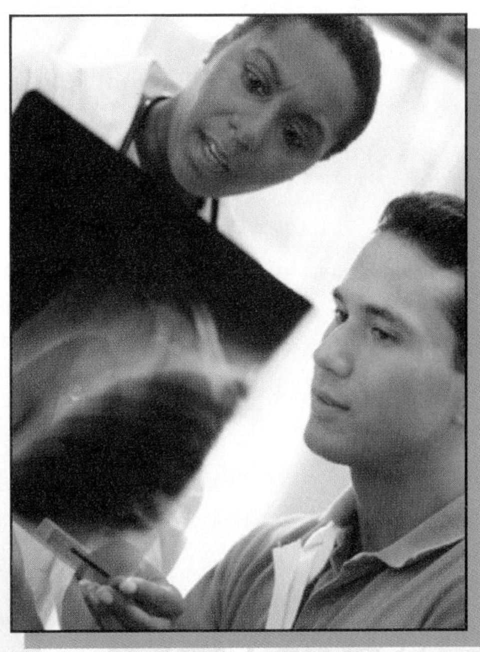

OBJECTIVES

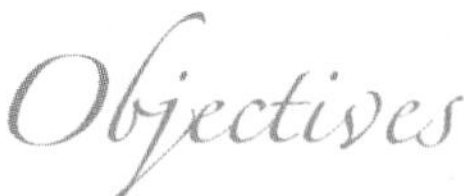

- Explain the levels of organization of the body.
- Match the parts of the cell with their functions.
- List the tissue types and recognize their functions.
- Match organs to body systems.
- Identify anatomic terms for parts of organs.
- Define, modify, and appropriately use directional terms.
- Recognize and label body cavities. Name appropriate organs for body cavities.
- Recognize and label abdominopelvic regions.
- Name and describe the various planes of the body.
- Recognize and recall combining forms, prefixes, and suffixes in this chapter.
- Demonstrate the ability to change singular terms to plural and vice versa.

ORGANIZATION OF THE HUMAN BODY

The human body and its general state of health and disease may be understood by studying the various **body systems**, such as the digestive and respiratory systems. Each body system is composed of different **organs**, such as the stomach and lungs. These organs are made up of combinations of **tissues**, such as epithelial and muscular tissue, which are in turn composed of various **cells** that have very specialized functions.

All of these levels of organization are involved in a continual process of sensing and responding to conditions in the organism's environment. A negative change at one level of one system may cause a reaction throughout the entire body. **Homeostasis** (hoh mee oh STAY sis) is the normal dynamic process of balance needed to maintain a healthy body. When the body can no longer compensate for trauma or pathogens, disease, disorder, and dysfunction result.

> **DID YOU KNOW?**
>
> The terms *disease*, *malaise* (mah LAYZ), and *dysfunction* all have prefixes meaning *not*, *bad*, or *abnormal*.

Cells

The smallest unit of the human body is the cell. Although there are a number of different types of cells, all of them share certain characteristics, one of them being **metabolism** (muh TAB boh lih zum). Metabolism is the act of converting energy by continually building up substances by **anabolism** (an NAB boh lih zum) and breaking down substances by **catabolism** (kuh TAB boh lih zum) for use by the body. Metabolism can be described as an equation:

$$\text{Metabolism} = \text{Anabolism} + \text{Catabolism}$$

Every cell has a nucleus within its cytoplasm. The nucleus contains the information needed to replicate itself and the directions to keep the cell functioning by directing the various organelles (cell parts). See Fig. 2-1 for a picture of a cell and the corresponding table below for a brief description of the pictured organelle and its function.

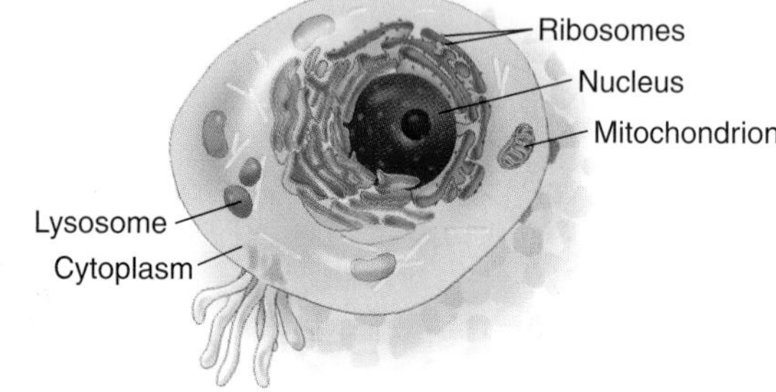

Fig. 2-1 The cell.

Cell Parts

CELL PART	FUNCTION
Nucleus (*pl.* nuclei) NOO klee us	Control center of cell; contains DNA, which carries genetic information
Cytoplasm SYE toh plaz um	Holds the organelles of the cell
Lysosome LYE soh sohm	Digestive bodies that break down foreign or damaged material in cell
Ribosome RYE boh sohm	Site of protein formation; contains RNA
Mitochondrion mye toh KON dree un (*pl.* mitochondria)	Converts nutrients to energy in the presence of oxygen

Tissues

There are four major categories of tissues. Within each type, the tissue is either supportive (**stromal** [STROH mull] tissue) or does the actual work (**parenchymal** [pair EN kuh mul] tissue) of the organ. For example, parenchymal nerve cells are the neurons that conduct the nervous impulse. Neuroglia are stromal nerve cells that enhance and support the functions of the nervous system. The four types of tissue include the following:

Epithelial (eh puh THEE lee ul): Acts as an internal or external covering for organs, for example, the outer layer of the skin or the lining of the digestive tract.
Connective: Includes a variety of types, all of which have an internal structural network. Examples include bone, blood, and fat.
Muscular: Includes three types, all of which share the unique property of being able to contract and relax. Examples include heart muscle, skeletal muscle, and visceral muscle.
Nervous: Includes cells which provide transmission of information to regulate a variety of functions, for example, neurons (nerve cells).

> **DID YOU KNOW?**
>
> Epithelial tissue originally referred to the membrane covering the nipple but now refers to the covering and lining of most of the body and its cavities.

Organs

Organs, also referred to as **viscera** (VIH sur ah) (*sing.* viscus), are arrangements of various types of tissue to accomplish specific purposes. The heart, for example, is made up of muscle tissue, called **myocardium** (mye oh KAR dee um), and it is lined with epithelial tissue known as **endocardium** (en doh KAR dee um). Organs are grouped within body systems but do have specific terms to describe their parts.

Parts of Organs

Organs can be divided into parts and have a set of terms that describe these various parts.

Antrum (AN trum): Any nearly closed cavity or chamber (e.g., gastric antrum).
Apex (A pecks): The pointed extremity of a conical structure (e.g., apex of the lung or heart).
Body: The largest or most important part of an organ (e.g., vertebral body).
Fornix (FOR nicks): Any vaultlike or arched body (e.g., vaginal fornix).
Fundus (FUN dis): The larger part, base, or body of a hollow organ that is farthest from the mouth of the organ (e.g., fundus of uterus).

Hilum (HYE lum): Recess, exit, or entrance of a duct into a gland or of nerves and vessels into an organ (e.g., hilum of kidney).
Lumen (LOO min): The space within an artery, vein, intestine, or tube (e.g., intestinal lumen, lumen of the arteries) (*pl.* lumina).
Sinus (SYE nus): A cavity or channel in bone, a dilated channel for blood, or a cavity to permit the escape of purulent (pus-filled) material (e.g., paranasal sinuses). Antrum and sinus are synonyms.
Vestibule (VES tih byool): A small space or cavity at the beginning of a canal (e.g., vestibule of the ear).

Combining Forms for Body Organization

Meaning	Combining Form
antrum	antr/o
apex	apic/o
blood	hem/o, hemat/o
body	som/o, somat/o
bone	oste/o, osse/o
cell	cyt/o
dissolve	lys/o
epithelium	epitheli/o
fat	adip/o
fornix	fornic/o
fundus	fund/o
heart muscle	myocardi/o
lumen	lumin/o
muscle	my/o
nerve	neur/o
nipple	thel/o
nucleus	kary/o, nucle/o
organ, viscera	organ/o, viscer/o
ribose	rib/o
sameness	home/o
sinus, cavity	sin/o, sinus/o
skeletal muscle	rhabdomy/o
smooth muscle	leiomy/o
system	system/o
tissue	hist/o
to cast	bol/o
vestibule	vestibul/o

Prefixes for Body Organization

Prefix	Meaning
ana-	up, apart
cata-	down
dis-	apart from
dys-	bad, difficult, painful, abnormal
endo-	within
epi-	above
mal-	bad, ill
meta-	change, beyond
para-	near, beside

Suffixes for Body Organization

Suffix	Meaning
-ia	condition
-ism	condition
-ium	structure
-plasm	formation
-stasis	controlling
-um	structure
-us	noun ending

COMBINING FORMS FOR ORGANS

MEANING	COMBINING FORM	MEANING	COMBINING FORM
bladder	cyst/o, vesic/o	nail	onych/o, ungu/o
blood	hem/o, hemat/o	ovary	oophor/o, ovari/o
bone	osse/o, oste/o	skin	cutane/o, derm/o, dermat/o
bone marrow, spinal cord	myel/o	small intestine	enter/o
hair	pil/o, trich/o	stomach	gastr/o
ileum	ile/o	testis	test/o, orchid/o
joint	arthr/o, articul/o	ureter	ureter/o
kidney	nephr/o, ren/o	urethra	urethr/o
muscle	my/o, myos/o		

Exercise 1: INTRACELLULAR FUNCTIONS

Match each cell part with its function.

____ 1. mitochondria
____ 2. ribosomes
____ 3. nucleus
____ 4. lysosomes
____ 5. cytoplasm

A. directs and replicates the cell
B. watery solution within cell, holds organelles
C. contain enzymes to digest material
D. responsible for energy production
E. synthesize proteins

Exercise 2: TYPES OF TISSUE

Match the characteristics of the tissue with its type.

____ 1. contracts tissue
____ 2. transmits information
____ 3. has an internal structural network
____ 4. is an internal/external body covering

A. nervous
B. epithelial
C. muscular
D. connective

Exercise 3: ORGAN PARTS

Match the organ part with its description.

____ 1. fundus
____ 2. lumen
____ 3. fornix
____ 4. hilum
____ 5. vestibule
____ 6. antrum
____ 7. body
____ 8. apex
____ 9. sinus

A. small space at beginning of canal
B. pointed extremity of conical organ
C. space within an artery
D. recess/exit/entrance of organ
E. larger part of a hollow organ farthest from the opening
F. cavity or channel
G. any nearly closed cavity
H. most important part of an organ
I. arched body

Fill in the blank with the correct organ part.

10. Fatty deposits may form in the ____________ (space within) the arteries, resulting in atherosclerosis.
11. Hector had a stone obstructing urine flow at the level of the ____________ (exit/entrance) of the right kidney.
12. The x-rays showed a blunted ____________ (tip) of the left lung.
13. The ____________ (largest part) of the stomach was described as being inflamed.
14. The paranasal ____________ (cavities in bone) were completely blocked.

Body Systems

The organs of the body systems work together to perform certain defined functions. For example, movement is a function of the musculoskeletal system. Although each system has a number of functions, one must remember that the systems interact, and problems with one system can affect the function of other systems. For example, in the condition called *secondary hypertension,* disease in one body system (usually the lungs) causes a pathologic increase in the blood pressure in the cardiovascular system. This hypertensive pressure is secondary to the primary cause (lung disease). Once the disorder of the initial system resolves, the hypertension disappears.

The following table lists each body system, its function, its related organs, and the combining forms used to describe conditions and disorders.

BE CAREFUL!

Do not confuse *my/o,* the combining form for muscle, and *myel/o,* the combining form for spinal cord.

Body Systems

BODY SYSTEM	FUNCTIONS	ORGANS	COMBINING FORMS
Musculoskeletal muss kyoo loh SKELL uh tul	support, movement, protection	muscles	my/o, myos/o
		bones	oste/o, osse/o
		joints	arthr/o, articul/o
		bone marrow	myel/o
Integumentary in teg yoo MEN tuh ree	protection	skin	derm/o, dermat/o, cutane/o
		hair	trich/o, pil/o
		nails	ungu/o, onych/o
Gastrointestinal gass troh in TESS tih nul	nutrition	stomach	gastr/o
		intestines	ile/o, enter/o
Urinary YOOR ih nair ee	elimination of nitrogenous waste	kidneys	ren/o, nephr/o
		bladder	cyst/o, vesic/o
		ureters, urethra	ureter/o, urethr/o
Reproductive	reproduction	ovaries	oophor/o, ovari/o
		testes	test/o, orchid/o
Blood/Lymphatic/ Immune lim FAT tick	transportation, protection	blood cells	erythrocyt/o, leukocyt/o, thrombocyt/o
		lymph glands	lymphaden/o, immun/o

Body Systems—cont'd

BODY SYSTEM	FUNCTIONS	ORGANS	COMBINING FORMS
Cardiovascular kar dee oh VASS kyoo lur	transportation	heart	cardi/o, coron/o
		vessels	arteri/o, ven/o, phleb/o
Respiratory RESS pur ah tore ee	delivers oxygen to cells and removes carbon dioxide	lungs	pulmon/o, pneumon/o
		bronchi	bronch/o
		trachea	trache/o
Nervous/Behavioral NER vus	receive/process information	brain	encephal/o cerebr/o
		nerves	neur/o
		mind	ment/i, phren/o
Special senses	information gathering	eyes	ophthalm/o, ocul/o, opt/o
		ears	ot/o, aur/o
Endocrine EN doh krin	effects changes through chemical messengers	pancreas	pancreat/o
		thyroid	thyroid/o

Case Study Continued

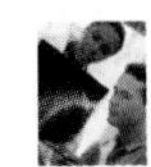

As the doctor on call in the emergency department examines John, she observes a moderately distressed young man favoring his left shoulder and with extensive soft tissue swelling in the left wrist area. She orders wrist and shoulder x-ray studies because she suspects John has a Colles' fracture of the wrist and possibly a shoulder separation.

Exercise 4: BODY SYSTEMS

Match the function with the appropriate body system.

____ 1. thyroid
____ 2. kidneys
____ 3. lungs
____ 4. brain
____ 5. testes
____ 6. intestines
____ 7. skin
____ 8. bones
____ 9. ovaries
____ 10. eyes
____ 11. liquid organs
____ 12. heart

A. integumentary
B. digestive
C. male reproductive
D. musculoskeletal
E. endocrine
F. special senses
G. blood and lymphatic
H. respiratory
I. female reproductive
J. nervous
K. urinary
L. cardiovascular

Exercise 5: Organs and Their Combining Forms

Match the following organ with its correct combining form.

____ 1. windpipe

____ 2. brain

____ 3. skin

____ 4. vein

____ 5. stomach

____ 6. pancreas

____ 7. bladder

____ 8. testis

____ 9. blood

____ 10. ovary

____ 11. ear

____ 12. bone

A. gastr/o
B ot/o
C. pancreat/o
D. cutane/o, derm/o, dermat/o
E. phleb/o, ven/o
F. cyst/o, vesic/o
G. encephal/o
H. oste/o
I. orchid/o, test/o
J. trache/o
K. oophor/o, ovari/o
L. hemat/o, hem/o

Fill in the blank with the correct term using an organ combining form.

13. A patient with phlebitis has a disorder of the __________ system.
14. A patient with orchiditis has an __________ of his __________.
15. An endotracheal tube is inserted in the __________.
16. An otoscope is used to examine a patient's __________.
17. Betty had blood in her urine. The physician advised that she undergo a __________ (visual examination of the bladder).

POSITIONAL AND DIRECTIONAL TERMS

Positional and directional terms are used in healthcare terminology to describe up and down, middle and side, and front and back. Because people may be lying down, raising their arms, and so on, standard English terms cannot be used to describe direction. The following table lists directional and positional terms as opposite pairs, with their respective combining forms or prefixes and illustrations. For example, x-rays may be taken from the front of the body to the back—an anteroposterior (AP) view—or from the back to front—a posteroanterior (PA) view (Figs. 2-2 and 2-3).

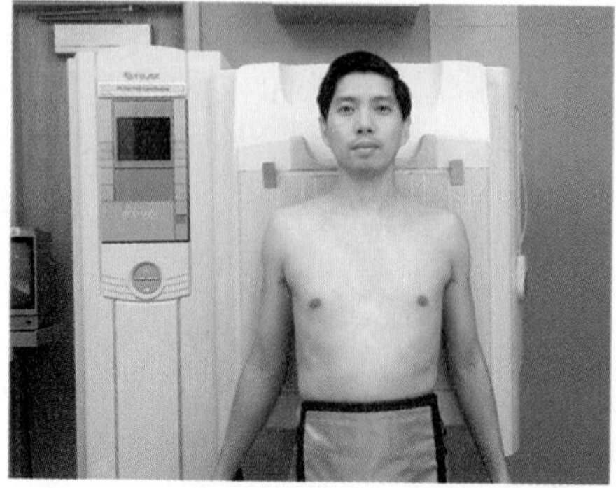

Fig. 2-2 Patient positioned for anteroposterior x-ray of the chest.

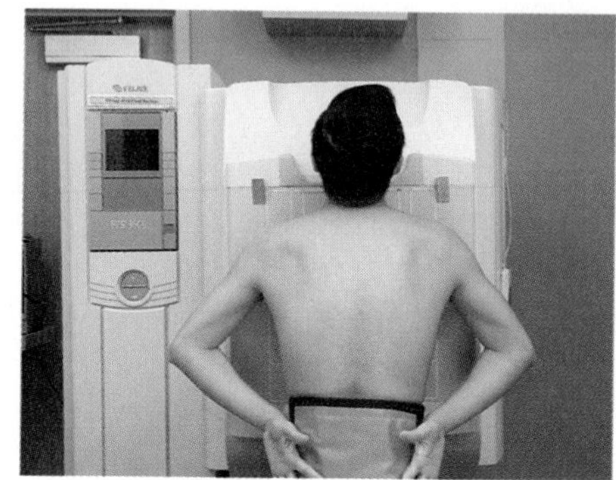

Fig. 2-3 Patient positioned for posteroanterior x-ray of the chest.

Positional and Directional Terms

Anterior (anter/o),
Ventral (ventr/o)
Front or belly side

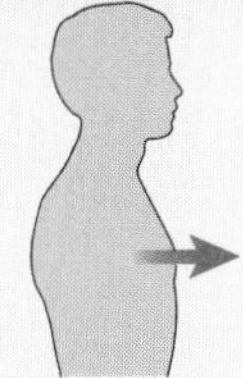

Posterior (poster/o),
Dorsal (dors/o)
Back of body

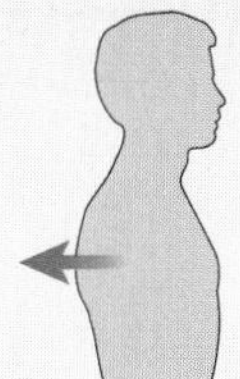

Superior, Cephalad (cephal/o)
Toward the head, up

Inferior, Caudad (caud/o)
Toward the tail, down

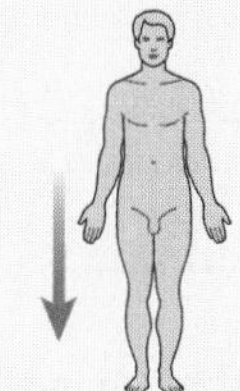

Medial (medi/o)
Toward the midline

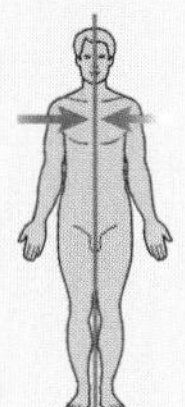

Lateral (later/o)
Toward the side

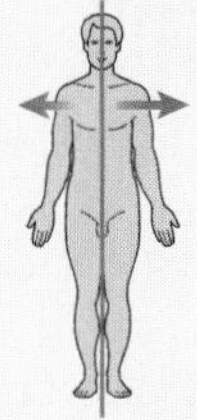

Ipsilateral (ipsi-)
On the same side
Unilateral (uni-)
On one side
Superficial
Towards the surface
Proximal (proxim/o)
Close or nearer to the point of attachment

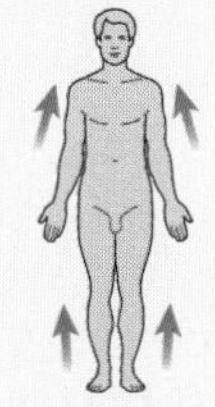

Contralateral (contra-)
On the opposite side
Bilateral (bi-)
On two (both) sides
Deep
Away from the surface
Distal (dist/o)
Far, farther from the point of attachment

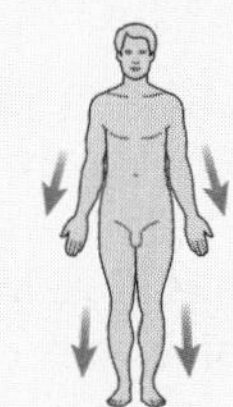

Supine
Lying on one's back

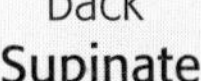

Supinate
Turn the palm upward
Palmar
Pertaining to the palm of the hand
Dextrad (dextr/o)
To the right
Afferent
Toward an organ

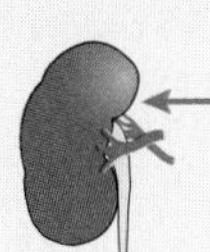

Prone
Lying on one's belly
Pronate
Turn the palm downward
Plantar
Pertaining to the sole of the foot
Sinistrad (sinistr/o, levo-)
To the left
Efferent
Away from an organ

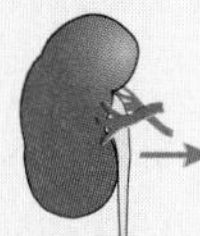

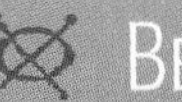

BE CAREFUL!

Do not confuse *anter/o,* meaning *anterior,* and *antr/o,* meaning *antrum.*

DID YOU KNOW?

Because most animals are four-legged, describing front, back, up and down becomes more difficult. That is why veterinarians use the directional terms *cephalad, caudal, ventral,* and *dorsal* to describe positions on their four-legged patients.

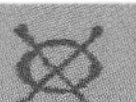

BE CAREFUL!

Do not confuse *bi-,* meaning *two,* and *bi/o-,* meaning *life.*

Case Study Continued

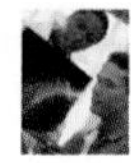

The radiologic technologist, Tisa Tanai, takes lateral and anteroposterior x-rays of John's left wrist and shoulder. The x-rays show a comminuted fracture of the dorsal aspect of the distal radius (Colles' fracture), but the shoulder x-rays are negative. John is interested in seeing his x-rays, so Tisa shows them to him and listens as he muses about how he is going to work around this unexpected complication.

Exercise 6: Positional and Directional Terms

Match the definition with the correct term.

_____ 1. medial
_____ 2. inferior
_____ 3. distal
_____ 4. anterior
_____ 5. dorsal
_____ 6. supine
_____ 7. plantar
_____ 8. deep
_____ 9. contralateral
_____ 10. ipsilateral
_____ 11. afferent
_____ 12. efferent

A. downward, away from the head
B. away from an organ
C. toward the midline
D. the opposite side
E. away from the surface
F. farther away from point of attachment
G. toward an organ
H. on the same side
I. toward the back
J. on one's back
K. toward the front
L. on the bottom of the foot

Fill in the blank with the correct directional or positional term.

13. After a stroke on the right side of her brain, Mrs. Bingham experiences paralysis on her contralateral side. Which side is that? _______________
14. The patient was placed in a supine position to examine her abdomen. How was she positioned? _______________
15. The nurse practitioner diagnoses a wart on the plantar surface of Jessy's left foot. What part of the foot was the wart on? _______________
16. Which end of the esophagus attaches to the stomach? _______________
17. Which nerves carry the nervous impulse towards the brain? _______________

BODY CAVITIES

The body is divided into five cavities (Fig. 2-4). Two of these five cavities are in the back of the body and are called the **dorsal** (DOOR sul) **cavities.** The other three cavities are in the front of the body and are called the **ventral** (VEN trul) **cavities.** Most of the body's organs are in one of these five body cavities.

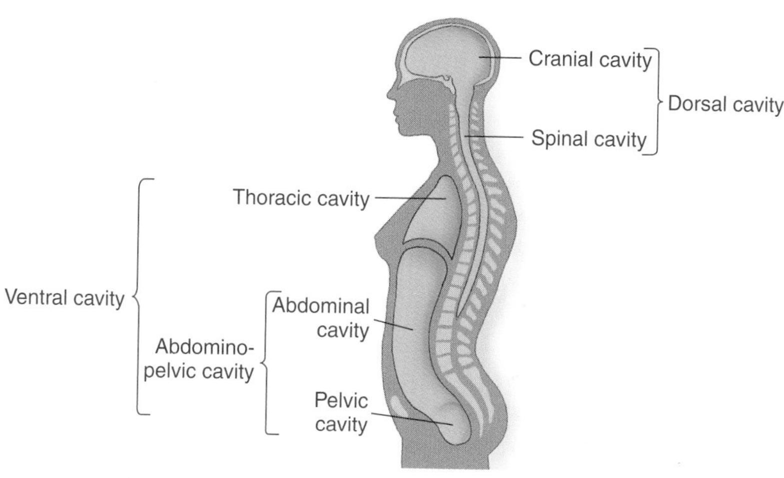

Fig. 2-4 Body cavities.

Dorsal Cavities

The **cranial** (KRAY nee ul) **cavity** contains the brain and is surrounded and protected by the cranium, or skull. The **spinal** (SPY nul) **cavity** contains the spinal cord and is surrounded and protected by the bones of the spine, or vertebrae.

Ventral Cavities

The **thoracic** (thoh RASS ick) **cavity** contains the heart and the lungs. This cavity is surrounded and protected by the ribs, sternum (breastbone), and the vertebrae. Within this cavity is the **mediastinum** (mee dee uh STY num) the space between the lungs and the **pleural** (PLOOR ul) **cavity,** the space between double-folded membrane that surrounds the lungs.

The **abdominal** (ab DOM ih nul) **cavity** contains the stomach, liver, and intestines. It is separated from the thoracic cavity by the muscle called the **diaphragm** (DYE uh fram) and lined by a highly vascular membrane called the **peritoneum** (pair uh tuh NEE um).

The **pelvic** (PELL vick) **cavity,** although sometimes listed together with the abdominal cavity, contains the bladder and reproductive organs. These organs are cradled on the sides and in the back by the pelvic bones. Because there is nothing that physically separates them, sometimes the abdominal and pelvic cavities are collectively referred to as the **abdominopelvic** (ab dom ih noh PELL vick) **cavity.**

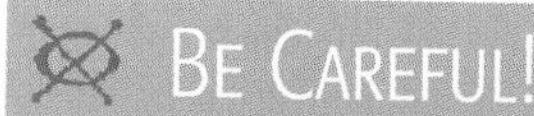

The term *abdomen* refers to a region, whereas the *stomach* is an organ.

COMBINING FORMS FOR BODY CAVITIES

MEANING	COMBINING FORM	MEANING	COMBINING FORM
abdomen	abdomin/o, celi/o, lapar/o	peritoneum	peritone/o
cranium, skull	crani/o	pleura	pleur/o
diaphragm	diaphragm/o, diaphragmat/o, phren/o	spine	spin/o
dorsal	dors/o	sternum	stern/o
mediastinum	mediastin/o	thorax	thorac/o
pelvis	pelv/i	ventral	ventr/o
		vertebra	vertebr/o

Exercise 7: Body Cavities

Match the organ with the appropriate body cavity.

____ 1. cranial
____ 2. abdominal
____ 3. pelvic
____ 4. spinal
____ 5. thoracic

A. spinal cord
B. bladder
C. stomach
D. brain
E. heart

Fill in the blank.

6. The surgeon performed a/an ____ (incision of the skull).
7. A patient undergoing a laparotomy would be undergoing an operative procedure of the ____ cavity.
8. To view the space between the lungs, the physician performed a/an ____ (visual examination of the space between the lungs).
9. ____ (inflammation of the membrane that surrounds the abdominal cavity) is a complication of appendicitis, in which the appendix ruptures and the lining of the abdominal cavity becomes inflamed.
10. In a regional spread of cervical cancer, removal of the contents of the ____ cavity (bladder, uterus, fallopian tubes, ovaries, rectum, vagina) may be indicated.

Be Careful!

Do not confuse *hypo-*, meaning *under* or *lack*, and *hyper-*, meaning *over* or *excess*.

Be Careful!

Do not confuse *ile/o*, meaning *ileum*, and *ili/o*, meaning *ilium*.

Did You Know?

The term *hypochondriac* usually refers to a person who complains of illnesses that he or she does not have. This connotation came to us from the Greeks, who believed a disorder of the spleen (located in the left hypochondriac region) caused this behavior.

ABDOMINOPELVIC REGIONS

The abdominopelvic regions are the nine regions that lie over the abdominopelvic cavity (Fig. 2-5). The area in the center of the abdominopelvic region is called the **umbilical** (um BILL ih kul) area. Laterally, to the left and right of this area, are the **lumbar** (LUM bar) regions. They are called the lumbar regions because they are bound by the lumbar vertebrae. Superior to lumbar regions, and below the ribs, are the **hypochondriac** (hye poh KON dree ack) regions. Medial to the hypochondriac regions, and superior to the umbilical region is the **epigastric** (eh pee GASS trick) region. Inferior to the umbilical region is the **hypogastric** (hye poh GASS trick) region, and lateral to the sides of the hypogastric region are, respectively, the right and left **iliac** (ILL ee ack) regions, sometimes referred to as the **inguinal** (ING gwih nul) regions.

ABDOMINOPELVIC QUADRANTS

A simpler method of naming a location in the abdominopelvic region is to divide the area into quadrants, using the navel as the intersection. These quadrants are referred to as either right or left, upper or lower (Fig. 2-6). In the right upper quadrant (RUQ) lies the liver. In the left upper quadrant (LUQ) lie the stomach and the spleen. The appendix is in the right lower quadrant (RLQ). If a patient complains of pain in the area of **McBurney's point**, the area that is approximately two thirds of the distance between the navel and the hip bone in the RLQ, appendicitis is suspected. Except for the appendix, the left lower quadrant (LLQ) contains organs similar to the lower right. In the LLQ, halfway between the navel and the hipbone, is **Munro's point.** This is a standard site of entrance for surgeons performing laparoscopic surgery.

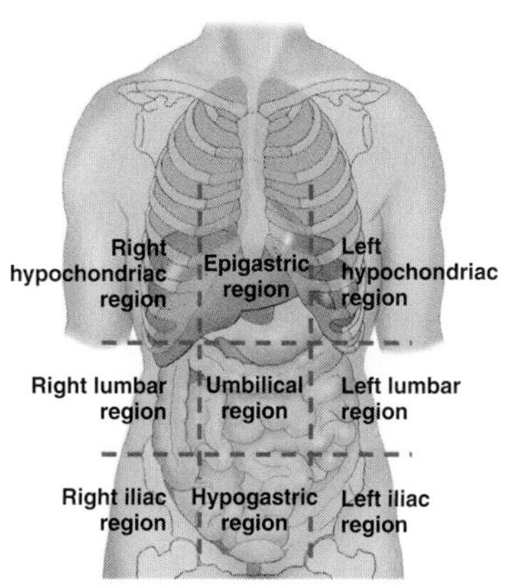

Fig. 2-5 Abdominopelvic regions.

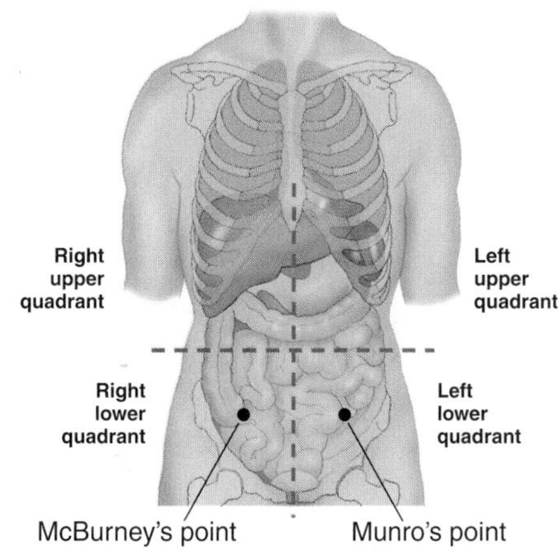

Fig. 2-6 Abdominopelvic quadrants with Munro's and McBurney's points.

PLANES OF THE BODY

Another way of describing the body is by dividing it into planes, or flat surfaces that are imaginary cuts or sections through the body. The use of plane terminology is common when describing imaging of internal body parts by computed tomography (CT) scans, magnetic resonance images (MRIs), positron emission tomography (PET) scans, or other imaging techniques. Figs. 2-7 to 2-9 show the three body planes and corresponding views of the brain.

Sagittal (SAJ ih tul) planes are vertical planes that separate the sides from each other (Fig. 2-7). A **midsagittal** plane separates the body into equal right and left halves. The **frontal** (or **coronal** [koh ROH nul]) plane divides the body into front and back portions (Fig. 2-8). The **transverse** plane divides the body horizontally into an upper part and a lower part (Fig. 2-9).

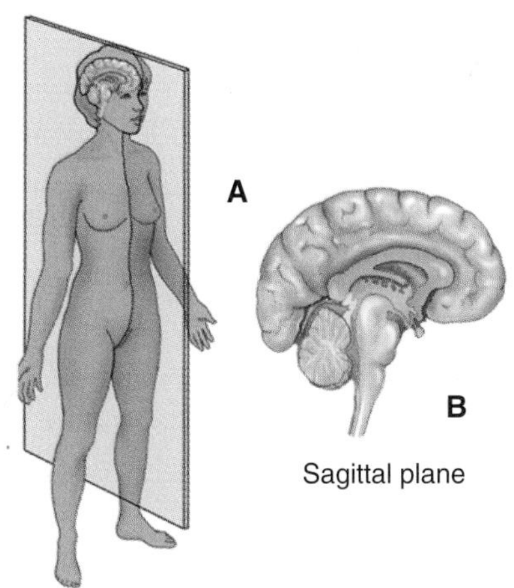

Fig. 2-7 **A,** Sagittal plane. **B,** Sagittal section of the brain.

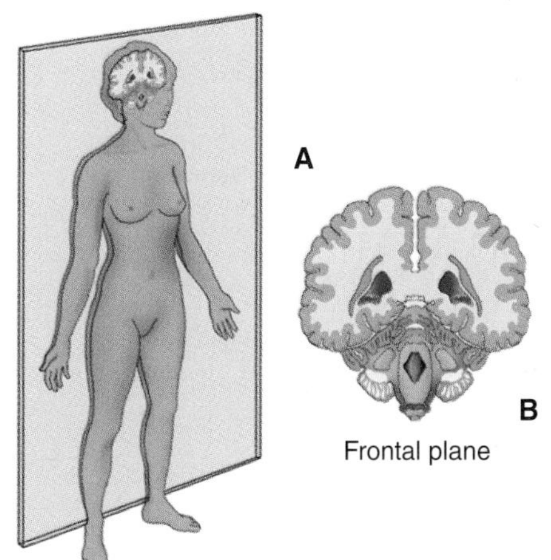

Fig. 2-8 **A,** Frontal plane. **B,** Frontal section of the brain.

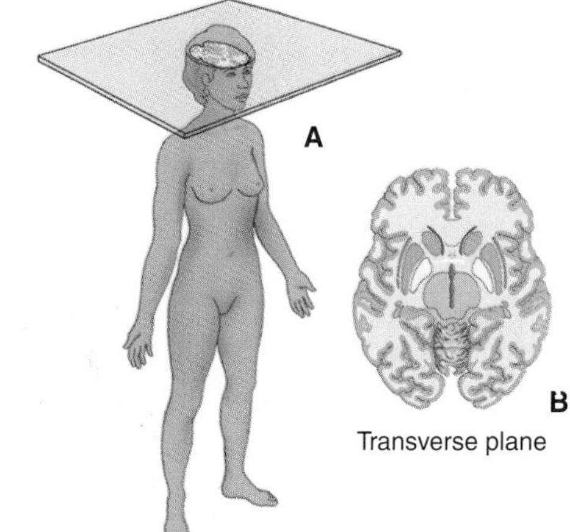

Fig. 2-9 **A,** Transverse plane. **B,** Transverse section of the brain.

COMBINING FORMS FOR ABDOMINOPELVIC REGIONS AND PLANES

MEANING	COMBINING FORM	MEANING	COMBINING FORM
abdomen	lapar/o	heart	coron/o
arrow	sagitt/o	ileum	ile/o
cartilage	chondr/o	ilium	ili/o
front	front/o	loin	lumb/o
groin	inguin/o	umbilicus	omphal/o, umbilic/o

PREFIXES FOR ABDOMINOPELVIC REGIONS AND PLANES

PREFIX	MEANING
epi-	above
hyper-	above, excessive
hypo-	below, deficient
mid-	middle

SUFFIXES FOR ABDOMINOPELVIC REGIONS AND PLANES

SUFFIX	MEANING
-iac	pertaining to
-ic	pertaining to
-scopy	process of visual examination

Exercise 8: ABDOMINOPELVIC REGIONS

Using your knowledge of directional terms and the nine abdominopelvic regions, answer the following questions.

1. Superior to the umbilical region is the ______________ region.
2. Lateral to the umbilical region are the left and right ______________ regions.
3. Medial to the left and right inguinal regions is the ______________ region.
4. Inferior to the lumbar regions are the left and right ______________ regions.
5. Lateral to the epigastric region are the right and left ______________ regions.

Exercise 9: PLANES OF THE BODY

1. Which plane divides the body into superior and inferior portions? ______________
2. Which plane divides the body into equal left and right sections? ______________
3. Which plane divides the body into anterior and posterior sections? ______________

Case Study Continued

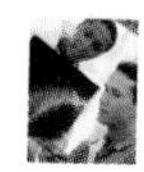

After John's x-rays were read, his wrist was put in a cast with a sling, and he was sent home with directions to take ibuprofen prn (as needed) for his discomfort. Although he would rather not have a broken wrist, he considers himself extremely lucky not to have injured himself more seriously. He looks forward to getting the cast off in 4 weeks and working on getting his wrist back in shape for tennis.

Abbreviations

Abbreviation	Definition	Abbreviation	Definition
LLQ	Lower left quadrant	ULQ	Upper left quadrant
LRQ	Lower right quadrant	URQ	Upper right quadrant
prn	As needed		

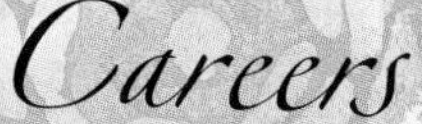

Careers

Radiologic Technologists

Diagnostic medical imaging is predicted to grow faster than most other healthcare professions because of the demographic increase in middle-aged and older individuals. Those individuals who cross-train in other imaging methods (e.g., ultrasounds, CT scans, MRI scans) will be increasingly more valuable in the job market.

Radiologic technologists produce x-rays for diagnostic purposes according to physician orders. They are responsible for positioning patients, preventing unnecessary radiation exposure, taking the films, and developing them. They may also be required to keep patient records and to adjust and maintain equipment.

Two-year associate's degree training programs are most prevalent, although 1- to 4-year programs exist. Hospitals are still the major employer for this field. Most programs require courses in anatomy and physiology, healthcare terminology, positioning of patients, medical ethics, radiation physics, radiobiology, and pathology.

Individuals interested in more career information can access the American Society of Radiologic Technologists Website at http://www.asrt.org/asrt.htm.

For a current list of accredited programs, contact the Joint Review Committee on Education in Radiologic Technology, 20 N. Wacker Dr., Suite 600, Chicago, IL 60606-2901 (Website: http://www.jrcert.org).

http: INTERNET PROJECT

The National Library of Medicine has a complete set of healthy male and female three-dimensional image models provided through the Visible Human Project. Frontal, coronal, and sagittal views of the entire body for both sexes are available. Go to http://www.nlm.nih.gov/research/visible_human.html to complete one of the following:

- Provide an annotated listing of five sites that are linked to this site.
- Determine the source of these bodies of healthy individuals.
- Choose a transverse, coronal, or sagittal section to view and describe.
- Explain the process of the cryosurgery imaging through the use of the following address: http://www.madsci.org/~lynn/VH/planes.html

Chapter Review

A. Organization of the Body

Fill in the blank.

1. Starting from the most complex to the least complex, list the levels of organization in the body.

   ____

   ____

2. Describe the role of homeostasis in the body.

   ____

   ____

3. Which part of the cell is responsible for:

   A. protein formation ______________________

   B. converting nutrients to energy ______________________

   C. holding the organelles ______________________

   D. digesting material ______________________

   E. controlling cell functions ______________________

Fill in the blank with the correct type of tissue.

4. ______________ includes three types of tissue, all of which share the unique property of being able to contract and relax.

5. ______________ includes a variety of types of tissue, all of which have an internal structural network.

6. ______________ acts as an internal or external covering for organs.

7. ______________ includes cells which provide transmission of information to regulate a variety of functions.

Fill in the blank with the correct body system.

8. The function of the ______________ system is to keep the human species on this planet.

9. The main function of the ______________ system is to cover and protect the body.

10. The primary function of the ______________ system is to supply fuel for the body in a form that the body can use.

11. The ______________ system functions to transport nutrients and oxygen to the tissues and to remove waste products.

12. The main function of the ______________ system is to eliminate poisonous waste from the body.

13. Two separate systems, the ____________ and the ____________ are grouped together because they are both "liquid" organs. The functions of the first system are to carry vital substances, regulate others, and protect the body against pathogens. The second system is responsible for returning fluid to the blood and also helping to destroy pathogens that invade the body.

14. The ____________ system provides support, movement, and protection. It also contains red bone marrow and provides a storage site for calcium.

15. The ____________ system keeps our supply of oxygen coming into the body and removes the waste products of respiration (carbon dioxide) from it.

16. The ____________ system receives and processes sensory information and effects movement in the body through neurochemical stimulation.

17. The ____________ system is a variety of organs that share the function of secreting chemical messengers called *hormones* into the bloodstream. These hormones effect changes elsewhere in the system.

18. Through the ____________ system, we gather information about the world around us and process it with our brains through our nervous system.

B. Directional Terms

19. List the opposite of each term.

A. superior ____________

B. prone ____________

C. medial ____________

D. supinate ____________

E. anterior ____________

F. distal ____________

G. caudal ____________

H. deep ____________

I. ventral ____________

J. afferent ____________

K. ipsilateral ____________

Circle the answer that correctly describes the phrase in parentheses.

20. When the basketball player *turned his hand palm down,* he experienced pain. *(supination, pronation)*
21. Tommy had a cut that just broke *the surface* of the skin. *(superficial, deep)*
22. The patient's bruise appeared on the part of her thigh *closest* to her hip. *(proximal, distal)*
23. The *front* of Kelly's body was sunburned. *(anterior, posterior)*
24. The x-ray showed that the *patient's heart was displaced to the left* in his chest cavity. *(sinistrocardia, dextrocardia)*

C. Body Cavities

Fill in the blank with the correct body cavity.

25. The brain and spinal cord are in the ____________ body cavities because they are in the ____________ of the body.

26. The heart, stomach, and bladder are in the ____________ body cavities because they are in the ____________ of the body.

27. The cavity that holds the brain is called the ____________ cavity.

28. The cavity that holds the spinal cord is called the ______________ cavity.

29. The cavity that holds the bladder is the ______________ cavity.

30. The cavity that holds the lungs is the ______________ cavity.

31. The heart and esophagus are located in the ______________.

32. The double-folded membrane that surrounds the lungs is the ______________.

33. The diaphragm is the muscle that separates the ______________ and the ______________ cavities.

34. The liver is in the ______________ cavity.

35. The highly vascular lining of the abdominal cavity is called the ______________.

D. Abdominopelvic Regions

36. Draw a torso below and label the nine abdominopelvic regions.

37. Label the quadrants on the torso provided and label them appropriately. Name an organ which could be found in each quadrant. Sketch in the location of Munro's and McBurney's points and explain in the margin what they signify.

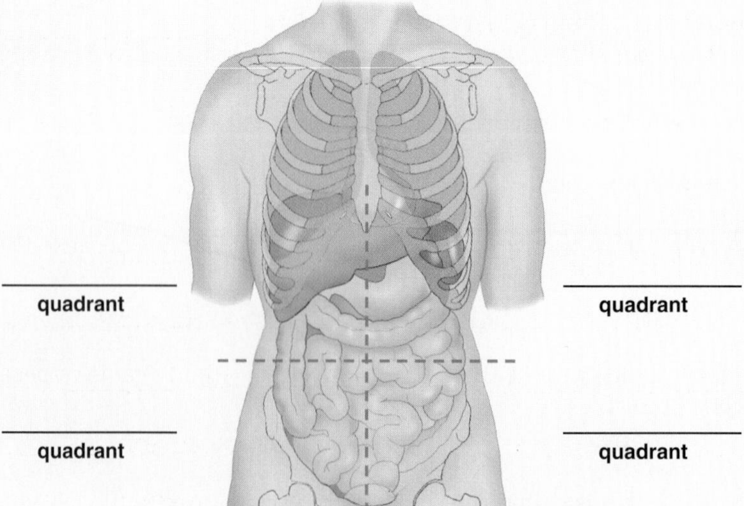

E. Planes of the Body

38. Label the planes provided on the diagram below.

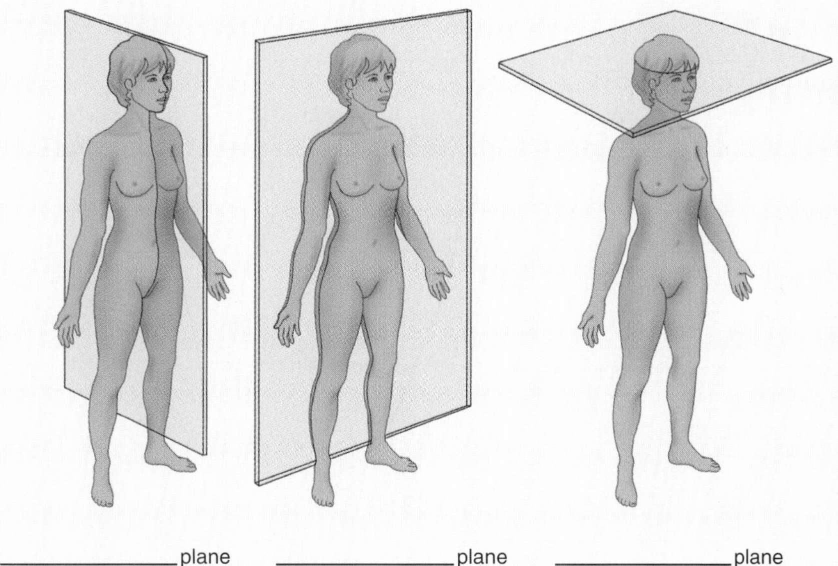

______________ plane ______________ plane ______________ plane

F. Combining Forms, Prefixes, and Suffixes

Using the Operating Schedule given below, answer the following questions. (Note that "SDS" refers to "same-day surgery.")

8:00 AM	colonoscopy	SDS
9:00 AM	EGD	SDS
9:30 AM	lt. knee arthroscopy	SDS
11:30 AM	rt. breast biopsy	SDS
12:30 PM	cystoscopy	SDS

39. What time did a patient have tissue removed for diagnostic purposes? ______________

40. What was the procedure that a patient had done to his/her knee? ______________

41. What time did a patient have his/her bladder visually examined? ______________

42. What is the definition of an EGD? ______________

43. Which procedure examined the large intestine? ______________

G. Singulars and Plurals

Make the following terms plural using the rules from Chapter One.

44. fornix ______________

45. lumen ______________

46. apex ______________

47. fundus ______________

48. larynx ______________

49. uterus ______________

50. hilum ______________

51. nucleus ______________

52. pleura ______________

53. cranium ______________

54. mitochondrion ______________

55. viscus ______________

H. Be Careful

Define the following.

56. ile/o and ili/o

57. my/o and myel/o (both definitions)

58. cyt/o and cyst/o

59. hyper- and hypo-

60. anter/o and antr/o

61. bi- and bi/o

Community Memorial Diagnostic Imaging Center
4545 Freedom Drive
St. Louis, MO 63118

DIAGNOSTIC REPORT

Examination Date: 4/25/03
Date Reported: 4/25/03
Physician: Sandra Robbins, MD
Hospital No. 234567

Patient: John Greco
Age: 29
X-ray #: 8937

Wrist Studies: Multiple views of the left hand were obtained and reveal a slight comminuted, compacted fracture of the dorsal aspect of the distal radius at about the level of its epiphysis with slight adjacent soft tissue swelling and a slight posteriorly displaced fracture across the articular surface of the radius. No other abnormalities were noted.

Impression: Colles' fracture, left wrist

Radiologist ______________________________
Samuel J. Morita, M.D.

I. Healthcare Report

62. Which end of the radius was fractured? The end closest to the wrist or the end nearest the elbow?

____

63. Was the bone displaced backwards or forwards? ______________________________

64. The term *articular* means pertaining to the ______________________________.

65. What does *dorsal* mean? ______________________________

CHAPTER 3

MUSCULOSKELETAL SYSTEM

"People are healed by different kinds of healers and systems because the real healer is within." **—George Goodheart**

Quote

Case Study

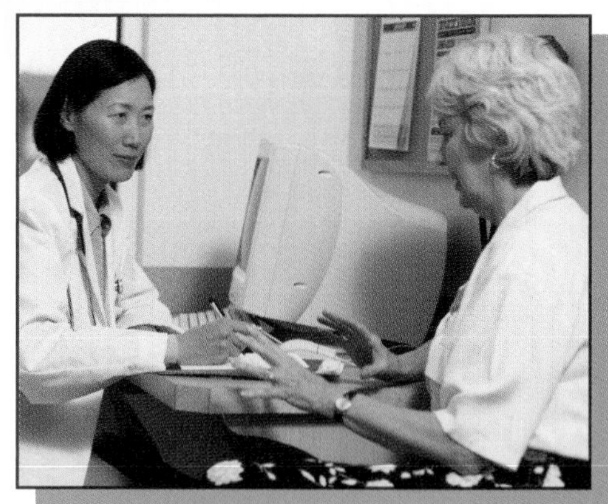

Amelia Long and Evelyn Auden have just met for the first time in the examining room of an orthopedic surgeon. Ms. Auden has an appointment to be evaluated for a possible total knee replacement (TKR) because of her worsening osteoarthritis. Although she has had some success in controlling the pain through the use of acupuncture, Ms. Auden's physician feels that it might be time to consider surgery. Amelia recently graduated from a medical assistant/office management program and is anxious to use her skills. She begins her assessment of Ms. Auden by taking her medical history and entering the information on the computer.

OBJECTIVES

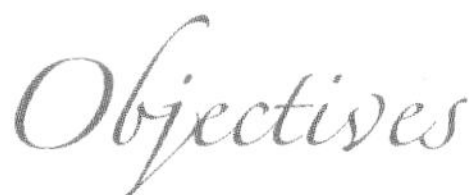

- In your own words, explain the functions of the musculoskeletal system.
- Recognize, recall, and apply healthcare terms related to the anatomy and physiology of the musculoskeletal system.
- Recognize, recall, and apply healthcare terms related to pathology of the musculoskeletal system.
- Recognize, recall, and apply healthcare terms related to diagnostic procedures introduced in this chapter.
- Recognize, recall, and apply healthcare terms related to the therapeutic interventions introduced in this chapter.
- Recognize, recall, and apply the pharmacology introduced in this chapter.
- Recognize, recall, and apply the abbreviations introduced in this chapter.
- Recognize and recall word components used in this chapter to build and decode healthcare terms relevant to the musculoskeletal system.
- Demonstrate the ability to change singular musculoskeletal system terms to plural terms and vice versa.
- Recognize, recall, and apply material learned in previous chapters.

FUNCTIONS OF THE MUSCULOSKELETAL SYSTEM

The **musculoskeletal** (muss skyoo loh SKELL uh tul) **system (MS)** consists of three interrelated parts: **bones, articulations (joints)**, and **muscles.** Bones are connected to one another by fibrous bands of tissue called **ligaments** (LIH gah ments). Muscles are attached to the bone by bands of tissue called **tendons** (TEN duns). The tough fibrous covering of the muscles (as well as some nerves and blood vessels) is called the **fascia** (FASH ee ah). Articular **cartilage** (KAR tih lij) covers the ends of many bones and serves a protective function.

Imagine a body without bones and muscles! Where would the organ systems be placed? What would protect the vital organs? And how would a person move? The musculoskeletal system meets these needs by:

1. Acting as a framework for the organ systems
2. Protecting many of the body's organs
3. Providing the organism the ability to move

Along with these functions, some bones are responsible for storage of minerals (calcium [Ca] and phosphorus [P]) and the continual formation of blood, a process called **hematopoiesis** (hee mah toh poh EE sis), in the bone marrow.

Combining forms for the major parts of this system are listed as follows:

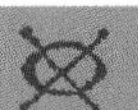

BE CAREFUL!

The abbreviation for the musculoskeletal system, MS, is the same as the abbreviation for mitral stenosis and multiple sclerosis.

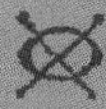

BE CAREFUL!

The word part *os* means *a mouth* or *an opening;* do not confuse it with the combining forms for bone.

COMBINING FORMS FOR THE MUSCULOSKELETAL SYSTEM

MEANING	COMBINING FORM	MEANING	COMBINING FORM
blood	hemat/o, hem/o	ligament	ligament/o, syndesm/o
bone	oste/o, oss/i, osse/o	muscle	muscul/o, my/o, myos/o
calcium	calc/o	phosphorus	phosph/o, phosphat/o
cartilage	chondr/o, cartilag/o	tendon	tendin/o, tend/o, ten/o
fascia	fasci/o		
joint (also called an articulation)	arthr/o, articul/o		

Exercise 1: COMBINING FORMS

Match all correct combining forms with their meaning. More than one answer may be correct.

_____ 1. joint	_____ 6. fascia	A. fasci/o	G. tendin/o
_____ 2. bone	_____ 7. cartilage	B. hemat/o	H. ligament/o
_____ 3. muscle	_____ 8. blood	C. oste/o	I. myos/o
_____ 4. tendon	_____ 9. calcium	D. calc/o	J. articul/o
_____ 5. ligament	_____ 10. phosphorus	E. arthr/o	K. syndesm/o
		F. chondr/o	L. phosph/o

DID YOU KNOW?

The term *skeleton* is derived from the Greek *skeletos,* meaning *dried up, parched,* or *withered.* Greeks used this word to describe mummies and dried-up bodies. The current use of the term, meaning the bones only, began in the 1500s.

ANATOMY AND PHYSIOLOGY

BONES

Types of Bones

Most adult bodies contain 206 bones. These bones are categorized as belonging either to the **axial** (ACK see ul) **skeleton,** which consists of the skull, rib cage, and spine or the **appendicular** (ap pen DICK yoo lur) **skeleton,** which consists of the shoulder bones, collar bones, pelvic bones, arms, and legs (Fig. 3-1). Human bones appear in a variety of shapes that suit their function in the body. See Fig. 3-1 and the following table for the location and the description of these bones.

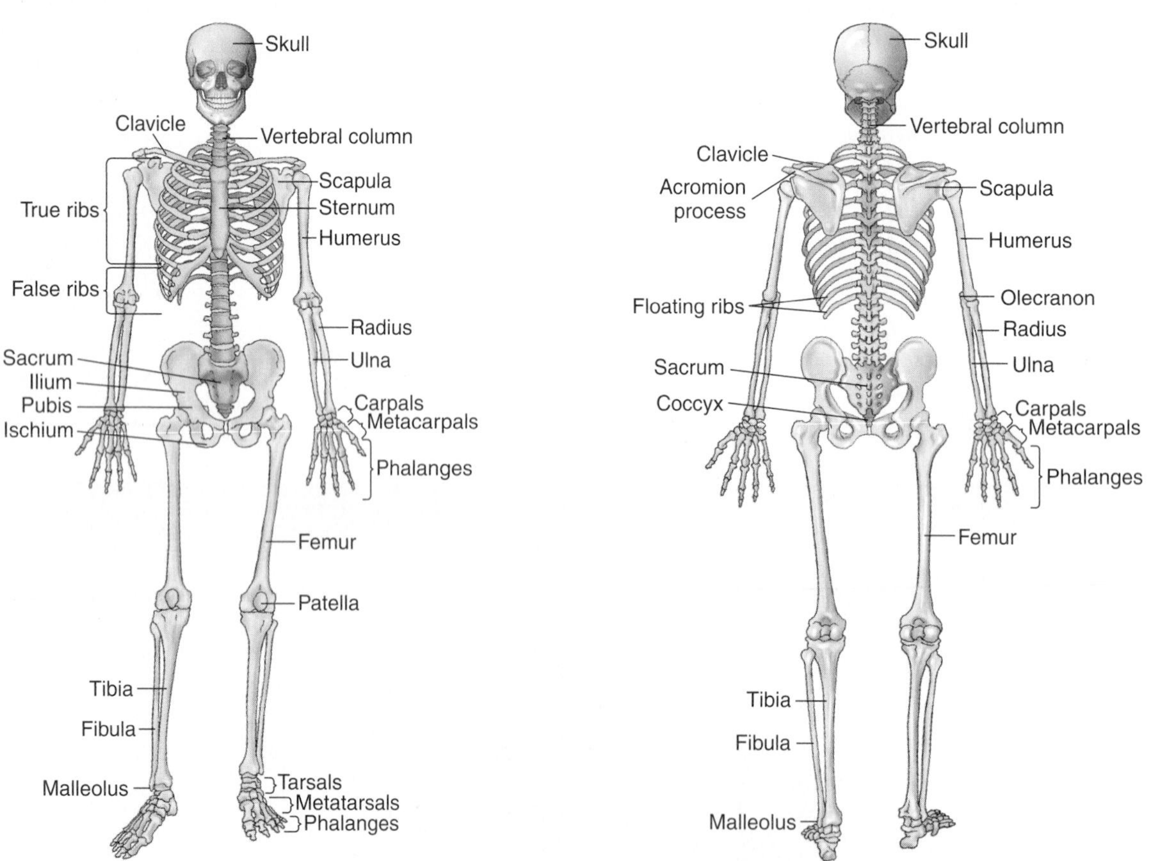

Fig. 3-1 Axial and appendicular skeleton.

Shapes of Human Bones

TYPES	EXAMPLES
long bones	humerus (upper arm bone), femur (thigh bone)
short bones	carpal (wrist bone), tarsal (ankle bone)
flat bones	sternum (breastbone), scapula (shoulder blade)
irregular bones	vertebra (backbone), stapes (a bone of the ear)
sesamoid (SEH sah moyd)	patella (knee cap) bones

Bone Structure

All bones are composed of mature bone cells, called **osteocytes** (OS tee oh sytes), and the material between the cells, called the **matrix** (MAY tricks). The matrix stores calcium and phosphorus for the body to use as needed in the form of mineral salts. Other types of bone cells include **osteoblasts,** cells that build bone, and **osteoclasts,** cells that break down bone cells to transform them as needed. The osteocytes and matrix together make up the hard, outer layer of bone known as **compact bone.** Within the compact bony tissue is a second layer of bone tissue called **spongy** or **cancellous** (KAN seh lus) **bone.** This spongy bone is composed of the same osteocytes and matrix, but, as its name implies, it is less dense. Within the spongy layer lie the medullary cavity and the red bone marrow, which produces all of the blood cells needed by the body.

Each long bone (Fig. 3-2) is composed mainly of a long shaft called the **diaphysis** (dye AFF ih sis). Each end of the bone is called an **epiphysis** (eh PIFF ih sis) (*pl.* epiphyses). Underneath the epiphyses are the **epiphyseal** (eh pee FIZZ ee ul) **plates,** the areas where bone growth normally occurs. Around the ages from 16 to 25, the plates close, and bone growth stops. The epiphysis and epiphyseal plates together form the **metaphysis** (meh TAFF ih sis).

The outer covering of the bone is called the **periosteum** (pair ee OS tee um) and the inner aspect of the bone is known as the **endosteum** (en DOS tee um). These two coverings hold the cells responsible for bone remodeling: the osteoblasts and osteoclasts. The shape of a bone enables practitioners to speak very specifically about a particular area on that bone. For instance, any groove, opening, or hollow space is called a **depression.** Depressions provide an entrance and exit for vessels, as well as protection for the organs they hold. Raised or projected areas are called **processes.** These are often areas of attachment for ligaments or muscles. The tables that follow give examples of bone depressions and processes.

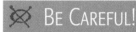

BE CAREFUL!

Remember that the ends of the long bones closest to the points of attachment (hips and shoulders) would be described as *proximal,* whereas those furthest from the points of attachment (feet and hands) would be described as *distal.*

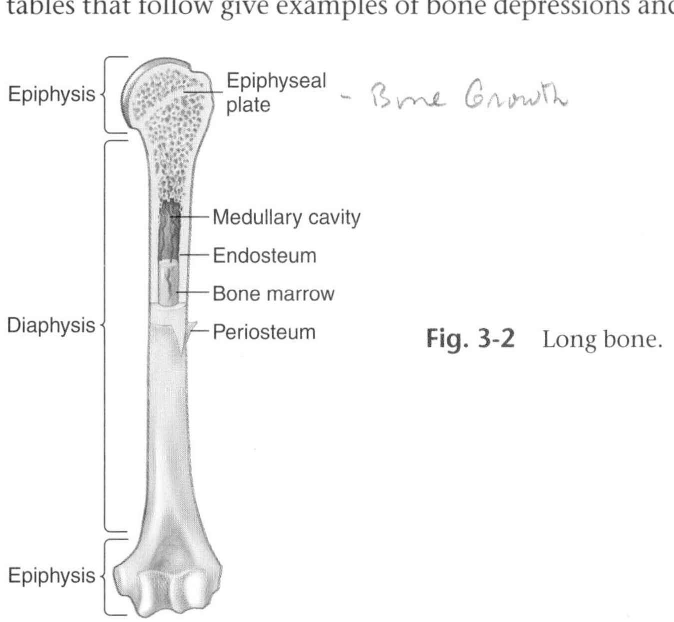

Fig. 3-2 Long bone.

Bone Depressions

DEPRESSION	MEANING
fissure (FISH ur)	A fairly deep cleft or groove.
foramen (foh RAY men) (*pl.* foramina)	An opening or hole, such as the foramen magnum in the skull.
fossa (FAH sah)	A hollow or depression, especially on the surface of the end of a bone, such as the olecranon fossa.
sinus (SYE nus)	A cavity or channel lined with a membrane such as the paranasal sinuses. Also called an *antrum.*
sulcus (SULL kus) (*pl.* sulci)	A general term that refers to a groove or depression in an anatomic structure, usually not as deep as a fissure.

Bone Processes

PROCESS	MEANING
condyle (KON dyle)	A rounded projection at the end of a bone that anchors ligaments and articulates with adjacent bones.
crest	A narrow elongated elevation, such as the iliac crest.
epicondyle (eh pee KON dyle)	A projection on the surface of the bone above the condyle.
head	A rounded, usually proximal portion of some long bones.
spine	A thornlike projection, such as the spinous process of a vertebra.
trochanter (troh KAN tur)	One of two bony projections on the proximal ends of the femurs that serve as points of attachment for muscles.
tubercle (TOO bur kul)	A nodule or small raised area.
tuberosity (too bur OSS ih tee)	An elevation or protuberance, larger than a tubercle.

Combining Forms for the Skeletal System

MEANING	COMBINING FORM	MEANING	COMBINING FORM
antrum	antr/o	elbow	olecran/o
bone	oste/o, osse/o	epicondyle	epicondyl/o
bone marrow	myel/o	nose	nas/o
condyle	condyl/o	sinus	sin/o, sinus/o

Prefixes for the Skeletal System

PREFIX	MEANING
dia-	through, complete
endo-, end-	within
epi-	above
meta-	change, beyond
peri-	surrounding

Suffixes for the Skeletal System

SUFFIX	MEANING
-blast	embryonic
-clast	breaking down
-cyte	cell
-physis	growth
-poiesis	formation
-um	structure, thing

Exercise 2: BONE BASICS

Match the following word components with their meanings.

K 1. myel/o
I 2. -physis
J 3. epi-
D 4. endo-
G 5. -poiesis
H 6. -cyte
E 7. peri-
C 8. meta-
L 9. oste/o
F 10. -um
A 11. -blast
B 12. -clast

A. embryonic
B. breakdown
C. change, beyond
D. within
E. surrounding
F. structure
G. formation
H. cell
I. growth
J. above
K. bone marrow
L. bone

Fill in the blank.

13. Osteoblasts Build bone, whereas osteoclasts Breakdown bone.

14. The shaft of a long bone is called a/an Diaphysis; the ends of a long bone are called epiphyses (plural!).

15. The outer covering of bone is the Periosteum, whereas the inner lining is the endosteum.

16. A foramen, a sulcus, and a fossa are examples of bone Depressions. A condyle, a trochanter, and a tuberosity are examples of bone Processes.

17. A synonym for a sinus is a/an Antrum.

The Axial Skeleton

The axial skeleton includes the skull, spine, and ribcage (see Fig. 3-1).

Skull

The skull is made up of two parts: the **cranium** (KRAY nee um) that encloses and protects the brain, and the **facial bones** (Fig. 3-3).

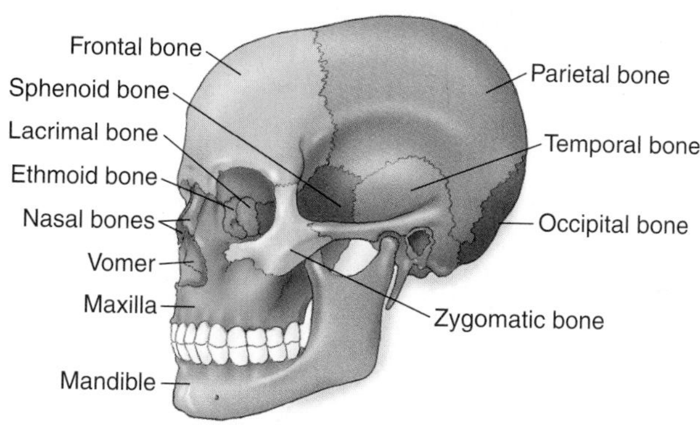

Fig. 3-3 Skull and facial bones.

Cranium

Frontal bone: Forms the anterior part of the skull and the forehead.
Parietal (puh RYE uh tul) **bones:** Form the sides of the cranium.
Occipital (ock SIP ih tul) **bone:** Forms the back of the skull. Notable is a large hole at the ventral surface in this bone, the foramen magnum (meaning *large*), which allows the brain communication with the spinal cord.
Temporal (TEM poor ul) **bones:** Form the lower two sides of the cranium.
Ethmoid (EHTH moyd) **bone:** Forms the roof and walls of the nasal cavity.
Sphenoid (SFEE noyd) **bone:** Anterior to the temporal bones and the basilar part of the occipital bone.

The last three bones of the skull, the ossicles, are tiny bones within the ear. These will be discussed in Chapter 14.

Facial Bones

Use Fig. 3-3 to locate the names and locations of the majority of the following facial bones:

Zygoma (zye GOH mah): Cheekbone. Also called the *zygomatic* (zye goh MAT tick) *bone.*
Lacrimal (LACK rih mul) **bones:** Paired bones at the corner of each eye that cradle the tear ducts.
Maxilla (MACK sill ah): Upper jaw bone. Also called the **maxillary bone.**
Mandible (MAN dih bul): Lower jaw bone. Also called the **mandibular bone.**
Vomer (VOH mur): Bone that forms the posterior/inferior part of the nasal septal wall between the nostrils.
Palatine (PAL eh tyne) **bones:** Make up part of the roof of the mouth.
Inferior nasal conchae (KON kee): Make up part of the interior of the nose.

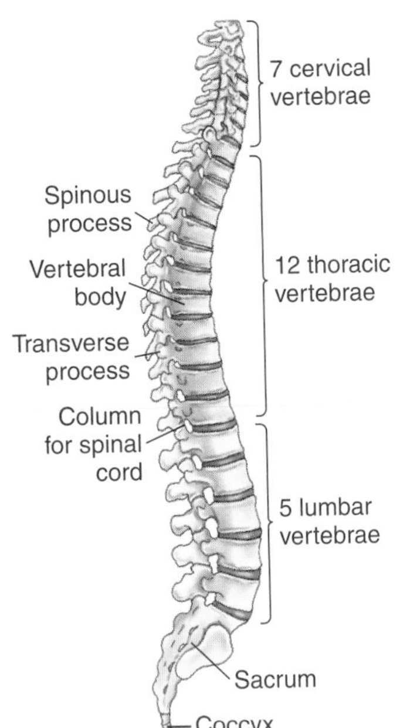
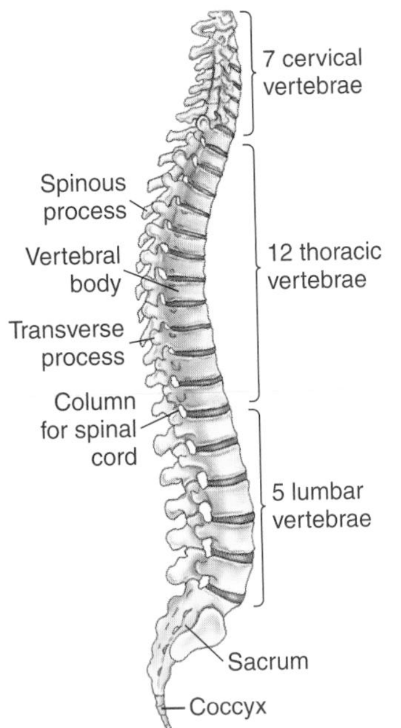

Fig. 3-4 Spine.

Spine

The **spinal**, or **vertebral**, column is divided into five regions from the neck to the tailbone. It is composed of 26 bones called the **vertebrae** (VUR teh bray). Fig. 3-4 and the following table list and illustrate the bones in the spine.

BE CAREFUL!

Do not confuse *sacr/o* with *sarc/o* (meaning *flesh*).

Bones of the Spine

REGION	TYPE AND ABBREVIATION
Cervical (SUR vih kul)	Neck bones (C1-C7)
Thoracic (thoh RAS ick)	Upper back (T1-T12)
Lumbar (LUM bar)	Lower back (L1-L5)
Sacral (SAY krul)	Sacrum (S1-S5) (5 bones, fused)
Coccygeal (kock sih JEE ul)	Coccyx (KOCK sicks) or tailbone

Ribcage

The **ribs** consist of 12 pairs of thin, flat bones attached to the thoracic vertebrae in the back and by costochondral (kost toh KON drul) tissue in the front (see Fig. 3-1). The ribs can be categorized as follows:

- True ribs: Seven pairs attached directly to the breastbone (sternum) in the front of the body

COMBINING FORMS FOR THE AXIAL SKELETON

Meaning	Combining Form	Meaning	Combining Form
back of body	dors/o	parietal	pariet/o
cervical (neck)	cervic/o	rib	cost/o
coccyx (tailbone)	coccyg/o	sacrum	sacr/o
ethmoid	ethmoid/o	skull	crani/o
frontal	front/o	sphenoid	sphenoid/o
jaw	gnath/o	spinal column	rachi/o, spin/o, vertebr/o
lamina	lamin/o	sternum	stern/o
lower back	lumb/o	temporal	tempor/o
mandible	mandibul/o	thorax	thorac/o
maxillary	maxill/o	vertebra	vertebr/o, spondyl/o
occipital	occipit/o	vomer	vomer/o
palatine	palat/o	zygoma	zygom/o, zygomat/o

- False ribs: Five pairs attached to the sternum by cartilage
- Floating ribs: Two pairs of false ribs not attached in the front of the body at all

In addition to ribs, the rib cage includes the **sternum** (STUR num), also known as the *breastbone.* The sharp point at the most inferior aspect of the sternum is called the **xiphoid** (ZIH foyd) **process.**

Exercise 3: BONES OF THE CRANIUM

Using the diagram provided below, label the bones of the cranium and face.

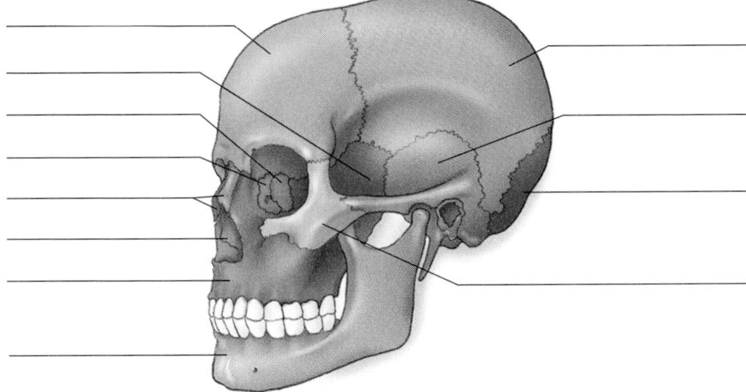

Exercise 4: FACIAL BONES

Choose the correct terms from the following list to fill in the blanks.

lacrimal, mandible, maxilla, vomer, zygoma

1. cheekbone ________________
2. upper jaw bone ________________
3. lower jaw bone ________________
4. bones that hold tear ducts ________________
5. bone that forms the wall between the nostrils ________________

Exercise 5: Bones of the Spine

1. Draw a sagittal view of the spine, filling in the spinal sections from top to bottom with the number of vertebrae in each. Use the stated abbreviations where appropriate. The following terms, although not in order, are the five spinal sections: **thoracic, coccygeal, sacral, cervical, lumbar.**

2. Build a term meaning *pertaining to the lumbar and sacral vertebrae.*

____

Exercise 6: Bones of the Rib Cage

Match the combining form or its meaning with the corresponding description.

C 1. true ribs

D 2. chondr/o

E 3. sternum

A 4. xiphoid

B 5. cost/o

A. process at end of sternum
B. rib
C. 7 pairs
D. cartilage
E. breastbone

Appendicular Skeleton

The appendicular skeleton is composed of the upper appendicular and the lower appendicular skeletons.

Upper Appendicular

The upper appendicular skeleton includes the shoulder girdle, which is composed of the **scapula, clavicle,** and the **upper extremities.** Refer to Fig. 3-1 for a correlation of each bone's description with its location.

Scapula (SKAP yoo lah): The scapulae, or shoulder blades, are flat bones that help to support the arms. The **acromion** (ack ROH mee un) **process** is the lateral protrusion of the scapula that forms the highest point of the shoulder.
Clavicle (KLA vih kul): The clavicle, or collarbone, consists of a pair of long, curved horizontal bones above the first ribs that attach to the sternum at one end and the acromion process of the scapula at the other. These bones help to stabilize the shoulder anteriorly.

The upper extremities consist of the following:

Humerus (HYOO mur us): Upper arm bone.
Radius (RAY dee us): Lower lateral arm bone parallel to the ulna. The distal end articulates with the thumb side of the hand.
Ulna (UL nuh): Lower medial arm bone. The distal end articulates with the little finger side of the hand.
Olecranon (oh LECK ruh non): A proximal projection of the ulna that forms the tip of the elbow.
Carpal (KAR pul): One of eight wrist bones.
Metacarpal (meh tuh KAR pul): One of the five bones that form the middle part of the hand.
Phalanx (FAY lanks): One of the 14 bones that comprise the fingers of the hand, two in the thumb and three in each of the other four fingers (*pl.* phalanges).

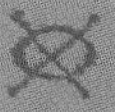

BE CAREFUL!

Do not confuse *ilium* with its homonym, *ileum,* which is a part of the digestive system.

DID YOU KNOW?

Archaeologists can often tell a male from a female skeleton by examining the pelvic outlets. The female pelvis is wider.

Lower Appendicular

The lower half of the appendicular skeleton can be divided into the **pelvis** (***pl.*** **pelves)** and the **lower extremities** (see Fig. 3-1). The pelvic bones (also called the *pelvic girdle*) consist of the following three bones:

Ilium (ILL ee um): The superior and widest bone of the pelvis.
Ischium (ISS kee um): The lower portion of the pelvic bone.
Pubis (PYOO bis) **or pubic bone:** The lower anterior part of the pelvic bone.

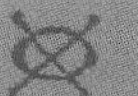

BE CAREFUL!

Do not confuse *perone/o,* meaning *fibula,* and *peritone/o,* meaning *the abdominal wall.*

The lower extremities include the following:

Femur (FEE mur): Thighbone.
Patella (puh TELL uh): Kneecap.
Tibia (TIB ee uh): Shin.
Fibula (FIB yuh luh): Smaller, lateral leg bone.
Malleolus (muh LEE uh lus): Process on the distal ends of tibia and fibula.
Tarsal (TAR sul): One of the seven bones of the ankle, hindfoot, and midfoot.
Metatarsal (met uh TAR suhl): One of the five foot bones between the tarsals and the phalanges.
Phalanx: One of the 14 toe parts, two in the great toe and three in each of the other four toes.

Combining Forms for the Appendicular Skeleton

Meaning	Combining Form	Meaning	Combining Form
carpal	carp/o	metatarsal	metatars/o
clavicle (neck)	cleid/o	patella	patell/o
femur	femor/o	phalanx (part of finger, toe)	phalang/o
fibula	fibul/o, perone/o	pubis or pubic bone	pub/o
finger, toe (whole)	dactyl/o	radius	radi/o
humerus	humer/o	scapula	scapul/o
ilium	ili/o	tarsal	tars/o
ischium	ischi/o	tibia	tibi/o
malleolus	malleol/o	ulna	uln/o
metacarpal	metacarp/o		

Exercise 7: Appendicular Skeleton

Classify the following bones or bone parts as belonging to the shoulder girdle, arm, leg, or pelvic girdle.

1. femur ______
2. patella ______
3. olecranon ______
4. clavicle ______
5. pubis ______
6. ilium ______
7. acromion process ______
8. tarsal ______

Exercise 8: Upper Appendicular Skeleton

Match the following.

____ 1. upper arm bone
____ 2. collarbone
____ 3. finger bones
____ 4. hand bones
____ 5. lower arm bones
____ 6. elbow
____ 7. shoulder blades
____ 8. wrist bones

A. olecranon
B. radius and ulna
C. metacarpals
D. humerus
E. carpals
F. phalanges
G. clavicle
H. scapulae

Exercise 9: Lower Appendicular Skeleton

1. Build a term for the joint between a metatarsal and a phalanx.

______

2. Name the three bones in the pelvis, paying attention to the correct spelling of each.

______

3. Fill in the blanks with one of the following healthcare terms.

tarsals, femur, fibula, patella, phalanges, metatarsals, tibia

A. shin bone ______________ E. foot bones ______________

B. kneecap ______________ F. lower lateral leg bone ______________

C. thigh bone ______________ G. ankle bones ______________

D. toe bones ______________

4. The malleolus is a structure that appears on the ______________ end of the fibula and tibia.

Joints

Joints, or *articulations* as they are sometimes called, are the parts of the body where two or more bones of the skeleton join. Examples of joints include the knee, which joins the tibia and the femur, and the elbow, which joins the humerus with the radius and ulna. Joints provide **range of movement (ROM)**, the range through which a joint can be extended and flexed. Different joints have different ROM, ranging from no movement at all to full range of movement. Categorized by ROM, they are as follows:

No ROM: Most **synarthroses** (sin ar THROH sees) are immovable joints held together by fibrous cartilaginous tissue. The suture lines of the skull are examples of synarthroses.

Limited ROM: Amphiarthroses (am fee ar THROH sees) are joints joined together by cartilage that are slightly movable, like the vertebrae of the spine or the pubic bones.

Full ROM: Diarthroses (dye ar THROH sees) are joints that have free movement. The most commonly known are ball-and-socket joints (like the hip) and hinge joints (like the knees). Other examples of diarthroses include the elbows, wrists, shoulders, and ankles. See Fig. 3-5 for an illustration of a knee joint.

Diarthroses, or **synovial** (sih NOH vee ul) **joints**, as they are frequently called, are the most complex of the joints. Because these joints help a person move around for a lifetime, they are designed to efficiently cushion the jarring of the bones and to minimize friction between the surfaces of the bones. Many of the synovial joints have **bursae** (BURR see) (*sing.* bursa), which are sacs of fluid that are located between the bones of the joint and the tendons that hold the muscles in place. Bursae help cushion the joints when they move. Synovial joints also have joint capsules that enclose the ends of the bones, a synovial membrane that

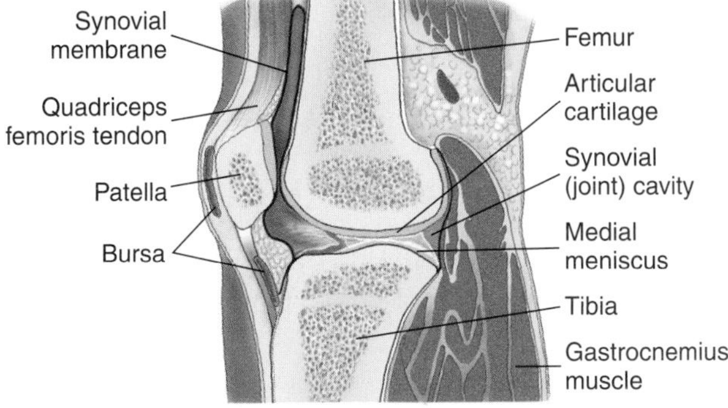

Fig. 3-5 Knee joint.

lines the joint capsules and secretes fluid to lubricate the joint, and articular cartilage that covers and protects the bone.

DID YOU KNOW?

The word *muscle* comes from the Latin *musculus,* the diminutive of *mus,* meaning *a mouse;* hence, literally, *a little mouse,* usually explained by the allusion to rippling of muscles under the skin as the scurrying of little mice.

Muscles

A muscle is a tissue that is composed of cells that are able to contract, resulting in movement. Muscles move the body in more ways than most people might imagine. Three specialized types of muscle and muscle movement include:

- Skeletal movement (skeletal, striated, or voluntary muscle)
- Movement of the smooth muscles of the body (visceral muscle)
- Contraction of the heart muscle (myocardium)

Muscle tissue has only the ability to contract and relax. Most skeletal muscles work in pairs that oppose each other, called *antagonistic muscles.* As one muscle relaxes, the other contracts, and together these effect a given action. Synergistic muscles are those that contract together.

Muscle Actions

ACTION	DESCRIPTION
Extension	to increase the angle of a joint
Flexion	to decrease the angle of a joint
Abduction	to move away from the midline
Adduction	to move towards the midline
Supination	to turn the palm or foot upward
Pronation	to turn the palm or foot downward
Dorsiflexion	to raise the foot, pulling the toes toward the shin
Plantar flexion	to lower the foot, pointing the toes away from the shin

Muscle Actions—cont'd

ACTION	DESCRIPTION
Eversion	to turn outward
Inversion	to turn inward
Protraction	to move a part of the body forward
Retraction	to move a part of the body backward
Rotation	to revolve a bone around its axis

Although the naming of all the muscles in the body is too intense an undertaking for this text, there are a few helpful rules that can be followed. Often points of attachment are key in naming the muscle in question. For example, the **sternocleidomastoid** (stur noh kly doh MASS toyd) muscle (Fig. 3-6) attaches to the sternum, the clavicle, and the mastoid process. Other muscles get their names from their general location. For instance, the pectoralis major is a large muscle in the chest.

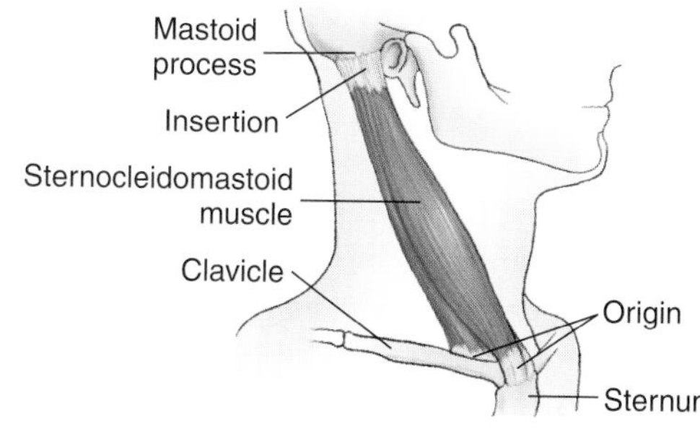

Fig. 3-6 Sternocleidomastoid muscle.

COMBINING FORMS FOR JOINTS AND MUSCLES

MEANING	COMBINING FORM	MEANING	COMBINING FORM
bursa	burs/o	muscle (heart)	myocardi/o
chest	pector/o	muscle (striated)	rhabdomy/o
clavicle	cleid/o	muscle (smooth)	leiomy/o
joint	arthr/o, articul/o	muscle	my/o
mastoid process	mastoid/o	sternum	stern/o

PREFIXES FOR JOINTS AND MUSCLES

PREFIX	MEANING	PREFIX	MEANING
ab-	away from	in-	in
ad-	towards	pro-	before, forward
amphi-	both	re-	back
di-	through, two	syn-	together
e-	out		

Exercise 10: JOINTS

1. What is the term for the following type of joint?

   A. immovable: ____________________

   B. full movement: ____________________

   C. limited movement: ____________________

2. What are the sacs of fluid that are designed to cushion the joints?

   ____

3. Explain three characteristics of synovial joints that assist in healthy joint function.

   ____

Exercise 11: MUSCLE ACTIONS

Fill in the blanks with the correct terms from the following list. There are more answers than questions.

abduction, adduction, dorsiflexion, eversion, extension, flexion, inversion, plantar flexion, pronation, protraction, retraction, rotation, supination

1. What is the process of turning outward called? ____________
2. What is the process of turning the palm upward called? ____________
3. What is the process of revolving a bone around its axis called? ____________
4. What is the process of moving away from the midline? ____________
5. What is the process of pointing the toes away from the shin called? ____________
6. What is the name for moving a body part forward? ____________
7. What is the name for decreasing the angle between the bones of a joint? ____________

8. What is the process of turning inward? _____________

9. What is the process of moving towards the midline called? _____________

10. What is the process of increasing the angle of a joint called? _____________

Match the type of muscle with its combining form.

_____ 11. rhabdomy/o

_____ 12. cardiomy/o

_____ 13. leiomy/o

A. heart muscle
B. smooth muscle
C. striated muscle

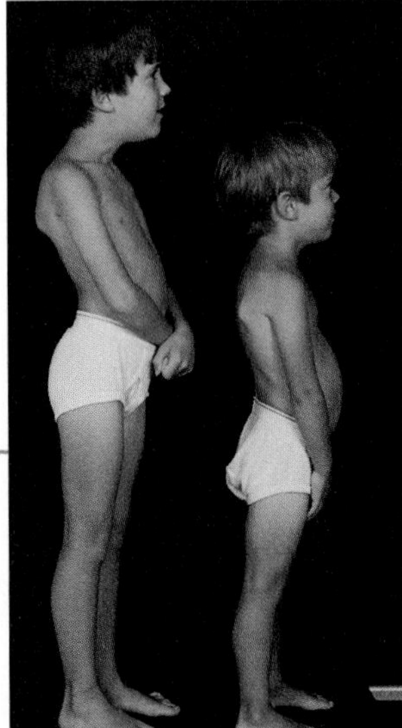

Fig. 3-7 Muscular dystrophy. These brothers show typical stance, lumbar lordosis, and forward thrusting of the abdomen.

Exercise 12: Joint and Muscle Prefix Practice

Match the prefixes with their correct meanings.

_____ 1. ab-

_____ 2. ad-

_____ 3. e-

_____ 4. in-

_____ 5. pro-

_____ 6. syn-

_____ 7. amphi-

_____ 8. di-

A. away from
B. out
C. through, two
D. in
E. before, forward
F. together
G. both
H. toward

PATHOLOGY

Terms Related to Congenital Conditions

Term	Word Origin	Definition
Achondroplasia ah kon droh PLAY zha	*a-* without *chondr/o* cartilage *-plasia* development	Disorder of the growth of cartilage at the epiphyses of the long bones and skull, resulting in dwarfism.
Muscular dystrophy MUSS kyoo lur DISS troh fee	*muscul/o* muscle *-ar* pertaining to *dys-* bad, abnormal *-troph/o* nourishment *-y* condition	Group of disorders characterized as an inherited progressive atrophy of skeletal muscle without neural involvement (Fig. 3-7).
Polydactyly pall ee DACK tih lee	*poly-* many, much *dactyl/o* fingers, toes *-y* condition, process	Condition of more than five fingers or toes on each hand or foot.
Spina bifida occulta SPY nah BIFF ih dah oh KULL tah	*spin/o* spine *bi-* two *-fida* to split *occulta* hidden	Congenital malformation of the bony spinal canal without involvement of the spinal cord.

Continued

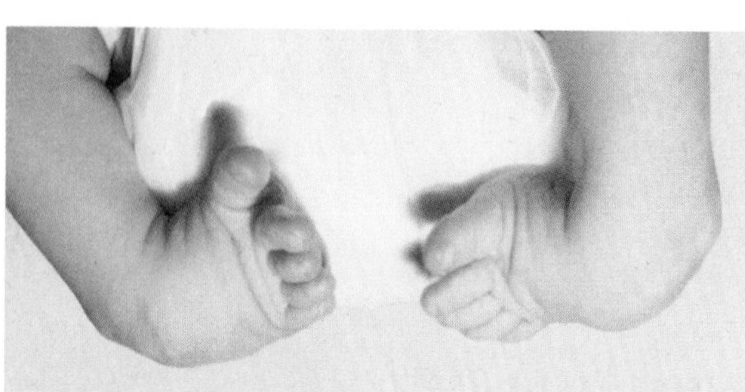

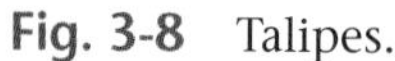

Fig. 3-8 Talipes.

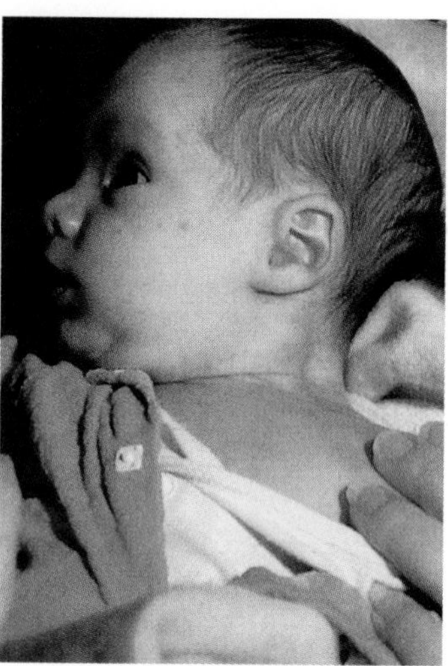

Fig. 3-9 Torticollis.

Terms Related to Congenital Conditions—cont'd		
TERM	**WORD ORIGIN**	**DEFINITION**
Syndactyly sin DACK tih lee	*syn-* together, with *dactyl/o* fingers, toes *-y* condition	Condition of the joining of the fingers or toes, giving them a webbed appearance.
Talipes TALL ih peez		Deformity resulting in an abnormal twisting of the foot. Also called **clubfoot** (Fig. 3-8).
Torticollis tore tih KOLL lis		Congenital or acquired condition that manifests itself as a contraction of the muscles of the neck. Also called **wryneck** (Fig. 3-9).

Exercise 13: Congenital Disorders

Match the congenital disorder with its description.

_____ 1. syndactyly

_____ 2. muscular dystrophy

__A__ 3. torticollis

__E__ 4. talipes

_____ 5. spina bifida occulta

__B__ 6. achondroplasia

_____ 7. polydactyly

A. wryneck
B. dwarfism resulting from lack of cartilage development
C. extra fingers or toes
D. progressive muscle weakening without involvement of nerves
E. clubfoot
F. malformation of the spinal canal
G. webbed fingers or toes

Trauma

Fractures

Put simply, a fracture is a broken bone. However, there are a number of types of breaks, each with its own name. Most fractures occur as a result of trauma, but some can result from an underlying disease like osteoporosis or cancer; these **pathologic fractures** are also sometimes called *spontaneous fractures*. All fractures may be classified into simple (closed) or compound (open) fractures. The break in a simple fracture does not rupture the skin, but a compound fracture splits open the skin, which allows more opportunity for infection to take place. See Fig. 3-10 and the following table for different types of fractures.

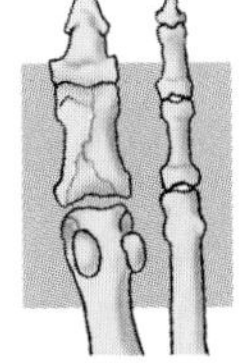

Comminuted

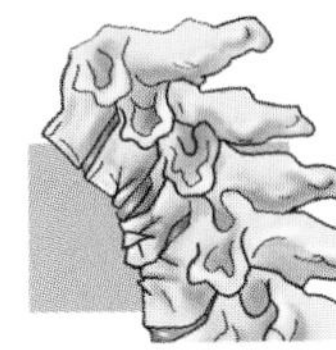

Compression

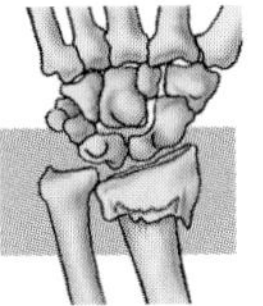

Colles'

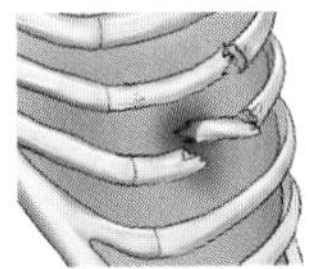

Complicated

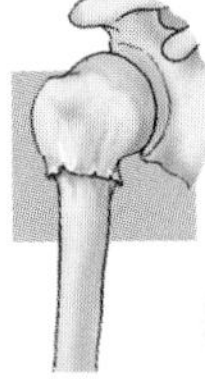

Impacted

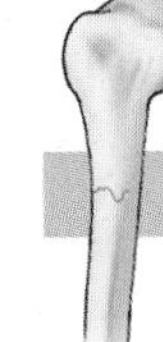

Hairline

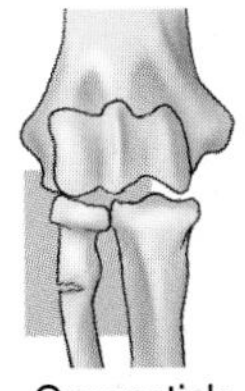

Greenstick

Fig. 3-10 Fractures.

Types of Fractures

FRACTURE	DEFINITION
Comminuted	The bone is crushed and/or shattered into many pieces.
Compression	The fractured area of bone collapses on itself.
Colles'	This break of the distal end of the radius at the epiphysis often occurs when the patient has attempted to break his or her fall.
Complicated	The bone is broken and pierces an internal organ.
Impacted	The bone is broken, and the ends are driven into each other.
Hairline	A minor fracture appears as a thin line on x-ray and may not extend completely through the bone.
Greenstick	The bone is partially bent and partially broken; this is a common fracture in children because their bones are still soft.
Pathologic	Any fracture occurring spontaneously as a result of disease.

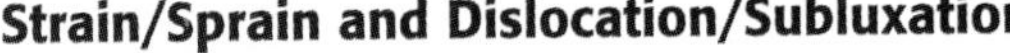

Strain/Sprain and Dislocation/Subluxation

A **sprain** is a traumatic injury to a joint involving the soft tissue: muscles, ligaments, and tendons. Swelling, pain, and discoloration of the skin may be present. The severity of the injury is measured in grades. A **strain** is a lesser injury, usually described as an overuse or overstretching of a muscle.

A bone that is completely out of its place in a joint is called a **dislocation.** If the bone is partially out of the joint, it is considered to be a **subluxation** (sub luck SAY shun). This can be a congenital or an acquired condition.

Exercise 14: FRACTURES

Match the fracture with its definition.

____ 1. complicated

____ 2. greenstick

____ 3. Colles'

____ 4. impacted

__I__ 5. comminuted

____ 6. simple/closed

____ 7. compound/open

____ 8. hairline

____ 9. pathologic

A. broken bone pierces internal organ
B. broken bone pierces skin
C. spontaneous fracture as a result of disease
D. bone is partially bent and partially broken
E. bone is broken, skin is closed
F. distal end of radius is broken
G. ends of broken bone are driven into each other
H. fracture appears as a line on the bone and fracture may not be completely through bone
I. bone is crushed

Exercise 15: SPRAINS/STRAINS AND DISLOCATIONS/SUBLUXATIONS

1. A partial displacement of a bone at a joint is a SUBLUXATION
2. An injury that can be described in grades and involves the soft tissue of a joint is a SPRAIN.
3. An overstretching of a muscle is a STRAIN.
4. A limb that is displaced from its normal position in a joint is an example of a DISLOCATION.

Terms Related to Bone Disease

TERM	WORD ORIGIN	DEFINITION
Osteomalacia os tee oh mah LAY sha	*oste/o* bone *-malacia* softening	Softening of bone caused by a loss of minerals from the bony matrix as a result of vitamin D deficiency.
Osteomyelitis os tee oh mye eh LYE tis	*oste/o* bone *myel/o* bone marrow *-itis* inflammation	Infection of the bone and bone marrow.
Osteoporosis os tee oh poor OH sis	*oste/o* bone *por/o* passage *-osis* abnormal condition	Loss of bone mass, which results in the bones being fragile and at risk for fractures (Fig. 3-11).
Rickets RICK etts		Osteomalacia occurring during childhood.

Terms Related to Joint Disease

TERM	WORD ORIGIN	DEFINITION
Bunion BUN yun	See **Did You Know?** box	Fairly common, painful enlargement and inflammation of the first metatarsophalangeal joint (the base of the great toe).
Carpal tunnel syndrome (CTS) KAR pul TUN ul	*carp/o* wrist bone *-al* pertaining to *syn-* together *-drome* to run	Compression injury that manifests itself as fluctuating pain, numbness, and paresthesias of the hand due to compression of the median nerve at the wrist.
Temporomandibular joint disorder (TMJ) tem pore oh man DIB byoo lur	*tempor/o* temporal bone *mandibul/o* lower jaw *-ar* pertaining to	Dysfunctional temporomandibular joint, accompanied by **gnathalgia,** jaw pain. Usually a congenital condition.
Osteoarthritis (OA) os tee oh arth RYE tis	*oste/o* bone *arthr/o* joint *-itis* inflammation	Joint disease characterized by degenerative articular cartilage and a wearing down of the bones' edges at a joint; considered a "wear-and-tear" disorder. Also called **degenerative joint disease (DJD)** (Fig. 3-12).
Rheumatoid arthritis (RA) ROO mah toyd arth RYE tis	*rheumat/o* watery flow *-oid* full of, like *arthr/o* joint *-itis* inflammation	Inflammatory joint disease believed to be autoimmune in nature; occurs in a much younger population (ages 20 to 45) than OA (Fig. 3-13).

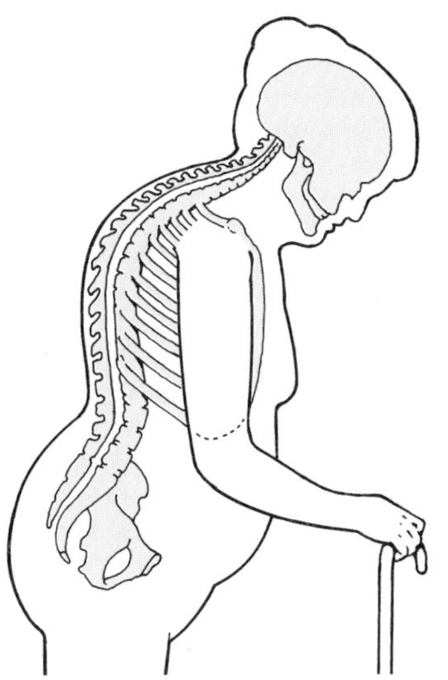

Fig. 3-11 The hallmark of osteoporosis: the dowager hump. Affected persons lose height, have a bent spine, and appear to sink into their hips.

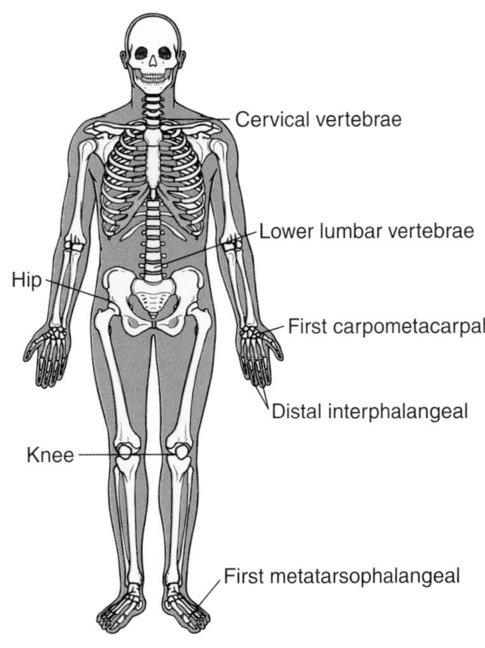

Fig. 3-12 Joints most frequently involved in osteoarthritis.

DID YOU KNOW?

Bunion comes from a Greek word that means *turnip.*

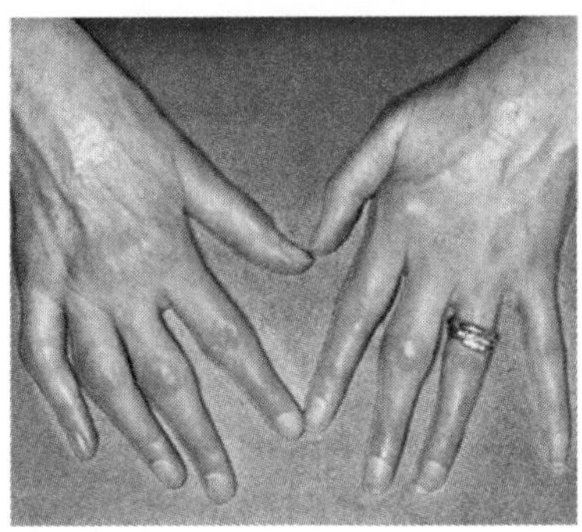

Fig. 3-13 Rheumatoid arthritis of the hands. Moderate involvement.

Case Study Continued

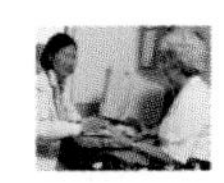

Amelia listens and takes notes as Ms. Auden tells her that she has been experiencing pain in her knees for several months, a common symptom of osteoarthritis, also called "the wear-and-tear" disease. Ms. Auden also says that she has been taking an assortment of medications, but because she has stomach irritation with these drugs, she has sought help from an acupuncturist recommended by a friend. Unfortunately, this has not relieved her pain either.

After taking Ms. Auden's history, Amelia takes her vital signs, including blood pressure, pulse, and temperature. She enters the results on computer and prints out a hard copy for the orthopedic surgeon to review when he examines Ms. Auden.

Spinal Malcurvatures

Back pain accounts for the greatest number of musculoskeletal complaints in the United States. In healthcare terminology, those complaints are classified as **dorsalgia** (door SAL zsa), upper back pain, and **lumbago** (lum BAY goh), lower back pain.

The spine has natural curves that allow support and flexibility; however, sometimes these curves become exaggerated and cause pain and disfigurement. The following are the most common types of disorders and malcurvatures of the spine. Occasionally combinations of these disorders occur.

Terms Related to Spinal Disorders

TERM	WORD ORIGIN	DEFINITION
Ankylosing spondylitis ang kih LOH sing spon dill LYE tis	***ankyl/o*** crooked or stiff ***spondyl/o*** vertebra ***-itis*** inflammation	Chronic inflammatory disease of idiopathic origin, which causes a fusion of the spine.
Herniated intervertebral disk	***inter-*** between ***vertebr/o*** vertebra ***-al*** pertaining to	Protrusion of the central part of the disk that lies between the vertebrae, resulting in compression of the nerve root and pain.
Kyphosis kye FOH sis	***kyph/o*** humpback ***-osis*** condition	Extreme posterior curvature of the thoracic area of the spine, commonly known as **humpback** or **hunchback.**
Lordosis lore DOH sis	***lord/o*** swayback ***-osis*** condition	Swayback; exaggerated anterior curve of the lumbar vertebrae (lower back).
Sciatica sye AT tih kah		Inflammation of the sciatic nerve, usually marked by pain and tenderness along the course of the nerve through the thigh and leg; may result in a wasting of the muscles of the lower leg (Fig. 3-14).
Scoliosis skoh lee OH sis	***scoli/o*** curvature ***-osis*** abnormal condition	Lateral S curve of the spine that can cause an individual to lose inches in height.
Spinal stenosis SPY nul steh NOH sis	***spin/o*** spine ***-al*** pertaining to ***stenosis*** abnormal condition of narrowing	Abnormal condition of narrowing of the lumbar spinal canal with attendant pain, sometimes caused by osteoarthritis or spondylolisthesis (Fig. 3-15).
Spondylolisthesis spon dih loh liss THEE sis	***spondyl/o*** vertebra ***-listhesis*** slipping	Condition resulting from the partial forward dislocation of one vertebra over the one beneath it.
Spondylosis spon dih LOH sis	***spondyl/o*** vertebra ***-osis*** abnormal condition	A stiffening of the vertebral joints.

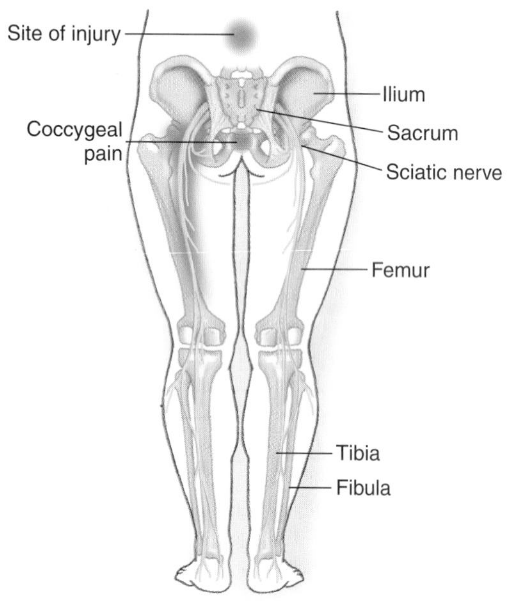

Fig. 3-14 Sciatica.

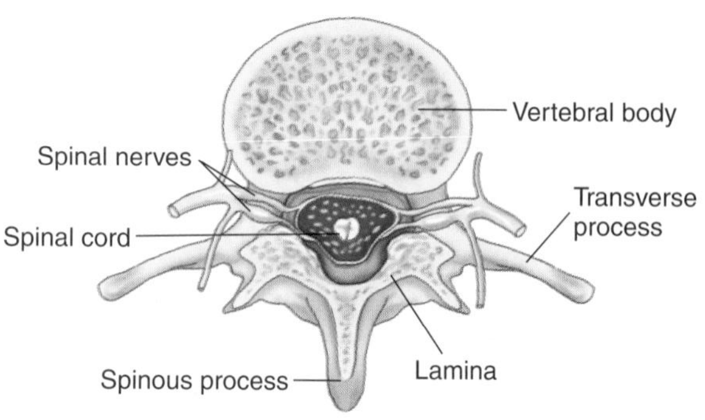

Fig. 3-15 Spinal stenosis. Bony overgrowth has narrowed the spinal canal and pinched the spinal nerves.

Terms Related to Muscle Disorders

TERM	WORD ORIGIN	DEFINITION
Contracture kun TRACK chur	***contractur/o*** a pulling together	Chronic flexion and fixation of a joint caused by atrophy and shortening of muscle fibers after a long period of disuse.
Fibromyalgia fye broh mye AL jah	***fibr/o*** fiber ***my/o*** muscle ***-algia*** pain	Disorder characterized by musculoskeletal pain, fatigue, muscle stiffness and spasms, and sleep disturbances (Fig. 3-16).
Myasthenia gravis mye ah STHEE nee ah GRAV us	***my/o*** muscle ***a-*** without ***-sthenia*** condition of strength ***gravis*** severe	Usually severe condition characterized by fatigue and a progressive muscle weakness, especially of the face and throat.

Exercise 16: SPINAL AND OTHER MUSCULOSKELETAL DISORDERS

Match the following.

___ 1. osteoarthritis
___ 2. osteoporosis
___ 3. spinal stenosis
___ 4. sciatica
___ 5. carpal tunnel syndrome
___ 6. bunion
___ 7. lumbago
___ 8. contracture
___ 9. fibromyalgia
___ 10. rickets
___ 11. rheumatoid arthritis
___ 12. spondylosis
___ 13. osteomyelitis
___ 14. osteomalacia
___ 15. spondylolisthesis
___ 16. myasthenia gravis

A. softening of the bone
B. compression of median nerve of wrist, leading to dysfunction
C. chronic flexion of a joint caused by muscle atrophy
D. stiffening of the vertebral joints
E. muscle disorder characterized by musculoskeletal pain, fatigue, and sleep disorders
F. osteomalacia during childhood
G. inflammation of nerve in lower back with pain radiating down legs
H. narrowing of the spinal canal
I. degenerative joint disease
J. usually severe disease characterized by muscular weakness
K. enlargement at base of the great toe
L. autoimmune type of arthritis
M. lower back pain
N. infection of bone and bone marrow
O. partial forward dislocation of adjacent vertebrae
P. loss of bone mass

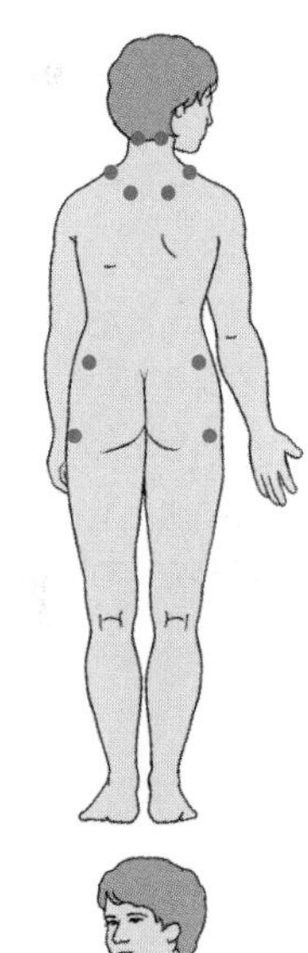

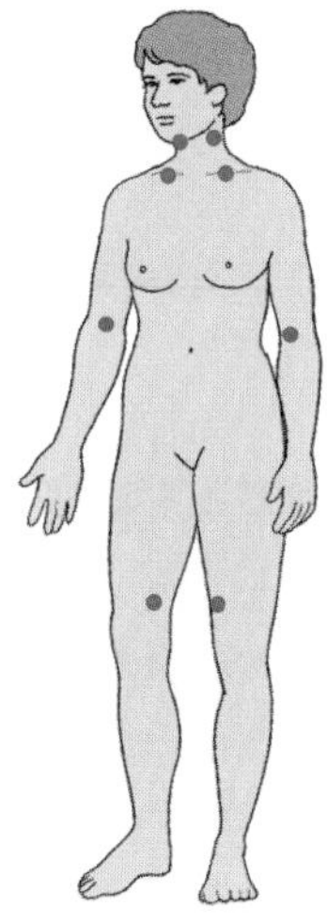

Fig. 3-16 Fibromyalgia tender points.

Match the three malcurvatures of the spine.

_____ 17. scoliosis

_____ 18. lordosis

_____ 19. kyphosis

A. hunchback
B. swayback
C. lateral S curve of the spine

DIAGNOSTIC PROCEDURES

Terms Related to Imaging

TERM	WORD ORIGIN	DEFINITION
Arthrography ar THRAH gruh fee	*arthr/o* joint *-graphy* process of recording	X-ray recording of a joint.
Arthroscopy ar THRAHS kuh pee	*arthr/o* joint *-scopy* visual examination	Visual examination of a joint, accomplished by use of an arthroscope (Fig. 3-17).
Computed tomography (CT) scan	*tom/o* section *-graphy* process of recording	Imaging technology that records transverse planes of the body for diagnostic purposes.
DEXA scan DECK suh		Dual-energy x-ray absorptiometry, a procedure that measures the density of bone at the hip and spine. Also called **DXA** (Fig. 3-18).
Electromyography ee leck troh mye AH gruh fee	*electro-* electrical *my/o* muscle *-graphy* process of recording	Procedure that records the electrical activity of muscles. Also known as **EMG.**
Magnetic resonance imaging (MRI)		Procedure that uses magnetic properties to record detailed information about internal structures.
Myelogram MYE eh loh gram	*myel/o* spinal cord *-gram* record, recording	X-ray of spinal canal done after injection of contrast medium.
Ultrasonography (US)	*ultra-* beyond *son/o* sound *-graphy* process of recording	Procedure in which high-frequency sound waves form an image of the body.
X-ray		Imaging technique using electromagnetic radiation for recording internal structures.

Laboratory Tests

TERM	WORD ORIGIN	DEFINITION
Rheumatoid factor test ROO mah toyd	*rheumat/o* watery flow *-oid* resembling	Lab test that looks for rheumatoid factor (RF) present in the blood of those who have rheumatoid arthritis.
Serum calcium (Ca)		Test to measure the amount of calcium in the blood.

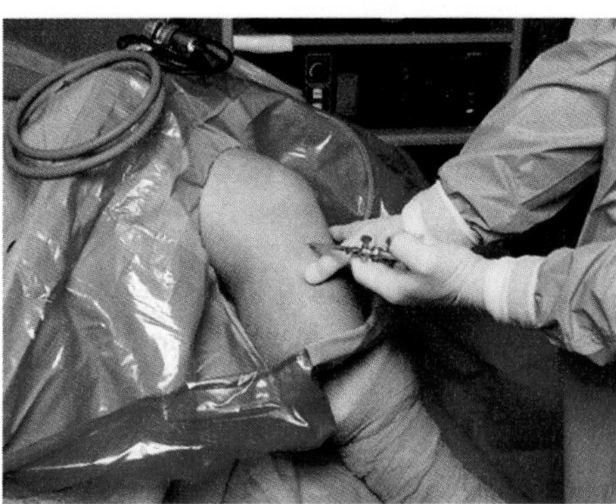

Fig. 3-17 Arthroscopy of the knee.

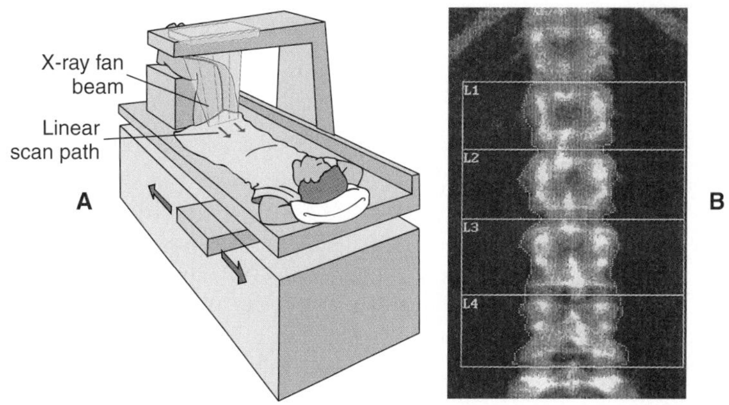

Fig. 3-18 Dual x-ray absorptiometry (DEXA). **A,** DEXA system. **B,** Scan of lumbar vertebrae.

Exercise 17: DIAGNOSTIC IMAGING AND LABORATORY PROCEDURES

Match the following.

____ 1. US

____ 2. MRI

____ 3. DXA

____ 4. arthrography

____ 5. x-ray

____ 6. arthroscopy

____ 7. RF

____ 8. serum calcium

____ 9. EMG

____ 10. CT scan

A. x-ray recording of a joint
B. test for rheumatoid arthritis
C. visual exam of a joint
D. imaging technique using electromagnetic radiation
E. imaging of a plane of the body
F. blood test for Ca
G. test to measure bone density, using dual-energy x-ray
H. imaging using magnetic resonance
I. ultrasonography
J. electromyography

Case Study Continued

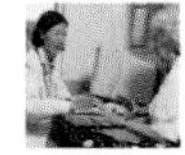

Ms. Auden has undergone a follow-up arthroscopy that shows extensive deterioration of the joint since her last visit. After reviewing the results of the arthroscopy, x-rays, and an MRI, her orthopedic surgeon advises a total knee replacement. Ms. Auden is nervous but decides she can no longer put up with the pain. She agrees to have the surgery.

THERAPEUTIC INTERVENTIONS

Setting Fractures

Broken bones must be "set"—that is, aligned and immobilized; the most common method is with a plaster cast. If a bone does not mend and realign correctly, it is said to be a **malunion.** If no healing takes place, it is a **nonunion.** A piece of bone that does not have a renewed blood supply will die; this tissue is then called **sequestrum** (seh KWES trum). Removal of dirt, damaged tissue, or foreign objects from a wound is one of the first steps in repairing an open fracture. This removal of debris is called **debridement** (de breed MON). Methods of fixation and alignment are described as follows:

External fixation: Noninvasive stabilization of broken bones in which no opening is made in the skin; instead, the stabilization takes place mainly through devices external to the body that offer traction.

Internal fixation: Stabilization of broken bones in their correct position, using pins, screws, plates, and so on, which are fastened to the bones to maintain correct alignment.

Reduction: Alignment and immobilization of the ends of a broken bone. Open reduction requires incision of the skin; closed reduction does not require incision.

Terms Related to Therapeutic Interventions

TERM	WORD ORIGIN	DEFINITION
Amputation am pyoo TAY shun		Removal of a limb when there are no feasible options to save it.
Arthrocentesis ar thruh sen TEE sis	*arthr/o* joint ***-centesis*** surgical puncture	Surgical puncture of a joint to remove fluid.
Arthrodesis ar thruh DEE sis	*arthr/o* joint ***-desis*** binding	Binding or stabilization of a joint by operative means.
Arthroplasty ar thruh PLAS tee	*arthr/o* joint *-plasty* surgical repair	General term meaning *surgical repair of a joint.*
Bunionectomy bun yun ECK toh mee	*bunion/o* bunion *-ectomy* excision, resection	Removal of a bunion (Fig. 3-19).
Kyphoplasty KYE foh plas tee	*kyph/o* hump *-plasty* surgical repair	Minimally invasive procedure designed to address the pain of fractured vertebrae resulting from osteoporosis or cancer (Fig. 3-20). A balloon is used to inflate the area of fracture before a cementlike substance is injected. The substance hardens rapidly, and pain relief is immediate in most patients.
Laminectomy lam ih NECK tuh mee	*lamin/o* lamina *-ectomy* excision, resection	Removal of the bony arches of one or more vertebrae to relieve compression of the spinal cord (Fig. 3-21).
Myorrhaphy mye ORE rah fee	*my/o* muscle *-rrhaphy* suture	Suture of a muscle.

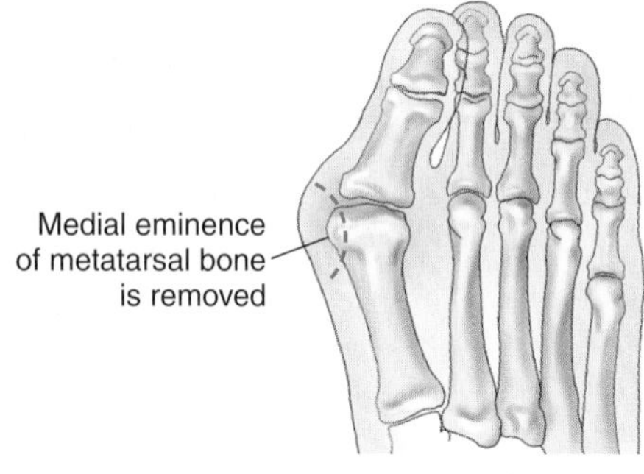

Fig. 3-19 Bunionectomy.

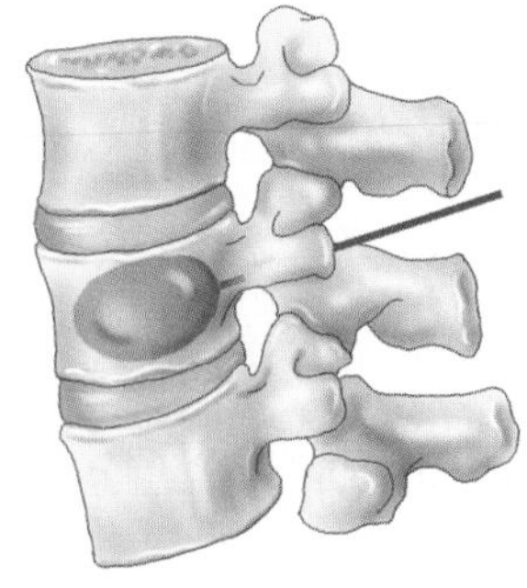

Fig. 3-20 Kyphoplasty.

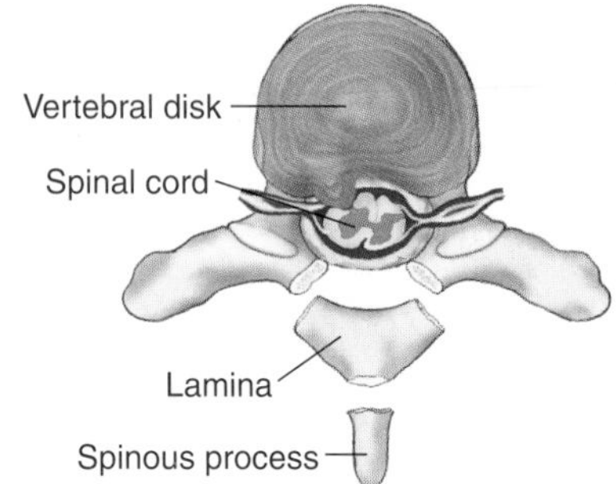

Fig. 3-21 Laminectomy.

Terms Related to Therapeutic Interventions—cont'd

TERM	WORD ORIGIN	DEFINITION
Operative ankylosis AH pur ah tiv ang kih LOH sis	*ankyl/o* stiffening *-osis* condition	Procedure used in the treatment of spinal fractures or after diskectomy or laminectomy for the correction of a herniated vertebral disk; also used to describe surgical fixation of a joint
Osteoclasis OS tee oh klay sis	*oste/o* bone *-clasis* intentional fracture	Refracture of a bone, usually done if a bone has a malunion.
Osteoplasty OS tee oh plas tee	*oste/o* bone *-plasty* surgical repair	Surgical repair of a bone.
Prosthesis pros THEE sis	*prosthes/o* addition	An artificial body part that is constructed to replace missing limbs, eyes, and other body parts (*pl.* prostheses) (Fig. 3-22).
Spondylosyndesis spon dih loh sin DEE sis	*spondyl/o* vertebra *syn-* together *-desis* binding	Fixation of an unstable segment of the spine by skeletal traction, immobilization of the patient in a body cast, or stabilization with a bone graft or synthetic device. Also called **spinal fusion** and **spondylodesis.**
Tenomyoplasty ten oh MYE oh plas tee	*ten/o* tender *my/o* muscle *-plasty* surgical repair	Surgical repair of a muscle and a tendon
Total hip replacement (THR)		Replacement of the femoral head and the acetabulum of the hip with either plastic or metal appliances.
Total knee replacement (TKR)		Extensive surgical procedure that involves the replacement of the entire knee joint, either unilaterally or bilaterally. (Fig. 3-23).

A

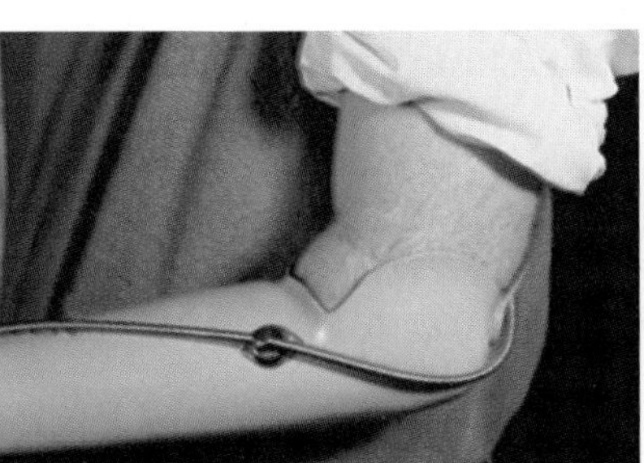

B

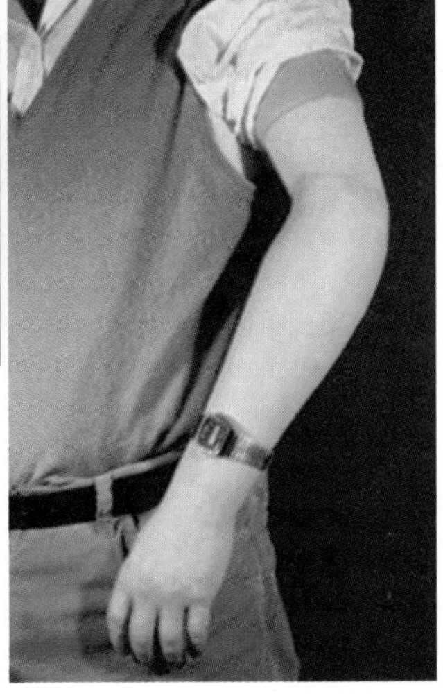

Fig. 3-22 Two types of arm prosthesis. **A,** Traditional fiberglass. **B,** New materials and techniques have made possible fabrication of prosthetic sockets that are light, soft, flexible, and secure.

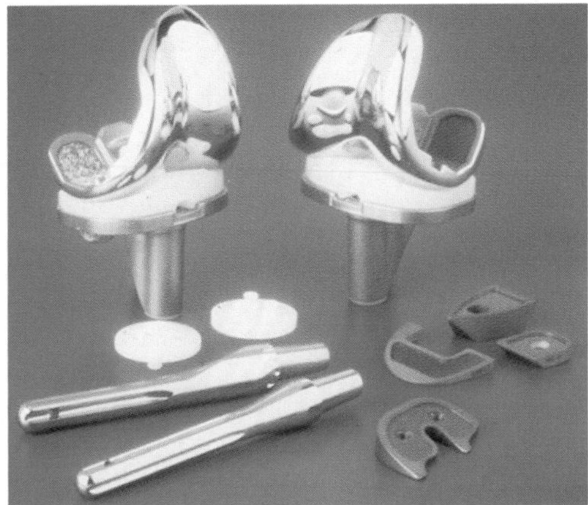

Fig. 3-23 Total knee replacement hardware.

Case Study Continued

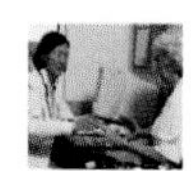

Ms. Auden has her TKR done 2 weeks after her appointment. Immediately after surgery, a compression bandage is attached to completely immobilize her knee in extension. By the time she goes home from the hospital, this is removed and replaced by a plastic shell. Almost immediately, Ms. Auden begins physical therapy to strengthen the joint muscles and give the new joint mobility. At-home exercises include ROM exercises, muscle strengthening, and stationary bicycling. Her recovery time takes several weeks, but on follow-up she says, "I just wish I had done this sooner!"

Exercise 18: THERAPEUTIC INTERVENTIONS

1. Build a term that means:

   A. surgical repair of a joint ____________

   B. surgical fracture of a bone ____________

   C. excision of a bunion ____________

   D. surgical repair of a muscle and a tendon ____________

Match the following.

____ 2. debridement

____ 3. open reduction

____ 4. sequestrum

____ 5. myorrhaphy

____ 6. osteoclasis

____ 7. arthrodesis

____ 8. prosthesis

____ 9. spondylosyndesis

____ 10. arthrocentesis

____ 11. closed reduction

A. suture of muscle
B. intentional fracture of bone
C. alignment of ends of bone with incision
D. alignment of ends of bone without incision
E. surgical puncture of a joint
F. artificial body part
G. dead bone
H. removal of debris
I. spinal fusion
J. fixation of a joint

PHARMACOLOGY

Analgesics/antiinflammatories: Used to treat inflammation and pain. Examples include steroidal and nonsteroidal antiinflammatory drugs (NSAIDs). Prednisolone (Delta-Cortef) is an example of a steroid; ibuprofen (Advil) and acetaminophen (Tylenol) are examples of NSAIDs.

Rheumatoid arthritis drugs: Examples include leflunomide (Arava), etanercept (Enbrel), and infliximab (Remicade).

Osteoarthritis drugs: Examples include COX-2 inhibitors (Celebrex), a new "stomach-friendly" NSAID.

Osteoporosis drugs: Examples include alendronate (Fosamax) and risedronate (Actinel).

Exercise 19: PHARMACOLOGY

1. Osteoporosis may be treated pharmacologically with ______________ or ______________.
2. Rheumatoid arthritis may be treated with ______________.
3. NSAIDs are used to treat what kinds of symptoms? ____________________________
4. Cox-2 inhibitors are used to treat ______________.

Abbreviations

Abbreviation	Meaning	Abbreviation	Meaning
C1-C7	First cervical through seventh cervical vertebrae	MD	Muscular dystrophy
Ca	Calcium	MRI	Magnetic resonance imaging
CAM	Complementary and alternative medicine	MS	Musculoskeletal
CT	Computed tomography	NSAID	Nonsteroidal antiinflammatory drug
CTS	Carpal tunnel syndrome	OA	Osteoarthritis
D1-D12	First dorsal through twelfth dorsal vertebrae	P	Phosphorus
DEXA, DXA	Dual energy x-ray absorptiometry	RA	Rheumatoid arthritis
DJD	Degenerative joint disease	RF	Rheumatoid factor
EMG	Electromyography	ROM	Range of motion
Fx	Fracture	S1-S5	First sacral through fifth sacral segments
L1-L5	First lumbar through fifth lumbar vertebrae	T1-T12	First thoracic through twelfth thoracic vertebrae
MA/OM	Medical assistant/office manager	THR	Total hip replacement
		TKR	Total knee replacement
		US	Ultrasonography

Exercise 20: ABBREVIATIONS

Explain the meanings of the abbreviations used in the following examples.

1. Greta was an 83-year-old white female with a compression Fx of L5.

   Fx = Fracture
   ____
2. The patient had been self-medicating her joint pain with NSAIDs.

   ____
3. Bursitis caused a limited ROM of the shoulder joint for Paul.

   ____
4. Which of the following is not an imaging procedure—CT, CTS, MRI, US? US = ultrasound

   CTS = Carpal Tunnel Syndrome
   ____
5. Acupuncture is one type of therapeutic intervention categorized as CAM.

   ____

Careers

Medical Assistants

One of the 10 fastest growing professions through the year 2010 is that of a medical assistant (MA). MAs are trained in both clinical and clerical duties and are a necessary part of healthcare teams as they treat a growing and aging population. Although some MAs are trained on the job, job prospects are best for medical assistants with formal training or experience.

Typical duties of the MA depend on the setting (e.g., size of the practice, hospital, location, and state laws governing the range of allowable duties) but may include reception, billing, scheduling, taking and recording vital signs, readying patients for examination, assisting the physician throughout the examination, performing laboratory tests, and sterilizing equipment.

Information on educational programs and the Certified Medical Assistant examination is available from The American Association of Medical Assistants at http://www.aama-ntl.org.

http: INTERNET PROJECT

The Agency for Healthcare Research and Quality has an interesting site for students interested in the healthcare field. Go to http://www.ahcpr.gov and use HCUPnet: an Interactive Tool for Hospital Statistics under the Data & Surveys menu. Choose Start HCUPnet, use the national sample, then choose from either a diagnosis or procedure category to make a list of the top 10 diagnoses or procedures in the musculoskeletal system (including connective tissue). A user's first choice must be "specific diagnoses or procedures." Once these selections are complete, print the choices, choose the top 10 most common diagnoses or procedures, and define each.

Chapter Review

A. Functions of the Musculoskeletal System

In your own words, explain what functions may be lost or disrupted when the musculoskeletal system is diseased or injured.

____

____

B. Anatomy and Physiology

1. Label the parts of the long bone on the diagram provided.

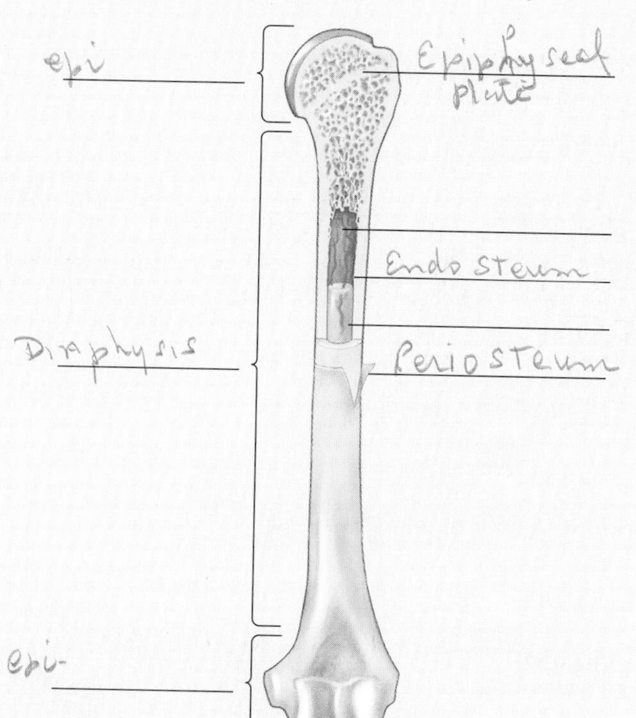

2. Decode the following terms.

A. endosteum ______________________

B. periosteum ______________________

C. diaphysis ______________________

D. epiphysis ______________________

E. metaphysis ______________________

F. osteoblast ______________________

G. osteoclast ______________________

H. osteocyte ______________________

Classify the following bones as parts of the cranium, face, spine, or ribcage.

3. occipital bone ________
4. sternum ________
5. zygoma ________
6. costa ________
7. frontal bone ________
8. maxilla ________
9. sacrum ________
10. T1 ________
11. temporal ________

12. What are the anatomic structures designed to cushion joints and what are their combining forms?

____

13. How do the prefixes in the terms *adduction* and *abduction* explain their possible muscle actions?

____

____

C. Pathology

Decode the following terms.

14. polydactyly ________
15. achondroplasia ________
16. spina bifida occulta ________
17. muscular dystrophy ________
18. syndactyly ________
19. osteomalacia ________
20. osteomyelitis ________
21. myasthenia gravis ________
22. spondylolisthesis ________
23. spinal stenosis ________

Fill in the blank with the type of trauma described.

24. Martin broke his collarbone while jumping on the bed. It did not pierce the skin, so what type of fracture is it? (give two names) ________
25. After dropping a bowling ball on her foot, Rena was treated for metatarsal bones that were shattered. What kind of fracture is this? ________
26. Darnell fell off a piece of playground equipment and sustained a fracture in which his bones were partially bent and partially broken. What type of fracture is this classified as?

    ____
27. Advanced cancer to the bone caused a spontaneous hip fracture in a patient living in an assisted care facility. This patient presents with which type of fracture? ________
28. Slipping on a spilled soda that hadn't been cleaned up, Javier tried to catch himself and ended up fracturing the distal end of his right radius. This is called which type of fracture?

    ____

29. Catching a football improperly may result in a finger bone that is partially disarticulated. In this case, the injury would be described as a/an ________________.
30. During the playoffs, the point guard ruptured a ligament in his ankle and damaged the soft tissue to that joint. The injury would be termed a/an ________________.
31. Rickets is osteomalacia that occurs during which stage of life? ________________
32. A data input clerk and a bus driver who had just visited their doctors discovered that they both had the same diagnosis—pain and numbness in their fingers due to compression of the median nerve of the wrist. This diagnosis was ________________.
33. The newly hired coder at a local community hospital was surprised to see the large number of patients with DJD. He knows that this is an abbreviation for ________________, which also means the same thing as ________________.
34. Inflammation of the joints is a characteristic of the autoimmune disorder ________________ arthritis.
35. Ms. Ralston presented with an enlargement and inflammation of the joint at the base of her great toe on her left foot. This was diagnosed as a/an ________________.
36. The name of the joint affected by the disorder described in question 35 is the ________________ joint.
37. Pain in the lower back is called ________________.
38. Inflammation of the sciatic nerve, usually accompanied by lower back pain and pain that travels through the buttocks and down the legs is called ________________.
39. Name the three malcurvatures of the spine and explain the differences among them.

____

____

____

40. Chronic pain, fatigue, muscle spasms and sleep disorders characterize which disorder?

____

41. A chronic fixation and flexion of a joint is called a/an ________________.

D. Diagnostic Procedures

42. Decode the following terms.

A. myelogram ________________

B. arthroscopy ________________

C. electromyography ________________

D. arthrography ________________

Fill in the blank.

43. Because Raymond had been having trouble with weakness in one arm, he had a procedure that records the electrical activity of muscles called a/an ____________.
44. One of the patients had an x-ray of the spinal canal using a contrast medium to assess damage sustained during a car accident. The procedure is termed a/an ____________.
45. The soccer player had an x-ray of his shoulder joint after injuries sustained in the championship match. The procedure is termed a/an ____________.
46. Ms. Wright was suspected to have osteoporosis. A procedure that measures density of bone is ____________.
47. Tyara had a lab test that reveals the presence or absence of a substance found in the blood of those with rheumatoid arthritis. The substance is called the ____________.

E. Therapeutic Interventions

48. Decode the following terms.

A. myorrhaphy ____________

B. kyphoplasty ____________

C. spondylosyndesis ____________

D. operative ankylosis ____________

E. laminectomy ____________

F. tenomyoplasty ____________

G. osteoclasis ____________

H. arthrodesis ____________

I. arthrocentesis ____________

J. osteoplasty ____________

49. Moving the ends of broken bones into alignment is called ____________.
50. If an incision is necessary, the process above is described as ____________.
51. Fastening sections of bone with pins is known as ____________.
52. External fixation is considered a non-____________ procedure, meaning that an incision is not necessary.
53. An imperfect healing of a broken bone is a ____________.
54. A piece of dead bone is called ____________.
55. Removal of a limb is called ____________, and the artificial appliance that replaces the limb is called a/an ____________.
56. The synonyms for spinal fusion are ____________ and ____________.

F. Pharmacology

57. Anna was prescribed Actonel to treat her ____________.

58. Methotrexate is used to treat which type of arthritis? ____________

59. COX-2 inhibitors are used to treat ____________.

60. NSAIDs are used to treat ____________.

G. Abbreviations

Spell out the abbreviation in the following sentences.

61. Mrs. Jones was advised to eat more Ca-rich foods. ____________

62. Johnna had a Fx of one of her metatarsals. ____________

63. Jason fell off a horse and sustained a fracture of his C2. ____________

64. Painful bursitis resulted in limited ROM of the patient's left shoulder. ____________

65. Robert was treated for DJD with a regimen of weight loss and NSAIDs before surgery was discussed.

____

H. Singulars and Plurals

Change the following singular terms to plural.

66. foramen ____________

67. bursa ____________

68. prosthesis ____________

69. phalanx ____________

70. sulcus ____________

71. vertebra ____________

72. ilium ____________

73. pelvis ____________

74. arthroscopy ____________

75. costa ____________

I. Translations

Rewrite the following to explain the underlined terms.

76. An x-ray revealed a <u>greenstick Fx</u> of the child's right <u>humerus</u>.

____

77. Ms. Burton-Smith was treated for <u>bursitis</u> secondary to an injury with heat, rest, and <u>NSAIDs</u>.

____

78. The basketball player had an <u>osteoclasis</u> for a <u>malunion</u> of one of his <u>metacarpals</u>.

____

79. The patient was sent for a <u>US</u> of her <u>calcaneus</u> to assess her <u>osteoporosis</u>.

____

80. The patient complained of <u>lumbago</u> resulting from his <u>spinal stenosis</u>.

____

81. <u>Electromyography</u> was used to confirm the child's <u>muscular dystrophy</u>.

____

J. Cumulative Review

Circle the correct answer.

82. Ms. Auden has been having problems with her knees. If she was to have a TKR done on both, it would be considered to be *(bilateral, bimedial).*
83. A fracture of the femoral head is at its *(proximal, distal)* end.
84. Lying on her back for an MRI, Ms. Auden was in a *(supine, prone)* position.
85. CT scans record *(sagittal, frontal, transverse)* planes of the body.
86. The *(abdominal, cranial, spinal, pelvic, thoracic)* cavity was jeopardized by multiple fractures of the ribs.
87. The area of the neck of the spine is referred to as the *(lumbar, sacral, cervical)* region.

K. Be Careful

Circle the correct answer.

88. Which is a person more likely to experience—*sarcoiliac* or *sacroiliac* pain?
89. Is the suturing of a muscle spelled *myorhaphy* or *myorrhaphy?*
90. In this chapter, does the abbreviation MS refer to *multiple sclerosis, musculoskeletal,* or *mitral stenosis?*
91. Is part of the hip bone called the *ileum* or the *ilium?*
92. It is possible to break which kind of bone—the *peritoneal* or *peroneal* bone?
93. Is the tough, outer covering of the bone called the *paraosteum, perosteum,* or *periosteum?*
94. Do the minerals in bone consist of *calcium and potassium* or *calcium and phosphorus?*
95. Is the socket in the hip the *acromion* or the *acetabulum?*
96. A Colles' fracture occurs to which bone: *radius, ulna,* or *humerus?*
97. The bone marrow is key in *hematopoiesis* or *hematoporosis?*

Anchorage Memorial Hospital
1247 Inuit Blvd.
Anchorage, AK 99506

Operating Room Report

Patient: Evelyn Auden
MR#: 23 45 67
Physician: John Redmond, MD
Date: 2/2/03

Preoperative Diagnosis: Degenerative Joint Disease, Right Knee
Postoperative Diagnosis: Degenerative Joint Disease, Right Knee
Name of Operation: Total Knee Replacement

Components: Zimmer NextGen LPS
Femur: size G
Tibia: 6
Articulating Surface: 10 mm
Patella: 38

Assistant: Dr. Sorda
Anesthesia: Spinal
Estimated Blood Loss: 150 cc
Antibiotics: Vancomycin 1 gm
Tourniquet: 350 mm Hg
Complications: none

Procedure

The patient was properly identified in the OR, and the leg was prepped and draped in the routine fashion. The leg was exsanguinated and the tourniquet inflated. A standard anterior approach was made along with the median parapatellar arthrotomy. The patella was everted. The fat pad was partially removed, the knee flexed, and all joint surfaces prepared in the conventional manner to the size needed. The surface was prepared with pulse irrigating system followed by antibiotic irrigation. They were then dried. All components were cemented simultaneously. Any excess cement was removed with curettes and/or osteotomes.

The knee was placed in full extension, if not slight hyperextension, while the cement cured. The patient tolerated the procedure well and left the operating room in stable condition.

____
Mae-Li Chong (surgeon)

L. Healthcare Report

98. How much blood was lost? ____________________
99. An "anterior approach" to the knee would be through which part of the knee?

____

100. What is the patella? ____________________
101. What is the parapatellar? ____________________
102. What is an arthrotomy? ____________________
103. If the patella were everted, how would it be placed? ____________________
104. What is an osteotome? ____________________
105. What would hyperextension be? ____________________

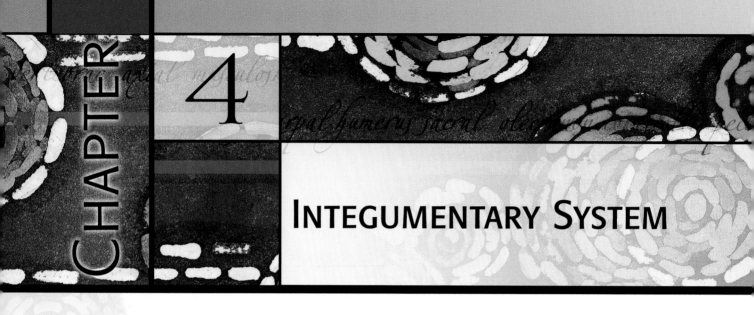

CHAPTER 4 INTEGUMENTARY SYSTEM

"Genius is one percent inspiration and ninety-nine percent perspiration." ***—Thomas Edison***

Quote

Case Study

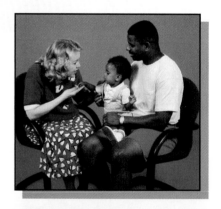

Eleven-month-old Ben Warner was enjoying himself as he practiced walking in his family's living room. His training circuit consisted of pulling up on the coffee table, edging around to the side near the couch, and then launching himself for a wobbly step before collapsing on the carpet. Unfortunately, Ben's dad left his newspaper and a fresh cup of hot coffee on the table when he went to answer the phone. It only took seconds for Ben to pull the newspaper and coffee onto himself, and his resulting howls brought his father running back to find his little boy with a nasty burn on his arm. Ben was taken to the emergency department (ED) of their local hospital.

In the Health Information Management department the following day, Olivia Crawford, Registered Health Information Technician (RHIT), Certified Coding Specialist (CCS), assigned codes to Ben's ED record.

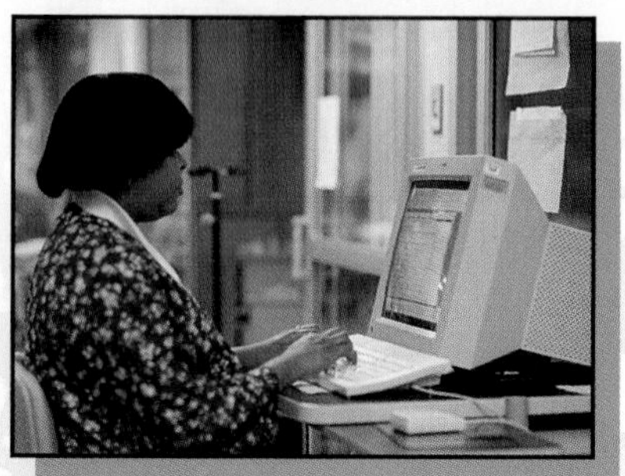

OBJECTIVES

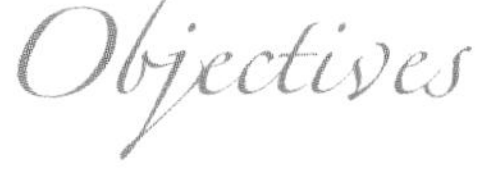

- In your own words, explain the functions of the integumentary system.
- Recognize, recall, and apply healthcare terms related to the anatomy and physiology of the integumentary system.
- Recognize, recall, and apply healthcare terms related to the pathology of the integumentary system.
- Recognize, recall, and apply healthcare terms related to the diagnostic procedures introduced in this chapter.
- Recognize, recall, and apply healthcare terms related to therapeutic interventions introduced in this chapter.
- Recognize, recall, and apply the pharmacologic terms introduced in this chapter.
- Recognize, recall, and apply the abbreviations introduced in this chapter.
- Recognize and recall word components used in this chapter to build and decode healthcare terms relevant to the integumentary system.
- Demonstrate the ability to change singular integumentary terms to plural forms and vice versa.
- Recognize, recall, and apply material learned in previous chapters.

FUNCTIONS OF THE INTEGUMENTARY SYSTEM

The most important function of the skin (integument) is that it acts as the first line of defense in protecting the body from disease by providing an external barrier. It also helps regulate the temperature of the body, provides information about the environment through the sense of touch, assists in the synthesis of vitamin D (essential for the normal formation of bones and teeth), and helps eliminate waste products from the body. It is the largest organ of the body and accomplishes its diverse functions with assistance from its accessory structures, which include the hair, nails, and two types of glands: sebaceous (oil) and sudoriferous (sweat). Any impairment of the skin has the potential to lessen its ability to carry out these functions, the result of which can lead to disease.

COMBINING FORMS FOR THE INTEGUMENTARY SYSTEM

MEANING	COMBINING FORM	MEANING	COMBINING FORM
gland	aden/o	skin	derm/o, dermat/o and cutane/o
hair	trich/o, pil/o	sudoriferous gland	hidraden/o
nails	onych/o, ungu/o	sweat	hidr/o
sebum, oil	seb/o		

Exercise 1: FUNCTIONS OF THE INTEGUMENTARY SYSTEM

Fill in the blanks.

1. The functions of the integumentary system are as follows:

   A. To help eliminate __________ from the body.

   B. To protect the body from disease by providing an external 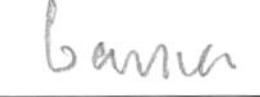 __________.

C. To provide information about the external environment through the sense of ________________.

D. To regulate ________________.

E. To synthesize vitamin D, which is essential for the normal formation of ________________ and ________________.

Match the combining forms for the integumentary system with their meanings.

_____ 2. cutane/o, dermat/o

_____ 3. ungu/o, onych/o

_____ 4. hidraden/o

_____ 5. trich/o, pil/o

_____ 6. hidr/o

_____ 7. seb/o

A. hair
B. sweat
C. oil
D. nail
E. sweat gland
F. skin

ANATOMY AND PHYSIOLOGY

Skin

The skin is composed of two layers: the **epidermis** (eh pih DUR mis), which forms the outermost layer, and the **dermis** or **corium** (KORE ee um), the inner layer (Fig. 4-1). The dermis is attached to a layer of connective tissue called the **hypodermis** or the **subcutaneous** (sub kyoo TAY nee us) layer, which is mainly composed of adipose (fatty) tissue.

> **BE CAREFUL!**
> Don't confuse *strata,* meaning *layers,* with *striae,* meaning *stretch marks.*

Epidermis

The top layer, the epidermis, is composed of several different layers, or strata, (*sing.* stratum) of epithelial (eh pih THEE lee ul) tissue. Epithelial tissue covers many of the external and internal surfaces of the body. Because the type of epithelial tissue that covers the body has a microscopic scaly appearance, it is referred to as **stratified squamous epithelium** (SKWAY muss eh pih THEE lee um).

> **BE CAREFUL!**
> Don't confuse *papill/o* and *papul/o,* which means *pimple.*

Although there is a limited blood supply to the epidermis (it is **avascular** [a VAS kyoo lur]—that is, it contains no blood vessels), constant activity is taking place. New skin cells are formed in the **basal** (BAY sul) (bottom) layer of the epidermis: the **stratum germinativum** (STRA tum jur mih nuh TIH vum). These cells then move outward toward the **stratum corneum** (top layer). During the transition, from the lowest layer to the outer layer, the cells become filled

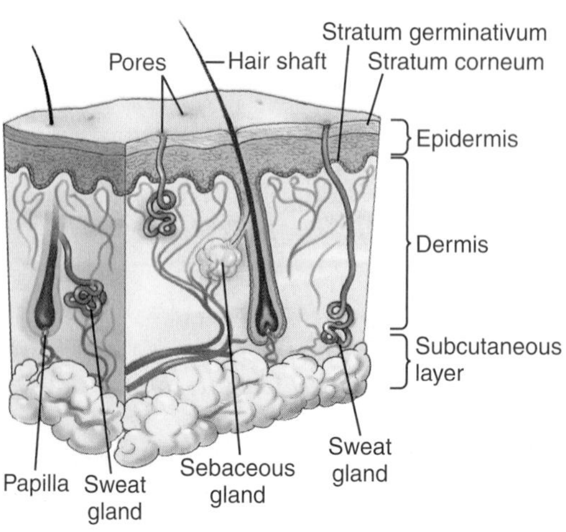

Fig. 4-1 Diagram of the skin.

with **keratin** (KAIR ah tin), which is a hard protein material. The nature of the keratin adds to the protective nature of the skin, giving it a waterproof property that helps retain moisture within the body.

The epidermis also protects the body by producing **melanocytes** (MEL an oh sites), the cells that produce pigment. When the skin is exposed to ultraviolet light, the melanocytes secrete more **melanin** (MELL ah nin) (pigment) to protect the layers underneath from radiation. People have different skin colors because of the varying amounts of melanin.

Dermis

The dermis, or corium, is the thick, underlying layer of the skin composed of vascular connective tissue. This layer houses the skin's blood supply, lymphatics, nervous tissue, hair follicles, and glands.

Accessory Structures

Glands. The **sudoriferous** (soo dur IF uh rus), or sweat, glands are located in the dermis and provide one means of thermoregulation for the body. They secrete sweat through tiny openings in the surface of the skin called **pores.** The secretion of sweat is called **perspiration.** These glands are present throughout the body but are especially abundant in the following areas: the soles of the feet, the palms of the hands, the armpits or axillae (*sing.* axilla), the upper lip, and the forehead.

The **sebaceous** (seh BAY shus) glands secrete an oily, acidic substance called **sebum** (SEE bum), which helps to lubricate hair and the surface of the skin. The acidic nature of sebum is key in inhibiting the growth of bacteria.

Hair. The hair has its roots in the dermis; these roots, together with their coverings, are called **hair follicles** (FALL ih kuls). The visible part is called the hair **shaft.** Underneath the follicle is a structure that encloses the capillaries called the **papilla** (pah PILL ah) (*pl.* papillae). The epithelial cells on top of the papilla are responsible for the formation of the hair shaft. When these cells die, the hair can no longer regenerate, and hair loss occurs. The main function of hair is to assist in thermoregulation by holding heat near the body. When cold, the hair stands on end, holding a layer of air as insulation near the body.

Nails. Nails cover and thus protect the dorsal surfaces of the distal bones of the fingers and toes (Fig. 4-2). The part that is visible is the **nail body**, whereas the **nail root** is in a groove under a small fold of skin at the base of the nail. The **nail bed** is the highly vascular tissue under the nail that appears pink when the blood is oxygenated or blue/purple when it is oxygen deficient. The moonlike white area at the base of the nail is called the **lunula** (LOON yoo lah), beyond which new growth occurs. The small fold of skin surrounding the lower part of the nail is called the **cuticle** (KYOO tih kul) or **eponychium** (eh puh NEE kee um).

DID YOU KNOW?

As the ability to see smaller and smaller body structures became possible, early anatomists named them according to what they resembled that was already named. For example, the nipple was the first structure called a papilla. Later, the term *papilla* was also used to name the projecting capillaries at the bottom of a hair shaft, the conical-shaped entrance to the optic nerve, and the taste buds on the tongue.

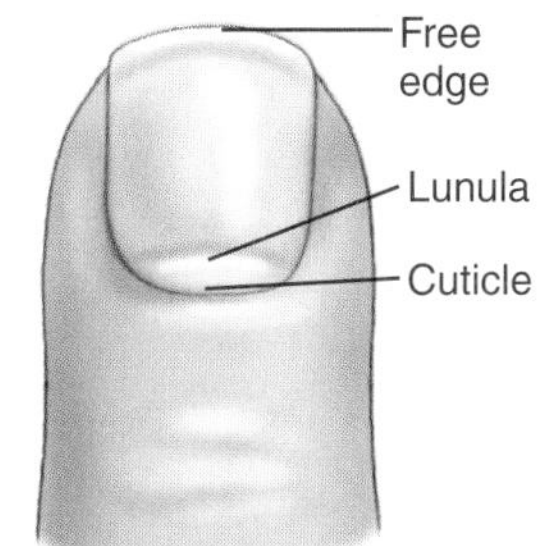

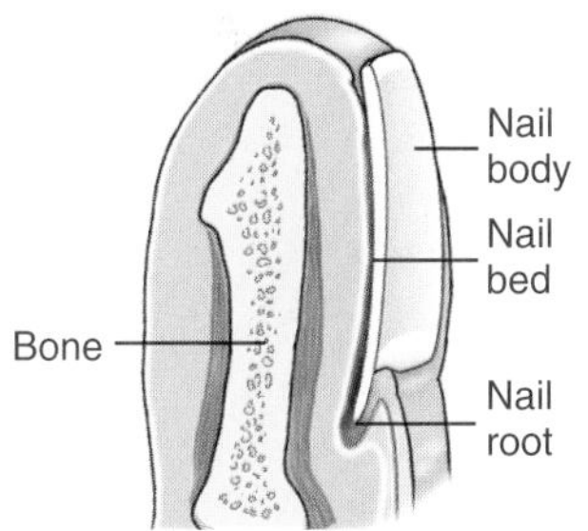

Fig. 4-2 The nail.

COMBINING FORMS FOR ANATOMY AND PHYSIOLOGY

MEANING	COMBINING FORM	MEANING	COMBINING FORM
base	bas/o	horny	corne/o
black	melan/o	papilla	papill/o
fat	adip/o	scaly	squam/o
follicle	follicul/o	sebum	seb/o
hard, horny	kerat/o	vessel	vascul/o

Exercise 2: ANATOMY AND PHYSIOLOGY

Match the combining forms with their meanings. More than one answer may be correct.

_____ 1. vessel	_____ 4. scaly	A. bas/o
_____ 2. fat	_____ 5. base	B. melan/o
_____ 3. black	_____ 6. horny	C. corne/o
		D. vascul/o
		E. squam/o
		F. adip/o
		G. kerat/o

Circle the correct term in parentheses.

7. The healthcare term for the sweat glands is the *(sebaceous, sudoriferous)* glands.
8. Perspiration is excreted through *(pores, papillae).*
9. The acidic nature of the skin helps to inhibit *(perspiration, bacteria).*
10. The hair root and its covering is called the *(follicle, adipose tissue).*
11. When hair stands on end, it is performing one of the functions of the skin called *(thermoregulation, elimination).*
12. The small fold of skin surrounding the base of the nail is called the *(lunula, cuticle).*
13. The pigment produced by cells in the epidermis that gives skin its color is *(melanocytes, melanin).*
14. A hard protein material that adds to the protective nature of the skin is *(keratin, eponychium).*
15. The highly vascular tissue under the nail is the nail *(bed, body).*

PATHOLOGY

Skin Lesions

A skin **lesion** (LEE zhun) is any visible, localized abnormality of skin tissue. It can be described as either primary or secondary. **Primary lesions** (Fig. 4-3) are early skin changes that have not yet undergone natural evolution or change caused by manipulation. **Secondary lesions** (Fig. 4-4) are the result of a natural evolution or manipulation of a primary lesion.

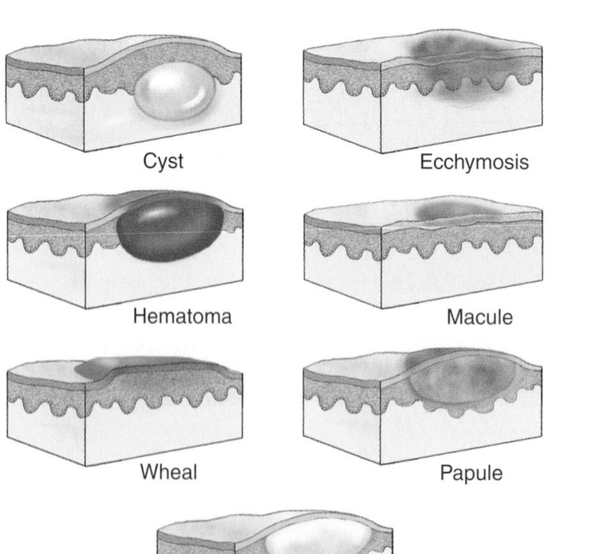

Fig. 4-3 Primary lesions.

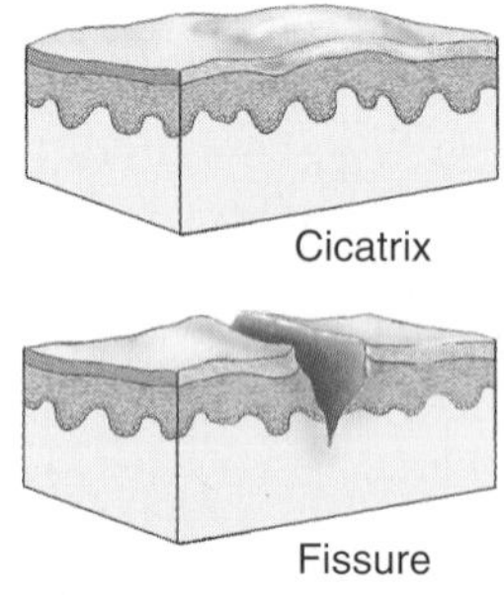

Fig. 4-4 Secondary lesions.

Terms Related to Primary Lesions

TERM	WORD ORIGIN	DEFINITION
Bulla (*pl.* **bullae**) BULL ah		Vesicle larger than ½ cm; seen with second-degree burns.
Cyst sist		Nodule filled with a semisolid material, such as a keratinous cyst (see Fig. 4-3).
Ecchymosis (*pl.* **ecchymoses**) eck ih MOH sis	*ec-* out *chym/o-* juice *-osis* abnormal condition	Hemorrhage or extravasation of blood into the subcutaneous tissue as a result of trauma to the underlying blood vessels or fragility of the vessel walls. The resultant darkening is commonly described as a **bruise** (see Fig. 4-3).
Hematoma hee mah TOH mah	*hemat/o* blood *-oma* mass, swelling	Collection of extravasated blood trapped in the tissues and palpable to the examiner (see Fig. 4-3).
Macule MACK yool	*macul/o* spot	Flat blemish or discoloration less than 1 cm, such as a freckle (see Fig. 4-3).
Nodule NOD yool	*nod/o* knot *-ule* diminutive	Palpable, solid lesion that may or may not be elevated less than 2 cm, such as a small lipoma.
Papule PAP yool	*papul/o* pimple	Solid skin lesion raised less than 1 cm, such as a pimple (see Fig. 4-3).
Patch		Large, flat, nonpalpable macule, larger than 1 cm.
Petechiae (*sing.* **petechia**) peh TEEK ee ee		Tiny ecchymoses within the dermal layer.
Plaque plack		Raised plateaulike papule greater than 1 cm, such as a psoriatic lesion or seborrheic keratosis.
Purpura PUR pur ah	*purpur/o* purple	Massive hemorrhage into the tissues under the skin.
Pustule PUS tyool	*pustul/o* pustule	Superficial, elevated lesion containing pus that may be the result of an infection, such as acne.
Telangiectasia tell an jee eck TAY zsa	*tele/o-* distant *angi/o* vessel *-ectasia* dilation	Permanent dilation of groups of superficial capillaries and venules.
Tumor TOO mur		Nodule over 2 cm; any mass or swelling, including neoplasms.
Vesicle VESS ih kul	*vesicul/o* blister or small sac	Circumscribed, elevated lesion containing fluid and smaller than ½ cm, such as an insect bite (see Fig. 4-3).
Wheals wheels		Circumscribed, elevated papules caused by localized edema, commonly resulting from an allergic reaction, called **urticaria.** Also called **hives** (see Fig. 4-3).

Terms Related to Secondary Skin Lesions		
Term	**Word Origin**	**Definition**
Atrophy AT troh fee	*a-* no, not, without *troph/o* nourishment *-y* process	Paper-thin, wasted skin often occurring in the aged or as stretch marks (**striae,** *sing.* stria) (STRY ay) from rapid weight gain.
Cicatrix (*pl.* cicatrices) SICK ah tricks		Scar—an area of fibrous tissue that replaces normal skin after destruction of some of the dermis (see Fig. 4-4).
Crust		Dried serum, blood, and/or pus. May occur in inflammatory and infectious diseases, such as impetigo. Also called a **scab.**
Erosion eh ROH zhun		Destruction of the surface layer of the skin by physical or inflammatory processes, such as that seen with herpes virus.
Excoriation ecks kore ee A shun		Hollowed-out or linear crusted area caused by traumatic scratching, abrasion, or burning. The sensation of itching is called **pruritus** (pyoor RYE tus).
Fissure FISH ur		Cracklike lesion of the skin, such as an anal fissure (see Fig. 4-4).
Keloid KEE loyd		Type of scar that is an overgrowth of tissue at the site of injury in excess of the amount of tissue necessary to repair the wound. The extra tissue is partially due to an accumulation of collagen at the site (Fig. 4-5).
Lichenification lye ken ih fih KAY shun		Thickening and hardening of the skin, often resulting from the irritation caused by repeated scratching of a pruritic lesion.
Scales		Small, thin flakes of keratinized epithelium frequently seen in rashes such as psoriasis.
Ulcer UL sur		Circumscribed craterlike lesion of the skin or mucous membrane resulting from **necrosis** (neck KROH sis), or tissue death, that can accompany an inflammatory, infectious, or malignant process. An example is the **decubitus ulcer** (deh KYOO bih tis) seen sometimes in bedridden patients.

Did You Know?

The term *extravasation* means the process of a substance (blood or lymph) leaking outside of a vessel into surrounding tissues. Petechia, ecchymosis, hematoma, and purpura are examples of extravasation. The term is easy to analyze. *Extra-* means *outside, vas/o* is a combining form for *a vessel,* and *-tion* means *the process of.*

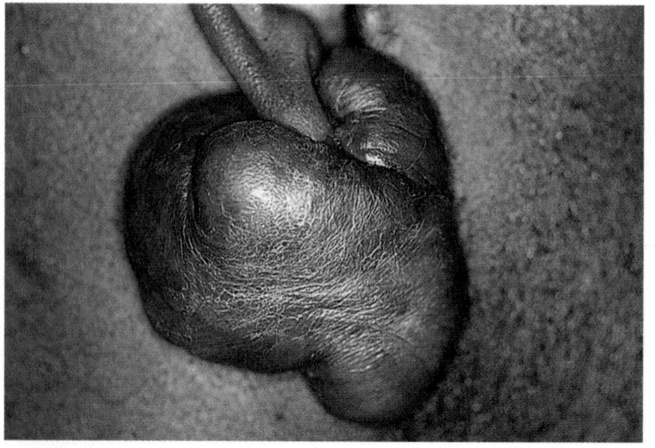

Fig. 4-5 Keloid caused by ear piercing.

Exercise 3: SKIN LESIONS

1. What is the term that means *an itching sensation?* (And be careful to spell it correctly!)

____

2. What is the difference between primary and secondary lesions?

____

____

Match the primary lesions with their definitions.

____ 3. vesicle
____ 4. papule
____ 5. wheals
____ 6. ecchymosis
____ 7. macule
____ 8. pustule

A. extravasated blood into subcutaneous tissue due to trauma
B. flat blemish or discoloration
C. circumscribed, raised papules
D. superficial, elevated lesion containing pus
E. circumscribed, raised lesion containing fluid
F. solid, raised skin lesion

Match the smaller version of a primary skin lesion with the larger version.

____ 9. petechia
____ 10. vesicle
____ 11. papule
____ 12. macule
____ 13. nodule

A. plaque
B. tumor
C. ecchymosis
D. bulla
E. patch

Match the following secondary lesions with their definitions.

____ 14. ulcer
____ 15. cicatrix
____ 16. fissure
____ 17. excoriation
____ 18. lichenification
____ 19. crust
____ 20. atrophy
____ 21. erosion

A. paper-thin, wasted skin
B. scab
C. destruction of the surface layer
D. cracklike lesion
E. hollowed-out crusted area
F. circumscribed, craterlike lesion
G. scar
H. thickening and hardening of the skin

Terms Related to Dermatitis and Bacterial Infections

TERM	WORD ORIGIN	DEFINITION
Atopic dermatitis a TOP ick dur mah TYE tis	*a-* without *top/o* place *-ic* pertaining to *dermat/o* skin *-itis* inflammation	Chronic, pruritic superficial inflammation of the skin usually associated with a family history of allergic disorders.
Carbuncle KAR bun kul		Furuncle with interconnecting subcutaneous pockets; commonly located on the back of the neck and the buttocks.

Continued

Terms Related to Dermatitis and Bacterial Infections—cont'd

TERM	WORD ORIGIN	DEFINITION
Cellulitis sell yoo LYE tis	*cellul/o* cell *-itis* inflammation	Diffuse, spreading, acute inflammation within solid tissues. The most common cause is a *Streptococcus pyogenes* infection (Fig. 4-6).
Contact dermatitis	*dermat/o* skin *-itis* inflammation	Irritated or allergic response of the skin that can lead to an acute or chronic inflammation (Fig. 4-7).
Eczema ECK suh muh		Superficial inflammation of the skin, characterized by vesicles, weeping, and pruritis. Also called **dermatitis.**
Folliculitis foh lick yoo LYE tis	*follicul/o* follicle *-itis* inflammation	Inflammation of the hair follicles, which may be superficial or deep, acute or chronic.
Furuncle FYOOR ung kul		Localized, suppurative staphylococcal skin infections originating in a gland or hair follicle and characterized by pain, redness, and swelling.
Impetigo im peh TYE goh		Superficial vesiculopustular skin infection, normally seen in children, but possible in adults.
Paronychia pair ah NICK ee ah	*par-* near, beside *onych/o* nail *-ia* condition	Infection of the fold of the skin at the margin of the nail.
Seborrheic dermatitis seh boh REE ick	*seb/o* sebum *-rrheic* pertaining to discharge *-dermat/o* skin *-itis* inflammation	Inflammatory scaling disease of the scalp and face. In newborns, this is known as *cradle cap.*

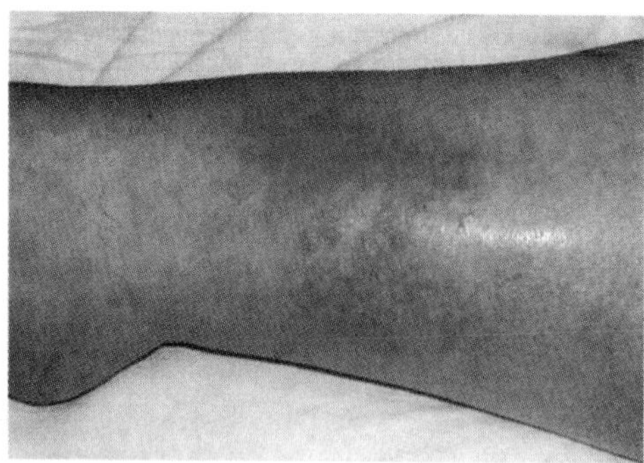

Fig. 4-6 Cellulitis of the lower leg.

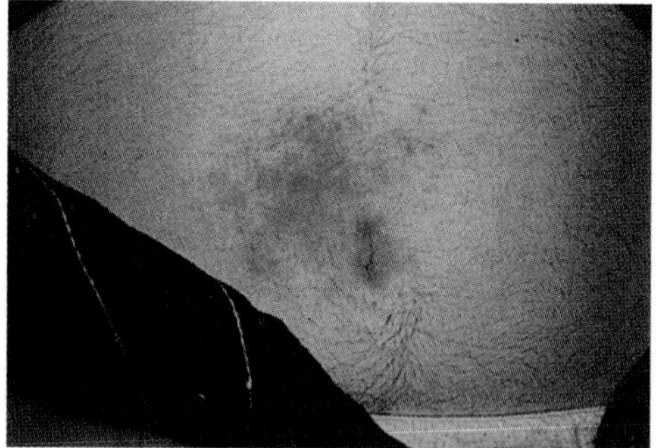

Fig. 4-7 Contact dermatitis caused by allergy to metal snap.

Exercise 4: Dermatitis and Bacterial Infections

Circle the correct term.

1. Another term for dermatitis is *(eczema, carbuncle).*
2. A chronic, pruritic superficial inflammation of the skin associated with a family history of allergic disorders is called *(atopic dermatitis, seborrheic dermatitis).*
3. An irritated or allergic response of the skin that can lead to an acute or chronic inflammation is called *(cellulitis, contact dermatitis).*

4. An inflammatory scaling disease of the scalp and face is termed *(impetigo, seborrheic dermatitis)*.
5. An infection of the fold of the skin at the margin of the nail is called *(onychomycosis, paronychia)*.
6. A diffuse, spreading, acute inflammation within solid tissues as a result of a streptococcal infection describes *(cellulitis, dermatitis)*.
7. A superficial vesiculopustular skin infection normally seen in children is called *(contact dermatitis, impetigo)*.
8. A localized, suppurative staphylococcal skin infection in a gland or hair follicle is called a *(carbuncle, furuncle)*.
9. Inflammation of the hair follicles is called *(trichomycosis, folliculitis)*.
10. A series of furuncles interconnected by subcutaneous pockets is called *(carbuncles, cellulitis)*.

Terms Related to Yeast and Fungal Infections

TERM	WORD ORIGIN	DEFINITION
Candidiasis kan dih DYE ah sis		Yeast infection in moist, occluded areas of the skin (armpits, inner thighs, underneath pendulous breasts) and mucous membranes. Also called **moniliasis** (mah nih LYE ah sis).
Dermatomycosis dur muh toh mye KOH sis	*dermat/o* skin *myc/o* fungus *-osis* abnormal condition	Fungal infection of the skin.
Onychomycosis on ih koh mye KOH sis	*onych/o* nail *myc/o* fungus *-osis* abnormal condition	Fungal infection of the nails.
Tinea capitis TIN ee ah KAP ih tis	*capit/o* head *-is* noun ending	Fungal infection of the scalp; also known as **ringworm.**
Tinea corporis TIN ee ah KOR poor is	*corpor/o* body *-is* noun ending	Ringworm of the body, manifested by pink to red papulosquamous annular (ringlike) plaques with raised borders; also known as **ringworm** (Fig. 4-8).
Tinea cruris TIN ee ah KROO ris	*crur/o* leg *-is* noun ending	A fungal infection that occurs mainly on external genitalia and upper legs in males, particularly in warm weather; also known as **jock itch.**
Tinea pedis TIN ee ah PEH dis	*ped/o* foot *-is* noun ending	Fungal infection of the foot; also known as **athlete's foot.**
Tinea unguium TIN ee ah UN gwee um	*ungu/o* nail *-ium* noun ending	Fungal infection of the nails; also known as **onychomycosis.**

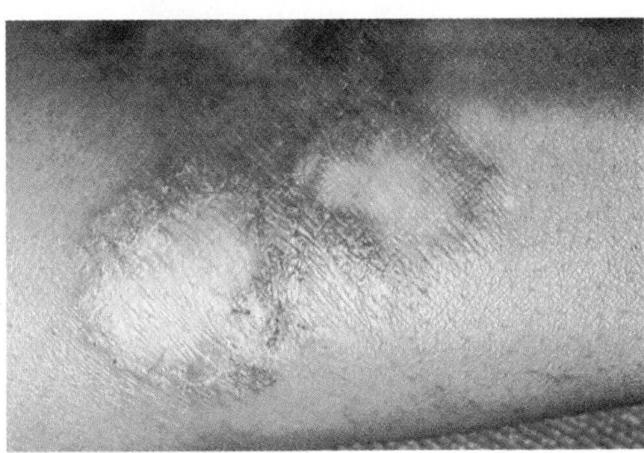

Fig. 4-8 Tinea corporis.

Terms Related to Parasitic Infestations

TERM	WORD ORIGIN	DEFINITION
Pediculosis peh dick yoo LOH sis	*pedicul/o* louse *-osis* abnormal condition	Parasitic infestation with lice, involving the head, body, or genital area (Fig. 4-9).
Scabies SKAY bees		Parasitic infestation caused by mites; characterized by pruritic papular rash.

Terms Related to Viral Infections

TERM	WORD ORIGIN	DEFINITION
Herpes simplex virus (HSV) HUR peez SIM plecks		Viral infection characterized by clusters of small vesicles filled with clear fluid on raised inflammatory bases on the skin or mucosa. HSV-1 causes fever blisters (herpetic **stomatitis**) and **keratitis,** an inflammation of the cornea. HSV-2 is more commonly known as **genital herpes.**
Herpes zoster HUR peez ZAH stur		Acute, painful, infectious rash caused by reactivation of the latent varicella-zoster virus. Also known as **shingles.**
Verruca (*pl.* **verrucae**) veh ROO kah		Common, contagious epithelial growths usually appearing on the skin of the hands, feet, legs, and face; can be caused by any of 60 types of the human papilloma virus (HPV) (Fig. 4-10). Also called **warts.**

BE CAREFUL!

The combining form *stomat/o* means *mouth,* not *stomach.*

DID YOU KNOW?

Kerat/o, which is the combining form for the hard property of the skin, is also the combining form for the cornea of the eye.

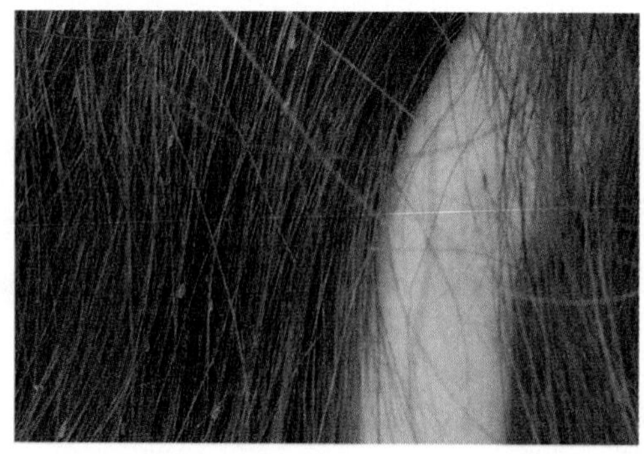

Fig. 4-9 Lice in hair.

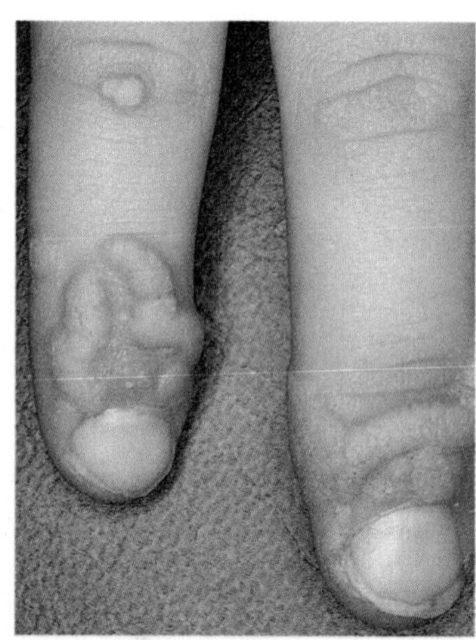

Fig. 4-10 Verrucae (warts).

Exercise 5: YEAST, FUNGAL, PARASITIC, AND VIRAL INFECTIONS

Match these fungal or yeast infections with their definitions or synonyms.

____ 1. athlete's foot

____ 2. ringworm of scalp

____ 3. moniliasis

____ 4. jock itch

____ 5. onychomycosis

____ 6. ringworm of body

A. tinea corporis
B. tinea cruris
C. tinea capitis
D. tinea pedis
E. tinea unguium
F. candidiasis

Name the healthcare term.

7. infestation with lice ________________.

8. shingles ________________.

9. warts (be sure to use plural spelling) ________________.

10. virus causing stomatitis ________________.

11. infestation with mites ________________.

12. fungal infection of the skin ________________.

Terms Related to Disorders of Hair Follicles and Sebaceous Glands

TERM	WORD ORIGIN	DEFINITION
Acne ACK nee		Inflammatory disease of the sebaceous glands characterized by papules, pustules, inflamed nodules, and **comedones** (kah mih DOH neez) (*sing.* comedo), which are plugs of sebum that partially or completely block a pore. Blackheads are open comedones, and whiteheads are closed comedones.
Alopecia al oh PEE shee ah		Baldness, or hair loss, resulting from genetic factors, aging, or disease (Fig. 4-11).

Continued

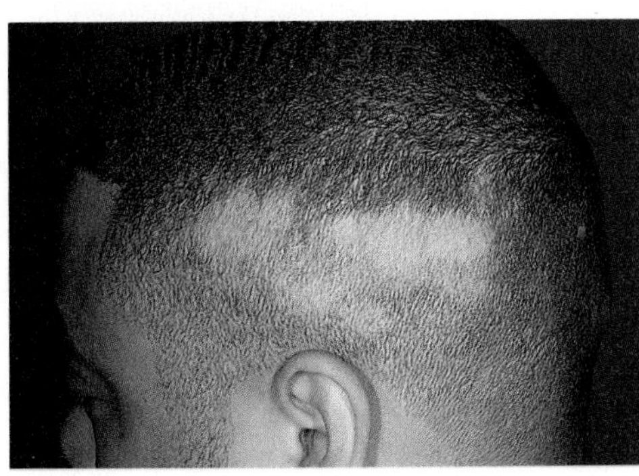

Fig. 4-11 Alopecia.

DID YOU KNOW?

Alopecia comes from the Greek term *alopekia*, meaning *fox mange*. Mange is an animal disease in which the hair comes out in clumps.

Terms Related to Disorders of Hair Follicles and Sebaceous Glands—cont'd

TERM	WORD ORIGIN	DEFINITION
Hypertrichosis hye pur trih KOH sis	*hyper-* excessive *trich/o* hair *-osis* abnormal condition	Abnormal excess of hair; also known as **hirsutism** (HER soo tih zum).
Keratinous cyst kur AT tin us	*kerat/o* hard, horny	Benign cavity lined by keratinizing epithelium and filled with sebum and epithelial debris.
Milia MILL ee ah		Tiny superficial keratinous cysts caused by clogged oil ducts.
Rosacea roh ZAY shah		Chronic inflammatory disorder that occurs in fair-skinned individuals and is characterized by telangiectasia, erythema, papules, and pustules on the face.
Trichotillomania trick oh till oh MAY nee ah		Disorder characterized by an impulsive tendency to pull one's hair out.

Term Related to Scaling Papular Diseases

TERM	WORD ORIGIN	DEFINITION
Psoriasis sur EYE ah sis		Common chronic skin disorder characterized by circumscribed, salmon-red patches covered by thick, dry, silvery scales that are the result of excessive development of epithelial cells (Fig. 4-12).

Terms Related to Cornification and Pressure Injuries

TERM	WORD ORIGIN	DEFINITION
Callus KAL us		Common painless thickening of the stratum corneum at locations of external pressure or friction.
Corn		Horny mass of condensed epithelial cells overlying a bony prominence resulting from pressure or friction; also referred to as a **clavus** (KLA vuhs).
Decubitus ulcer deh KYOO bih tus		Inflammation, ulcer, or sore in the skin over a bony prominence. Most often seen in aged, debilitated, cachectic (wasted), or immobilized patients, pressure sores or ulcers are graded by stages of severity. The highest stage, stage 6, involves muscle, fat, and bone. Also known as a **bedsore, pressure ulcer,** or **pressure sore** (Fig. 4-13).
Ichthyosis ick thee OH sis	*ichthy/o* fish *-osis* abnormal condition	Category of dry skin that has the scaly appearance of a fish. It ranges from mild to severe. The mild form is known as **xeroderma** (zir uh DUR mah).

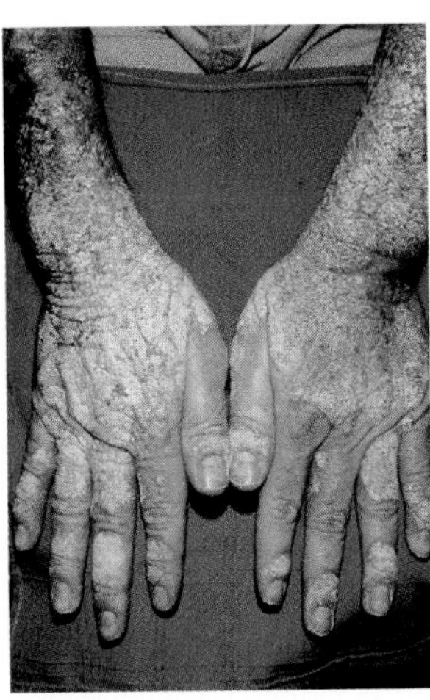

Fig. 4-12 Psoriasis.

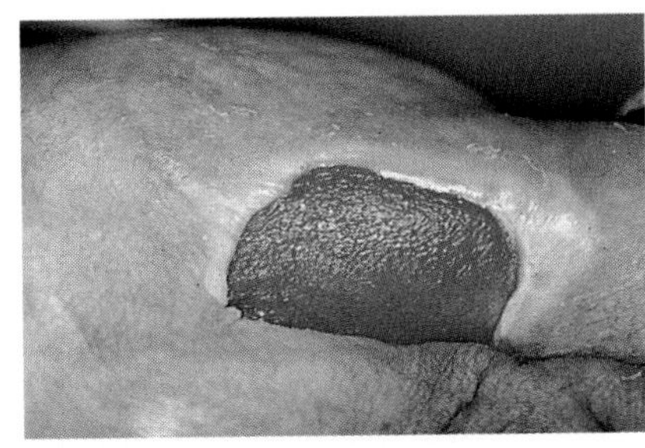

Fig. 4-13 Stage III pressure (decubitus) ulcer.

DID YOU KNOW?

The term *decubitus* comes from a Latin noun meaning *a lying down* and the adjective, *related to the elbow.* Romans rested on their elbows when reclining. One assumes they eventually suffered pressure sores on their elbows from this constant position.

Exercise 6: DISORDERS OF HAIR FOLLICLES AND SEBACEOUS GLANDS, SCALING PAPULAR DISEASES, AND PRESSURE INJURIES

Fill in the blanks with the correct terms from the list below.

acne, alopecia, clavus, decubitus ulcer, hypertrichosis, keratinous cyst, milia, pressure sore, psoriasis, rosacea, trichotillomania, xeroderma

1. What is a chronic inflammatory disorder characterized by telangiectasia, erythema, papules, and pustules on the face? Rosacea
2. What is a disorder of circumscribed salmon-red patches covered with thick, silvery scales? Psoriasis
3. What is another name for hirsutism? hypertrichosis
4. What is the term for the tendency to pull one's hair out? trichotillomania
5. What is the term for baldness? Alopecia
6. What is the term for a benign cavity filled with sebum and epithelial debris, and lined with keratinized epithelium? Keratinous cyst
7. What is the common inflammatory disease of the sebaceous glands characterized by comedones, papules, pustules, and inflamed nodules? acne
8. What is another term for a corn? clavus
9. What are two alternative terms for bedsores? pressure sore / decubitus ulcer
10. What are tiny, superficial keratinous cysts? milia
11. What is the term for mildly dry skin? Xeroderma

Terms Related to Pigmentation Disorders

Term	Word Origin	Definition
Albinism AL bih niz um	***albin/o*** white ***-ism*** condition	Complete lack of melanin production by existing melanocytes, resulting in pale skin, white hair, and pink irides (*sing.* iris).
Hyperpigmentation	***hyper-*** excessive ***pigment/o*** paint ***-ation*** condition	Abnormally increased pigmentation.
Hypopigmentation	***hypo-*** deficient ***pigment/o*** paint ***-ation*** condition	Congenital or acquired decrease in melanin production.
Melasma mah LAZ mah		Hyperpigmentation of the forehead, cheeks, and/or nose as a result of the effect of pregnancy or oral contraceptives. The pigmentation recedes gradually, although sometimes incompletely, when the pregnancy concludes or the oral contraceptives are discontinued. Also called **chloasma** (kloh AZ muh).
Vitiligo vih tih LYE goh		Benign acquired disease of unknown origin, consisting of irregular patches of various sizes lacking in pigment (Fig. 4-14).

Terms Related to Disorders of Sweating

Term	Word Origin	Definition
Hyperhidrosis hye pur hye DROH sis	***hyper-*** excessive ***hidr/o*** sweat ***-osis*** abnormal condition	Excessive perspiration caused by heat, strong emotion, menopause, hyperthyroidism, or infection.
Miliaria mill ee AIR ee uh		Minute vesicles and papules, often with surrounding **erythema,** (redness), caused by occlusion of sweat ducts during times of exposure to heat and high humidity.

Exercise 7: Pigmentation Disorders and Disorders of Sweating

Build the term.

1. an abnormal condition of excessive perspiration ________________
2. an abnormal condition of deficient pigmentation ________________

Fill in the blank.

3. An acquired disorder of irregular patches of various sizes lacking in pigment is ________________.
4. A patient whose body produces no melanin has a diagnosis of ________________.
5. Minute vesicles and papules caused by occlusion of sweat ducts are called ________________.
6. Hyperpigmentation of the face during pregnancy or while taking oral contraceptives is called ________________ or ________________.

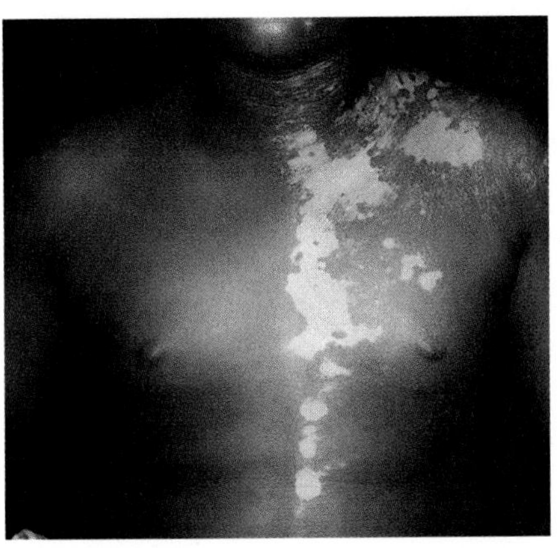

Fig. 4-14 Vitiligo.

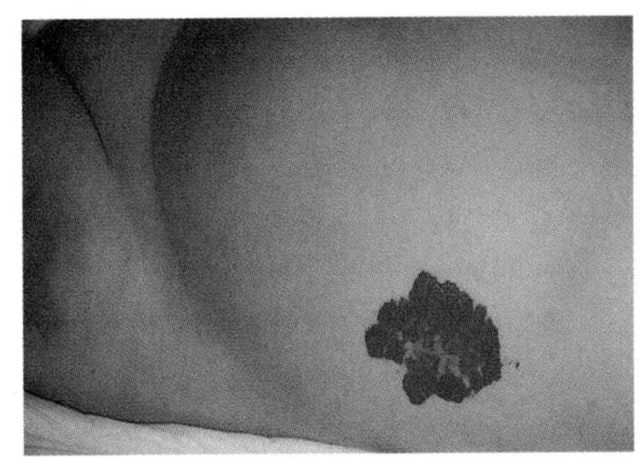

Fig. 4-15 Hemangioma.

BE CAREFUL!

Hidr/o- with an *i* means *sweat; hydr/o-* with a *y* means *water.* Both are pronounced HYE droh.

BE CAREFUL!

Don't confuse *milia,* a condition resulting from oil-filled ducts, with *miliaria,* a condition resulting from sweat-filled ducts.

Terms Related to Benign (Noncancerous) Skin Growths

TERM	WORD ORIGIN	DEFINITION
Angioma an jee OH mah	***angi/o*** vessel ***-oma*** swelling, mass	Localized vascular lesion that includes hemangiomas, vascular nevi, and lymphangiomas (Fig. 4-15).
Dermatofibroma dur mat toh fye BROH mah	***dermat/o*** skin ***fibr/o*** fiber ***-oma*** swelling, mass	Skin nodule that is painless, round, firm, red or gray, elevated, and usually found on the extremities.
Dysplastic nevus (*pl.* **nevi**) dis PLAS tick NEE vus	***dys-*** abnormal ***plast/o*** formation ***-ic*** pertaining to	Various abnormal changes of a pigmented congenital skin blemish that give rise to a concern for progression to malignancy. Changes of concern are categorized as ABCD: **a**symmetry **b**orders, irregular **c**olors, changes or uneven pigmentation **d**iameter, increasing size or >6 mm
Lipoma lih POH mah	***lip/o*** fat ***-oma*** mass, swelling	Fatty tumors that are soft, movable, subcutaneous nodules.
Nevus		Pigmented lesion often present at birth. Also called a **mole.**
Seborrheic keratosis seh boh REE ick kair ah TOH sis	***seb/o*** sebum ***-rrheic*** pertaining to discharge ***kerat/o*** hard, horny ***-osis*** abnormal condition	Benign, circumscribed, pigmented, superficial warty skin lesion that may be accompanied by pruritus.
Skin tags		Small, soft, pedunculated lesions that are harmless outgrowths of epidermal and dermal tissue, usually occurring on the neck, eyelids, armpits, and groin; usually occur in multiples. Also known as **acrochordons** (ack roh KORE dons).

Exercise 8: BENIGN SKIN GROWTHS

Matching.

_____ 1. pigmented lesion

_____ 2. acrochordon

_____ 3. fatty tumor

_____ 4. painless skin lesion

_____ 5. benign warty skin lesion

_____ 6. vascular nevus

A. skin tag
B. lipoma
C. seborrheic keratosis
D. mole
E. dermatofibroma
F. angioma

Burns

Burns are injuries to tissues that result from exposure to thermal, chemical, electrical, or radioactive agents. They may be classified into four different degrees of severity, depending on the layers of the skin that are damaged. Coders must categorize burns higher than second degree according to the "rule of nines" (Fig. 4-16) that divides the body into percentages that are, for the most part, multiples of nine: the head and neck equaling 9%, each upper limb 9%, each lower limb 18%, the front and back of the torso 36%, and the genital area 1%. Fig. 4-17 is an illustration of the different degrees of burns.

- **First degree:** Burn in which only the first layer of the skin, the epidermis, is damaged; also known as a *superficial burn.* Characterized by redness (erythema), tenderness, and hyperesthesia, with no scar development.
- **Second degree:** Burn in which the first and second layers of the skin (epidermis and part of the dermis) are affected; sometimes called a *partial-thickness burn.* Characterized by redness, blisters, and pain, with possible scar development.
- **Third degree:** Burn that damages the epidermis, dermis, and subcutaneous tissue; also known as a *full-thickness burn.* Pain is not present because the nerve endings in the skin have been destroyed. Skin appearance may be deep red, pale gray, brown, or black. Scar formation is likely.

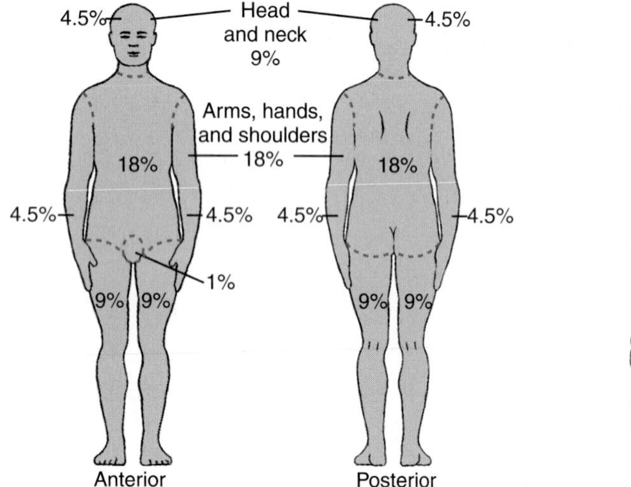

Fig. 4-16 Rule of nines for estimating extent of burns.

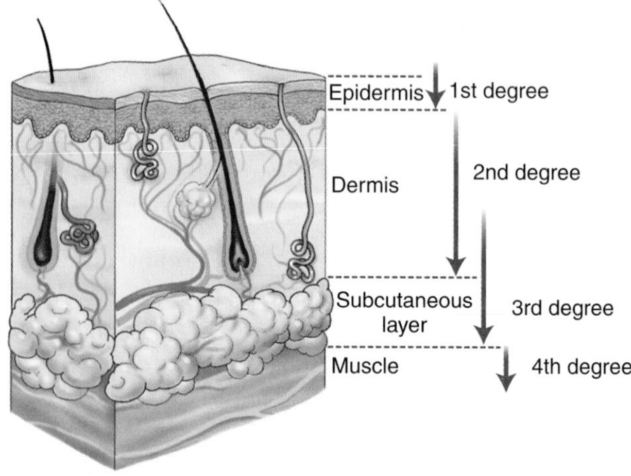

Fig. 4-17 Degree of burns and depth of tissue involvement.

- **Fourth degree:** Although not a universally accepted category, some burn specialists use this category to describe a rare burn that extends beyond the subcutaneous tissue into the muscle and bone.
- **Eschar** (ESS kar): Scab or dry crust that results from a burn, trauma, or infection.

Exercise 9: BURNS

Match the characteristics of the burns listed with their degree.

_____ 1. first degree
_____ 2. second degree
_____ 3. third degree
_____ 4. fourth degree

A. Ironing a blouse for work, Rhonda burned her hand, resulting in blisters and erythema.
B. John suffered burns over two thirds of his body with many areas of tissue burned to the bone.
C. Because Kristin forgot to reapply her sunblock, she sustained a sunburn that resulted in painful reddened skin.
D. Smoking in bed resulting in burns that destroyed the epidermis, dermis, and extended through the hypodermis on the victim's chest and shoulders.

Fill in the blank.

5. The healthcare term for a crust or scab especially related to burns is _______________.
6. The rule of nines is used to categorize the _______________ of a burn, depending on the body surfaces affected.

Case Study Continued

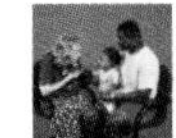

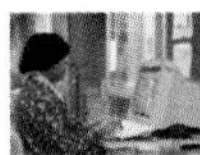

The coffee that scalded Ben caused a mottled, sensitive, and painful area on his arm that soon developed a large blister. He was diagnosed as having a second-degree (partial thickness) burn. His dad was told that he would need to try to keep Ben from picking at the blister, because patients with this type of burn are at risk for developing scar tissue.

DIAGNOSTIC PROCEDURES

Terms Related to Biopsies

TERM	WORD ORIGIN	DEFINITION
Excisional biopsy		Biopsy in which the entire tumor may be removed with borders as a means of diagnosis and treatment.
Exfoliation ecks foh lee A shun		Scraping or shaving off samples of friable (easily crushed) lesions for a laboratory examination called **exfoliative cytology.**
Incisional biopsy		Biopsy in which larger tissue samples may be obtained by excising a wedge of tissue and suturing the incision.
Needle aspiration		Aspiration of fluid from lesions to obtain samples for culture and examination.
Punch biopsy		Biopsy in which a tubular punch is inserted through to the subcutaneous tissue, and the tissue is cut off at the base (Fig. 4-18).

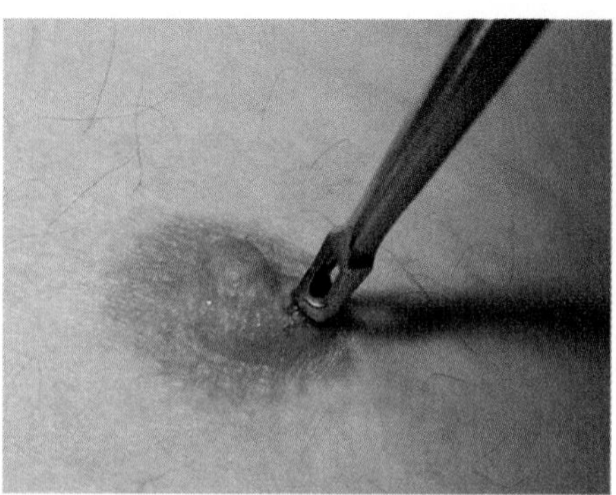

Fig. 4-18 Punch biopsy.

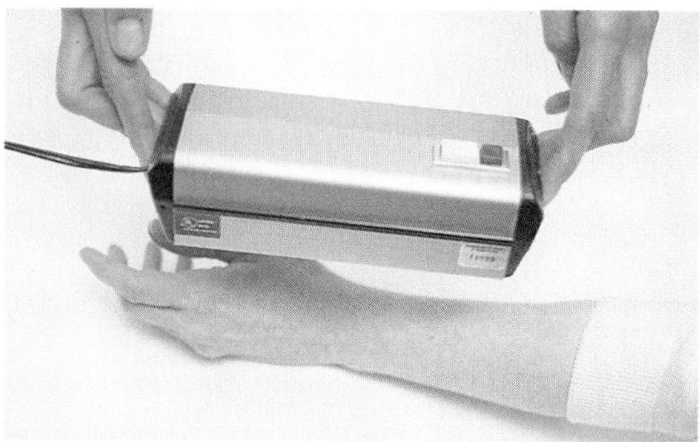

Fig. 4-19 Wood's lamp. The purple color on the skin indicates that no fungal infection is present.

Terms Related to Laboratory Tests

Term	Word Origin	Definition
Bacterial analyses		Culture and serology of lesions to help diagnose such disorders as impetigo.
Fungal tests		Cultures of scrapings of lesions used to identify fungal infections such as tinea pedis, tinea capitis, and tinea cruris.
Sweat tests		Laboratory procedure test for abnormally high levels of sodium and chloride present in the perspiration of persons with cystic fibrosis.
Tuberculosis (TB) skin tests		Intradermal test (e.g., Mantoux test) using purified protein derivative (PPD) to test for either dormant or active tuberculosis; much more accurate test than the multiple puncture tine test, which has been used for screening purposes.
Tzanck test tzahnk		Microscopic examination of lesions for the purpose of diagnosing herpes zoster and herpes simplex.
Viral culture		Sampling of vesicular fluid for the purpose of identifying viruses.
Wood's light examination		Method to identify a variety of skin infections through the use of a Wood's lamp, which produces ultraviolet light; tinea capitis and pseudomonas infections in burns are two of the disorders it can reveal (Fig. 4-19).
Wound and abscess cultures		Lab samplings that can identify pathogens in wounds such as diabetic or decubitus ulcers, postoperative wounds, or abscesses.

Exercise 10: Diagnostic Procedures

Fill in the blanks with the correct terms from the list below.

excisional, exfoliation, incisional, needle aspiration, punch

1. An entire tumor is removed in a/an _______________ biopsy.

2. Fluid from a lesion is aspirated to obtain samples for culture in a/an _______________ biopsy.

3. A wedge of tissue is removed and the incision is sutured in a/an ______________ biopsy.

4. Samples of friable lesions are scraped or shaved off in ______________.

5. A cylindrical punch is inserted into the subcutaneous tissue layer, and the tissue is cut off at the base in ______________ biopsy.

Match the following disorders with the tests that may be used to diagnose them.

F 6. ringworm	G 10. herpes zoster, herpes simplex	A. Wood's light examination
C 7. impetigo	A 11. tinea capitis, pseudomonas	B. Mantoux
E 8. cystic fibrosis	D 12. bedsore, infection	C. bacterial analysis
B 9. tuberculosis		D. wound abscess culture
		E. sweat test
		F. fungal test
		G. Tzanck test

THERAPEUTIC INTERVENTIONS

Terms Related to Grafting Techniques and Other Therapies

TERM	WORD ORIGIN	DEFINITION
Allograft AL oh graft	*all/o* other	Harvest of skin from another human donor for temporary transplant until an autograft is available.
Autograft AH toh graft	*auto-* self	Harvest of the patient's own skin for transplant (Fig. 4-20).
Dermatome DUR mah tohm	*dermat/o* skin *-tome* instrument to cut	Instrument used to remove split skin grafts.
Flap		Section of skin transferred from one location to an immediately adjacent one.
Full-thickness graft		Free skin graft using full portions of both the epidermis and dermis.
Laser therapy		Procedure to repair or destroy tissue, particularly in the removal of tattoos, warts, port wine stains, and psoriatic lesions.
Occlusive therapy	*occlus/o* to close *-ive* pertaining to	Use of a nonporous occlusive dressing to cover a treated area to increase the absorption and effectiveness of a medication; used to treat psoriasis, lupus erythematosus, and chronic hand dermatitis.

Continued

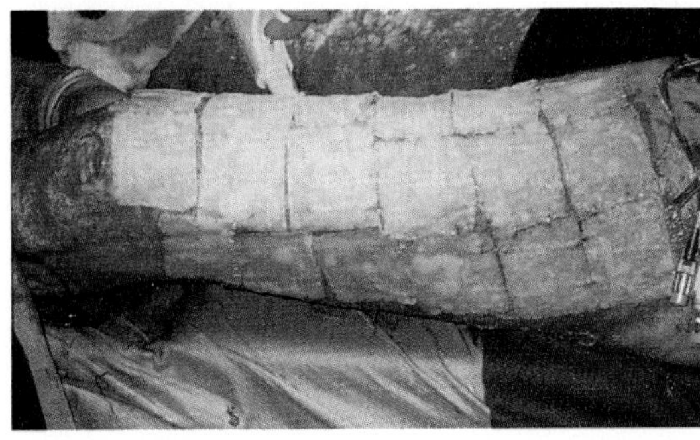

Fig. 4-20 Epithelial autografts. Thin sheets of skin are attached to gauze backing.

DID YOU KNOW?

The term *dermatome* also describes an area on the surface of the body that receives innervation from afferent fibers of a spinal root.

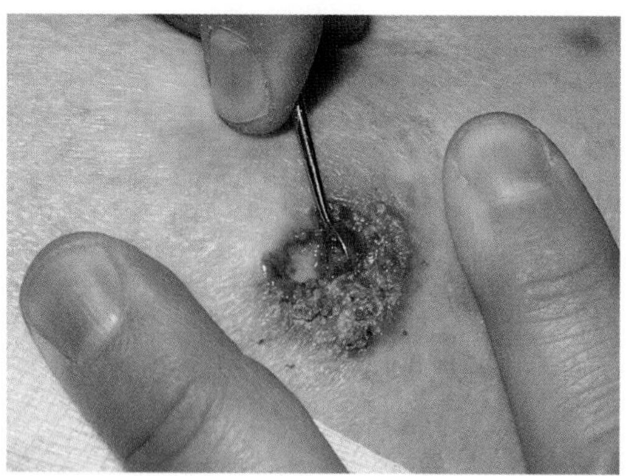

Fig. 4-21 Curettage.

Terms Related to Grafting Techniques and Other Therapies—cont'd

TERM	WORD ORIGIN	DEFINITION
Psoralen ultraviolet A (PUVA) therapy SORE ah lin		Directing of one of the types of ultraviolet light on psoriatic lesions.
Skin grafting (SG)		Skin transplant performed when normal skin cover has been lost due to burns, ulcers, or operations to remove cancerous tissue.
Split-thickness skin graft (STSG)		Skin graft using the epidermis and parts of the dermis.
Xenograft ZEE noh graft	*xen/o* foreign	Temporary skin graft from another species, often a pig, used until an autograft is available.

Terms Related to Tissue Removal

TERM	WORD ORIGIN	DEFINITION
Cauterization kah tur rye ZAY shun	*cauter/o* burn *-zation* process of	Destruction of tissue by burning with thermal heat.
Cryosurgery KRY oh sur juh ree	*cryo-* extreme cold	Destruction of tissue through the use of extreme cold, usually liquid nitrogen.
Curettage KYOOR uh tahz		Scraping material from the wall of a cavity or other surface to obtain tissue for microscopic examination; this is done with an instrument called a **curette** (Fig. 4-21).
Debridement dah breed MON		First step in wound treatment, involving removal of dirt, foreign bodies (FB), damaged tissue, and cellular debris from the wound or burn to prevent infection and to promote healing.
Escharotomy ess kar AH tuh mee	*eschar/o* scab *-tomy* incision	Surgical incision into necrotic tissue resulting from a severe burn. This may be necessary to prevent edema leading to ischemia (loss of blood flow) in underlying tissue.
Incision and drainage (I&D)		To cut open and remove the contents of a wound, cyst, or other lesion.
Shaving (paring)		Slicing of thin sheets of tissue to remove lesions.

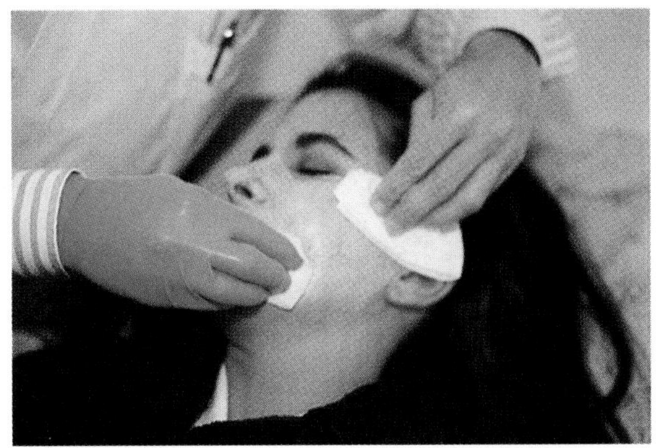

Fig. 4-22 Application of a chemical peel.

Terms Related to Cosmetic Procedures

TERM	WORD ORIGIN	DEFINITION
Blepharoplasty BLEF ar oh plas tee	*blephar/o* eyelid *-plasty* surgical repair	Surgical restructuring of the eyelid.
Chemical peel		Use of a mild acid to produce a mild, superficial burn; normally done to remove wrinkles (Fig. 4-22).
Dermabrasion dur mah BRAY zhun	*derm/o* skin *-abrasion* scraping	Surgical procedure to resurface the skin; used to remove acne scars, nevi, wrinkles, and tattoos.
Dermatoplasty dur mat toh PLAS tee	*dermat/o* skin *-plasty* surgical repair	Transplant of living skin to correct effects of injury, operation, or disease.
Lipectomy lih PECK toh mee	*lip/o* fat *-ectomy* removal	Resection of fatty tissue.
Liposuction LIP oh suck shun	*lip/o* fat	Technique for removing adipose tissue with a suction pump device.
Rhytidectomy rye tih DECK tuh mee	*rhytid/o* wrinkle *-ectomy* removal	Surgical operation to remove wrinkles. Commonly known as a "face-lift."

Exercise 11: THERAPEUTIC INTERVENTIONS

1. Explain the differences among the following.

   A. autograft ______________________________

   B. allograft ______________________________

   C. xenograft ______________________________

2. Which type of graft includes the epidermis and the dermis? ______________________________

3. What instrument is used to cut skin for grafting? ______________________________

Fill in the blanks with the correct terms from the list below.

cauterization, cryosurgery, curettage, debridement, incision and drainage, laser therapy, occlusive therapy, shaving

4. _______________ is used to destroy tattoos.
5. Removing dirt, foreign bodies, damaged tissue, and cellular debris from a wound is called _______________.
6. The destruction of tissue by burning with thermal heat is called _______________.
7. The destruction of tissue through the use of extreme cold is called _______________.
8. Scraping of material from the wall of a cavity is called _______________.
9. I&D is _______________.
10. Another term for paring is _______________.
11. A covered treatment area is called _______________.

Matching.

_____ 12. resection of fatty tissue

_____ 13. excision of wrinkles

_____ 14. resurfacing the skin

_____ 15. restructuring of eyelids

_____ 16. therapeutic superficial burn

_____ 17. suction of adipose tissue

_____ 18. transplant of skin

A. chemical peel
B. liposuction
C. blepharoplasty
D. rhytidectomy
E. lipectomy
F. dermabrasion
G. dermatoplasty

Case Study Continued

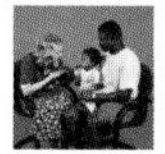

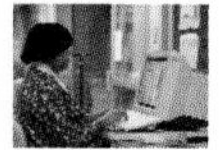

If Ben's burn had been more serious, he might have needed a grafting procedure, possibly harvesting of some of his own tissue from his buttocks. Fortunately, the burn did not appear to be severe enough to warrant the need for grafting. If the wound does not heal properly and a disfiguring scar develops, he may be a candidate for revision of the scar at a later date.

PHARMACOLOGY

Routes of Administration

Several medications are administered on, within, or through the skin. The most common of these routes of administration include the following:

Hypodermic (H): General term that refers to any injection under the skin.
Intradermal (ID): Route of injection within the dermis (Fig. 4-23, *A*). Also called **intracutaneous.**
Subcutaneous: Route for injection into the fat layer beneath the skin (Fig. 4-23, *B*).

BE CAREFUL!

ID means *intradermal;* I&D means *incision and drainage.*

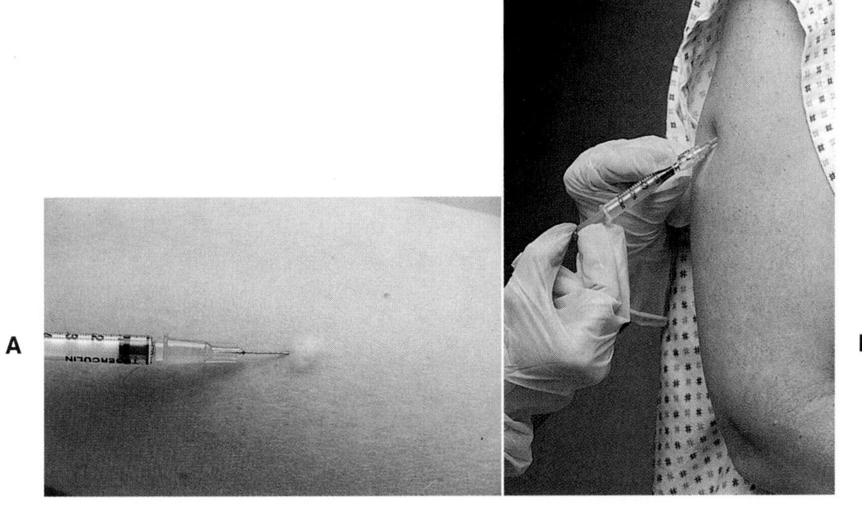

Fig. 4-23 **A,** Intradermal injection. **B,** Subcutaneous injection.

Topical: Type of drug applied directly on the skin as a cream, gel, lotion, or ointment.

Transdermal therapeutic system (TTS): Use of a transdermal patch; involves placing medication in a gel-like material that is applied to the skin, allowing for a specified, timed release of the medicine. Examples are nitroglycerin for angina pectoris and Nicoderm for smoking cessation.

Dermatologic Drugs

Traditional Pharmacology

Anesthetic agents: Drugs to reduce pain and discomfort; can be given topically in an affected area. Examples include lidocaine and Solarcaine.

Antiacne drugs: Medications containing benzoyl peroxide. Some topical agents are available over the counter (OTC). Prescription medications may be topical (e.g., erythromycin, metronidazole, tretinoin [Retin-A]) or oral (e.g., tetracycline, minocyline, or isotretinoin [Accutane]).

Antibacterial agents: Drugs that target bacteria. Topical agents include erythromycin, gentamicin, metronidazole, silver sulfadiazine (Silvadene), and mupirocin.

Antifungal agents: Drugs that attack fungi, such as nystatin, triamcinolone, butenafine (Mentax), ciclopirox olamine (Loprox), or econazole (Spectazole).

Antiinflammatory agents: Drugs that reduce inflammation and its resulting pain. Aspirin is the most common oral agent in this category. Topical corticosteroids in this group include fluocinonide (Lidex), triamcinolone, and hydrocortisone.

Antipruritic agents: Drugs that lessen itching. Examples include diphenhydramine OTC, available in oral or topical formulations. Those available by prescription include cyproheptadine, hydroxyzine HCl, and hydroxyzine pamoate.

Antipsoriatics and antieczema drugs: Agents that treat diseases such as psoriasis and eczema. Examples include chloroxine, tazarotene (Tazorac), and methotrexate.

Antiseptic agents: Topical drugs used to prevent infection by destroying pathogens. An example is methyolate (Timersol).

Antiviral agents: Drugs designed to lessen the effects of viruses. Examples include valacyclovir (Valtrex) and acyclovir (Zovirax).

Emollients (ih MOLL yents): Topical substances that soften the skin. A well-known example is Lubriderm.

> **DID YOU KNOW?**
>
> Many dermatologic drugs share the prefixes *anti-*, meaning that they are against whatever is named, *-lytics,* meaning that they destroy or break down something, or *-cides,* meaning that they are intended to kill something.

Keratolytics (kair ah toh LIT icks): Topical substances used to break down hardened skin, such as that seen on warts, corns, and calluses. Examples include salicylic acid and combinations, cantharidin, and podofilox (Condylox).

Parasiticides (pair ah SIH tih sydes): Agents that attack a variety of parasites. For instance, within this group of drugs, **scabicides** destroy mites, and **pediculicides** destroy lice.

Protectives: Topicals with sun protection factors (SPFs) to protect the skin against ultraviolet A and B in sunlight. A wide variety of these are available OTC.

Alternative and Complementary Methods of Treatment

Herbal medicine: Drugs from minimally altered plant sources, such as aloe vera (to treat sunburn and stomach ulcers) or tea tree oil (used for its antibacterial, antiviral, and antifungal properties to treat boils, wound infections, and acne). Also, therapeutic use of essential oils, useful in treating dry flaky skin, decubitus ulcers, diabetic ulcers, herpes zoster, and herpes simplex type 1.

Exercise 12: PHARMACOLOGY

Build terms to describe the following.

1. Medication injected "within the dermis" is given by the ______________ route.
2. Medications applied "in place" directly to the skin are given by the ______________ route.
3. A general term meaning *under the skin* is ______________.
4. Medications delivered via a patch through the skin are given by ______________.
5. Medication applied to an affected area to reduce pain and discomfort is called a/an ______________.
6. An herbal medicine used for sunburn and stomach ulcers is called ______________.
7. Erythromycin, tretinoin, tetracycline, and isotretinoin are all used to treat ______________.
8. Medications that target bacteria are called ______________.
9. Triamcinolone, nystatin, and econazole are all ______________ medications.
10. Give three examples of antiinflammatory medications:

____

Match the following pharmaceutical agents with their actions.

____ 11. softens the skin

____ 12. breaks down hardened skin

____ 13. lessens itching

____ 14. prevents infection

____ 15. treats HSV-2

____ 16. treats lice

____ 17. treats mites

A. antipruritic
B. antiseptic
C. keratolytic
D. emollient
E. antiviral
F. scabicide
G. pediculicide

Case Study Continued

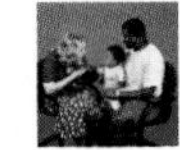
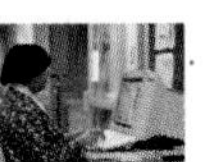

Ben's forearm was treated with Silvadene cream, an antibiotic, and covered with a loose dressing. His dad was advised to keep the burn covered with sterile bandages and to return in a week to have it checked.

Abbreviations

Abbreviation	*Meaning*	*Abbreviation*	*Meaning*
Bx	Biopsy	I&D	Incision and drainage
CCA	Certified coding associate	ID	Intradermal
CCS	Certified coding specialist	NKDA	No known drug allergy
CCS-P	Certified coding specialist—physician's office	OTC	Over the counter
CPC	Certified professional coder	PPD	Purified protein derivative
CPC-H	Certified professional coder—hospital	PUVA	Psoralen ultraviolet A
Decub	Pressure ulcer	RHIA	Registered health information administrator
DRG	Diagnosis-related group	RHIT	Registered health information technician
ED	Emergency department	SG	Skin graft
FB	Foreign body	SPF	Sun protection factor
H	Hypodermic	STSG	Split-thickness skin graft
HPV	Human papilloma virus	TB	Tuberculosis
HSV-1	Herpes simplex virus 1	TTS	Transdermal therapeutic system
HSV-2	Herpes simplex virus 2	Ung	Ointment
Hx	History	UV	Ultraviolet

Exercise 13: ABBREVIATIONS

Write the abbreviation for each of the following.

1. a route of administration within the dermis: ID
2. radiation from sunlight: UV
3. skin graft: SG
4. pressure ulcer: ____________
5. example of material removed from a wound during debridement: ____________
6. nonprescription: ____________
7. biopsy: Bx
8. history: Hx
9. patch to deliver medicine: TTS
10. ointment: UNG

Careers

Health Information Technicians

Projected to be one of the 20 fastest growing occupations by the U.S. Government Bureau of Labor Statistics, health information technician (HIT) is one of the few healthcare professions in which little or no physical contact with patients may be expected. The work environment is usually a pleasant, comfortable, "electronic" office setting, in which the technician organizes and evaluates patient records, ensuring that they remain complete and up-to-date. Employment opportunities are usually in hospitals, with an increasing number of openings in physician clinics/offices, nursing facilities, and home healthcare agencies.

Some HITs may choose to specialize in various areas of health information. In particular demand is the coder. These technicians assign a code to each diagnosis and procedure, using classification manuals via printed or electronic media. The classification of the codes, along with their placement into diagnosis-related groups (DRGs), determines the amount of reimbursement a hospital may expect to receive for patients covered by Medicare or other insurance programs that adhere to the DRG system.

HITs must have a strong knowledge of healthcare terminology, anatomy and physiology, disease process, coding procedures, statistics, supervision methods, and the legal aspects of maintaining healthcare records. A nationally recognized credential is available from the American Health Information Management Association (AHIMA) after successful completion of a program in health information technology and a passing score on the registered health information technician's (RHIT) examination.

If the student is interested in specializing in coding only, the AHIMA offers three separate credentials, the Certified Coding Associate (CCA), the Certified Coding Specialist (CCS), and Certified Coding Specialist–Physician's Office (CCS-P), which are attainable by sitting for a national examination. To be eligible, an applicant must have a high school diploma (from a U.S. high school) or its educational equivalent. AHIMA strongly recommends coding experience before attempting the examination.

Another organization that certifies coders is the American Academy of Professional Coders (AAPC). The two credentials that are offered are the Certified Professional Coder–Hospital (CPC-H) for facility coding and the Certified Professional Coder (CPC) for physician coding.

Those wishing to advance themselves through further study may pursue a bachelor's degree in Health Information Management and its credential of a Registered Health Information Administrator (RHIA), gained by sitting for its requisite examination.

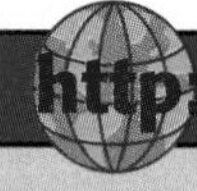

INTERNET PROJECT

Olivia Crawford, our TCS coder, found out about health information careers by searching online. She visited the Website for the U.S. Government's Bureau of Labor Statistics *Occupational Outlook Handbook.* Once there, she was able to investigate the current "hottest jobs" and "occupations with most job growth" under their Employment Projections section. After she had identified several professions that sounded interesting, she searched for more information under Professional and Related Occupations by choosing "health diagnosing and treating occupations" and "health technologists and technicians."

For the first part of this assignment, visit the Website at http://www.bls.gov/oco and choose "Employment Projections" to find either the five "hottest" jobs in healthcare or the five healthcare "occupations with most job growth" projected in the next few years. You will need to choose health-related careers from the list, as others will also appear.

The second part of the assignment is to choose a healthcare field from the Professional and Related Occupations menu and write a 4-page, double-spaced summary, including the following:

- Title of profession
- Nature of work
- Employment
- Training, other qualifications, and advancement
- Job outlook
- Earnings
- Related occupations
- Sources of additional information
- Contact information for the programs nearest to you. Include addresses, phone numbers, and names of program directors.

Chapter Review

A. Functions of the Integumentary System

1. In your own words, describe the functions of the integumentary system.

____

____

____

B. Anatomy and Physiology

2. Label the following diagram. pg 82

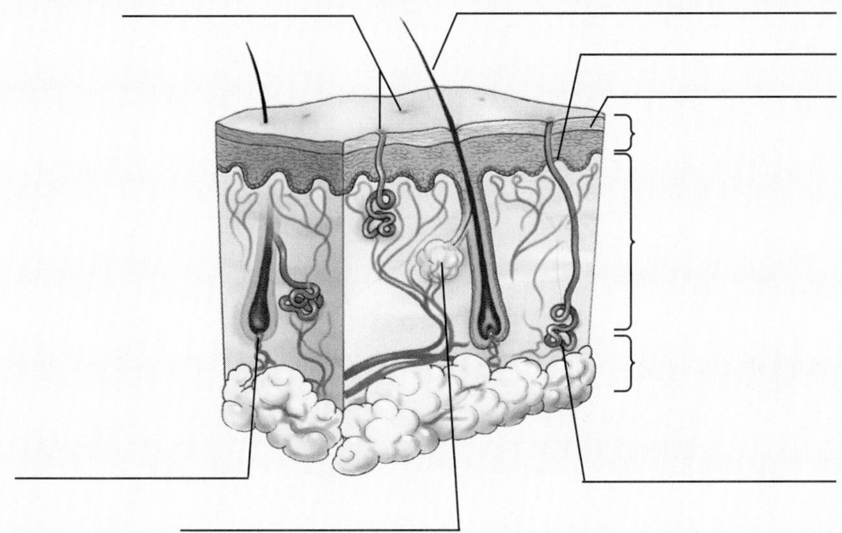

3. Fill in the combining forms for the following anatomic structures.

   A. skin ______________

   B. hair ______________

   C. nails ______________

   D. sudoriferous glands ______________

   E. oil (glands) ______________

   F. hair root and covering ______________

4. The term for the layers that compose the epidermis is STRATA.

5. The epidermis is the AVAScular layer, meaning that it does not have a rich blood supply.
6. The nerve endings, hair follicles, and sebaceous glands are located in the layer of the skin called the dermis or Corium.
7. Fatty tissue is stored in the adipose or the hypodermis layer.

C. Pathology

Decode the following terms.

8. dermatitis ____________________
9. folliculitis ____________________
10. onychomycosis ____________________
11. angioma Tumor of vessel
12. hyperhidrosis ____________________
13. hypertrichosis ____________________
14. seborrheic keratosis ____________________
15. lipoma ____________________
16. dysplastic nevus Mole
17. xeroderma ____________________
18. Define "lesion."

____

____

19. What is the difference between a primary and secondary lesion?

____

____

____

20. Define the following.

A. petechia ____________________

B. ecchymosis ____________________

C. purpura ____________________

D. hematoma ____________________

E. telangiectasia ____________________

Blood vessel disruption

21. What do the terms in Question 20 have in common?

____

22. Given the following examples, name the type of lesion:

A. 0.4-cm blister ________________

B. scab ________________

C. freckle ________________

E. scar ________________

E. bruise ________________

F. bedsore ________________

G. stria ________________

23. Jeremy presented with a localized suppurative staph infection in hair follicles on his neck. What type of infection did he have? ________________

24. Manuel developed athlete's foot after showering in his local gym without shower shoes. The healthcare term for athlete's foot is ________________.

25. Irene developed a yeast infection after she had been on a course of antibiotics. The healthcare term for one type of yeast infection is ________________.

26. Shri had to send home notices about a child who had lice in his classroom. The term for a lice infestation is pedi culosis.

27. A parasitic infection caused by mites is ________________.

28. Roseanne had verrucae on the plantar surface of her feet. Verrucae are WARTS.

29. Shingles is the common name for Herpis Zoster.

30. Roberta went to see her dermatologist because of thinning hair. She was diagnosed with ________________.

31. Extremely dry skin, named for its scaly appearance is called ________________.

32. What is the difference between a corn and a callus?

____

____

33. Give an example of hypopigmentation: ________________

34. Give an example of hyperpigmentation: ________________

35. What is eschar? Scar over a Burn

36. List the depth of skin or body tissue affected and the observable changes for each of the four degrees of burns listed.

    A. first degree ______________________________

    B. second degree ______________________________

    C. third degree ______________________________

    D. fourth degree ______________________________

D. Diagnostic Procedures

37. The entire tumor is removed in a/an _______________ biopsy.

38. Fluid from a lesion is aspirated to obtain samples for culture in a/an

    ______________________________ biopsy.

39. A wedge of tissue is removed and the incision is sutured in a/an _______________ biopsy.

40. Samples of friable lesions are scraped or shaved off in _______________.

41. A tubular punch is inserted into the subcutaneous tissue layer, and the tissue is cut off at the base in

    a/an _______________ biopsy.

42. A test to diagnose herpes zoster or herpes simplex is _______________.

43. Tinea capitis and pseudomonas infections are two disorders tested by

    ______________________________.

44. The Mantoux test is used to diagnose _______________.

45. A test for cystic fibrosis is the _______________ test.

46. Postoperative wound drainage would indicate the need for _______________ and _______________ cultures.

47. Vesicular fluid can be tested through a/an _______________ culture.

48. Impetigo is tested by a/an _______________ analysis.

49. Tinea pedis is tested by a/an _______________ test.

E. Therapeutic Interventions

50. Decode the following terms.

    A. dermatome ____

    B. dermatoplasty ____

    C. escharotomy ____

    D. cryosurgery ____

E. lipectomy ____

F. rhytidectomy ____

G. dermabrasion ____

51. Explain the differences among the following.

A. autograft ________________________

B. allograft ________________________

C. xenograft ________________________

52. The difference between cryosurgery and cauterization is that the first uses extreme ____________ to destroy tissue, whereas the latter uses ____________ to destroy tissue.

53. Differentiate among the following.

A. shaving ________________________

B. debridement ________________________

C. curettage ________________________

54. Covering a treated area with a nonporous dressing to increase absorption and effectiveness is ____________ therapy.

F. Pharmacology

55. Medications injected within the dermis are given by ____________ route.

56. Medications applied directly on the skin are given by ____________ route.

57. Essential oils used to treat disease are part of a discipline called ____________.

58. Aloe is a type of ____________ medicine.

59. Samantha applied a medication to reduce the pain and discomfort of her sunburn. It is classified as a/an ____________.

60. Keratolytics are designed to ________________________.

61. Dr. Wong prescribed a ____________ to treat a lice infestation.

62. Monica was prescribed a type of medication to lessen itching classified as ________________________

63. Topical substances that soften skin are ____________.

G. Abbreviations

Write out the abbreviations for the following questions.

64. If Paula had a Bx, she had a/an ____________.

65. An STSG means that someone has had a/an ____________.

66. NKDA in a patient's chart means that the patient has ________________.

67. A fever blister is caused by ________________.

68. I&D performed on a cyst is ________________ and ________________.
69. Darius had the abbreviation "Decub" recorded on his chart. What does that mean?

____

70. A patient's treatment includes TTS, which means ________________________________.

71. A type of light treatment for psoriasis is called ________________________________.

72. Past diseases and procedures would be mentioned in a patient's ________________.

H. Singulars and Plurals
Change the following singular terms to plural.

73. stria ________________________________

74. bulla ________________________________

75. onychomycosis ________________________________

76. decubitus ________________________________

77. ecchymosis ________________________________

78. petechia ________________________________

79. comedo ________________________________

80. verruca ________________________________

81. stratum ________________________________

I. Translations
Rewrite the following to explain the underlined terms.

82. The patient had a verruca on the plantar surface of his foot removed with cryosurgery.

____

____

83. The elderly patient developed a decubitus ulcer from lack of proper care during an extended hospital stay.

____

____

84. The patient bought a wig to cover her alopecia caused by trichotillomania.

____

____

85. Mr. Hassan complained of intense pruritus from urticaria.

____

____

86. The burn patient was in for an escharotomy and a consultation for a possible allograft.

____

____

J. Cumulative Review

Circle the correct answer.

87. The nails protect the *(proximal, dorsal)* surfaces of the fingers.
88. A first-degree burn is a *(superficial, deep)* burn.
89. The *cutane* in *subcutaneous* is a *(prefix, suffix, word root, combining form)*.
90. During debridement of a compound fracture, sequestrum was removed. What, in lay terms, was removed? _______________
91. Write the synonyms for the following terms.

    A. acrochordon _______________

    B. clavus _______________

    C. nevus _______________

    D. hirsutism _______________

    E. verruca _______________

    F. cicatrix _______________

    G. pressure sore _______________

K. Be Careful

Explain the difference between these paired terms.

92. hidro and hydro _______________
93. milia and miliaria _______________
94. stria and strata _______________
95. ID and I&D _______________
96. papillo and papulo _______________

Selvidge Memorial Hospital
17201 Northridge Drive
St. Paul, MN 55407

ED RECORD

Patient Name: Benjamin Warner
Allergies: NKDA

Physician Name: Dr. James
Med Report: #59776

Patient Complaint: Second-degree burns on forearm of African-American male, 11 months. Father states that child pulled hot coffee off table onto arm. Denies other injuries. + erythema, 3 cm bulla
Impression: 2-degree burn to right arm, 1%

Rx: Silvadene dressing, Children's Advil prn
Condition on Discharge: Stable

ICD-9-CM Codes Assigned:
943.21—Burn of forearm: blisters, epidermal loss (second degree)
948.00—Burns classified according to extent of body surface involved: less than 10% or unspecified
E924.0—Accident caused by hot substance or object, caustic or corrosive material, and steam; hot liquids and vapors, including steam

L. Healthcare Report

97. What type of burn is described?
    A. superficial
    B. partial thickness
    C. full thickness
98. What are the characteristics present that make this a second-degree burn?

    ____
99. E codes categorize the external cause of the injury. What did the E code describe in this case?

    ____
100. How big was the blister on the child's arm?

    ____

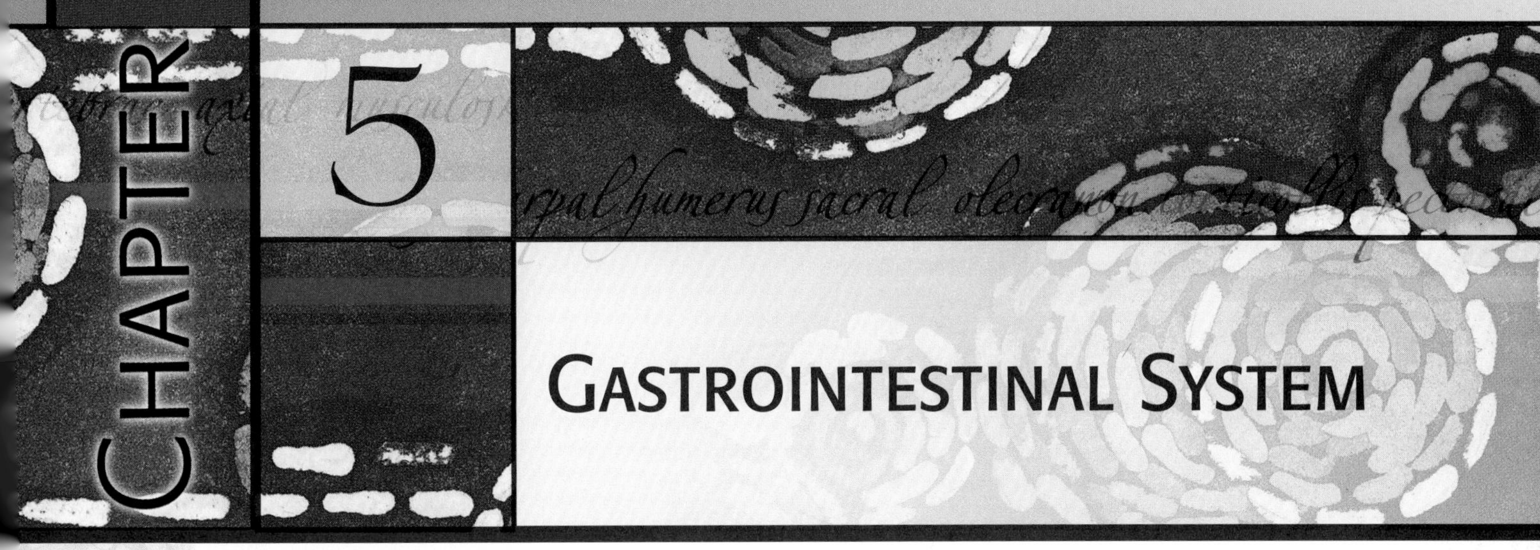

Chapter 5 Gastrointestinal System

"Good health is a serious business. Like life itself, it has to be worked at and it takes on added meaning with effort." **—Norman Cousins**

Quote

Case Study

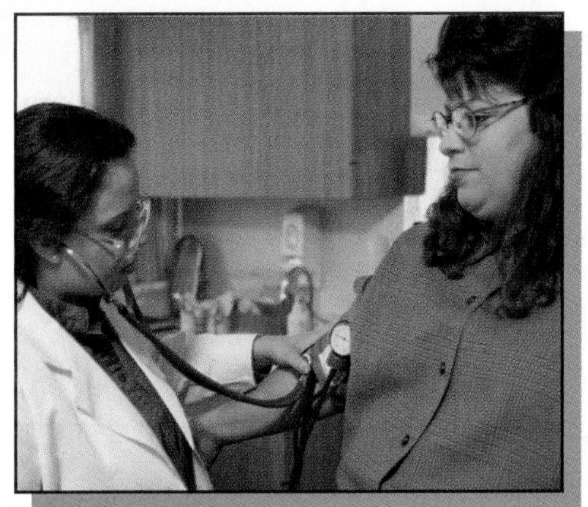

For the past 2 weeks, every time Mariah Hopkins has eaten a heavy meal she has had upper right quadrant (URQ) pain and occasional nausea and vomiting. The pain would last for a couple of hours and then subside. However, after a night of unremitting pain, Mariah can stand it no longer and calls her physician. He does a quick examination at his office and, suspecting cholelithiasis, sends her to the local hospital for immediate testing and admission. Elena Sanchez, one of the medical-surgical nurses on the floor that afternoon, helps Mariah get settled for her admission and notices that the patient's skin has a yellowish hue.

OBJECTIVES

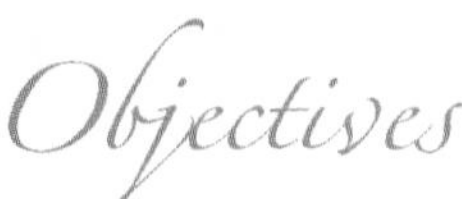

- In your own words, explain the functions of the gastrointestinal system.
- Recognize, recall, and apply healthcare terms related to the anatomy and physiology of the gastrointestinal system.
- Recognize, recall, and apply healthcare terms related to the pathology of the gastrointestinal system.
- Recognize, recall, and apply healthcare terms related to the diagnostic procedures introduced in this chapter.
- Recognize, recall, and apply healthcare terms related to therapeutic interventions of the gastrointestinal system.
- Recognize, recall, and apply the pharmacology introduced in this chapter.
- Recognize, recall, and apply the abbreviations introduced in this chapter.
- Recognize and recall all word components used in this chapter to build and decode healthcare terms relevant to the gastrointestinal system.
- Demonstrate the ability to change terms from singular gastrointestinal terms to plural forms.
- Recognize, recall, and apply material learned in previous chapters.

FUNCTIONS OF THE GASTROINTESTINAL SYSTEM

The digestive system (Fig. 5-1) provides the nutrients needed for cells to replicate themselves continually and build new tissue. This is done through several distinct processes: **ingestion**, the intake of food; **digestion**, the breakdown of food; **absorption**, the process of extracting nutrients; and **elimination**, the excretion of any waste products. Other names for the system are the **gastrointestinal (GI) tract**, which refers to the two main parts of the system, and the **alimentary** (al ih MEN tair ee) **canal**, which refers to the tubelike nature of the digestive system, starting at the mouth and continuing in varying diameters to the anus.

The healthcare term for the process of chewing is **mastication** (mass tih KAY shun); the term for swallowing is **deglutition** (deh gloo TIH shun). The wavelike movement that propels food through the alimentary canal is known as **peristalsis** (pair ih STALL sis). The combining form *phag/o* means *to eat* or *to swallow;* hence, difficulty with deglutition could be termed **dysphagia** (dis FAY zsa). The term **hyperalimentation** (hye pur al ih men TAY shun) refers to the process of taking in more nutrients than the body optimally needs.

DID YOU KNOW?

The alimentary canal acquires its name from the Latin term *alimentum,* which refers to food or nourishment. Its influence is currently seen in contemporary words such as *adult,* meaning *grown up or nourished, alimony,* meaning *an allowance for sustenance,* and *alma mater,* meaning *a nourishing mother.*

COMBINING FORMS FOR THE DIGESTIVE SYSTEM

MEANING	COMBINING FORM
eat or swallow	phag/o
intestines	intestin/o
nutrition	aliment/o
stomach	gastr/o

PREFIXES AND SUFFIXES FOR THE DIGESTIVE SYSTEM

PREFIX/SUFFIX	MEANING
dys-	difficult
hyper-	excessive
peri-	surrounding
-stalsis	contraction

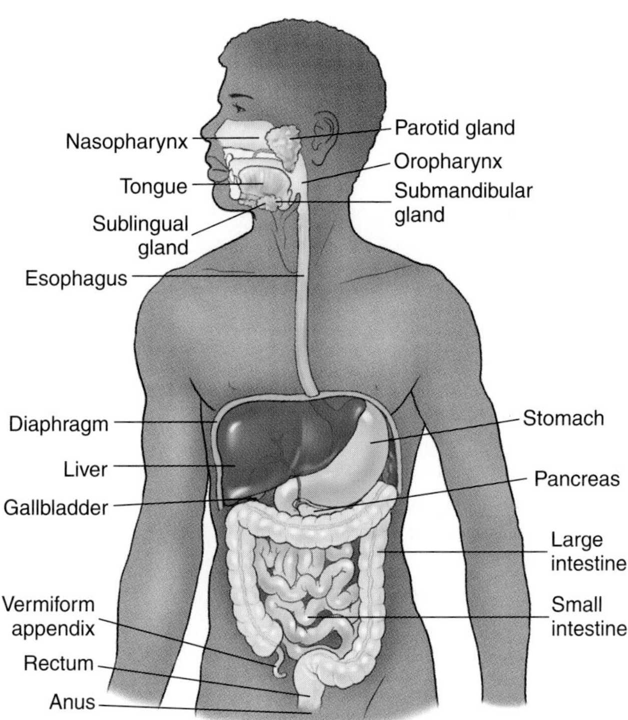

Fig. 5-1 The gastrointestinal system.

Exercise 1: FUNCTIONS OF THE DIGESTIVE SYSTEM

Fill in the blanks.

1. Alternative terms for the digestive system are the __________ canal and __________ system.
2. The digestive system provides __________ needed for __________ to replicate themselves and build new tissue.

Identify the GI function described using one of the following terms.

absorption, ingestion, elimination, digestion

3. If the body were not able to break down food, mechanically or chemically, it would not be able to accomplish which process of the GI system? __________
4. Problems with taking nutrients into the body's cells *after* food has been broken down within the digestive tract have to do with the process of __________.
5. A patient who has difficulty getting rid of the waste products of the digestive process has problems with which function of the GI system? __________
6. The process of taking in food is called __________.

Matching.

C 7. deglutition

D 8. peristalsis

F 9. dysphagia

B 10. alimentary canal

A 11. mastication

E 12. hyperalimentation

A. process of chewing
B. GI tract
C. process of swallowing
D. wavelike movement through the GI system
E. excessive nutrient intake
F. difficulty swallowing

ANATOMY AND PHYSIOLOGY

Oral Cavity

Food normally enters the body through the mouth, or **oral cavity** (Fig. 5-2, *A*). The function of this cavity is initially to break down the food mechanically by chewing (mastication) and lubricate the food to ease in swallowing (deglutition).

The oral cavity begins at the **lips**, the two fleshy structures surrounding its opening. The inside of the mouth is bounded by the **cheeks**, the **tongue** at the floor, and an anterior **hard palate** (PAL it) and posterior **soft palate**, which form the roof. The upper and lower jaws hold 32 permanent **teeth** that are set in the flesh of the **gums.** The **uvula** (YOO vyoo lah) is the tag of flesh that hangs down from the medial surface of the soft palate. The three pairs of **salivary** (SAL ih vair ee) **glands** provide **saliva**, a substance that moistens the oral cavity, initiates the digestion of starches, and aids in chewing and swallowing. The glands are named for their locations: **parotid** (pair AH tid), near the ear; **submandibular** (sub man DIB yoo lur), under the lower jaw; and **sublingual** (sub LEENG gwul), under the tongue.

Throat

The throat, or **pharynx** (FAIR inks), is a tube that connects the oral cavity with the esophagus. It can be divided into three main parts: the nasopharynx, the oropharynx, and the hypopharynx. The **nasopharynx** (nay soh FAIR inks) is the most superior part of the pharynx, located behind the nasal cavity. The **oropharynx** (oh roh FAIR inks) is the part of the throat directly adjacent to the oral cavity, and the **hypopharynx** (hye poh FAIR inks) is the part of the throat directly below the oropharynx (Fig. 5-2, *B*).

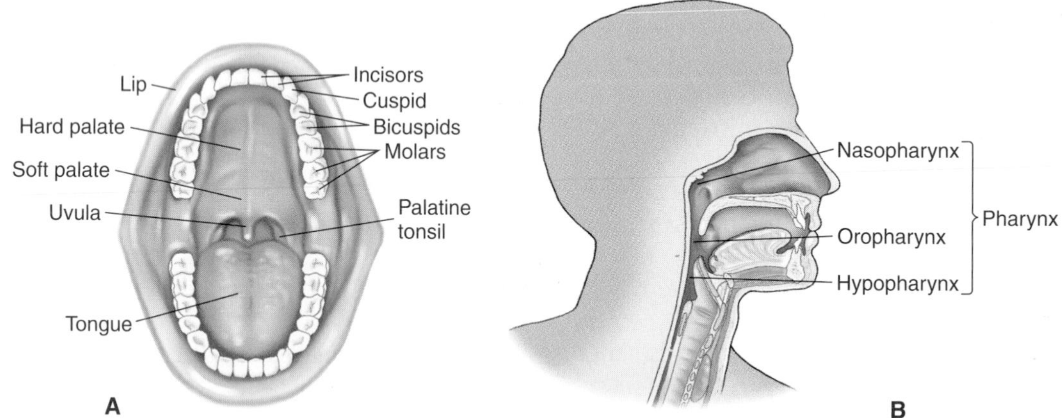

Fig. 5-2 **A**, The oral cavity. **B**, The pharynx.

Esophagus

The **esophagus** (eh SAH fah gus) is a muscular, mucus-lined tube that extends from the throat to the stomach. It carries a masticated lump of food, a **bolus** (BOH lus), from the oral cavity to the stomach by means of peristalsis. The glands in the lining of the esophagus produce mucus, which aids in lubricating and easing the passage of the bolus to the stomach. The muscle that must relax before the food enters the stomach is known by three names: the **lower esophageal** (eh sah fah JEE ul) **sphincter** (SFINK tur) **(LES)**, the **gastroesophageal sphincter**, or the **cardiac sphincter**, which gets its name because of its proximity to the heart.

> **DID YOU KNOW?**
>
> A **sphincter** is a ringlike muscle; sphincters appear in other parts of the body as well, for example, in the urinary system and the eye.

COMBINING FORMS FOR THE ORAL CAVITY, THROAT, AND ESOPHAGUS

MEANING	COMBINING FORM	MEANING	COMBINING FORM
cheek	bucc/o	nose	nas/o
ear	ot/o	oral cavity	or/o
esophagus	esophag/o	pharynx	pharyng/o
gums	gingiv/o	saliva	sial/o
hard and soft palates	palat/o	salivary glands	sialaden/o
heart	cardi/o	teeth	dent/i, odont/o
jaw bone (lower)	mandibul/o	throat	pharyng/o
jaw bone (upper)	maxill/o	tongue	lingu/o, gloss/o
lips	labi/o, cheil/o	uvula	uvul/o
mouth	or/o, stom/o, stomat/o		

PREFIXES FOR ANATOMY AND PHYSIOLOGY

PREFIX	MEANING
hypo-	below
par-	near, beside
sub-	below

Exercise 2: ORAL CAVITY, THROAT, AND ESOPHAGUS

Match the combining forms with the following definitions. There may be more than one combining form for a given definition.

____ 1. teeth	____ 7. cheek	A. esophag/o	I. gloss/o
____ 2. gums	____ 8. salivary gland	B. bucc/o	J. sial/o
____ 3. roof of mouth	____ 9. saliva	C. cheil/o	K. stomat/o
____ 4. tongue	____ 10. uvula	D. or/o	L. pharyng/o
____ 5. mouth	____ 11. throat	E. lingu/o	M. dent/i, odont/o
____ 6. lips	____ 12. esophagus	F. palat/o	N. uvul/o
		G. labi/o	O. sialaden/o
		H. gingiv/o	

Fill in the blanks with the following choices.

sphincter, esophagus, hypopharynx, bolus, nasopharynx, oropharynx, pharynx

13. What is the general term for the throat? ____________________
14. What is the term for the part of the throat that is behind the mouth?

____

15. What is the part of the throat that is behind the nasal cavity? ____________________
16. What is the name for the section of the throat that is *below* the oral cavity?

____

17. What is the name of the tube that extends from the throat to the stomach?

____

18. What is the term for a ringlike muscle? ____________________

19. What is the name for a chewed mass of food that is swallowed? ____________________

Name the salivary gland.

20. The one that is "near the ear": ____________________

21. The one that is "under the tongue": ____________________

22. The one that is "under the lower jaw bone": ____________________

List the three names for the ringlike muscle between the esophagus and the stomach.

23. ________________ 24. ________________ 25. ________________

Stomach

DID YOU KNOW?

The suffix *-ase* is used to form the name of an enzyme. It is added to the name of the substance upon which the enzyme acts: for example, *lipase,* which acts on lipids, or *amylase,* which acts on starches. *-ose* is a chemical suffix indicating that a substance is a carbohydrate, such as *glucose.*

The stomach, an expandable vessel, is divided into three sections: the **fundus** (FUN dus), the **body**, and the **pylorus** (pye LORE us) (Fig. 5-3). The portion of the stomach that surrounds the esophagogastric connection is the fundus (*pl.* fundi), which is also referred to as the **cardia** (KAR dee ah). This section of the stomach has no acid-producing cells, unlike the remainder of the stomach. The body is the central part of the stomach, and the pylorus (*pl.* pylori) is at the distal end of the stomach, where the small intestine begins. A small muscle, the **pyloric sphincter,** regulates the gentle release of food from the stomach into the small intestine. When the stomach is empty, it has an appearance of being lined with many ridges. These ridges, or wrinkles, are called **rugae** (ROO jee) (*sing.* ruga).

The function of the stomach is to store temporarily the chewed food that it receives from the esophagus. This food is mixed with gastric juices and hydrochloric acid to further the digestive process chemically. This mixture is called **chyme** (kyme). The smooth muscles of the stomach contract to aid in the mechanical digestion of the food. A continual coating of mucus protects the stomach, as well as the rest of the digestive system, from the acidic nature of the gastric juices.

Small Intestine

Once the chyme has been formed in the stomach, the pyloric sphincter relaxes a bit at a time to release portions of it into the first part of the **small intestine,** called the **duodenum** (doo AH deh num). The small intestine gets its name, not because of its length (it is about 20 feet long), but because of the diameter of its **lumen**

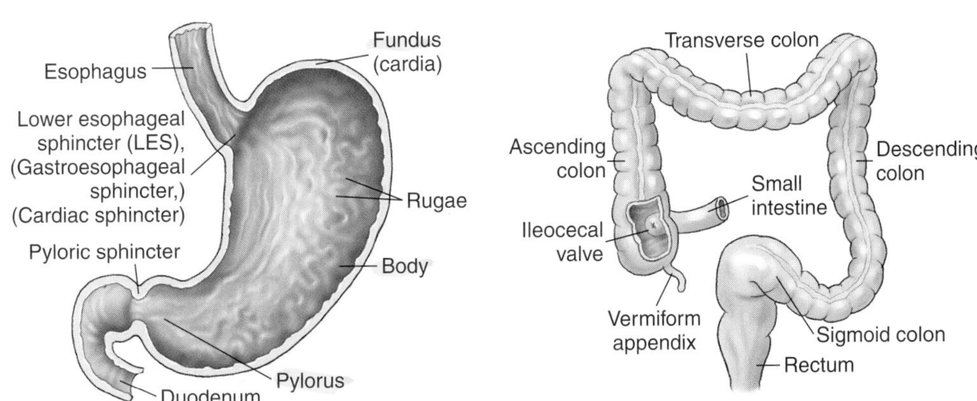

Fig. 5-3 The stomach.

Fig. 5-4 The large intestine (colon).

(LOO mun) (a tubular cavity within the body). The remaining two sections of the small intestine are the **jejunum** (jeh JOO num) and **ileum** (ILL ee um).

Multiple circular folds in the small intestines, called **plicae** (PLY see), contain thousands of tiny projections called **villi** (VILL eye) (*sing.* villus), which contain blood capillaries that absorb the products of carbohydrate and protein digestion. The villi also contain lymphatic vessels known as **lacteals** (LACK tee uls) that absorb **lipid** (LIH pid) substances from the chyme.

Large Intestine

In contrast to the small intestine, the **large intestine** (Fig. 5-4) is only about 5 feet long, but it is much wider in diameter. The primary function of the large intestine is the elimination of the waste products from the body. Some synthesis of vitamins occurs in the large intestine, but unlike the small intestine, the large intestine has no villi and is not well suited for absorption. The **ileocecal** (ILL ee oh SEE kul) valve is the exit from the small intestine and entrance to the colon. The first part of the large intestine, the **cecum** (SEE kum), has a wormlike appendage, called the **vermiform appendix** (VUR mih form ah PEN dicks) dangling from it. Although this organ does not seem to have any direct function related to the digestive system, it is thought to have a possible immunologic defense mechanism.

No longer called chyme, whatever has not been absorbed by the small intestines is now called **feces** (FEE sees). The feces pass from the cecum to the **ascending colon** (KOH lin), through the **transverse colon**, the **descending colon**, the **sigmoid colon**, and on to the **rectum**, where they are held until released from the body completely, through the anal sphincter. The process of releasing feces from the body is called **defecation.**

BE CAREFUL!

Don't confuse the term *ilium,* meaning *part of the hip bone,* with *ileum,* meaning *part of the small intestine.*

BE CAREFUL!

The combining form *gastr/o* refers only to the *stomach.* The combining forms *abdomin/o, lapar/o,* and *celi/o* refer to the *abdomen.*

BE CAREFUL!

Do not confuse *-cele,* the suffix meaning *herniation,* with *celi/o,* the combining form for *abdomen.*

BE CAREFUL!

Do not confuse *an/o,* the combining form for *anus; ana-,* the prefix meaning *up* or *apart;* and *an-,* the prefix meaning *no* or *not.*

COMBINING FORMS FOR THE STOMACH AND INTESTINES

MEANING	COMBINING FORM	MEANING	COMBINING FORM
abdomen	abdomin/o, celi/o, lapar/o	jejunum	jejun/o
anus	an/o	lipid (fat)	lip/o
appendix	append/o, appendic/o	rectum	rect/o
cecum	cec/o	rectum and anus	proct/o
colon	col/o, colon/o	sigmoid colon	sigmoid/o
fold	plic/o	small intestines	enter/o
stomach	gastr/o	starch	amyl/o
ileum	ile/o	sweet, sugar	gluc/o

Exercise 3: THE STOMACH, SMALL INTESTINE, AND LARGE INTESTINE

Match the following combining forms and body parts with their terms.

____ 1. fat
____ 2. folds
____ 3. colon
____ 4. jejunum
____ 5. ileum
____ 6. starch
____ 7. rectum
____ 8. anus
____ 9. sugar
____ 10. duodenum
____ 11. stomach
____ 12. cecum
____ 13. sigmoid colon
____ 14. tubular cavity
____ 15. enter/o
____ 16. pylorus
____ 17. rectum and anus
____ 18. appendic/o, append/o

A. proct/o
B. first part of large intestines
C. structure hanging from cecum
D. small intestines
E. lumen
F. gluc/o
G. gastr/o
H. second part of small intestines
I. amyl/o
J. lip/o
K. plicae
L. first part of small intestines
M. muscle between stomach and first part of small intestines
N. last straight part of colon
O. large intestines
P. distal part of small intestines
R. final sphincter in GI tract
S. S-shaped part of large intestines

19. Place the following terms in anatomic order, starting with the small muscle between the stomach and the first part of the small intestine and going down the body.

descending colon, rectum, ileum, duodenum, pyloric sphincter, cecum and appendix, ileocecal valve, sigmoid colon, anal sphincter, transverse colon, ascending colon, jejunum

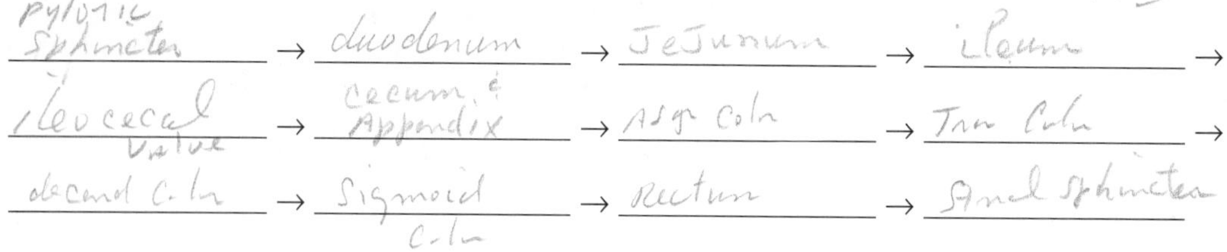

Circle the correct answer.

20. When chewed food is mixed with gastric juices and hydrochloric acid in the stomach, it becomes *(rugae, chyme)*. When this mixture enters the large intestine, it becomes *(urine, feces)*.
21. The villi and plicae are structures that serve to *(absorb nutrients, form waste products)*.
22. In which intestine are the majority of nutrients absorbed? *(large, small)*

Accessory Organs (Adnexa)

The accessory organs are the gallbladder, liver, and pancreas (Fig. 5-5). These organs secrete fluid into the GI tract but are not a direct part of the tube itself. Sometimes, these structures are referred to as **adnexa** (ad NECK sah).

The two lobes that form the **liver** (LIH vur) virtually fill the right upper quadrant of the abdomen and extend partially into the left upper quadrant. The liver forms a substance called **bile**, which **emulsifies** (ee MUL sih fyez), or mechanically breaks down, fats into smaller portions so that they can be chemically digested. Bile is composed of **bilirubin** (BILL ee ROO bin), the waste product formed by the normal breakdown of hemoglobin in red blood cells at the end of their life spans, and **cholesterol** (koh LESS tur all), a fatty substance found only in animal tissues. **Bile ducts** in the liver merge into the **hepatic** (heh PAT ick)

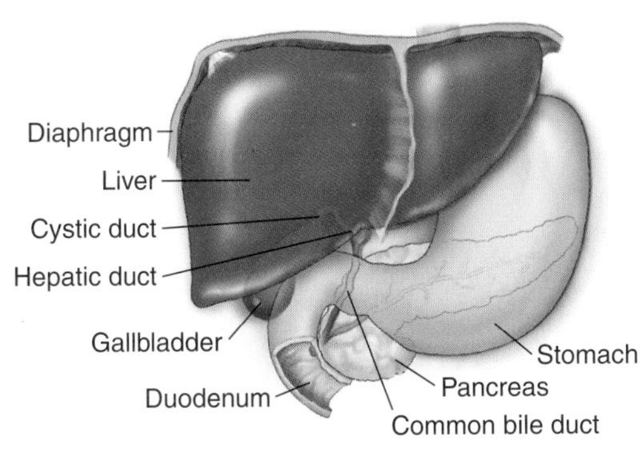

Fig. 5-5 Accessory organs.

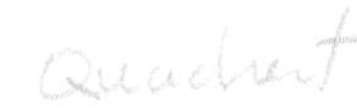

duct, which carries the bile out of the liver. The hepatic duct joins with the **cystic** (SISS tick) **duct** of the gallbladder, forming the **common bile duct**, which carries the bile to the duodenum. The bile is stored in the **gallbladder** (GALL blad ur), a small sac found on the underside of the right lobe of the liver. When fatty food enters the duodenum, a hormone called **cholecystokinin** (koh lee sis toh KYE nin) is secreted, causing a contraction of the gallbladder to move bile out into the cystic duct, then the common bile duct, and finally into the duodenum.

The **pancreas** (PAN kree us) is a gland located in the upper left quadrant. It is involved in the digestion of the three types of food molecules: carbohydrates, proteins, and lipids. The pancreatic enzymes are carried through the pancreatic duct that empties into the common bile duct. Pancreatic involvement in the food digestion is an **exocrine** (ECK soh krin) function. Pancreatic **endocrine** (EN doh krin) functions are discussed in Chapter 15.

COMBINING FORMS FOR THE ACCESSORY ORGANS

MEANING	COMBINING FORM	MEANING	COMBINING FORM
bile	chol/e, bil/i	liver	hepat/o
bile vessels	cholangi/o	lobe	lob/o
common bile duct	choledoch/o	pancreas	pancreat/o
gallbladder	cholecyst/o		

Exercise 4: ACCESSORY ORGANS

Match the combining forms with their terms.

G 1. pancreas
D 2. gallbladder
A 3. lobe
C 4. liver
B 5. bile
E 6. bile vessels
F 7. common bile duct

A. lob/o
B. chol/e, bil/i
C. hepat/o
D. cholecyst/o
E. cholangi/o
F. choledoch/o
G. pancreat/o

8. Name the quadrants in which each of the accessory organs is located.

   A. liver ______________________

   B. gallbladder ______________________

   C. pancreas ______________________

Fill in the blanks using the following terms.

emulsification, bilirubin, cholesterol, cholecystokinin, adnexa

9. Another word for GI accessory structures: ______________________

10. The process of breaking down fats into smaller portions: ______________________

11. The hormone that causes a contraction of the gallbladder to release bile:

    ____

12. The waste product left over from breakdown of red blood cells: ______________________

13. A fatty substance found in animal tissues: ______________________

Case Study Continued

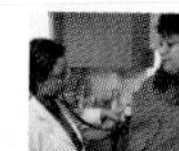

After recording Mariah's vital signs (pulse, blood pressure, respirations, and temperature), Elena observes that Mariah flinches as her upper abdomen is gently palpated. Mariah tells her that she had been eating pizza at her daughter's birthday party the night before and that the pain, now severe, is localized on her right side and has been accompanied by vomiting. On the patient's chart, Elena notes significant tenderness and a palpable gallbladder in the right hypochondrium. She also records a mildly elevated temperature. Mariah's doctor stops by her room to let her know that he has ordered blood and urine tests, along with imaging studies. He tells her that if what he suspects is true, she will be having surgery to remove her gallbladder.

PATHOLOGY

DID YOU KNOW?

Remember what onomatopoeia is? It means words like "pop" or "fizz" that imitate sounds. The term *hiccup* is a healthcare example of a word that was created to imitate the sound of the act.

DID YOU KNOW?

Nausea derives its name from the Greek word for seasickness. Notice the similarity between the words *nausea* and *nautical.*

DID YOU KNOW?

Heartburn is a misnomer, although an understandable one. When one experiences this burning sensation, it is in the chest area near the heart.

Terms Related to Upper Gastrointestinal Complaints

TERM	WORD ORIGIN	DEFINITION
Dyspepsia dis PEP see ah	*dys-* abnormal, bad *-pepsia* digestion	Feeling of epigastric discomfort that occurs shortly after eating. The discomfort may range from a feeling of nausea, fullness, heartburn, and/or bloating. Also called **indigestion.**
Eructation ee ruck TAY shun		Release of air from the stomach through the mouth. Eructation may be caused by rapid eating or intentionally or unintentionally swallowing air **(aerophagia).** Also called **burping** or **belching.**
Halitosis hal ih TOH sis	*halit/o* breath *-osis* abnormal condition	Bad-smelling breath.
Heartburn	See **Did You Know?** box	Painful burning sensation in esophagus usually caused by reflux of stomach contents, hyperactivity, or peptic ulcer. Also known as **pyrosis** (pye ROH sis).
Hiccup HICK up	See **Did You Know?** box	Involuntary contraction of the diaphragm, followed by a rapid closure of the glottis (which in turn causes the characteristic sound of a hiccup). Also known as **hiccough** or **singultus.**
Nausea NAH see ah	See **Did You Know?** box	Sensation that accompanies the urge to vomit but does not always lead to vomiting.
Regurgitation ree gur jih TAY shun		Return of swallowed food to the mouth. Regurgitation may, however, describe any backwards flow in the body, not just that of a GI nature.
Vomiting VAH mih ting		Forcible or involuntary emptying of the stomach through the mouth. The material expelled is called **vomitus** or **emesis.** The vomiting of blood is called **hematemesis** (hee mah TEM eh sis).

Terms Related to Lower Gastrointestinal Complaints

TERM	WORD ORIGIN	DEFINITION
Constipation kon stih PAY shun		Infrequent, incomplete, or delayed bowel movements.
Diarrhea dye ah REE ah	*dia-* through, complete *-rrhea* discharge, flow	Abnormal discharge of watery, semisolid stools.
Flatus FLAY tus		Gas expelled through the anus.
Hematochezia hee mat oh KEE zee ah	*hemat/o* blood *-chezia* condition of stools	Bright red, frank lower GI bleeding from the rectum that may originate in the distal colon. Passage of bloody stools.
Irritable bowel syndrome (IBS)		Abnormal increase in the activity of the small and large intestines, leading to diarrhea and flatus.
Melena mah LEE nah	*melan/o* black, dark	Black, tarry stools caused by the presence of partially digested blood.
Obstipation ob stih PAY shun		Extreme constipation, intestinal obstruction.

Exercise 5: Upper and Lower GI Complaints

Matching.

_____ 1. diarrhea

_____ 2. obstipation

_____ 3. flatus

_____ 4. melena

_____ 5. halitosis

_____ 6. IBS

_____ 7. constipation

_____ 8. nausea

_____ 9. hematochezia

_____ 10. regurgitation

A. bloody stools
B. bad breath
C. delayed defecation
D. feeling of need to vomit
E. gas passed through the anus
F. backward flow
G. black, tarry stools
H. loose, watery stools
I. extremely delayed defecation
J. diarrhea/gas/constipation resulting from stress with no underlying disease

Match the synonyms.

_____ 11. indigestion

_____ 12. singultus

_____ 13. pyrosis

_____ 14. eructation

_____ 15. emesis

A. vomit
B. hiccup
C. burping
D. dyspepsia
E. heartburn

Terms Related to Congenital Disorders		
Term	**Word Origin**	**Definition**
Cleft palate kleft PAL it		Failure of the palate to close during embryonic development, creating an opening in the roof of the mouth. Cleft palate is often accompanied by a cleft lip (Fig. 5-6).
Esophageal atresia eh soff uh JEE ul ah TREE zsa	***esophag/o*** esophagus ***-eal*** pertaining to ***a-*** not, without ***-tresia*** condition of an opening	Esophagus that ends in a blind pouch and therefore lacks an opening into the stomach.
Hirschsprung's disease HERSH sprungs		Congenital absence of normal nervous function in part of the colon, which results in an absence of peristaltic movement, accumulation of feces, and an enlarged colon. Also called **congenital megacolon.**
Pyloric stenosis pye LORE ick sten OH sis	***pylor/o*** pylorus ***-ic*** pertaining to ***-stenosis*** abnormal condition of narrowing	Condition in which the muscle between the stomach and the small intestine narrows or fails to open adequately to allow partially digested food into the duodenum.

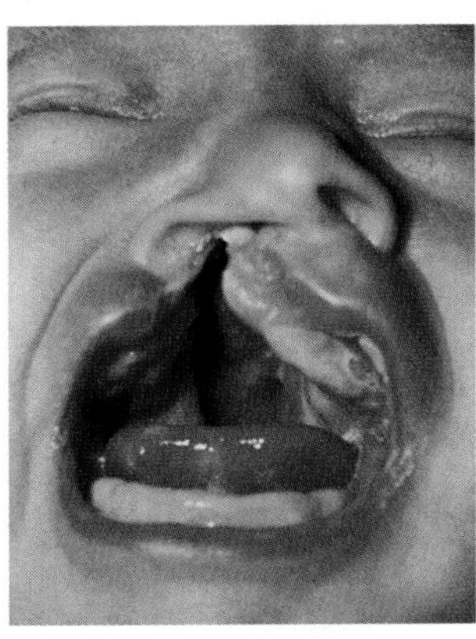

Fig. 5-6 Cleft palate and cleft lip.

Exercise 6: CONGENITAL DISORDERS

Fill in the blank with the correct term.

pyloric stenosis, cleft palate, esophageal atresia, Hirschsprung's disease, congenital megacolon

1. The term that refers to the lack of an opening between the tube that extends from the throat to the stomach is ______________________.
2. A congenital fissure in the roof of the mouth is called ______________________.
3. If the patient has a lack of normal nervous function in part of the large intestine, which results in an accumulation of feces, he or she may be diagnosed with ______________________.
4. Another name for the answer to question 3 is ______________________.
5. A narrowing of the muscle between the stomach and the duodenum is called ______________________.

Terms Related to Oral Cavity Disorders

TERM	WORD ORIGIN	DEFINITION
Aphthous stomatitis AFF thus stoh mah TYE tis	*aphth/o* ulceration *-ous* pertaining to *stomat/o* mouth *-itis* inflammation	Recurring condition characterized by small erosions (ulcers), which appear on the mucous membranes of the mouth. Also called a **canker sore.**
Cheilitis kye LYE tis	*cheil/o* lip *-itis* inflammation	Inflammation of the lips.
Cheilosis kye LOH sis	*cheil/o* lip *-osis* abnormal condition	Abnormal condition of the lips present in riboflavin (a B vitamin) deficiency.
Dental caries KARE ees	*dent/i* teeth *-al* pertaining to	Plaque disease caused by an interaction between food and bacteria in the mouth, leading to tooth decay. Also called **cavities.**
Dental plaque plack		Film of material that coats the teeth and may lead to dental decay if not removed.
Gingivitis jin jih VYE tis	*gingiv/o* gums *-itis* inflammation	Inflammatory disease of the gums characterized by redness, swelling, and bleeding (Fig. 5-7).

Continued

Terms Related to Oral Cavity Disorders—cont'd		
TERM	**WORD ORIGIN**	**DEFINITION**
Herpetic stomatitis hur PET ick stoh mah TYE tis	*stomat/o* mouth *-itis* inflammation	Inflammation of the mouth caused by the herpes simplex virus (HSV). Also known as a **cold sore** or **fever blister.**
Leukoplakia loo koh PLAY kee ah	*leuk/o* white *-plakia* condition	Condition of white patches that may appear on the lips and buccal mucosa (Fig. 5-8). It is usually associated with tobacco use and may be precancerous.
Malocclusion mal oh KLOO zhun	*mal-* bad, poor *-occlusion* condition of closure	Condition in which the teeth do not touch properly when the mouth is closed (abnormal bite).
Periodontal disease pair ee oh DON tul	*peri-* surrounding *odont/o* tooth *-al* pertaining to	Pathologic condition of the tissues surrounding the teeth.
Pyorrhea pye or REE yah	*py/o* pus *-rrhea* flow, discharge	Purulent discharge from the tissue surrounding the teeth; often seen with gingivitis.

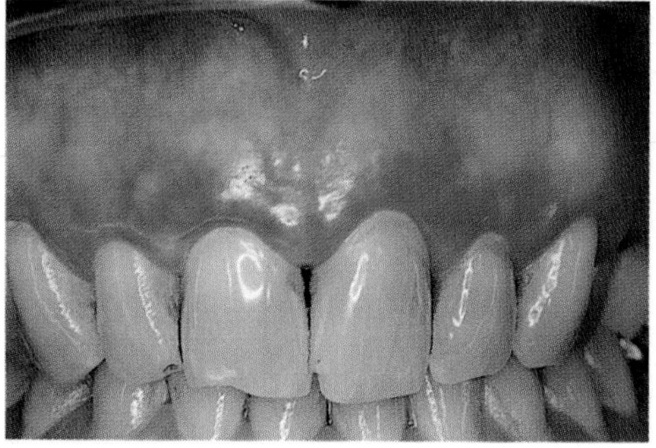

Fig. 5-7 Gingivitis.

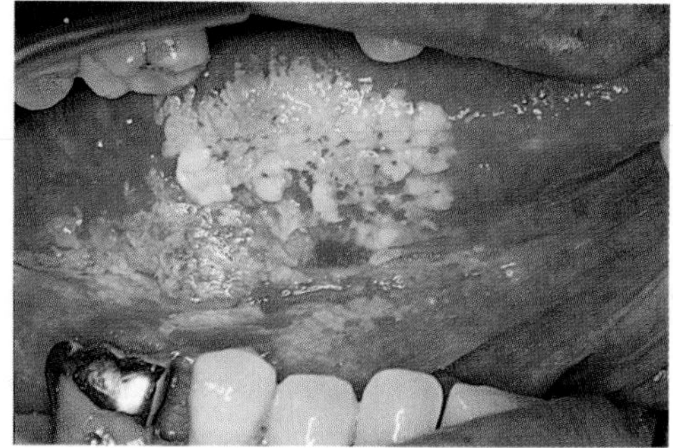

Fig. 5-8 Leukoplakia.

Exercise 7: ORAL CAVITY DISORDERS

Matching.

____ 1. dental caries

____ 2. gingivitis

____ 3. cheilitis

____ 4. cheilosis

____ 5. aphthous stomatitis

____ 6. herpetic stomatitis

____ 7. dental plaque

____ 8. leukoplakia

____ 9. malocclusion

____ 10. periodontal disease

A. tooth decay
B. disorder of tissue surrounding teeth
C. abnormal bite
D. canker sore
E. inflammation of the lips
F. inflammation of the gums
G. cold sore
H. abnormal condition of lips
I. material that coats teeth
J. white patches

Terms Related to Disorders of the Esophagus

TERM	WORD ORIGIN	DEFINITION
Achalasia ack uh LAY zsa	*a-* not, without *-chalasia* condition of relaxation	Impairment of esophageal peristalsis along with the lower esophageal sphincter's inability to relax. Also called **cardiospasm, esophageal aperistalsis** (ay per rih STALL sis), and **megaesophagus.**
Dysphagia dis FAY zsa	*dys-* bad, difficult *-phagia* condition of swallowing, eating	Difficulty with swallowing that may be due to an obstruction (e.g., a tumor) or a motor disorder (e.g., a spasm).
Gastroesophageal reflux disease (GERD) gass troh eh sah fah JEE ul	*gastr/o* stomach *esophag/o* esophagus *-eal* pertaining to *re-* back *-flux* flow	Flowing back, or return, of the contents of the stomach to the esophagus caused by an inability of the lower esophageal sphincter (LES) to contract normally; characterized by pyrosis with or without regurgitation of stomach contents to the mouth (Fig. 5-9).

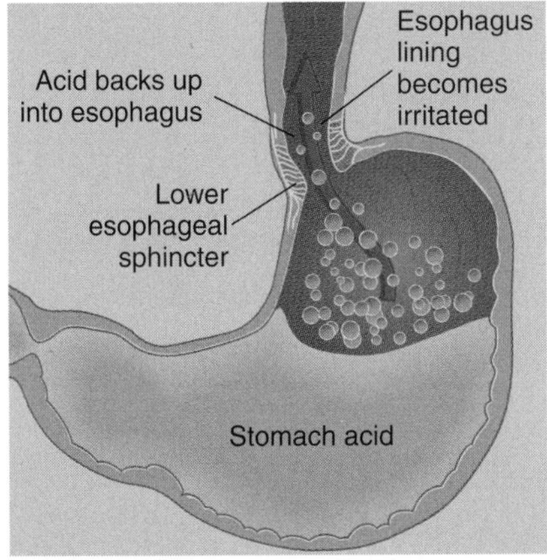

Fig. 5-9 GERD.

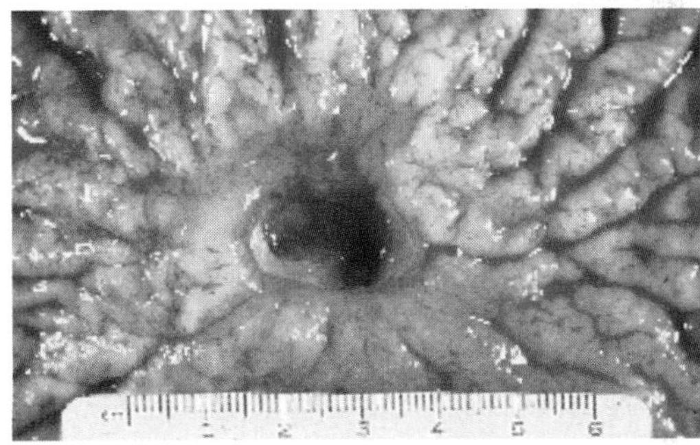

Fig. 5-10 Chronic peptic ulcer.

Terms Related to Disorders of the Stomach

TERM	WORD ORIGIN	DEFINITION
Gastralgia gass TRAL zsa	*gastr/o* stomach *-algia* pain	Gastric pain. Also called **gastrodynia** (gass troh DIH nee ah).
Gastritis gass TRY tis	*gastr/o* stomach *-itis* inflammation	Acute or chronic inflammation of the stomach that may be accompanied by anorexia, nausea and vomiting (N&V), or indigestion.
Peptic ulcer disease (PUD)		An erosion of the protective mucosal lining of the stomach or duodenum (Fig. 5-10). Also called a **gastric ulcer.**

Exercise 8: ESOPHAGEAL AND STOMACH DISORDERS

Matching. More than one answer may be correct.

____ 1. PUD
____ 2. gastralgia
____ 3. gastritis
____ 4. achalasia
____ 5. dysphagia
____ 6. GERD

A. cardiospasm
B. difficulty swallowing
C. inflammation of the stomach
D. stomach pain
E. gastrodynia
F. erosion of the gastric mucosa
G. return of the contents of the stomach to the esophagus
H. megaesophagus
I. esophageal aperistalsis

Terms Related to Intestinal Disorders

TERM	WORD ORIGIN	DEFINITION
Acute peritonitis pair ih tuh NYE tis	*periton/o* peritoneum *-itis* inflammation	Inflammation of the peritoneum that most commonly occurs when an inflamed appendix ruptures.
Anal fissure A nul FISH ur	*an/o* anus *-al* pertaining	Cracklike lesion of the skin around the anus.
Anorectal abscess an oh RECK tul AB ses	*an/o* anus *rect/o* rectum *-al* pertaining to	Circumscribed area of inflammation in the anus or rectum, containing pus.
Appendicitis ah pen dih SYE tis	*appendic/o* appendix *-itis* inflammation	Inflammation of the vermiform appendix (Fig. 5-11).
Colitis koh LYE tis	*col/o* colon *-itis* inflammation	Inflammation of the large intestine.
Crohn's disease krohns		Inflammation of the ileum or the colon that is of idiopathic origin. Also called **regional enteritis.**
Diverticulitis dye vur tick yoo LYE tis	*diverticul/o* diverticulum *-itis* inflammation	Inflammation occurring secondary to the occurrence of diverticulosis.
Diverticulosis dye vur tick yoo LOH sis	*diverticul/o* diverticulum *-osis* abnormal condition	Development of diverticula, pouches in the lining of the colon (Fig. 5-12).

 **BE CAREFUL!**

Don't confuse *peritone/o*, which is the *membrane lining of the abdominal cavity*, with *perone/o*, which is a combining form for the *fibula.*

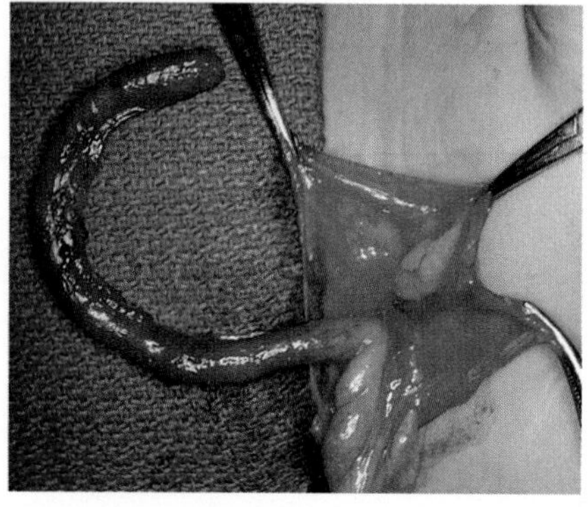

Fig. 5-11 Appendicitis. Note the darker pink color of the appendix, indicating the inflammation.

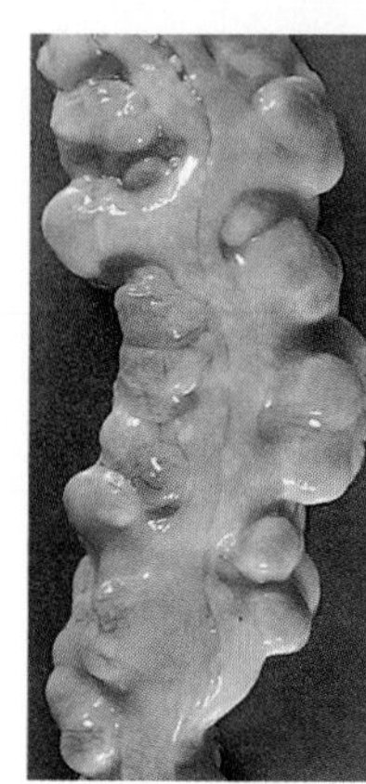

Fig. 5-12 Diverticulosis.

Terms Related to Intestinal Disorders—cont'd

TERM	WORD ORIGIN	DEFINITION
Fistula FIST yoo lah		Abnormal channel from an internal organ to the surface of the body.
Hemorrhoid HEM uh royd		Varicose veins in the lower rectum or anus.
Ileus ILL ee us		Obstruction.
Inflammatory bowel disease (IBD)		Ulceration of the lining of the intestine characterized by bleeding and diarrhea.
Intussusception in tuh suh SEP shun		Inward telescoping of the intestines.
Paralytic ileus pare uh LIH tick ILL ee us		Lack of peristaltic movement in the intestinal tract. Also called **adynamic ileus.**
Polyp PAH lip		Benign growth that may occur in the intestines.
Proctitis prock TYE tis	*proct/o* rectum and anus *-itis* inflammation	Inflammation of the rectum and anus (also called **rectitis**).
Pruritus ani proo RYE tis A nye		Common chronic condition of itching of the skin surrounding the anus.
Ulcerative colitis UL sur uh tiv koh LYE tis	*col/o* colon *-itis* inflammation	Chronic inflammation of the colon and rectum manifesting itself with bouts of profuse watery diarrhea.
Volvulus VOL vyoo lus		Twisting of the intestine.

Exercise 9: INTESTINAL DISORDERS

Matching.

____ 1. polyp

____ 2. colitis

____ 3. anal fissure

____ 4. volvulus

____ 5. proctitis

____ 6. paralytic ileus

____ 7. fistula

____ 8. intussusception

____ 9. acute peritonitis

____ 10. pruritus ani

____ 11. ulcerative colitis

____ 12. Crohn's disease

____ 13. hemorrhoids

____ 14. IBD

A. inflammation of the appendix
B. general term for an obstruction
C. a twisting of the intestines
D. inward telescoping of the intestines
E. idiopathic inflammation of ileum or colon
F. profuse watery diarrhea accompanies this condition
G. ruptured appendix puts a patient at risk for this
H. growth on mucous membranes
I. inflammation of pouches in the walls of GI tract
J. abnormal condition of pouches in GI tract

DID YOU KNOW?

Chronic liver disease, or cirrhosis, is the tenth leading cause of death in the United States.

____ 15. diverticulitis

____ 16. diverticulosis

____ 17. anorectal abscess

____ 18. appendicitis

____ 19. ileus

K. inflammation of the large intestine
L. inflammation of the anus and rectum
M. itching of the skin around the anus
N. varicosities around the anus and rectum
O. cracklike lesion in the skin around the anus
P. abnormal channel that forms between the inside and the outside of the body
Q. circumscribed area of purulent material in the distal end of the digestive tract
R. lack of peristaltic movement in intestines
S. erosion of intestinal lining accompanied by bleeding and diarrhea

Terms Related to GI Accessory Organ Disorders

TERM	WORD ORIGIN	DEFINITION
Cholangitis koh lan JYE tis	*cholangi/o* bile vessel *-itis* inflammation	Inflammation of the intrahepatic and extrahepatic bile ducts.
Cholecystitis koh lee sis TYE tis	*cholecyst/o* gallbladder *-itis* inflammation	Inflammation of the gallbladder.
Choledocholithiasis koh lee doh koh lih THY ih sis	*choledoch/o* common bile duct *lith/o* stones *-iasis* condition	Presence of stones in the common bile duct.
Cholelithiasis koh lee lih THY ih sis	*chol/e-* gall, bile *lith/o* stones *-iasis* condition	Presence of stones (calculi) in the gallbladder, sometimes characterized by right upper quadrant pain **(biliary colic)** with nausea and vomiting (Fig. 5-13).
Cirrhosis sur OH sis	*cirrh/o* orange-yellow *-osis* abnormal condition	Chronic degenerative disease of the liver, most commonly associated with alcohol abuse (Fig. 5-14).
Hepatitis heh pah TYE tis	*hepat/o* liver *-itis* inflammation	Inflammatory disease of the liver that is caused by an increasing number of viruses, alcohol, and drugs. Currently named by letter, **Hepatitis A-G,** the means of viral transmission is not the same for each form.
Hepatitis A	*hepat/o* liver *-itis* inflammation	Virus transmitted through direct contact with fecally contaminated food or water.
Hepatitis B	*hepat/o* liver *-itis* inflammation	Virus transmitted through contaminated blood or sexual contact.
Hepatitis C	*hepat/o* liver *-itis* inflammation	Virus transmitted through blood transfusion, percutaneous inoculation, or sharing infected needles.
Hepatitis D	*hepat/o* liver *-itis* inflammation	Form of hepatitis that manifests itself only in patients who have acquired hepatitis B.
Hepatitis E	*hepat/o* liver *-itis* inflammation	Strain of hepatitis virus that is transmitted through fecally contaminated food or water.
Hepatitis G	*hepat/o* liver *-itis* inflammation	Newer hepatitis virus that can be transmitted by blood.
Pancreatitis pan kree uh TYE tis	*pancreat/o* pancreas *-itis* inflammation	Inflammation of the pancreas.

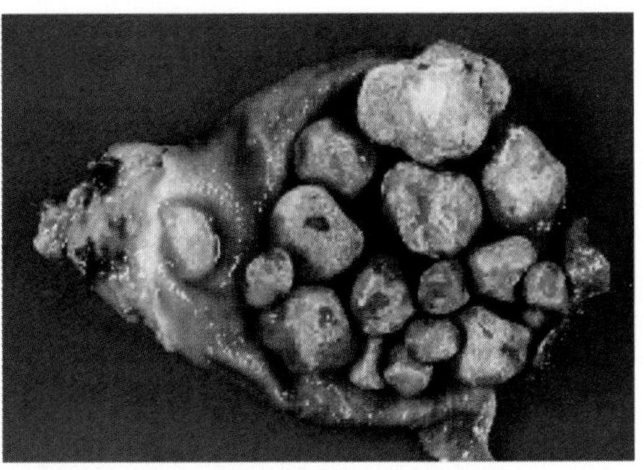

Fig. 5-13 Gallstones in the gallbladder.

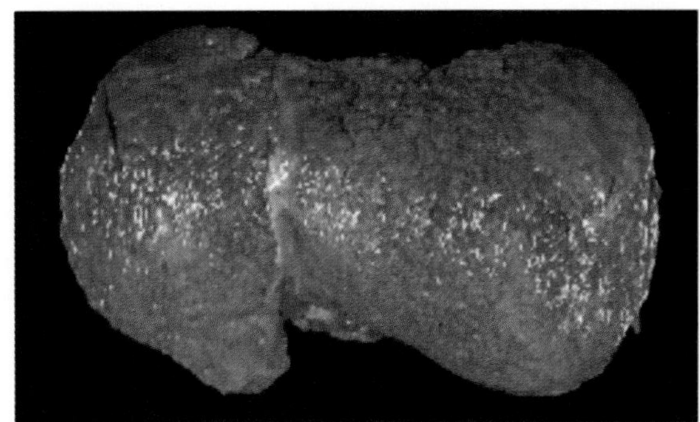

Fig. 5-14 Cirrhosis of the liver.

Exercise 10: GI ACCESSORY ORGAN DISORDERS

Fill in the blanks using the following terms.

pancreatitis, hepatitis, cholangitis, choledocholithiasis, cholelithiasis, cirrhosis, cholecystitis

1. What is a chronic degenerative disorder of the liver, usually caused by alcohol abuse?

   cirrhosis ________________

2. What is the term for the presence of stones in the gallbladder? cholelithiasis ________________
3. What is the term for an inflammation of the bile vessels? cholangitis ________________
4. What is the term for the presence of stones in the common bile duct?

   choledocholithiasis ________________

5. What is the term for an inflammation of the pancreas? ________________
6. What is an inflammatory disease of the liver that is named by letter?

   ____

7. What is the term for an inflammation of the gallbladder? cholecystitus ________________

Terms Related to Hernias

TERM	WORD ORIGIN	DEFINITION
Femoral hernia FEM uh rul HER nee ah	*femor/o* femur *-al* pertaining to	Protrusion of a loop of intestine through the femoral canal into the groin. Also called a **crural hernia.**
Hiatal hernia hye A tul HER nee ah	*hiat/o* an opening *-al* pertaining to	Protrusion of a portion of the stomach through the diaphragm. Also known as a **diaphragmatic hernia** and **diaphragmatocele** (dye uh frag MAT oh seel) (Fig. 5-15).
Incarcerated hernia in KAR sih ray tid HER nee ah	See **Did You Know?** box	Loop of bowel with ends occluded, so that solids cannot pass; herniated bowel can become strangulated. Also called an **irreducible hernia.**

Continued

DID YOU KNOW?

Incarcerated hernias acquire their name from the Latin term for *in prison,* meaning that the tissues described are confined, constricted, and *imprisoned.*

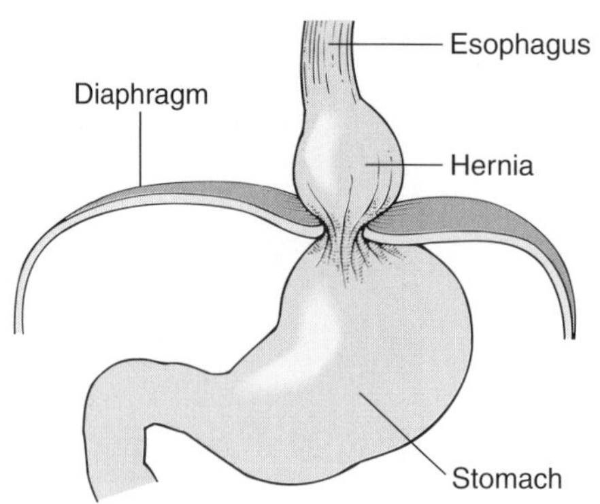

Fig. 5-15 Hiatal hernia.

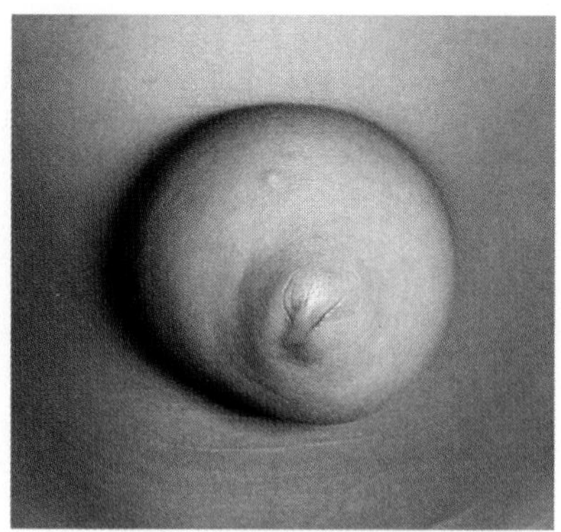

Fig. 5-16 Umbilical hernia.

Terms Related to Hernias—cont'd

TERM	WORD ORIGIN	DEFINITION
Inguinal hernia IN gwin nul HER nee ah	*inguin/o* groin *-al* pertaining to	Protrusion of a loop of intestine into the inguinal canal.
Strangulation		Constriction of a tubular structure, including intestines, leading to an impedance of circulation.
Umbilical hernia um BILL ih kul HER nee ah	*umbilic/o* umbilicus *-al* pertaining to	Protrusion of the intestine and omentum through a weakness in the abdominal wall (Fig. 5-16).

Exercise 11: HERNIAS

Matching.

A 1. hiatal hernia

B 2. umbilical hernia

F 3. strangulation

C 4. incarcerated hernia

D 5. inguinal hernia

E 6. femoral hernia

A. diaphragmatocele
B. protrusion of part of the intestines and omentum through the abdominal wall
C. irreducible hernia
D. protrusion of intestine in the inguinal canal
E. protrusion of intestine through the femoral canal
F. constriction of a tubular structure

DIAGNOSTIC PROCEDURES

Imaging

Visualizing the internal workings of the digestive system can be achieved with a wide variety of techniques but is usually accomplished through either radiographic imaging or endoscopy, or a combination of the two. Most of the procedures below are a form of radiography, or "taking x-rays." However, because the tissues of the digestive system are soft (as opposed to bone), a radiopaque contrast medium may be necessary to outline the digestive tract. This substance may be introduced into the body through the oral or anal openings or it may be injected. Fluoroscopy provides instant visual access to deep tissue structures.

DID YOU KNOW?

The term *enema* is derived from the Greek term meaning to *send in*—as in the intrarectal introduction of fluid for cleansing or medicinal purposes.

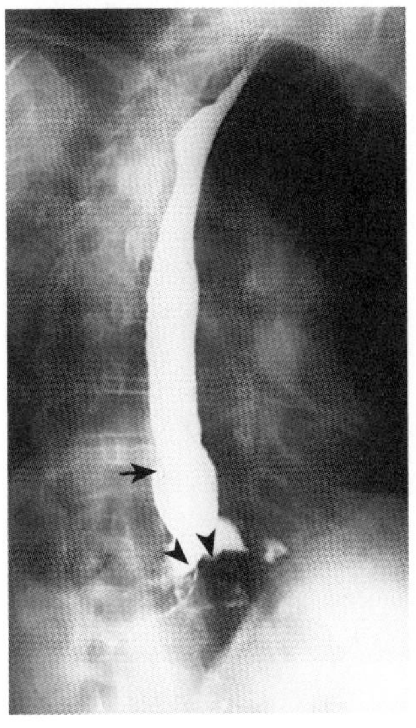

Fig. 5-17 Barium swallow.

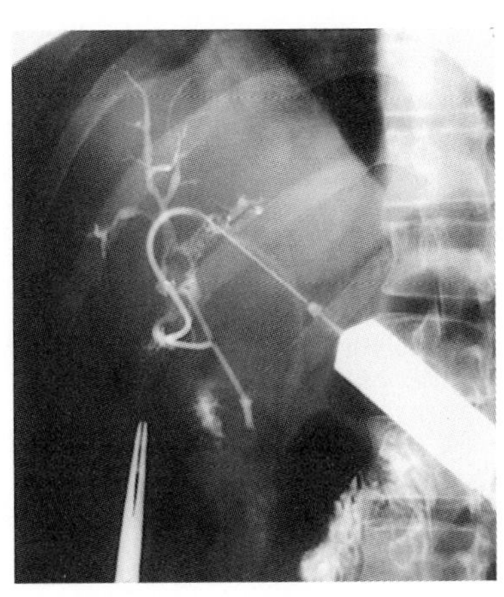

Fig. 5-18 Cholangiography.

DID YOU KNOW?

The combining form *man/o* refers to a Greek term meaning *scanty*. *Man/u* is Latin and refers to the hand. Manometry gets its name from a device that measures a lessening (scanty) amount of air pressure.

Terms Related to Imaging

TERM	WORD ORIGIN	DEFINITION
Barium enema BAIR ee um EN nuh mah	See **Did You Know?** box	Introduction of a barium sulfate suspension through the rectum for imaging of the lower digestive tract to detect obstructions, tumors, and other abnormalities.
Barium swallow		Radiographic imaging done after the oral ingestion of a barium sulfate suspension; used to detect abnormalities of the esophagus (Fig. 5-17).
Cholangiography koh lan jee AH gruh fee	*cholangi/o* bile vessels *-graphy* recording	Radiographic procedure that captures images of the common bile duct through the injection of a contrast medium into the bile duct, after which a series of digital images are taken (Fig. 5-18).
Cholecystography koh lee sis TAH gruh fee	*cholecyst/o* gallbladder *-graphy* process of recording	Contrast study in which iodine is ingested orally. The gallbladder is then imaged at different time intervals to assess its functioning; this procedure is used to diagnose cholecystitis, cholelithiasis, tumors, and other abnormalities of the gallbladder.
Computed tomography (CT) scan	*tom/o* section, cutting *-graphy* process of recording	Radiographic technique that produces detailed images of "slices" or cross-sections of the body; used in the digestive system to diagnose tumors or abnormal accumulations of fluid.

Continued

Terms Related to Imaging—cont'd

TERM	WORD ORIGIN	DEFINITION
Endoscopy en DAH skuh pee	*endo-* within *-scopy* process of visually examining	General term for any internal visualization of the body using an instrument called an **endoscope,** which has its own fiberoptic light source. The endoscope enters the GI tract through the oral cavity (esophagoscopy, gastroscopy, and esophagogastroduodenoscopy [EGD]); through the anus (proctoscopy, colonoscopy, sigmoidoscopy); or through an incision in the abdominal wall (laparoscopy).
Fluoroscopy floo RAH skuh pee	*fluor/o* to flow *-scopy* visually examine	Special kind of x-ray procedure that allows visualization of structures in real time directly on a monitor screen.
Manometry mah NAH met tree	*man/o* scanty *-metry* process of measurement	Test that measures the motor function (muscle pressure) of the esophagus.
Ultrasonography ul trah soh NAH gruh fee	*ultra-* beyond, excessive *son/o* sound *-graphy* process of recording	Use of high-frequency sound waves to image deep structures of the body; used in the digestive system to detect gallstones and tumors.

Terms Related to Laboratory Tests

TERM	WORD ORIGIN	DEFINITION
Biopsy BYE op see	*bi/o* life *-opsy* viewing	Removal and examination of living tissue from the body for either diagnostic or therapeutic purposes.
Gamma-glutamyl transferase (GGT) GAM uh GLOO tah mil TRANS fur ace		Blood test to detect increased enzymes that can indicate cirrhosis, hepatitis, acute pancreatitis, acute cholecystitis or nephrosis, and to test for *Helicobacter pylori* antibodies.
Stool culture		Fecal exam to test for microorganisms in the feces, such as worms, amoebae, bacteria, and protozoa.
Stool guaiac, hemoccult test GWEYE ack HEEM oh kult	*hem/o* blood	Fecal specimen exam to detect hidden blood, which may indicate gastrointestinal bleeding.
Total bilirubin BILL lee roo bin		Blood test to detect possible jaundice (yellowing of the skin), cirrhosis, or hepatitis.

Exercise 12: DIAGNOSTIC PROCEDURES

Fill in the blanks with the appropriate terms from the following list.

stool culture, hemoccult, total bilirubin, CT scan, barium swallow, cholecystography, guaiac, biopsy, gamma-glutamyl transferase, cholangiography, endoscopy, fluoroscopy, ultrasonography, manometry, barium enema

1. High-frequency sound waves detect a tumor. The imaging technique is called

ultra sonography ________________________.

2. The patient ingests a contrast medium, after which imaging of the esophagus is done. This is called ____________________.
3. An iodine compound is swallowed and a series of images of the gallbladder is taken. This is called ____________________.
4. A cross-sectional image of the abdomen is taken. This is called a/an ____________________.
5. The common bile duct is imaged radiographically after injection with a contrast medium. This is called ____________________.
6. A contrast medium was introduced into the patient's rectum and studies were done of the lower digestive tract. This is called a/an ____________________.
7. What test measures the motor function of the esophagus? ____________________
8. A fecal examination that tests for microorganisms is called a/an ____________________.
9. Examination for blood in the stool is done by performing a stool ____________________ or ____________________ test.
10. Removal of living tissue for diagnostic and/or therapeutic reasons is called ____________________.
11. What type of test is done to test for jaundice, cirrhosis, or hepatitis? ____________________
12. What is the test for elevated enzymes of *H. pylori* antibodies? ____________________
13. What is the general term for a visual examination within the body? ____________________
14. What is the special type of x-ray procedure that images internal structures in real time on a monitor screen? ____________________

Case Study Continued

When the laboratory results are reported, Mariah's white blood cell count and serum bilirubin are both well above normal limits. An oral cholecystography and an ultrasound both indicate that she indeed has cholelithiasis. Mariah is prepped for laparoscopic surgery.

THERAPEUTIC INTERVENTIONS

When building a therapeutic intervention term that includes the creation of a stoma, the anatomic structures must be named in the order they appear in the body system. For example, a **duodenoileostomy** is a new opening between the duodenum and the ileum. The duodenum is listed first because it occurs before the ileum in the digestive system. Other examples are **esophagogastrostomy** and **jejunocecostomy.** These "**ostomies**" may be either temporary or permanent. If, however, the opening is not between two structures, but is to the surface of the body, then the order is (obviously) irrelevant. An example would be a **colostomy**—a new opening of the colon to the surface of the abdomen.

Terms Related to Therapeutic Interventions

TERM	WORD ORIGIN	DEFINITION
Anastomosis ah nas tih MOH sis		New connection created between two (usually hollow) structures that did not previously exist.
Colostomy koh LOSS toh mee	*col/o* colon *-stomy* new opening	Surgical redirection of the bowel to a **stoma** (STOH mah), an artificial opening, on the abdominal wall (Fig. 5-19).
Enema EH nih mah		Method of introducing a solution into the rectum for therapeutic (relief of constipation) or hygienic (preparation for surgery) reasons.
Gastrectomy gass TRECK tuh mee	*gastr/o* stomach *-ectomy* removal	Surgical removal of all or part of the stomach.
Hemorrhoidectomy heh moh roy DECK tuh mee	*hemorrhoid/o* hemorrhoid *-ectomy* removal	Surgical excision of hemorrhoids.
Herniorrhaphy hur nee OR rah fee	*herni/o* hernia *-rrhaphy* suture	Hernia repair; suture of a hernia.
Laparoscopic surgery lap uh roh SCAH pick	*lapar/o* abdomen *-scopic* pertaining to visually examining	Surgery done through several small incisions in the abdominal wall with the aid of an instrument called a **laparoscope.** A **laparoscopic cholecystectomy** is the removal of the gallbladder (Fig. 5-20).
Laparotomy (lap) lap uh RAH tuh mee	*lapar/o* abdomen *-tomy* incision	Any surgical incision in the abdominal wall for the purpose of an operative approach or for exploratory purposes.
Ligation lye GAY shun	*ligat/o* tying *-tion* the process of	Tying off of a blood vessel or duct (e.g., the cystic duct is ligated when the gallbladder is removed during a cholecystectomy).
Lysis of adhesions LYE sis	*lys/o* breakdown *-is* noun ending	Surgical destruction of adhesions (scar tissue that binds two anatomic surfaces) e.g., in the peritoneal cavity.
Nasogastric intubation nay soh GASS trick in too BAY shun	*nas/o* nose *gastr/o* stomach *-ic* pertaining to	Placement of a tube from the nose, down the back of the throat, then into the stomach, for the purpose of removing gastric contents.
Paracentesis pair ah sen TEE sis	*para-* near, beside *-centesis* surgical puncture	Procedure for withdrawing fluid from a body cavity, most commonly to remove fluid accumulated in the abdominal cavity.
Resections		Excisions of structures.

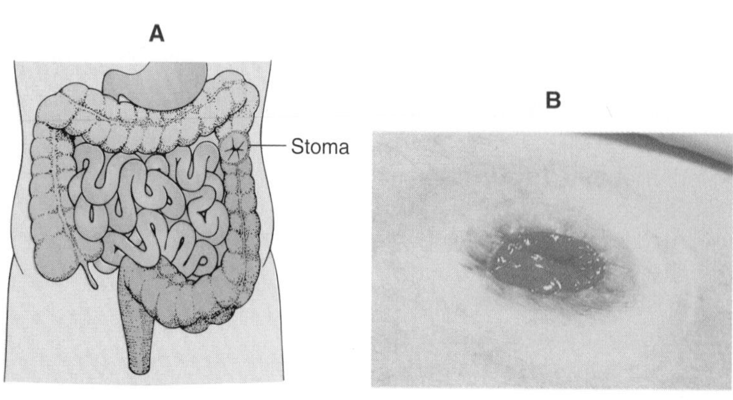

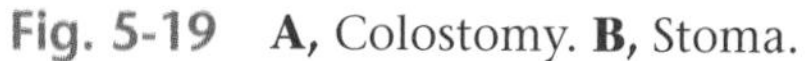
Fig. 5-19 **A,** Colostomy. **B,** Stoma.

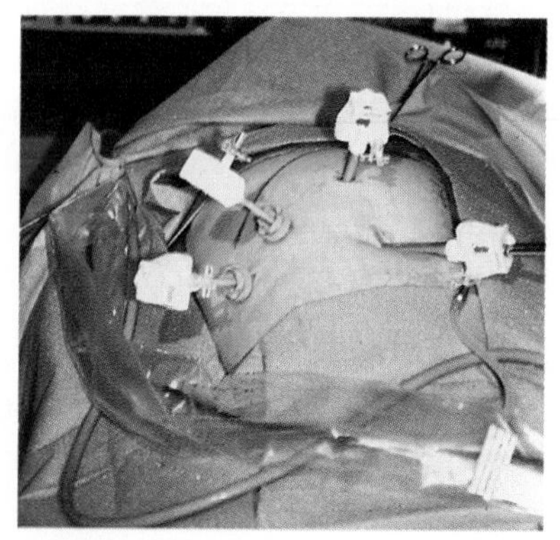
Fig. 5-20 Laparoscopic cholecystectomy.

 Exercise 13: THERAPEUTIC INTERVENTIONS

Matching.

_____ 1. removal of fluid from a body cavity

_____ 2. exploratory surgery of the abdomen

_____ 3. joining of two hollow tubes or organs

_____ 4. introduction of a solution in the rectum for cleansing or therapeutic purposes

_____ 5. tying off a vessel or a duct

_____ 6. destruction of adhesions

_____ 7. inserting a tube from the nose to the stomach

_____ 8. artificial opening

_____ 9. hernia repair

_____ 10. name of the instrument used to view the interior of the abdominal cavity

_____ 11. removal of hemorrhoids

_____ 12. removal of part of the stomach

_____ 13. opening of large intestine to the wall of the abdomen

_____ 14. surgery done through incisions on abdominal wall with aid of laparoscope

A. anastomosis
B. paracentesis
C. laparoscopic surgery
D. hemorrhoidectomy
E. laparotomy
F. enema
G. herniorrhaphy
H. ligation
I. hemigastrectomy
J. nasogastric intubation
K. colostomy
L. laparoscope
M. stoma
N. lysis of adhesions

PHARMACOLOGY

Most of the medications prescribed for the GI system are in drug classes that begin with the prefix *anti-*, because they are intended to be *against* the disorders they aim to treat.

Anorexiants (an nor RECK see unts): A class of appetite suppressants designed to aid in weight control, often in an attempt to treat **morbid obesity** (an amount of body fat that threatens normal health). Examples of anorexiants are sibutramine (Meridia) and xenical (Orlistat).

Antacids: A group of drugs or dietary substances that buffer (neutralize) or absorb hydrochloric acid in the stomach. Conditions that may be treated with antacids include GERD, pyrosis, and ulcers.

Antibiotics: Antimicrobial agents used to treat infections, a variety of which may be used in the digestive system, for example, to treat ulcers caused by the *H. pylori* bacterium.

Antidiarrheals: Drugs that provide relief from intestinal cramping and diarrhea by acting on the nerve supply of the digestive tract. The generic name, loperamide, is sold under a number of brand names (Imodium, Kaopectate II, Maalox Antidiarrheal).

Antiemetics: Drugs that prevent or alleviate nausea and vomiting, including drugs such as scopolamine that relieve motion sickness.

Cathartic (kuh THAR tick): Agent that causes evacuation of the bowel by stimulating peristalsis, increasing the fluidity or bulk of intestinal contents, softening the feces, or lubricating the intestines. Generally considered much stronger than laxatives. Also called a **purgative.**

DID YOU KNOW?

Laxative comes from the Latin word *laxare,* meaning *to loosen;* cathartic comes from the Greek word *katharsis,* meaning *a cleansing.*

> **DID YOU KNOW?**
>
> An FDA-approved food supplement, Cholestin, contains lovastatin, so patients must be queried as to their intake of OTC supplements to avoid possible overdose and interactions.

Cholesterol-reducing agents: Drugs that reduce total blood cholesterol and, in some cases, also increase LDL cholesterol. Examples are lovastatin (Mevacor), Simvastin (Zocor) and atorvastatin (Lipitor). Natural-based products include Benecol, a plant stanol ester that contains products that can lower total and LDL cholesterol. Soy products contain phytoestrogens that have led to an FDA-approved health claim for reducing risk of heart disease when containing 6.25 g of soy protein per serving.

Laxative: Mild medication that causes evacuation of the bowel by increasing the bulk of the feces, softening the stool, or lubricating the intestinal wall.

Exercise 14: PHARMACOLOGY

Match each disorder with the type of drug that is used to treat it.

____ 1. nausea and vomiting

____ 2. *H. pylori* infection

____ 3. pyrosis, dyspepsia

____ 4. high HDL and LDL

____ 5. excessive weight gain

____ 6. constipation

____ 7. intestinal cramping and loose, watery stools

A. laxative
B. antidiarrheal
C. antibiotic
D. antacid
E. cholesterol-reducing drug
F. antiemetic
G. anorexiant

Case Study Continued

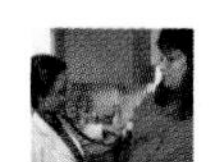

Elena Sanchez speaks to Mariah the afternoon after her laparoscopic cholecystectomy. All of her symptoms are gone, and she is relieved to have the cause of her illness treated. Elena advises Mariah that she might continue to have an intolerance to fatty foods and some discomfort at the surgical site, and that she might experience some flatulence, a normal occurrence after abdominal surgery. Mariah is relieved to find out that the symptoms will resolve in a couple of weeks.

Abbreviations

Abbreviation	*Definition*	*Abbreviation*	*Definition*
BE	Barium enema	HBV	Hepatitis B virus
BaS	Barium swallow	IBD	Inflammatory bowel disease
BM	Bowel movement	IBS	Irritable bowel syndrome
CT scan	Computed tomography scan	Lap	Laparoscopy
EGD	Esophagogastroduodenoscopy	LPN	Licensed practical nurse
GB	Gallbladder	N&V	Nausea and vomiting
GERD	Gastroesophageal reflux disease	NPO	Nothing by mouth (L. *nil per os*)
GGT	Gamma-glutamyl transferase	PUD	Peptic ulcer disease
GI	Gastrointestinal	RN	Registered nurse
HAV	Hepatitis A virus		

Exercise 15: ABBREVIATIONS

Spell out the abbreviations used in the following examples.

1. The 76-year-old patient complained of no BM in the last week. He had not had a/an

   ______________________.

2. The patient was admitted for suspected GB disease. ______________________
3. The nurse recorded the patient's symptoms as N&V, without a fever.

   ____

4. Constant heartburn for Phyllis may have been a result of GERD. ______________________
5. Stressful situations were made even more so for Bill when his IBS flared up.

   ____

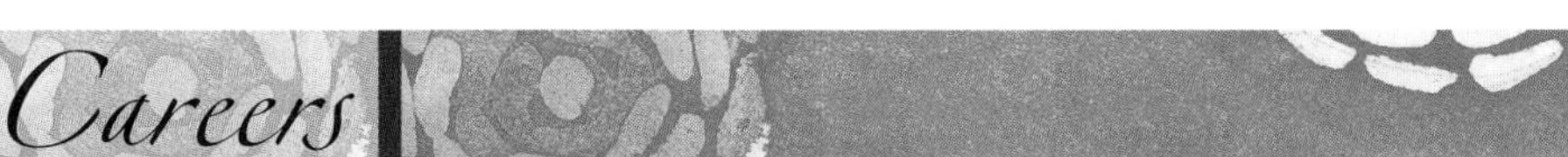

Medical-Surgical Nurses

Nursing is a career in high demand. Prospective students can choose between hospital schools that can provide them with either licensed practical nurse (LPN) or registered nurse (RN) credentials, or colleges that combine an associate- or bachelor-level degree with the RN credential. A master's or doctoral degree can also be earned in a number of different specialty areas.

Students interested in the nursing field are normally required to have had certain courses with satisfactory grades (usually a C or better) within a given time period specified by each nursing program. These courses normally include high school algebra, biology, and chemistry, or their university equivalents. On completion of a nursing program, students are required to take either a state licensing (for LPN) or registration (for RN) examination before they are permitted to practice.

Most nurses begin their careers as medical-surgical (med-surg) nurses, working in those respective areas for at least 2 years before they branch into a specialty area. Two specialized areas of nursing that require further study include nurse practitioners and certified nurse midwives. Nurse practitioners can conduct physical examinations, provide immunizations, diagnose and treat common illnesses and injuries, and order and interpret x-rays and lab tests. Certified nurse midwives are responsible for prenatal care of normally healthy women, delivering babies, and conducting follow-up care during the postpartum period.

Further information on nursing programs is available through several avenues. Your local library will have resources to help you locate nursing programs available in your area. Calling your nearby hospitals and universities may also provide information about local programs. If you choose to use the Internet, the following sites may be useful.

The Education and Career Center provides information on private schools, colleges and universities, graduate study, study abroad, summer programs and distance learning. Their address is http://www.petersons.com/professional/nurslist.html.

The National League for Nursing Accrediting Commission has links to a directory of accredited nursing programs at http://www.accrediting-comm-nlnac.org/1999directory-main.htm.

According to the U.S. Bureau of Labor Statistics, opportunities for careers in nursing through 2010 are very good, and employment opportunities are expected to grow faster than the average for all occupations. There is a current nationwide shortage in this largest of all healthcare occupations.

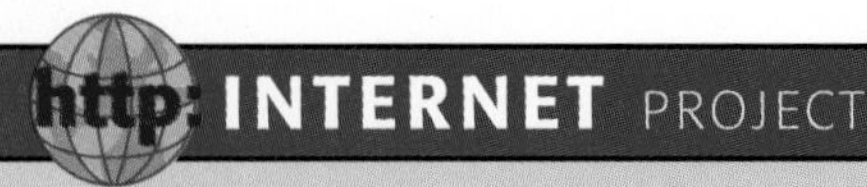

When Benjamin Franklin said, "In this world nothing can be said to be certain, except death and taxes," he might have been wise to add the word "change" as yet another certainty. Students studying healthcare terminology continually need to update their skills as new diseases, diagnostic techniques, treatments, and drugs are discovered. Using the following links applicable to hepatitis, research one of the following topics:

- Ways that healthcare workers can protect themselves from hepatitis C and other diseases spread by contact with human blood.
- The most recent statistics for "chronic liver disease and cirrhosis" as a leading cause of death in the United States, along with the death rate and number of cases reported for hepatitis A and B.
- The newest treatments for hepatitis C, including recent improvements in diagnostic techniques.
- An annotated list of five Websites (aside from these) that explain the differences among the different types of hepatitis. Be sure to include hepatitis D and E.

Assignment

Write a 2-page summary of all findings. Cite references using the formats listed at the Modern Language Association of America Website for citing World Wide Web sources at: http://www.mla.org.

Suggested Websites

World Health Organization Website: http://www.who.int/health-topics/hepatitis
CDC's National Center for Infectious Diseases Website: http://www.cdc.gov/ncidod/diseases/hepatitis
National Library of Medicine MEDLINEplus Health Information Website: http://www.nlm.nih.gov/medlineplus
CDC's National Center for Health Statistics: http://www.cdc.gov/nchs/fastats

Chapter Review

A. Functions of the Gastrointestinal System

1. Name and explain the functions of the digestive system.

____

____

2. Name one disorder that illustrates dysfunction of the system (e.g., if a patient has dyspepsia, he/she has problems [dys-] digesting food).

melena, IBS, Flatus p125

____

B. Anatomy and Physiology

3. Using the diagrams below, label the anatomic areas indicated, *along with combining forms,* where appropriate. Fig 5-1, 5-5 pgs 117 & 123

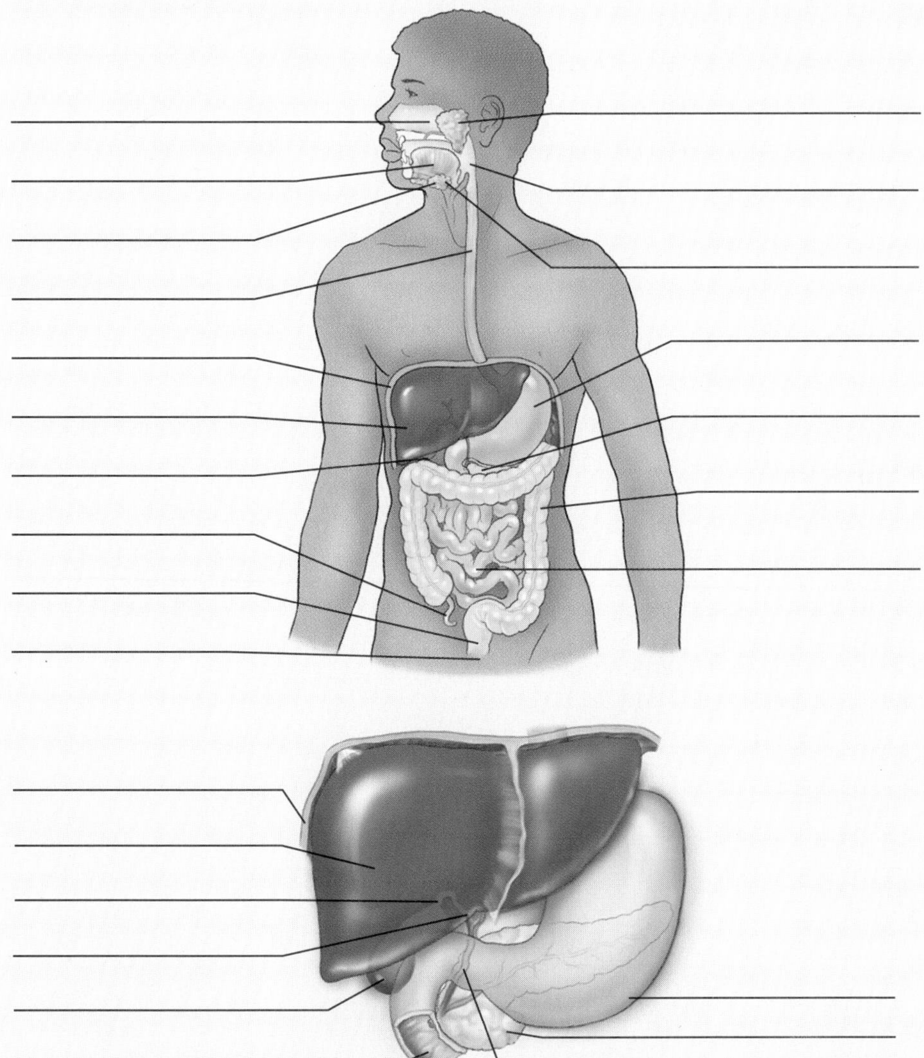

4. Follow the path of a food bolus as it passes from the lips through the intestinal tract, past the accessory organs, and out through the anus. List the organs it passes and use (at least one of) their combining forms. Begin this way—Lips: cheil/o, labi/o; Teeth: dent/i, odont/o, and so on.

____

____

____

____

____

____

____

5. What terms that end with *-tion* can be substituted for the following?

A. chewing: ______________

B. swallowing: deglutition

C. eliminating feces: ______________

D. breakdown of fats: ______________

Name the following structures.

6. Parts of organs marked by boundaries (the liver has two of these) ______________

7. Circular folds in the small intestines plicae

8. A tubular cavity within the body ______________

9. Thousands of tiny projections in the small intestine that contain blood capillaries that absorb the products of carbohydrate and protein digestion ______________

Fill in the blanks with the correct term for the following substances.

10. The suffix for enzymes -ase

11. The suffix for carbohydrates -ose

12. The waste product of the normal breakdown of hemoglobin bilirubin

13. A fatty substance found only in animal tissues and excreted in bile

cholesterol

14. Combination of gastric juices and hydrochloric acid chyme

Decode the following.

15. sublingual under tongue

16. hypopharynx lower throat

17. gastroesophageal ________________________________

18. ileocecal ________________________________

19. hepatobiliary ________________________________

C. Pathology
Build a term.

20. pertaining to the cheek ________________

21. inflammation of the gums ________________

22. inflammation of the gallbladder ________________

23. a condition of no opening of the distal esophagus ________________

24. inflammation of abnormal pouches in the digestive system ________________

25. bloody vomit ________________

Decode the term.

26. cheilitis ________________________________

27. pyloric stenosis ________________________________

28. choledocholithiasis ________________________________

29. proctalgia ________________________________

30. gastroenteritis ________________________________

31. achalasia ________________________________

32. leukoplakia ________________________________

33. pyorrhea ________________________________

34. malocclusion ________________________________

35. hematochezia ________________________________

36. dysphagia ________________________________

Recall the term.

37. telescoping of a portion of intestine within itself ________________

38. twisting of the intestines ________________

39. return of the contents of the stomach to the mouth ________________

40. condition involving varicose veins around the anus and rectum ________________

41. a chronic degenerative condition of the liver ________________

42. term for tooth decay ______________________

43. term for loose, watery feces ______________________

44. term for gas passed through the anus ______________________

45. a cracklike groove in the skin around the anus ______________________

46. itching of the skin around the anus ______________________

47. bad breath ______________________

48. belching or burping ______________________

Fill in the blank with the correct synonym.

49. congenital megacolon ______________________

50. fever blister ______________________

51. indigestion ______________________

52. heartburn ______________________

53. canker sore ______________________

54. diaphragmatocele ______________________

55. gastric ulcer ______________________

D. Diagnostic Procedures

56. The patient's symptoms indicate that he may have internal bleeding, but no blood is seen in the stool. What laboratory test would be performed to detect hidden blood? ______________________

57. In what procedure is an instrument used to view the inside of the body?

____

58. What procedure involves taking a piece of living tissue for diagnostic and/or therapeutic reasons?

____

59. Because Rafael has been having bouts of profuse diarrhea, his physician suspects a possible infection with amoebae. What laboratory test examines the feces for microorganisms?

____

60. A patient presents to the lab with an order for a laboratory test used to examine the increase in enzyme levels in, for example, cirrhosis or acute pancreatitis. What is this test?

____

61. The patient is given a radiopaque liquid to drink to coat her upper GI tract before an x-ray procedure to examine abnormalities. She is having a/an ______________________.

62. Hamid is given an enema with a radiopaque liquid during an x-ray exam of his lower GI tract. He is having a/an ______________________.

63. A patient with suspected gallstones has an x-ray procedure of her gallbladder. She has a/an cholecystography.

64. A patient with dysphagia and regurgitation problems is tested with manometry. What does this test do? test motor function of the esophagus

E. Therapeutic Interventions

Decode the term.

65. cholecystectomy ____________

66. gastroileostomy ____________

67. colostomy ____________

68. hemiglossectomy removal 1/2 tongue

Build a term.

69. hernia repair herniorrhaphy

70. incision of the abdominal cavity ____________

71. removal of stones from the gallbladder ____________

72. resection of part or all of the stomach ____________

73. removal of hemorrhoids ____________

74. new connection between the duodenum and jejunum ____________

Recall the term.

75. tying off ligation

76. destruction of adhesions lysis of adhesions

77. removal of fluid from the abdominal cavity paracentesis

78. joining two hollow tubes or organs anastomosis

79. an artificial opening stoma

80. introduction of solution into rectum for therapeutic reasons enema

F. Pharmacology

81. Ms. Ralston was given a drug to control nausea and vomiting. This type of drug is called a/an antiemetic.

82. Because Mr. McDowell had been constipated, he was given a drug to loosen stools and gently promote bowel movements. This is called a/an laxitive.

83. If the type of drug used in question 82 did not work, the patient could be given a drug that "cleanses" the bowel and creates a stronger urge to defecate. This is called a/an cathartic.

84. Patients with microbial infections may be given a type of drug called a/an antibiotic.
85. Changes in diet when traveling may cause some people to have loose, watery stools. The type of drug that may relieve this condition is known as a/an antidiarrhea.
86. Patients with high cholesterol that does not respond well to changes in diet and lifestyle may be prescribed a drug called a/an cholesterol-reducing agent.
87. Patients with severe problems controlling their weight may be prescribed a type of drug called a/an anorexiants.

G. Abbreviations

Write the meanings of the abbreviations.

88. The patient was treated for an UGI tract disorder that was suspected to be GERD or PUD. The patient's history has been positive for HAV in the last 5 years. An EGD and manometry confirmed the diagnosis.

UGI - upper Gastro Intestinal EGD - oscopy
GERD Gastro esophageal Reflux Disease
PUD Peptic Ulcer Disease HAV Hepatitis A virus

89. The patient complained of nonspecific abdominal pain, N&V, frequent BMs, and a low-grade fever. Reviewing her healthcare history, the physician saw that she had been evaluated for GB disease last year.

______

90. A GGT was ordered to rule out PUD. Gamma-glutamyl transferase
91. The surgical patient was cautioned to be NPO the night before surgery.

nothing by mouth

H. Singulars and Plurals

Change the following terms from singular to plural.

92. stoma STomata
93. fistula fistulae
94. endoscopy ______
95. esophagus esophagi
96. fundus fundi
97. ruga rugae
98. pharynx pharynges
99. anastomosis ______

100. lumen lumina

101. villus villi

I. Translations

Rewrite the following in your own words.

102. José underwent a colostomy as a treatment for advanced ulcerative colitis.

103. The 5-week-old patient had a pylorotomy to treat a case of pyloric stenosis.

104. After reporting hematemesis, melena, and gastralgia, the patient was found to have PUD.

105. The 35-year-old patient complained of URQ pain, N&V, and fever. After appendicitis and acute pancreatitis were ruled out, she was diagnosed with acute cholecystitis.

106. Hematochezia and proctalgia were the symptoms leading to an endoscopic examination that revealed hemorrhoids.

J. Cumulative Review

107. What is the structure at the distal end of the esophagus?

108. In what quadrant is the appendix?

109. What type of muscles are the stomach and intestines, and what is the combining form for this type of muscle? leiomy/o

110. Explain the rules for spelling the term for an anastomosis between the stomach and the ileum, then spell it.

111. What body cavity contains the esophagus? Thoracic

112. What is the abbreviation for a biopsy? Bx

Decode the term.

113. proctoplasty ________________

114. hypercholesterolemia ________________

115. sialolithiasis ________________

116. choledochotomy ________________

117. enterorrhaphy ________________

K. Be Careful

118. Define the following:

A. an/o ________________ C. an- ________________

B. ana ________________

119. Define the following:

A. -cele ________________ B. celi/o ________________

120. Define the following:

A. stom/o ________________ C. stomach ________________

B. stomat/o ________________

121. Define the following:

A. abdomin/o ________________ C. celi/o ________________

B. gastr/o ________________

122. Define the following:

A. ileus ________________ B. ileum ________________

123. Define the following:

A. perone/o ________________ B. peritone/o ________________

124. Give three examples of how the word root cardi can be used.

____

____

125. Explain the difference between -ase and -ose.

____

____

Synergy Hospital
781 Magnolia Blvd.
Atlanta, GA 30311

OPERATIVE REPORT

Patient Name: Mariah Hopkins
Physician: Alberta Jones, MD
Preoperative Diagnosis: Cholelithiasis
Postoperative Diagnosis: Same
Anesthesia: General, endotracheal

MR: 180031
Date: 4/22/02

Procedure

Before the induction of anesthesia, while in the operating room, the patient was identified as Mariah Hopkins. With the patient in a supine position, under general endotracheal anesthesia, with a Foley catheter and a nasogastric tube in place, the abdomen was scrubbed and painted with Betadine and draped in the usual manner.

An infraumbilical curvilinear incision was made, and the fascia was identified. It was grasped with an Allis forceps and incised. This allowed the peritoneal cavity to be entered under direct vision. A trocar was then placed, and a camera was inserted. The peritoneal cavity was identified, and the abdomen was insufflated with carbon dioxide. The chronic calculous cholecystitis was treated with a standard four-port laparoscopic cholecystectomy. The cystic duct was identified with certainty. It was traced to the common hepatic duct. It was ligated with surgical clips and divided. This allowed the cystic artery to be identified and likewise controlled. The gallbladder was then taken out from below upwards. Bleeding in the liver bed was controlled with Bovie electrocautery. Before removal of the gallbladder, the wound was irrigated until clear. The gallbladder was then removed through the umbilical port without incident.

The wounds were closed in the usual manner. The sponge and instrument counts were correct on two separate occasions. The patient tolerated the procedure well.

Samantha Schwartz (surgeon)

L. Operative Report

126. The bleeding was controlled using ______________________.

127. The route of the general anesthesia was ______________________.

128. The incision was made where in regard to the navel? ______________________

129. To say that the patient was in a supine position means that she was lying on her ______________________.

130. To ligate a structure means to ______________________.

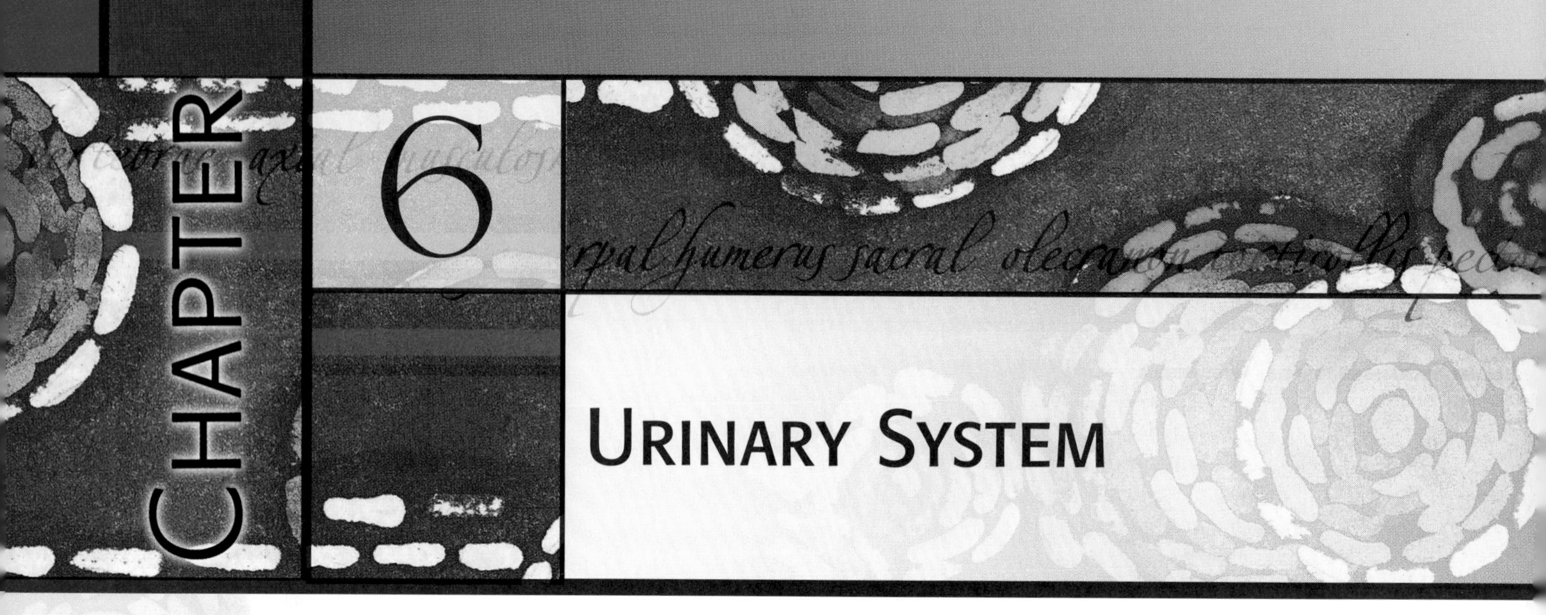

CHAPTER 6

URINARY SYSTEM

"What is man, when you come to think about him, but a minutely set, ingenious machine for turning with infinite artfulness, the red wine of Shiraz into urine?" **—Isak Dinesen**

Quote

Case Study

Brian Coulter has been experiencing sharp pain in his back, which has radiated to his lower left quadrant for the last few days. Now, Friday night, it seems worse than it has ever been, so he drives to his local emergency department hoping for some relief. Also in the emergency department is Margarette Anders, who has been feverish and has been having problems voiding. After reviewing the registrar's list of patient complaints, Tim Pao, the triage nurse, assesses Brian's complaints as more urgent than Margarette's (and the many others waiting to be seen) and calls him back to an evaluation area.

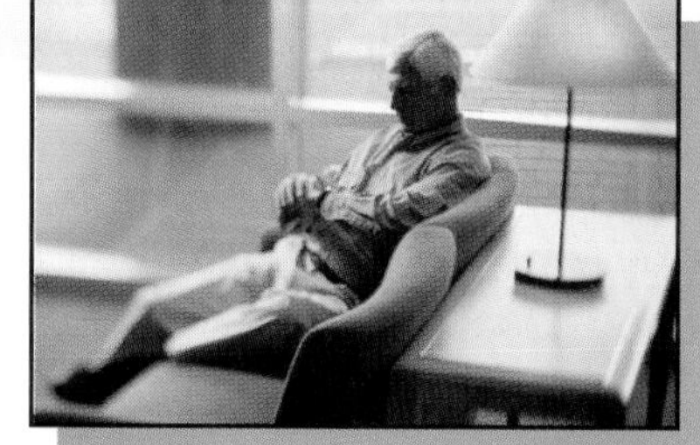

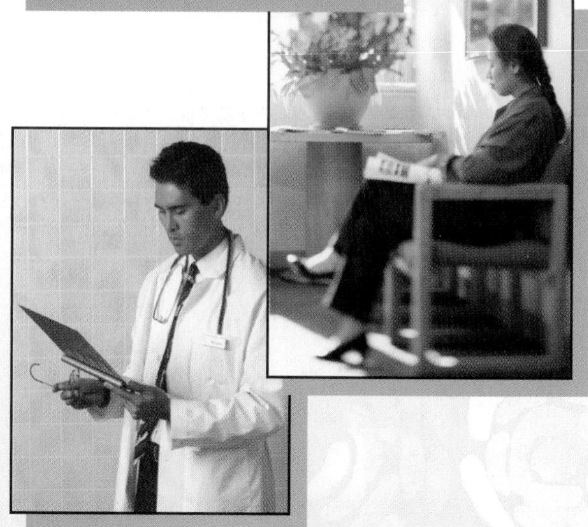

OBJECTIVES

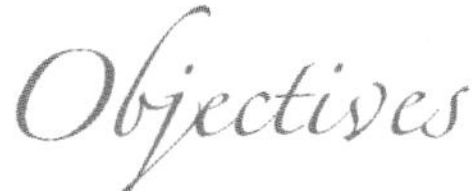

- In your own words, explain the functions of the urinary system.
- Recognize, recall, and apply healthcare terms related to the anatomy and physiology of the urinary system.
- Recognize, recall, and apply healthcare terms related to the pathology of the urinary system.
- Recognize, recall, and apply healthcare terms related to the diagnostic procedures related to the urinary system.
- Recognize and recall instruments as described relative to the urinary system.
- Recognize, recall, and apply healthcare terms related to therapeutic interventions introduced in this chapter.
- Recognize, recall, and apply the pharmacology introduced in this chapter.
- Recognize, recall, and apply the abbreviations in this chapter.
- Recognize and recall word components used in this chapter to build and decode healthcare terms relevant to the urinary system.
- Demonstrate the ability to change singular urinary terms to plural.
- Recognize, recall, and apply material learned in previous chapters.

FUNCTIONS OF THE URINARY SYSTEM

The major function of the urinary system is to maintain continually a healthy balance of the amount and content of **extracellular fluids** within the body. Biologists use the term *homeostasis* to describe this important process. The process of metabolism changes food and liquid (with its requisite fats, carbohydrates, and proteins) into building blocks, energy sources, and waste products. To operate efficiently, the body needs to monitor and rebalance the amounts of these substances constantly in the bloodstream. The breakdown of proteins and amino acids in the liver leaves chemical wastes such as urea, creatinine, and uric acid in the bloodstream. These wastes are toxic nitrogenous substances that must be excreted in the urine. The act of releasing urine is called **urination, voiding,** or **micturition** (mick ter RIH shun).

Succinctly phrased by Homer William Smith in 1939, "It is no exaggeration to say that the composition of the blood is determined not by what the mouth ingests but by what the kidneys keep; they are the master chemists of our internal environment, which, so to speak, they synthesize in reverse."

DID YOU KNOW?

During the day, the average person urinates about five times, usually 1.5 liters total.

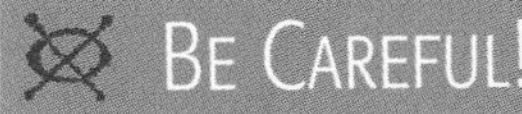

BE CAREFUL!

-uria is a suffix that means a condition of the urine; *urea* is a chemical waste product.

COMBINING FORMS FOR THE URINARY SYSTEM

MEANING	COMBINING FORM
cell	cellul/o, cyt/o
same	home/o
urine, urinary system	ur/o, urin/o

PREFIXES AND SUFFIXES FOR THE URINARY SYSTEM

PREFIX/SUFFIX	MEANING
extra-	outside
-stasis	controlling, stabilizing
-uria	condition of the urine

Exercise 1: Functions of the Urinary System

Circle the correct term.

1. Through the process of *(homeostasis, deglutition)* the body monitors the *(intracellular, extracellular)* fluid and removes the waste products of *(carbohydrates, proteins)* from the body called *(uria, urea)*, creatinine and uric acid. The process of *(forming, excreting)* urine is termed urination.

ANATOMY AND PHYSIOLOGY

The urinary system is composed of two kidneys, two ureters, a urinary bladder, and a urethra (Figs. 6-1 and 6-2). The work of the urinary system is done by a specialized tissue in the **kidneys** called **parenchymal** (pair EN kuh mul) **tissue.** The **ureters** (YOOR eh turs) are thin, muscular tubes that move urine in peristaltic waves from the kidneys to the bladder. The **urinary bladder** is the sac that stores the urine until it is excreted, and the **urethra** (yoo REE thrah) is the tube that conducts the urine out of the body. The opening of the urethra is called the **urinary meatus** (YOOR in nair ee mee ATE us). The triangular area in the bladder between the ureters' entrance and the urethral outlet is called the **trigone** (TRY gohn). The ureters, bladder, and urethra are all **stromal** (STROH mul) **tissue,** which is a supportive tissue.

The Kidney

Because the kidneys are primarily responsible for the functioning of the urinary system, it is helpful to look at them in more detail. Each of the two kidneys is located high in the abdominal cavity, tucked under the ribs in the back and behind the lining of the abdominal cavity (retroperitoneal). The normal human kidney is about the size of a fist. If a kidney were sliced open, the outer portion, the **cortex** (KORE tecks) (*pl.* cortices) and the inner portion, called the **medulla** (muh DOO lah) (*pl.* medullae) would be visible (Fig. 6-3). The **renal pelvis** and **calyces** (KAL ih seez) (*sing.* calyx) are an extension of the ureter inside of the kidney. The term **renal** means *pertaining to the kidneys.*

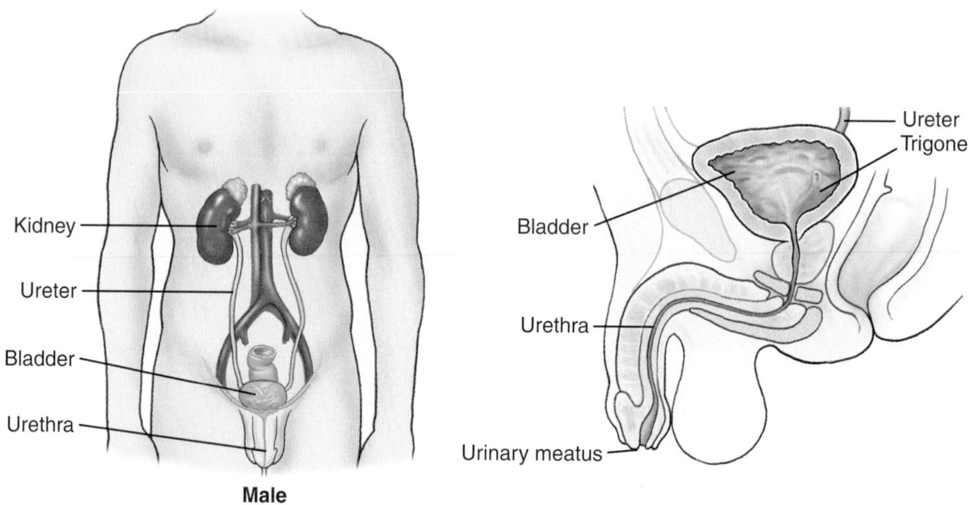

Fig. 6-1 Male urinary system.

The **hilum** (HYE lum) (*pl.* hila) is the location on the kidney where the ureter and renal vein leave the kidney and the renal artery enters. The cortex contains tissue with millions of microscopic units called **nephrons** (NEFF rons) (Fig. 6-4). Here in the tiny nephrons, blood passes through a continuous system of urinary filtration, reabsorption, and secretion that measures, monitors, and adjusts the levels of substances in the extracellular fluid.

The Nephron

The nephrons filter all of the blood in the body approximately every 5 minutes. The **renal afferent arteries** transport unfiltered blood to the kidneys. Once in the kidneys, the blood travels through small arteries called **arterioles** (ar TEER ree ohls) and finally into tiny balls of renal capillaries, called **glomeruli** (gloh MER yoo lye) (*sing.* glomerulus). These glomeruli cluster at the entrance to each nephron. It is here that the process of filtering the blood to form urine begins.

The nephron consists of four parts: (1) the **renal corpuscle** (KORE pus sul), which is composed of the glomerulus and its surrounding Bowman's capsule; (2) a **proximal convoluted tubule**; (3) the **nephronic loop**, also known as the Loop of Henle; and (4) the **distal convoluted tubule**. As blood flows through the capillaries, water, electrolytes, glucose, and nitrogenous wastes are passed through the glomerular membrane and collected. The most common electrolytes are

 **BE CAREFUL!**

Calic/o and *cali/o* are the combining forms for *calyx*, but *calc/o* is the combining form for *calcium*.

BE CAREFUL!

It is easy to confuse the combining forms *perone/o*, which means *fibula; perine/o*, which means *the space between external genitalia and the anus;* and *peritone/o*, which means *the abdominal lining*.

DID YOU KNOW?

The term *gross* in *gross anatomy* refers to those structures that can be seen with the naked eye as opposed to a microscope.

DID YOU KNOW?

The term *glomerulus* is derived from a Latin word that means *a little ball of yarn*, which does describe the appearance of a renal glomerulus.

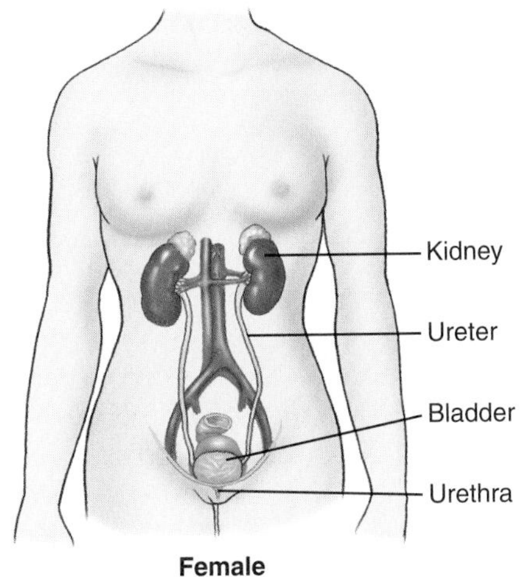

Fig. 6-2 Female urinary system.

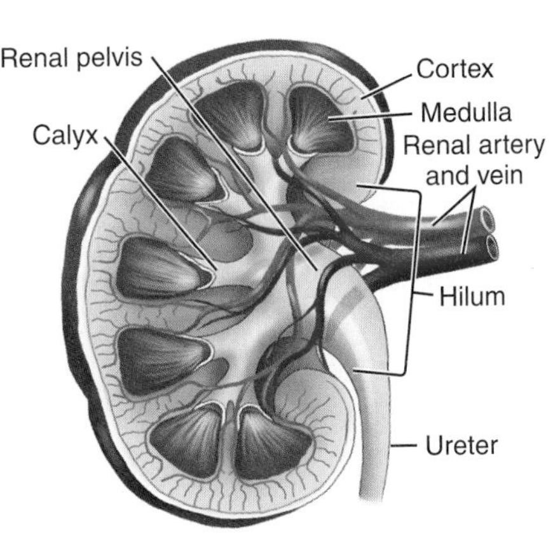

Fig. 6-3 Cross-section of a kidney.

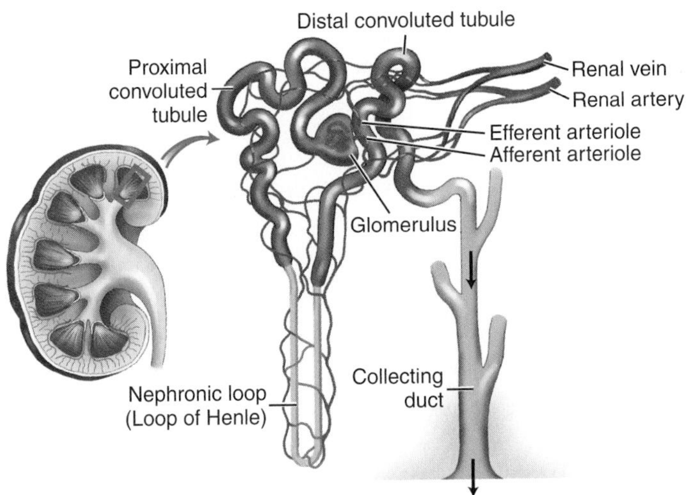

Fig. 6-4 The nephron.

sodium (Na), chloride (Cl), and potassium (K). Blood cells and proteins are too large to pass through the glomerular membrane. Selective filtration and reabsorption continues along the renal tubules, with the end result of urine concentration and subsequent dilution occurring in the renal medulla. From there, the urine flows to the calyces and exits the kidney, flowing through the ureter into the bladder, where it is stored until it can be expelled from the body through the urethra.

COMBINING FORMS FOR ANATOMY AND PHYSIOLOGY

MEANING	COMBINING FORM	MEANING	COMBINING FORM
calyx	calic/o, cali/o	peritoneum	peritone/o
chloride	chlor/o	potassium	potassi/o
cortex	cortic/o	renal pelvis	pyel/o
glomerulus	glomerul/o	sodium	natr/o
hilum	hil/o	trigone	trigon/o
kidney	nephr/o, ren/o	ureter	ureter/o
meatus	meat/o	urethra	urethr/o
medulla	medull/o	urinary bladder	cyst/o, vesic/o

Exercise 2: THE URINARY SYSTEM

Match the combining form with its term.

____ 1. opening of the urethra

____ 2. tubes connecting kidneys and bladder

____ 3. tube conducting urine out of the bladder

____ 4. same as ren/o

____ 5. sac that stores urine

____ 6. area between ureters coming in and urethra going out in the sac that stores urine

____ 7. urine, urinary system

____ 8. renal pelvis

____ 9. outer portion of the kidney

____ 10. inner portion of the kidney

____ 11. artery

____ 12. renal calyx

____ 13. location where ureter and renal vein leave kidney and renal artery enters

A. nephr/o
B. ur/o, urin/o
C. meat/o
D. urethr/o
E. cyst/o, vesic/o
F. ureter/o
G. trigon/o
H. medull/o
I. calic/o, cali/o
J. cortic/o
K. hil/o
L. pyel/o
M. arteri/o

Circle the correct term.

14. The basic working unit of the kidney is the *(hilum, nephron)*.
15. The nephron is located in the *(cortex, medulla)* of the kidney.
16. The name of the ball of capillaries within the nephron is the *(calyces, glomerulus)*.
17. The capsule that surround these capillaries is called *(Bowman's, Henle's)* capsule.
18. Blood is carried to the nephron through the *(afferent, efferent)* arteriole.
19. *(Water and electrolytes, Blood and proteins)* are normally too large to pass through the glomerular membrane into its surrounding capsule.

20. Place the following terms in order, showing the normal direction of the flow of urine from structures within the kidney to when it leaves the body.

ureter, renal pelvis, urinary meatus, renal cortex, urethra, urinary bladder, renal medulla

renal cortex → medulla → pelvis → ureter → urinary bladder →

urethra → meatus

Case Study Continued

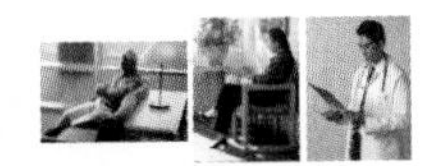

Tim takes Brian's vital signs and questions him for details regarding his complaint. In the past few minutes, Brian's pain has intensified. He is having a hard time sitting, seems agitated, and is obviously distressed. He apologizes, saying that on top of the severe pain, he also feels nauseous and may need to vomit. His pain is currently localized in the left upper quadrant but occasionally moves across the anterior abdomen.

Margarette recognizes the burning sensation and urgency to urinate as familiar symptoms of previous urinary tract infections. Although she has tried to "flush it out" by drinking copious amounts of cranberry juice, this time it did not work. She knew earlier today that she should call her physician, but she waited too long. Because her condition is not judged to be a true healthcare emergency, she is in for a lengthy wait.

PATHOLOGY

Terms Related to Urinary Conditions Ending in -uria

TERM	WORD ORIGIN	DEFINITION
Albuminuria al byoo mih NOOR ee ah	*albumin/o* protein *-uria* urinary condition	Albumin (a protein) in the urine. Also called **proteinuria** (pro teen NOOR ee ah).
Anuria A NOOR ee ah	*an-* without *-uria* urinary condition	Condition of no urine.
Azoturia a zoh TOOR ee ah	*az/o* nitrogen *-uria* urinary condition	Excessive nitrogenous compounds, including urea, in the urine.
Bacteriuria back tur ee YOOR ee ah	*bacteri/o* bacteria *-uria* urinary condition	Bacteria in the urine.
Dysuria dis YOOR ee ah	*dys-* painful, abnormal *-uria* urinary condition	Condition of painful urination.
Glycosuria gly kohs YOOR ee ah	*glyc/o* sugar *-uria* urinary condition	Sugar in the urine.
Hematuria hee mah TOOR ee ah	*hemat/o* blood *-uria* urinary condition	Blood in the urine.
Nocturia nock TOOR ee ah	*noct/i* night *-uria* urinary condition	Condition of excessive urination at night.
Oliguria ah lig GYOOR ee ah	*olig-* scanty, few *-uria* urinary condition	Condition of scanty urination.

Continued

Terms Related to Urinary Conditions Ending in -uria—cont'd		
TERM	**WORD ORIGIN**	**DEFINITION**
Polyuria pah lee YOOR ee ah	*poly-* profuse, excessive *-uria* urinary condition	Condition of excessive urination.
Pyuria pye YOOR ee ah	*py/o* pus *-uria* urinary condition	Pus in the urine.

Terms Related to Urinary Signs		
TERM	**WORD ORIGIN**	**DEFINITION**
Abscess AB ses		Cavity containing pus and surrounded by inflamed tissue.
Azotemia a zoh TEE mee ah	*az/o* nitrogen *-emia* blood condition	Condition of excessive urea in the blood indicating nonfunctioning kidneys.
Diuresis dye yoor EE sis	*di-* through, complete *ur/o* urine *-esis* state of	Condition of increased formation and excretion of urine, of large volumes of urine. Caffeine and alcohol are **diuretics** (dye yoor RET icks)—that is, they increase the amount of urine produced.
Edema eh DEE mah		Accumulation of fluid in the tissues; can result from kidney failure.
Enuresis en yoor EE sis	*en-* in *ur/o* urine *-esis* state of	Also commonly known as "bedwetting," enuresis can be **nocturnal** (at night) or **diurnal** (during the day).
Hypertension hye pur TEN shun	*hyper-* excessive	Condition of high blood pressure.
Incontinence in KON tih nense		Inability to hold urine.
Polydipsia pah lee DIP see ah	*poly-* excessive, many *-dipsia* thirst	Condition of excessive thirst (usually accompanied by polyuria).
Retention		Inability to release urine.
Urgency		Intense sensation of the need to urinate immediately.

Exercise 3: Urinary Conditions and Signs

Matching.

_____ 1. pus in the urine

_____ 2. no urine

_____ 3. blood in the urine

_____ 4. profuse urine

_____ 5. bacteria in the urine

_____ 6. excessive urea in the urine

_____ 7. scanty urine

_____ 8. protein in the urine

_____ 9. painful urination

_____ 10. sugar in the urine

A. dysuria
B. polyuria
C. oliguria
D. glycosuria
E. azoturia
F. pyuria
G. albuminuria
H. hematuria
I. anuria
J. bacteriuria

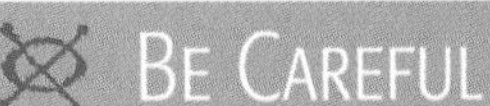

Circle the correct term.

11. Urinary *(incontinence, retention)* is the inability to release urine.
12. If a patient complains of an accumulation of fluid around her ankles, she may be exhibiting *(urgency, edema)*.
13. A patient with a renal *(abscess, diuresis)* has a cavity containing pus and surrounded by inflamed tissue in the kidneys.
14. A sign of kidney failure may be excessive urea in the blood, called *(anuria, azotemia)*.
15. A concerned parent calls in to discuss her 4-year-old son's inability to remain dry during the night. This bedwetting may be diagnosed as *(oliguria, enuresis)*.
16. Caffeine and alcohol are substances that cause an increase in the volume of fluids excreted from the body. They effect a/an *(enuresis, diuresis)*.
17. A feeling of a need to urinate immediately is called *(urgency, incontinence)*.
18. The elderly gentleman was seen by his physician because he was unable to control his urination. He was suffering from urinary *(incontinence, retention)*.

BE CAREFUL!

Py/o means *pus,* and *pyel/o* means *renal pelvis.* A dilation of the renal pelvis caused by an accumulation of pus would be pyopyelectasis.

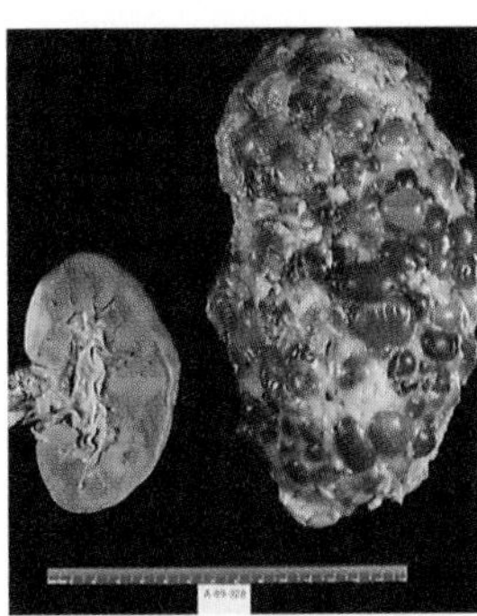

Fig. 6-5 Comparison of a polycystic kidney *(right)* with a normal kidney *(left)*.

DID YOU KNOW?

The term *diabetes* comes from the Greek word meaning to *pass through,* and an excessive production of urine is a symptom in both forms of diabetes. Insipidus refers to the "tasteless" nature of the urine of people with this disorder. Mellitus comes from the Latin word for honey.

Terms Related to Urinary System Disorders, Stones, and Diabetes

TERM	WORD ORIGIN	DEFINITION
Diabetes insipidus (DI) dye ah BEE teez in SIP ih dus	See **Did You Know?** box	Deficiency of antidiuretic (ADH) hormone, which causes the patient to excrete large quantities of urine **(polyuria)** and exhibit excessive thirst **(polydipsia).**
Diabetes mellitus (DM) dye ah BEE teez meh LYE tus	See **Did You Know?** box	Metabolic disease caused by an absolute or relative deficiency of insulin and characterized by hyperglycemia, glycosuria, water and electrolyte loss, ketoacidosis, and possible eventual coma.
Polycystic kidney disease pah lee SIS tick	*poly-* many *cyst/o* sac *-ic* pertaining to	Inherited disorder characterized by an enlargement of the kidneys caused by many bilateral renal cysts that reduce functioning of renal tissue (Fig. 6-5).
Renal colic REE nul KAH lick	*ren/o* kidney *-al* pertaining to	Severe pain associated with stones lodged in the ureter.
Urinary calculi YOOR ih nair ee KAL kyoo lye		Stones anywhere in the urinary tract, but usually in the renal pelvis or urinary bladder. Usually formed in patients with an excess of the mineral calcium. Also called **urolithiasis** (yoo roo lih THIGH uh sis) (Fig. 6-6).
Urinary tract infection (UTI)		Infection anywhere in the urinary system, caused most commonly by bacteria, but also by parasites, yeast, and protozoa (*sing.* protozoon). Most frequently occurring disorder in the urinary system.

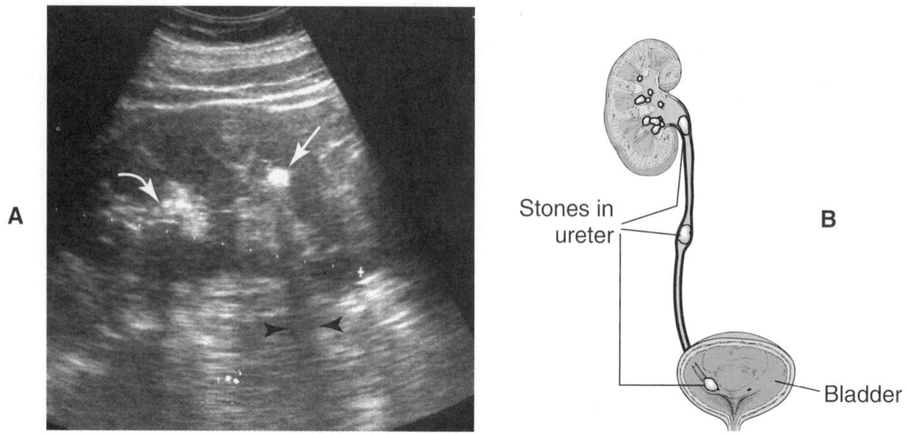

Fig. 6-6 **A,** Ultrasound of stones in the renal pelvis. **B,** Locations of ureteral calculi.

Exercise 4: Urinary Disorders, Stones, and Diabetes

Matching.

_____ 1. inherited congenital disorder of the kidneys

_____ 2. pain caused by a stone lodged in the ureter

_____ 3. disease caused by deficiency of insulin

_____ 4. infection anywhere in the urinary system

_____ 5. deficiency of antidiuretic hormone

_____ 6. stones in the urinary tract

_____ 7. excessive thirst

A. urolithiasis
B. polydipsia
C. polycystic kidney disease
D. diabetes mellitus
E. urinary tract infection
F. renal colic
G. diabetes insipidus

8. Build terms for the following:

A. stones in the kidney _______________

B. stones in the ureter _______________

C. stones in the bladder _______________

D. stones in the urethra _______________

Terms Related to Kidney Disorders		
Term	**Word Origin**	**Definition**
Acute renal failure (ARF)		Sudden inability of the kidneys to excrete wastes, resulting from hemorrhage, trauma, burns, toxic injury to the kidney, pyelonephritis or glomerulonephritis, or lower urinary tract obstruction. Characterized by oliguria and rapid azotemia.
Chronic renal failure (CRF)		Long-term inability of the kidney to excrete wastes.
Glomerulonephritis gloh MUR yoo loh neh FRY tis	*glomerul/o* glomerulus *nephr/o* kidney *-itis* inflammation	Inflammation of the glomeruli of the kidney characterized by proteinuria, hematuria, decreased urine production, and edema.
Hydronephrosis hye droh neh FROH sis	*hydro-* water *nephr/o* kidney *-osis* abnormal condition	Dilation of the pelvis and calices of one or both kidneys resulting from the obstruction of the flow of urine.

Terms Related to Kidney Disorders—cont'd

TERM	WORD ORIGIN	DEFINITION
Nephritic syndrome neh FRIH tick	*nephr/o* kidney *-itic* pertaining to *syn-* together *-drome* to run	Group of signs and symptoms of a urinary tract disorder, including hematuria, hypertension, and renal failure.
Nephritis neh FRY tis	*nephr/o* kidney *-itis* inflammation	Inflammation of the kidney; a general term that does not specify the location of the inflammation or its cause.
Nephropathy neh FROP ah thee	*nephr/o* kidney *-pathy* disease	Disease of the kidneys; a general term that does not specify a disorder.
Nephroptosis neh frop TOH sis	*nephr/o* kidney *-ptosis* drooping, prolapse	Prolapse or sagging of the kidney.
Nephrotic syndrome neh FRAH tick	*nephr/o* kidney *-tic* pertaining to	Abnormal group of symptoms in the kidney, characterized by proteinuria, hypoalbuminemia, and edema; may occur in glomerular disease and as a complication of many systemic diseases (e.g., diabetes mellitus). Also called **nephrosis** (neh FROH sis).
Pyelonephritis pye uh loh neh FRY tis	*pyel/o* renal pelvis *nephr/o* kidney *-itis* inflammation	Infection of the renal pelvis and parenchyma of the kidney, usually the result of lower urinary tract infection.
Renal failure	*ren/o* kidney *-al* pertaining to	Inability of the kidneys to excrete wastes, concentrate urine, and conserve electrolytes.
Renal hypertension	*ren/o* kidney *-al* pertaining to *hyper-* excessive *-tension* pressure	High blood pressure secondary to kidney disease.
Renal sclerosis REE nul sklih ROH sis	*ren/o* kidney *-al* pertaining to *sclerosis* a hardening	Hardening of the arteries of the kidneys. Also known as **nephrosclerosis** (neh froh sklih ROH sis).

Terms Related to Bladder, Ureter, and Urethra Disorders

TERM	WORD ORIGIN	DEFINITION
Cystitis sis TYE tis	*cyst/o* urinary bladder *-itis* inflammation	Inflammation of the urinary bladder.
Cystocele SIS toh seel	*cyst/o* urinary bladder *-cele* herniation	Herniation of the urinary bladder (Fig. 6-7).

Continued

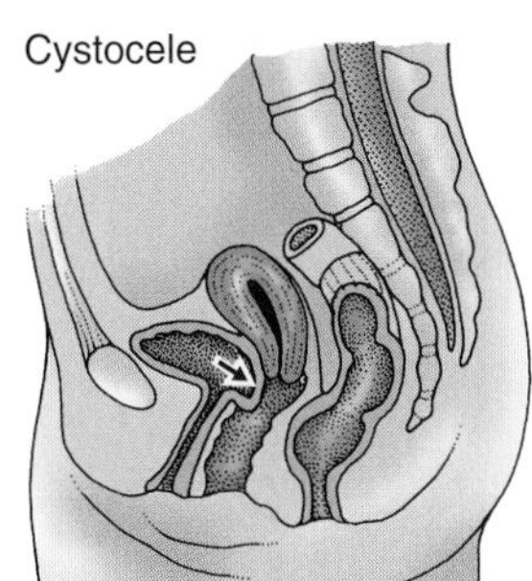

Fig. 6-7 Cystocele. The urinary bladder is displaced downward, which causes bulging of the anterior vaginal wall.

DID YOU KNOW?

Secondary hypertension is hypertension caused by another disorder; if the hypertension is without known cause, then it is called *essential hypertension.*

Terms Related to Bladder, Ureter, and Urethra Disorders—cont'd

TERM	WORD ORIGIN	DEFINITION
Ureterocele yoo REE tur oh seel	*ureter/o* ureter *-cele* herniation	Prolapse of the terminal end of the ureter into the bladder.
Urethral stenosis yoo REE thruhl sten NOH sis	*urethr/o* urethra *-al* pertaining to *stenosis* a narrowing	Narrowing of the urethra. Also called a **urethral stricture.**
Urethritis yoo ree THRY tis	*urethr/o* urethra *-itis* inflammation	Inflammation of the urethra.
Vesicoureteral reflux ves ih koh yoo REE tur ul REE flucks	*vesic/o* urinary bladder *ureter/o* ureter *-al* pertaining to *re-* back *-flux* flow	Abnormal backflow of urine from the bladder to the ureter.

Exercise 5: KIDNEY, URETER, BLADDER, AND URETHRAL DISORDERS

Matching.

_____ 1. -ptosis

_____ 2. hydro-

_____ 3. acute

_____ 4. chronic

_____ 5. syndrome

_____ 6. -cele

A. group of signs/symptoms with a common cause
B. long term
C. prolapse
D. herniation
E. water
F. sudden, severe

Matching.

_____ 7. inability of the kidneys to excrete wastes

_____ 8. a hardening of the arteries of the kidneys

_____ 9. prolapse of the kidney

_____ 10. inflammation of the renal parenchyma and the renal pelvis

_____ 11. disease of the kidney

_____ 12. inflammation of the kidney

_____ 13. hypertension, renal failure and hematuria characterize this syndrome

_____ 14. inflammation of the capillaries within the renal corpuscles

_____ 15. inflammation of the tube leading from the bladder to the outside of the body

_____ 16. inflammation of the bladder

_____ 17. herniation of the tube from the kidney to the bladder

_____ 18. backward flow of urine from the bladder toward the kidney

A. glomerulitis
B. cystitis
C. nephritis
D. nephroptosis
E. vesicourethral reflux
F. urethritis
G. pyelonephritis
H. nephritic syndrome
I. nephrosclerosis
J. nephropathy
K. ureterocele
L. renal failure

DIAGNOSTIC PROCEDURES

Urinalysis

Urinalysis (UA) is the physical, chemical, and/or microscopic examination of urine. The following table gives examples of the constituents examined, and the normal and abnormal findings, with their possible interpretations.

Urinalysis

Physical Examination

Appearance **(Fig. 6-8)**
Normal finding: Clear
Abnormal finding with interpretation: Cloudiness may indicate a UTI.

Color **(Fig. 6-9)**
Normal finding: Straw-colored or light amber
Abnormal findings with interpretations: Lighter color may indicate diabetes insipidus or overhydration. Darker colors may indicate a concentrated urine caused by dehydration, drugs or liver disease.

Quantity
Normal finding: Approximately 1½ liters per day
Abnormal findings with interpretations: Profusion may indicate diabetes insipidus or a variety of other conditions precipitating diuresis. Smaller than normal amounts may be a result of dehydration, blockages, or strictures.

Specific Gravity (SG): Measures the ability of the kidneys to regulate the concentration of urine.
Normal finding: Normal is a reading of 1.015-1.025, which is slightly more dense than the weight of water.
Abnormal findings with interpretations: Diabetes or kidney damage may be the cause of a low specific gravity.

Chemical Examination

Bilirubin
Normal finding: Not present
Abnormal finding with interpretation: Presence may indicate liver disease or biliary obstruction.

Blood
Normal finding: Not present
Abnormal findings with interpretations: Red blood cells may indicate an inflammation or trauma in the urinary tract. White blood cells may indicate a UTI.

Creatinine
Normal finding: 1-2.5 mg/24 hours
Abnormal findings with interpretations: An increase may indicate infection. A decrease may indicate kidney disease.

Glucose
Normal finding: Not present
Abnormal finding with interpretation: A presence may indicate diabetes mellitus.

Continued

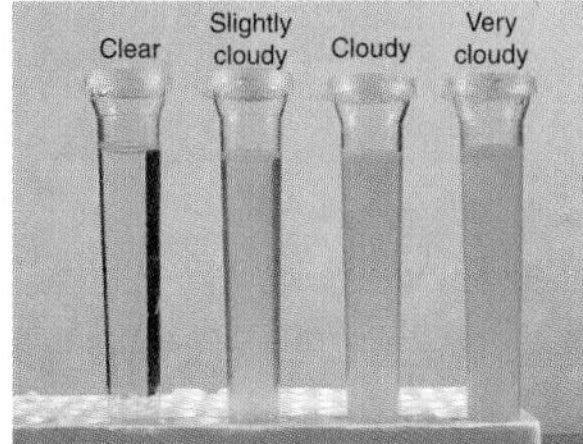

Fig. 6-8 Appearance of urine.

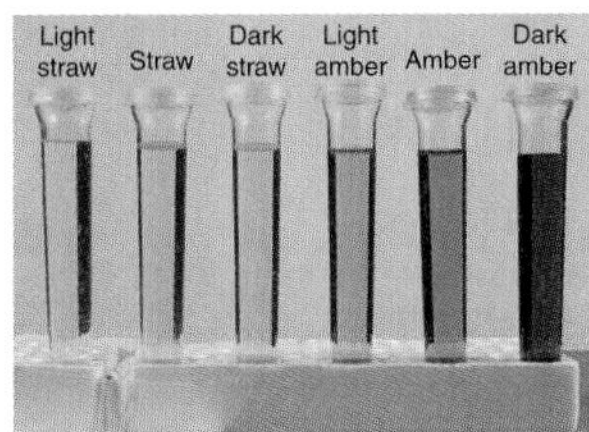

Fig. 6-9 Color of urine.

Urinalysis—cont'd

Chemical Examination—cont'd

Ketones
Normal finding: Not present
Abnormal finding with interpretation: Diabetes mellitus or starvation may be the cause.

pH
Normal finding: 5.0-7.0; slightly acidic is normal.
Abnormal findings with interpretations: pH increases in alkalosis, decreases in high-protein diets.

Protein
Normal finding: Not present
Abnormal findings with interpretations: Increased amounts present in kidney disease; albumin present when glomeruli are damaged.

Microscopic Examination

Bacteria
Normal finding: Not present
Abnormal finding with interpretation: Urinary tract infection

Pus
Normal finding: Not present
Abnormal finding with interpretation: Pyelonephritis

Terms Related to Laboratory Tests

Term	Word Origin	Definition
Blood urea nitrogen (BUN) YOOR ee ah		Blood test that measures the amount of nitrogenous waste in the circulatory system; an increased level is an indicator of kidney dysfunction.
Creatinine clearance test kree AT ih nin		Test of kidney function that measures the rate at which nitrogenous waste is removed from the blood by comparing its concentration in the blood and urine over a 24-hour period.

Terms Related to Imaging

Term	Word Origin	Definition
Computed tomography (CT) scan toh MAH gruh fee	*tom/o* section *-graphy* recording	Computerized image that shows a "slice" of the body.
Intravenous urography (IVU) in truh VEE nus yoo RAH gruh fee	*intra-* within *ven/o* vein *-ous* pertaining to *ur/o* urinary system *-graphy* process of recording	Radiographic imaging of the kidneys, ureters, and bladder done with a contrast medium (Fig. 6-10). Also called **intravenous pyelography (IVP).**

Terms Related to Imaging—cont'd

TERM	WORD ORIGIN	DEFINITION
Kidneys, ureters, and bladder (KUB)		Radiographic imaging of the kidney, ureters, and bladder without a contrast medium.
Nephrotomography neh froh toh MAH gruh fee	*nephr/o* kidney *tom/o* section *-graphy* process of recording	Sectional radiographic exam of the kidneys.
Voiding cystourethrography (VCUG) VOY ding sis toh yoor ee THRAH gruh fee	*cyst/o* bladder *urethr/o* urethra *-graphy* process of recording	Radiographic imaging of the urinary bladder and urethra done with a contrast medium while patient is urinating (Fig. 6-11).

Terms Related to Other Diagnostic Procedures

TERM	WORD ORIGIN	DEFINITION
Biopsy BYE op see	*bi/o* life, living *-opsy* viewing	Taking a piece of tissue for microscopic study. A **closed biopsy** is done by an endoscopy or aspiration (by suction through a fine needle). An **open biopsy** is done through an incision.
Cystoscopy sis TOSS koh pee	*cyst/o* bladder *-scopy* visual examination	Visual examination of the urinary bladder using a cystoscope (Fig. 6-12).

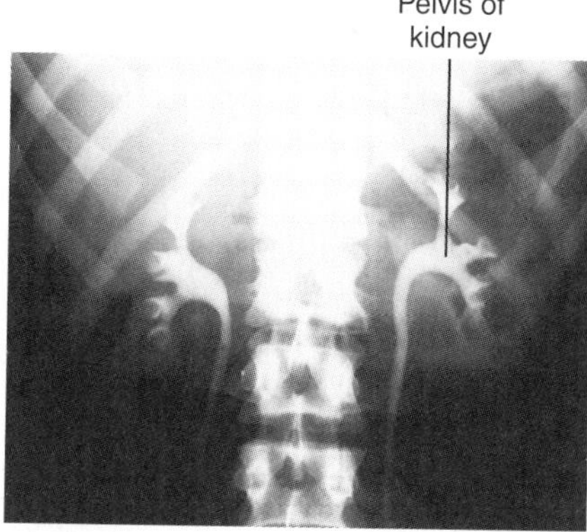

Fig. 6-10 Intravenous urogram (IVU).

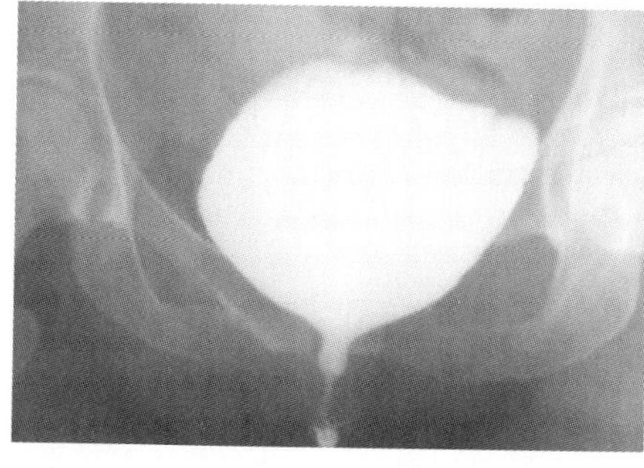

Fig. 6-11 Female voiding cystourethrogram (VCUG).

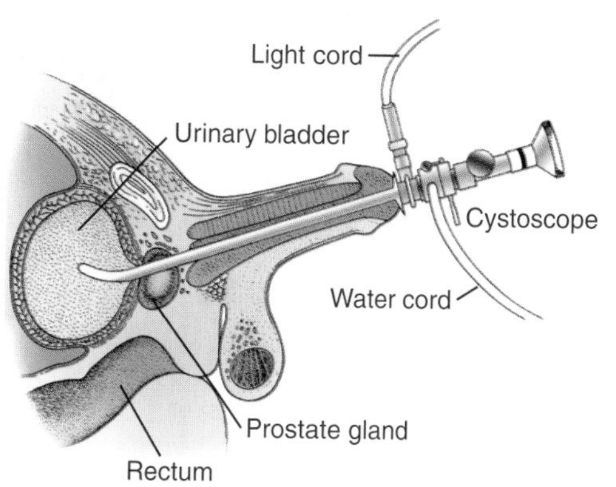

Fig. 6-12 Cystoscopy.

Terms Related to Instruments

TERM	WORD ORIGIN	DEFINITION
Catheter KATH uh tur		Hollow, flexible tube that can be inserted into a vessel, organ, or cavity of the body to withdraw or instill fluid, monitor types of various information, and visualize a vessel or cavity. Catheters can be inserted through the urethra into the bladder to drain urine (Fig. 6-13).
Cystoscope SIS toh skohp	*cyst/o* urinary bladder *-scope* instrument for visual examination	Instrument for visual examination of the inside of the bladder. (See Fig. 6-12 for a drawing of a cystoscope.)
Laparoscope LAP ur oh skohp	*lapar/o* abdomen *-scope* instrument for visual examination	Type of endoscope consisting of an illuminated tube with an optical system, inserted through the abdominal wall for examining the peritoneal cavity.
Lithotrite LITH oh tryte	*lith/o* stone *-trite* instrument to crush stones	Instrument used to crush a calculus in the urinary bladder; fragments may then be expelled or washed out.
Nephroscope NEFF roh skohp	*nephr/o* kidney *-scope* instrument for visual examination	Fiberoptic instrument used specifically for the disintegration and removal of renal calculi; an ultrasonic probe emitting high-frequency sound waves breaks up the calculi, which are removed by suction through the scope.
Stent stehnt		Tubular device for supporting hollow structures during surgical anastomosis or for holding arteries open after angioplasty.
Urinometer yoor ih NOM meh tur	*urin/o* urine *-meter* instrument to measure	Type of hydrometer used to measure the specific gravity (SG) of a urine sample. Also known as a **urometer.**

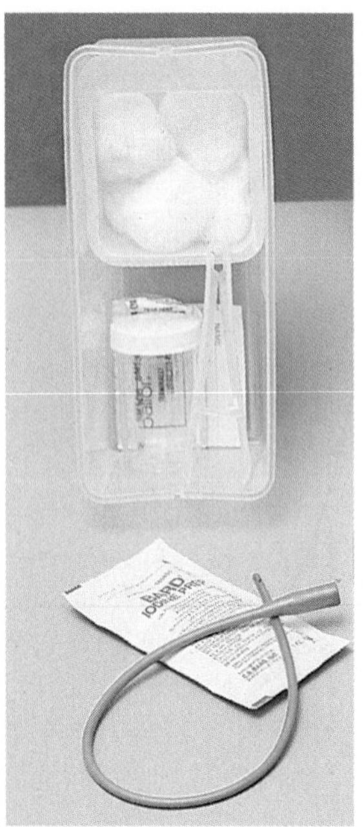

Fig. 6-13 *Top,* Indwelling catheter kit. *Bottom,* Straight catheter.

Exercise 6: DIAGNOSTIC PROCEDURES

Using the urinalysis table provided on pp. 163-164, answer the following.

If a urinalysis reveals:

1. a small amount of urine, then the patient may have

   ____________________.

2. pus in the urine, then the patient may have

   ____________________.

3. a low specific gravity, then the patient may have

   ____________________.

4. the presence of white blood cells, then the patient may have

   ____________________.

5. the presence of bacteria, then the patient may have

_______________________________.

6. the presence of ketones, then the patient may have _______________________________.

Fill in the blanks.

7. Both the BUN and creatinine clearance tests measure the function of the ______________ in their ability to remove waste from the blood.

8. BUN stands for _______________________________.
9. X-rays of the urinary system may take many forms. A radiographic technique that images the kidneys, ureters, and bladder using a contrast medium is called ______________.
10. A sectional radiographic exam of the kidney is called nephrotomography.
11. A radiographic technique that images the bladder and urethra while the patient is voiding is called VCUG.
12. Endoscopies are visual examinations of the interior of the body. Name a visual examination of the following:

    A. kidney _______________________________

    B. ureters _______________________________

    C. bladder _______________________________

    D. urethra _______________________________
13. If a biopsy is done through an incision, it is considered ______________.

Matching.

_____ 14. a tube for supporting structures

_____ 15. an instrument to measure SG of urine

_____ 16. a tube to insert in an organ

_____ 17. an instrument to crush stones

_____ 18. an instrument to view the bladder

E 19. an instrument to view the kidney and crush stones within it

A. catheter
B. stent
C. lithotrite
D. urinometer
E. nephroscope
F. cystoscope

Case Study Continued

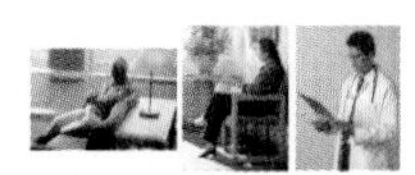

Consulting with the resident on call, Brian is immediately sent for imaging and lab studies. The imaging order calls for an x-ray of the abdomen, a renal ultrasound, and a spiral CT scan to rule out a suspected urinary calculus. The CBC is normal, but the urinalysis reveals a finding of blood in the urine and an abnormally low pH.

After 2 hours of dreary TV reruns and well-thumbed magazines, Tim calls Margarette, takes notes on her symptoms, and then leads her back to a bathroom, where she is instructed to give a urine sample.

THERAPEUTIC INTERVENTIONS

Terms Related to Therapeutic Interventions		
TERM	**WORD ORIGIN**	**DEFINITION**
Ileal conduit ILL ee ul KON doo it	*ile/o* ileum *-al* pertaining to	Channel, pipe, or tube that guides urine from the ureters to the ileum in the digestive system to be excreted through the large intestine, when the bladder is no longer available for storing the urine and releasing it through the urethra. Also known as a **ureteroileostomy** (yoo ree tur oh ill ee AH stuh mee).
Lithotripsy LITH oh trip see	*lith/o* stone *-tripsy* crushing	Process of crushing stones either to prevent or clear an obstruction in the urinary system; crushing may be manual, by high-energy shock waves, or by pulsed dye laser. In either case, the fragments may be expelled naturally or washed out (Fig. 6-14).
Nephrectomy neh FRECK tuh mee	*nephr/o* kidney *-ectomy* removal	Resection of the kidney.
Nephrolithotomy neh froh lith AH tuh mee	*nephr/o* kidney *-lithotomy* removal of a stone	Removal of a kidney stone.
Nephropexy neh froh PECK see	*nephr/o* kidney *-pexy* suspension	Suspension or fixation of the kidney.
Nephrostolithotomy neh frah stoh lith AH tuh mee	*nephr/o* kidney *stom/o* opening *-lithotomy* removal of a stone	Removal of a stone from the kidney through a preexisting nephrostomy.
Nephrostomy neh FRAH stuh mee	*nephr/o* kidney *-stomy* new opening	Opening made in the kidney so that a catheter can be inserted.
Nephrotomy neh FRAH tuh mee	*nephr/o* kidney *-tomy* incision	Incision of the kidney.
Transurethral procedure trans yoo REE thrul	*trans-* through *urethr/o-* urethra *-al* pertaining to	Any procedure conducted through the urethra.
Urethrolysis yoo ree THRAH lih sis	*urethr/o* urethra *-lysis* destruction of adhesions	Destruction of the adhesions of the urethra.
Vesicotomy vess ih KAH tuh mee	*vesic/o* bladder *-tomy* incision	Incision of the urinary bladder.

Subject: Unit 8 URL's Angie

Message no. 280

Author: Angela Fox

Date: Friday, November 7, 2003 1:39pm

The first website is carboxylic acids practice problems. These would be great to go over before a test or quiz. http://www.cem.msu.edu/~cem252/sp97/ch19/ch19practice.html The second website I found is about conductivity of carboxylic acids. It has a lot more information on there as well. It shows various kinds of expirments that would be helpful in a chemistry course. http://jchemed.chem.wisc.edu/JCESoft/CCA/CCA5/MAIN/1ORGANIC/ORG15/MENU.HTM Angie Fox

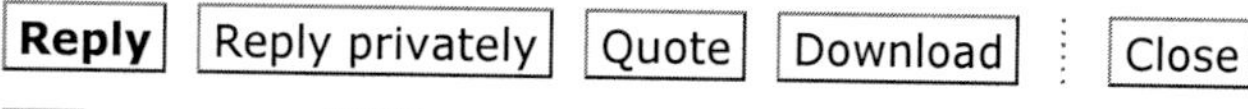

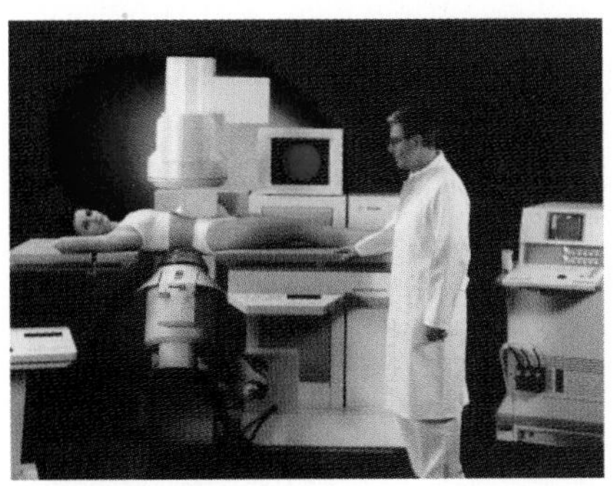

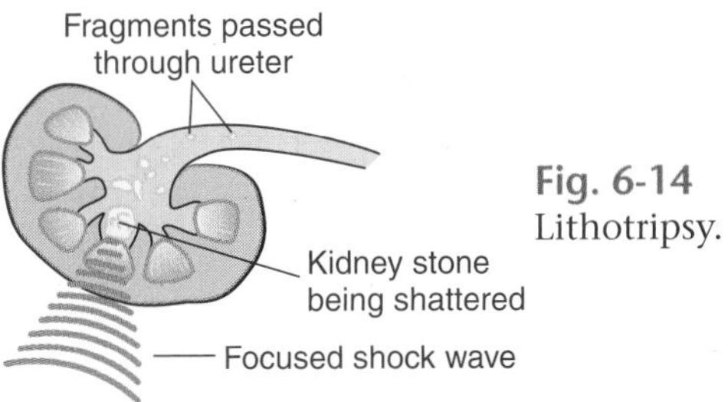

Fig. 6-14 Lithotripsy.

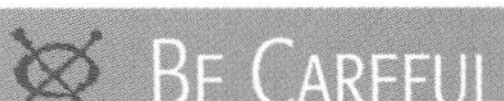

Do not confuse *ilium,* which is a *pelvic bone,* with *ileum,* which is a *part of the small intestine.*

Terms Related to Kidney Failure Treatment

TERM	WORD ORIGIN	DEFINITION
Continuous ambulatory peritoneal dialysis (CAPD) pair eh tuh NEE ul dye AL ih sis	*peritone/o* peritoneum *-al* pertaining to *dia-* through, complete *-lysis* separation, breakdown	Type of renal dialysis in which an indwelling catheter in the abdomen permits fluid to drain into and out of the peritoneal cavity to cleanse the blood.
Hemodialysis (HD) hee moh dye AL ih sis	*hem/o* blood *dia-* through, complete *-lysis* separation, breakdown	Type of renal dialysis that cleanses the blood by shunting it from the body through a machine for diffusion and ultrafiltration and then returning it to the patient's circulation.
Renal dialysis dye AL ih sis	*ren/o* kidney *-al* pertaining to *dia-* through, complete *-lysis* separation, breakdown	Process of diffusing blood across a semipermeable membrane to remove substances that a healthy kidney would eliminate, including poisons, drugs, urea, uric acid, and creatinine.
Renal transplantation	*ren/o* kidney *-al* pertaining to *trans-* across *-plant* a sprout or shoot	Surgical transfer of a complete kidney from a donor to a recipient (Fig. 6-15).

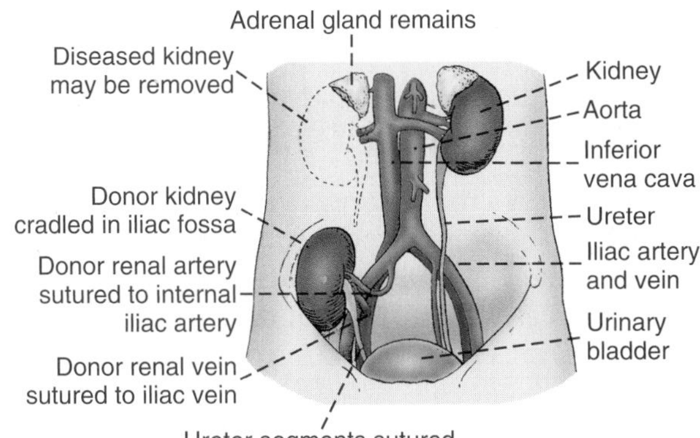

Fig. 6-15 Kidney transplant.

DID YOU KNOW?

Transplants are the grafting of an organ or tissue from one site to another and acquire their name from the process of grafting plants.

Exercise 7: URINARY THERAPEUTIC INTERVENTIONS

Matching.

____ 1. excision of a kidney

____ 2. incision of a kidney

____ 3. removal of a renal calculus

____ 4. fixation of a kidney

____ 5. new opening of a kidney

____ 6. removal of a stone from the kidney through a preexisting opening

A. nephrostolithotomy
B. nephrolithotomy
C. nephrectomy
D. nephrostomy
E. nephrotomy
F. nephropexy

Fill in the blank with one of the following choices.

lithotripsy, renal transplant, ileal conduit, urethrolysis, dialysis procedures

7. What is the healthcare term for the destruction of adhesions in the urethra?

____

8. What is another term for a ureteroileostomy? ____________________________
9. The patient with renal calculi was a candidate for a procedure in which the stones were crushed. This is called ____________________________.
10. What do CAPD and HD have in common? ____________________________
11. Roger experienced kidney failure and required the surgical transplantation of a complete kidney from a donor. This procedure is called a/an ____________________________.

Case Study Continued

Brian's CT scan shows a left distal ureteral stone and hydronephrosis. His physician tells him he needs to have a ureteroscopic stone extraction. Tim helps Brian contact his family and make arrangements for hospitalization.

PHARMACOLOGY

Acidifiers/Alkalinizers: Drugs that change the pH of the urine.
Antidiuretics: Drugs that suppress urine formation.
Antispasmodics: Drugs that help prevent muscle spasms in the bladder.
Diuretics: Drugs that increase the formation of urine.
Enuresis management: Drugs that help control urinary incontinence, especially bedwetting.
Stone prevention agents: Calcium oxalate or uric acid.
Urinary antiinfectives: Drugs that fight infection in the urinary system, such as antibiotics, and antifungals.

Exercise 8: PHARMACOLOGY

Matching.

_____ 1. diuretic

_____ 2. antispasmodic

_____ 3. antiinfective

_____ 4. stone prevention agent

_____ 5. enuresis management

_____ 6. acidifier, alkalinizer

_____ 7. antidiuretic

A. calcium oxalate, uric acid
B. suppresses urine formation
C. prevents muscle spasms
D. changes the pH of urine
E. increases formation of urine
F. antibiotics, antifungals
G. helps control urinary incontinence

Case Study Continued

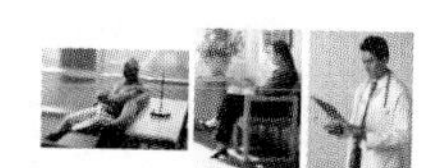

Margarette's lab results come back positive for the common type of uncomplicated urinary tract infection, *E coli*. Her physician prescribes an antibiotic. After Tim explains the need to take the entire prescription, she heads home after having the prescription filled at her local pharmacy.

Abbreviations

Abbreviation	Definition	Abbreviation	Definition
ADH	Antidiuretic hormone	IVU	Intravenous urography
ARF	Acute renal failure	K	Potassium
BUN	Blood urea nitrogen	KUB	Kidneys, ureters, bladder
CAPD	Continuous ambulatory peritoneal dialysis	L	Liter
CRF	Chronic renal failure	mg	Milligram
Cl	Chloride	Na	Sodium
CT	Computed tomography	pH	Acidity/alkalinity
cysto	Cystoscopy	SG	Specific gravity
DI	Diabetes insipidus	STD	Sexually transmitted disease
DM	Diabetes mellitus	UA	Urinalysis
ESRD	End stage renal disease	UTI	Urinary tract infection
ESWL	Extracorporeal shockwave lithotripsy	VCUG	Voiding cystourethrography
HD	Hemodialysis		

Exercise 9: ABBREVIATIONS

Write the meanings of the abbreviations.

1. The patient with DM had produced 3.0 L of urine in the last 24 hours.

____

2. The patient with CRF was treated with HD.

____

3. Ellen's UA noted a low SG. The diagnosis was DI.

4. Antonia was treated for a UTI.

5. A VCUG helped to confirm the patient's diagnosis of hydronephrosis.

Careers

Triage Nurses

Although many people would run from the possibility, some individuals crave the excitement of a career that demands decision making, often under tremendous pressure. One setting for that type of work is the emergency department (ED). Numerous television shows have drawn attention to the types of situations that employees may face in that kind of setting.

One potential career path to explore is that of triage nurse. The term *triage* is derived from an Old French term meaning *to sift.* The triage nurse sorts ED patients according to the urgency of their complaints and puts them in the order in which they will be seen by the physicians. The triage nurse is also responsible for an initial assessment, noting all pertinent information necessary for further evaluation and treatment of the patient.

Related to the ED triage nurse is the telephone triage nurse, a position that allows patients to be "sorted" over the phone as to the severity of their disorders. These nurses work in a specialty area that has grown in response to increasing healthcare costs and overutilized emergency departments.

Ideally, both the triage nurse and the telephone triage nurse would have experience in med-surg nursing practice dealing with a wide variety of patient disorders. The American Nurses Association has a series of links to specialty sites that include the Emergency Nurses Association (ENA), as well as Trauma Information Pages. The Website is http://nursingworld.org/rnindex/snp.htm. The ENA site has information on certification for this vocation.

http: INTERNET PROJECT

Bilateral kidney failure signifies the loss of the body's ability to filter toxins and fluids from the blood. Using the Websites listed as a starting point, answer the following questions:

- How prevalent are the three types of kidney failure in the United States?
- What are the main causes of kidney failure?
- What are the symptoms of kidney failure?
- What treatments are available?
- What, if any, clinical trials are available for treating kidney failure?
- What are the ways to prevent kidney failure?
- What are the demographic differences (e.g., sex, race, age) in kidney failure?

Here are a few Websites to get you started.
National Kidney Foundation: http://www.kidney.org
National Institute of Diabetes and Digestive and Kidney Diseases: http://www.niddk.nih.gov
MEDLINEplus: Kidney Failure and Dialysis: http://www.nlm.nih.gov/medlineplus/kidneyfailureanddialysis.html
Mayo Clinic: Kidney Failure: http://www.mayoclinic.com/invoke.cfm?id=DS00280

Chapter Review

A. Functions of the Urinary System

Fill in the blanks.

1. In your own words, describe the functions of the urinary system.

   ____

   ____

   ____

2. The urinary system removes protein wastes from the body called ______________, ______________, and ______________.

3. The term that means a *steady state* or state of equilibrium in the body is ______________.

4. The kidneys monitor the ______________-cellular fluid in the body.

5. Terms for the process of excreting urine are ______________, ______________, and ______________.

B. Anatomy and Physiology

6. Label the urinary system drawings below with the following terms: kidneys, ureters, bladder, urethra. Include their combining forms.

7. Label the cross-section of the kidney below, filling in the renal pelvis, renal medulla and cortex, calyx, hilum, ureter, and blood vessels entering and exiting. Include combining forms.

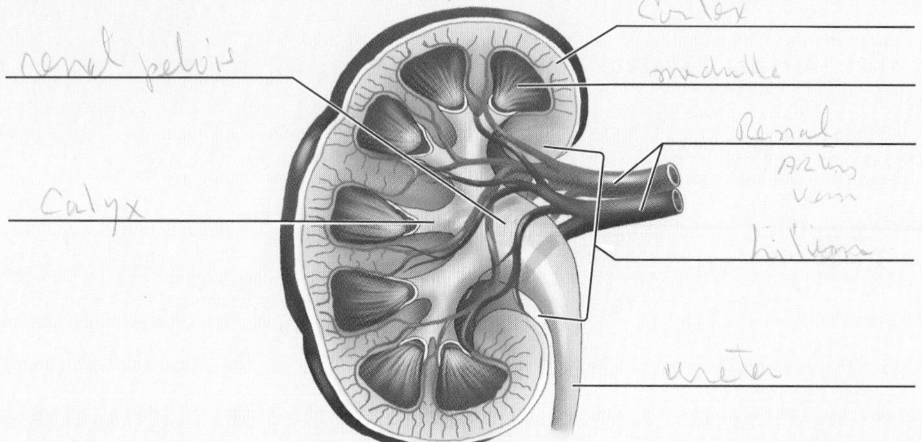

8. The ______________ is the working unit of the kidney. What is the name of the bundle of the capillaries in the nephron? ______________

9. What is the name of the capsule that encloses this bundle? ______________________

10. Name the substances that are normally filtered out of the bloodstream in the nephron.

____

____

____

C. Pathology

11. If someone cannot control urination, he or she is said to have urinary ______________.

12. If someone is unable to urinate, he or she is described as having urinary ______________.

13. An excessive excretion of urine is called ______________.

14. A healthcare term for "bedwetting" is ______________.

15. When the kidneys are not functioning correctly, they may be responsible for an accumulation of fluid in the tissues called ______________ and/or high blood pressure called ______________.

Build a term.

16. What is the term for inflammation of the kidneys? ______________________

17. What is the term for disease of the kidney? ______________________

18. What is a term for an abnormal condition of the kidneys? ______________________

19. What is the term for a prolapse of the kidneys? ______________________________

20. What is the term for "pertaining to the kidney"? (use ren/o) ______________________________

Decode the term.

21. urethral stenosis ______________________________

22. urethroplasty ______________________________

23. ureterocele ______________________________

24. pyelonephritis ______________________________

25. meatotomy ______________________________

26. nephrolithiasis ______________________________

27. glomerulonephritis ______________________________

28. pyuria ______________________________

29. hematuria ______________________________

30. oliguria ______________________________

31. anuria ______________________________

32. polyuria ______________________________

33. bacteriuria ______________________________

34. albuminuria ______________________________

D. Diagnostic Procedures
Circle the correct answers.

35. Patients with UTIs would be expected to have which of the following abnormal results on UA? *(glucose, protein, bacteria, appearance, quantity, blood, ketones)*
36. A patient with diabetes mellitus would normally have which abnormal results on UA? *(glucose, protein, bacteria, appearance, blood, creatinine, color)*
37. A patient with dehydration and starvation may be expected to have abnormal readings of which of the following on UA? *(bacteria, color, bilirubin, blood, quantity, ketones)*

Fill in the blank.

38. The test that measures the amount of urea in the blood is called a/an ______________.

39. A nephrotomogram is a ______________________________.

40. Patients who have a piece of living tissue removed through an incision, have a ______________.

41. An imaging technique of the kidneys, ureters, and bladder that uses a contrast medium is a/an ______________.

42. What is the difference between a stent and a catheter?

____

43. What does a urinometer do?

____

44. A lithotrite is an instrument to _______________________________________.

E. Therapeutic Interventions

Build a term.

45. a new opening of the ureter ____________________

46. removal of adhesions from the urethra ____________________

47. procedures via the urethra ____________________

48. incision of a kidney ____________________

Decode the term.

49. nephrolithotomy _______________________________________

50. urethrolysis _______________________________________

51. nephrostomy _______________________________________

52. nephrostolithotomy _______________________________________

53. vesicotomy _______________________________________

Fill in the blank.

54. Placement of a hollow tube for the purpose of removing urine is called urinary ______________.

55. A patient who has his blood cleansed by a machine undergoes ______________.

56. Donation and implantation of a kidney is a kidney ______________.

57. If a patient has nephrolithiasis, she might be a candidate for which type of procedure? ______________

58. Nephroptosis may be corrected by Nephropexy.

59. Ureteroileostomy is also known as ileal Conduit.

F. Pharmacology

60. Ms. Hartzel has been prescribed calcium oxalate because she needed a ______________ prevention agent for her nephrolithiasis.

61. Ms. Hancock has been prescribed a urinary ______________ for her cystitis.

62. Five-year-old Winston is on a course of drugs to control his bedwetting. They are designed to affect

______________ management.

63. Solomon Muntz dropped by to pick up his prescription to help him get rid of retained fluid. He is picking up a type of ________________.

64. Susan Small is behind Mr. Muntz in line. She has diabetes insipidus and needs her medication to control the symptom of profuse urination. It is a/an ________________.

G. Abbreviations

Give the appropriate abbreviation for the following.

65. A patient has stones removed through the use of high-frequency sound waves, or ________________.

66. A woman calls, complaining of fever, urinary urgency, and dysuria. She probably has a/an ________________.

67. A series of tests to examine a urine sample is ________________.

68. The acid/alkaline description of the urine is its ________________.

69. An abbreviation for a visual examination of the urinary bladder is called ________________.

70. While awaiting a kidney transplant, Ms. Jones goes 3 times a week to have impurities removed from her blood by machine. The abbreviation for this procedure is ________________.

71. The abbreviations for sodium, chloride, and potassium electrolytes are ________________, ________________ and ________________.

72. An ambulatory type of dialysis that uses an indwelling catheter that permits fluid to drain into and out of the peritoneal cavity to cleanse the blood is abbreviated ____CAPP____.

73. An abbreviation for an x-ray of the kidneys without a contrast medium is ____KUB____.

74. An abbreviation for an imaging technique of the patient as he/she is urinating is ____VCUG____.

75. An abbreviation for a long-term failure of the kidneys to function is ____CRF____.

H. Singulars and Plurals

Change the following terms from singular to plural.

76. nephrosis ________________________________

77. urethra ________________________________

78. kidney ________________________________

79. glomerulus ________________________________

80. calyx ____Calyeces____

81. nephropathy ________________________________

82. calculus ________________________________

83. urinalysis ________________________________

84. protozoon ______________________________

85. bacterium ______________________________

I. Translations

In your own words, rewrite the following sentences.

86. A 34-year-old patient was admitted with edema and hypertension. Her lab work showed that she had a high BUN and albuminuria.

____

____

87. The 88-year-old woman was admitted for severe dehydration, fainting, and anuria.

____

____

88. Mr. Samuels was treated for his nephrolithiasis with lithotripsy.

____

____

89. Once a UTI was ruled out, Rebecca was evaluated for ongoing enuresis.

____

____

90. A cystoscope was used to locate the site of a small urinary abscess in the patient's bladder.

____

____

J. Cumulative Review

Circle the correct answer.

91. The kidneys are *(inferior, superior)* to the bladder.
92. The *(distal, proximal)* end of the femur is at the patella.
93. The *(distal, proximal)* end of the stomach meets the esophagus.
94. The appendix is in the *(lower right, lower left)* quadrant.
95. Someone who has indigestion has *(dyspepsia, dysphagia)*.
96. There are *(five, seven, twelve)* bones in the cervical spine.
97. A *(compound, complicated)* fracture is a broken bone that pierces the skin.
98. A condition of excessive sweating is *(hyperhidrosis, hyperhydrosis)*.
99. The healthcare term for a wart is a *(nevus, verruca)*.
100. The healthcare term for a black and blue mark is a/an *(cicatrix, ecchymosis)*.

K. Be Careful

Circle the correct term or combining form.

101. One of the bones in the hip? *ileum* or *ilium*
102. The renal pelvis? *py/o* or *pyel/o*
103. The lining of the abdomen? *perone/o*, *peritone/o*, or *perine/o*
104. The suffix for urinary condition? *urea* or *uria*
105. Conducting away from a structure? *afferent* or *efferent*
106. The renal calyx? *calic/o* or *calc/o*

St. Mary's Hospital
999 Holyoke Drive
Boston, MA 01922

OPERATIVE REPORT

Patient: Brian Coulter MR#: 949 821
Physician: Alex Romanov Date: 6/17/01
Preoperative Diagnosis: Left ureteral calculus with hydronephrosis
Postoperative Diagnosis: Left ureteral calculus with hydronephrosis
Procedures: Cystoscopy, retrograde pyelogram, and ureteroscopic stone extraction
Anesthesia: General
Indications: This 59-year-old male with a 3-week history of left flank pain developed an acute exacerbation of LLQ pain, nausea, and vomiting, with subsequent appearance in the emergency room. A CT scan demonstrated a 0.9-cm stone in the distal left ureter, with a prominent hydronephrosis.
Procedure: Patient was brought to the OR, properly identified, and, following administration of general anesthesia, placed in a dorsal lithotomy position. The genitalia were prepared with Betadine and draped in a sterile manner.

Cystoscopy was performed, demonstrating a normal bladder. The left ureteral orifice was identified and a cone-tip catheter inserted. A retrograde pyelogram demonstrated a normal-caliber distal ureter with a faintly opacified stone present 2 cm from the distal ureter, with a proximal hydronephrosis.

A flexible-tip, movable-cord guide wire was inserted through the ureter and threaded adjacent to the stone and up to the level of the renal pelvis under fluoroscopic guidance. A balloon dilating catheter was inserted into the distal ureter and dilated to 12 atmospheres of pressure. After withdrawing the balloon dilating catheter, the #13 French Olympus ureteroscope was inserted atraumatically under direct vision into the distal ureter. Immediately on entering the ureter, the stone was identified tumbling free within the distal dilated ureter. The stone was engaged in a stone basket and delivered atraumatically through the distal ureter.

The specimen was sent to the laboratory for stone analysis. Inspection of the ureter revealed no residual fragments or strictures. The bladder was drained, the cystoscope removed, and the patient was sent to the recovery room in stable condition.

____
Gina Ramirez (surgeon)

L. Operative Report

107. What is a left ureteral calculus? ____________________
108. How do we know that there was no abnormal narrowing of the ureter?

____

109. What term describes the sudden onset of symptoms? ____________________

110. Did the ureteral calculus cause an obstruction? ____________________

How do you know? ____________________
111. What were all the instruments and/or procedures used to image the problem?

____

112. What term indicates that no further injury was caused by the surgery?

____

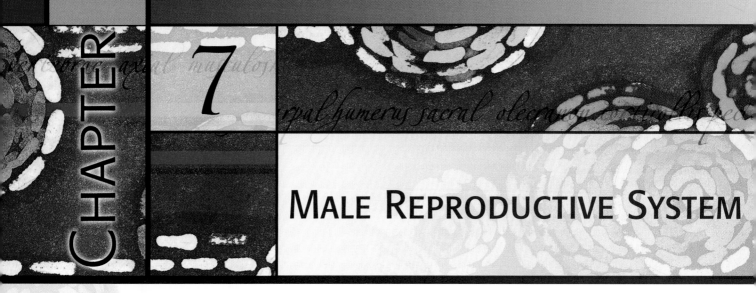

Chapter 7 Male Reproductive System

"Recognizing and preventing men's health problems is not just a man's issue. Because of its import on wives, mothers, daughters, and sisters, men's health is truly a family issue." **—Congressman Bill Richardson**

Quote

Case Study

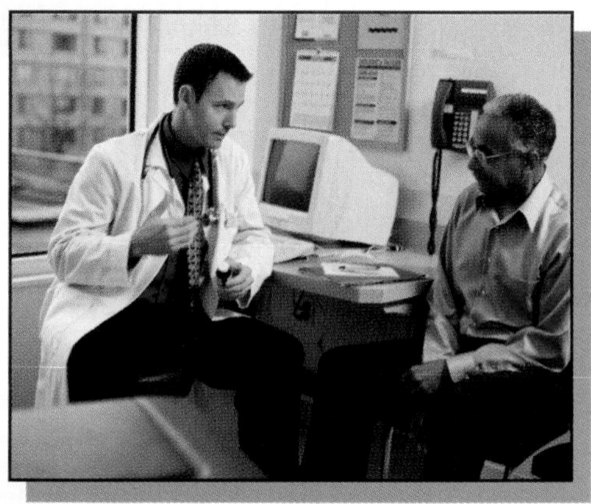

Sam Trudell, a 64-year-old retired postman, has come to see Adam Duncan, a physician's assistant (PA) in a family physician practice. Mr. Trudell has been suffering from decreased ability to urinate and suspects he has another urinary tract infection (UTI), the second in as many months. Adam tells Mr. Trudell that he suspects an enlarged prostate is causing his problem.

OBJECTIVES

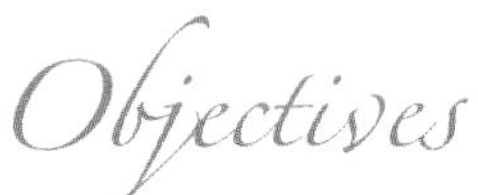

- In your own words, explain the functions of the male reproductive system.
- Recognize, recall, and apply healthcare terms related to the anatomy and physiology of the male reproductive system.
- Recognize, recall, and apply healthcare terms related to the pathology of the male reproductive system.
- Recognize, recall, and apply healthcare terms related to diagnostic procedures of the male reproductive system.
- Recognize, recall, and apply healthcare terms related to the therapeutic interventions of the male reproductive system.
- Recognize, recall, and apply the abbreviations introduced in this chapter.
- Recognize, recall, and apply word components used in this chapter to build and decode healthcare terms relevant to the male reproductive system.
- Recognize, recall, and apply material learned in previous chapters.

FUNCTIONS OF THE MALE REPRODUCTIVE SYSTEM

The function of the male reproductive system is to reproduce. In the process of providing half of the genetic material (in the form of spermatozoa) necessary to form a new person—and then successfully storing, transporting, and delivering this material to fertilize the female counterpart, the ovum—the species survives.

ANATOMY AND PHYSIOLOGY

Both the male and female anatomy can be divided into two parts: **parenchymal** (puh REN kih mul), or primary tissue, which produces sex cells for reproduction; and **stromal** (STROH mul), or secondary tissue, which includes all of the glands, nerves, ducts, and other tissues that serve a supportive function in producing, maintaining, and transmitting these sex cells. Together these types of reproductive tissue, in either sex, are called **genitalia** (jen ih TAIL ee ah). The parenchymal organs that produce the sex cells in either sex are called **gonads** (GOH nads). The sex cells themselves are called **gametes** (GAM eets).

In the male, the gonads are the **testes** (TESS teez) (*sing.* testis) or **testicles** (TESS tick kuls), paired organs that produce the gametes called **spermatozoa** (spur mat ah ZOH ah) (*sing.* spermatozoon). The testes are suspended in a sac called the **scrotum** (SKROH tum) (*pl.* scrota) outside the body (Fig. 7-1).

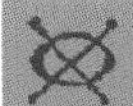

BE CAREFUL!

Don't confuse *vesic/o,* which means the *urinary bladder,* and *vesicul/o,* which means the *seminal vesicle.*

At **puberty** (PYOO bur tee), the stage in life in which males and females become functionally capable of sexual reproduction, the interstitial cells in the testicles begin to produce **testosterone** (tess TOSS tur rohn), a sex hormone responsible for the growth and development of male sex characteristics. The spermatozoa are formed in a series of tightly coiled tiny tubes in each testis called the **seminiferous tubules** (sem ih NIFF ur us TOO byools). The formation of sperm is called **spermatogenesis** (spur mat toh JEN ih sis). The serous membrane that surrounds the front and sides of the testicle is called the **tunica vaginalis testis** (TOON ih kah vaj ih NAL is TESS tis). From the seminiferous tubules, the formed spermatozoa travel to the **epididymis** (eh pih DID ih mis) (*pl.* epididymides), where they are stored.

When the seminal fluid is about to be ejected from the urethra **(ejaculation)**, the spermatozoa travel through the left and right **vas deferens** (vas DEH fur ens), also called the **ductus deferens** (DUCK tus DEH fur ens), from the epididymides,

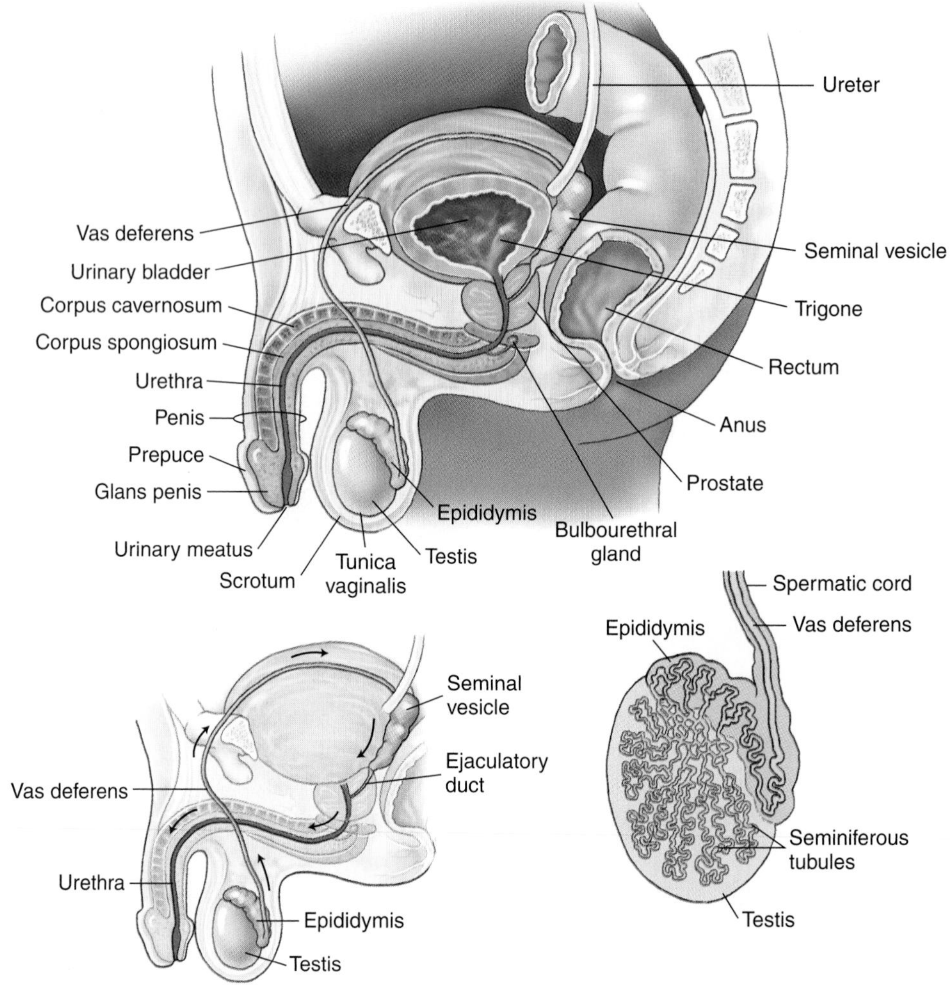

Fig. 7-1 Male reproductive system with inset of sperm production.

around the bladder. The **spermatic cord** is an enclosed sheath that includes the vas deferens, along with arteries, veins, and nerves.

In order to survive and thrive, the sperm are nourished by fluid from a series of glands. The **seminal vesicles** (SEM ih nul VESS ih kuls), **Cowper** (or **bulbourethral** [bul boh yoo REE thrul] glands, and **prostate** (PROS tate) gland provide fluid either to nourish or to aid in motility and lubrication. The sperm and the fluid together make up a substance called **semen** (SEE men). The **ejaculatory duct** (ee JACK yoo lah tore ee) begins where the seminal vesicles join the vas deferens, and this "tube" joins the urethra. Once the sperm reach the urethra, they travel out through the shaft, or body, of the **penis** (PEE nuss), which is composed of three columns of highly vascular erectile tissue. There are two columns of **corpora cavernosa** (KORE poor ah kav ur NOH suh) and one of **corpus spongiosum** (KORE puss spun jee OH sum) that fill with blood through the dorsal veins during sexual arousal. During ejaculation, the sperm exit through the enlarged tip of the penis, the **glans penis.** At birth, the glans penis is surrounded by a fold of skin called the **prepuce** (PREE pyoos), or **foreskin.** The removal of this skin is termed **circumcision** (sur kum SIH zhun).

When ejaculation occurs during sexual intercourse (**coitus** [KOH ih tus] or **copulation** [kop yoo LAY shun]), the sperm then race toward the female sex cell, or ovum. If a specific sperm penetrates and unites with the ovum, **conception** takes place, and formation of an embryo begins.

COMBINING FORMS FOR ANATOMY AND PHYSIOLOGY

MEANING	COMBINING FORM
epididymis	epididym/o
glans penis	balan/o
penis	pen/i, phall/o
prepuce	preputi/o
prostate	prostat/o
scrotum	scrot/o
semen	semin/i
seminal vesicle	vesicul/o
spermatozoon	sperm/o, spermat/o
testicle, testis	test/o, testicul/o, orch/o, orchi/o, orchid/o
urethra	urethr/o
vas deferens, ductus deferens	vas/o

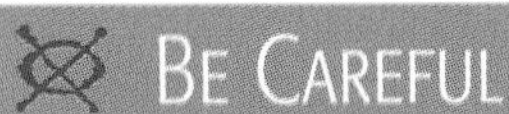

BE CAREFUL!

Don't confuse *phall/o,* which means *penis,* and *phalang/o,* which is a *bone in the finger and toe.*

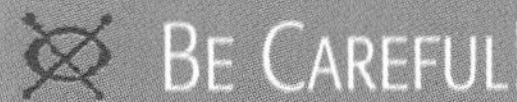

BE CAREFUL!

Don't confuse *urethr/o,* which means *urethra,* and *ureter/o,* which means the *ureter.*

Exercise 1: FUNCTION, ANATOMY, AND PHYSIOLOGY

Matching.

____ 1. penis
____ 2. prostate
____ 3. seminal vesicle
____ 4. scrotum
____ 5. foreskin
____ 6. semen
____ 7. urethra
____ 8. glans penis
____ 9. ductus deferens
____ 10. spermatozoon
____ 11. epididymis
____ 12. testis

A. vesicul/o
B. preputi/o
C. orchid/o
D. phall/o
E. epididym/o
F. spermat/o
G. scrot/o
H. vas/o
I. semin/i
J. urethr/o
K. prostat/o
L. balan/o

Fill in the blanks with one or more of the following.

genitalia, gonads, gametes, copulation, puberty, ejaculation, conception, spermatogenesis, coitus, parenchymal, stromal

13. What are the terms for sexual intercourse? ____________
14. What is the term for sex cells? ____________
15. What is the term for the release of sperm? ____________
16. What is a combination of stromal and parenchymal tissue in the reproductive system? ____________
17. What are the organs that produce sex cells? ____________
18. What is the term for the production of spermatozoa? ____________
19. At what stage of life does the capability for sexual reproduction take place? ____________
20. What is the term for the process of union of the sperm and the ovum? ____________

21. The gonads are which type of tissue? parenchymal
22. The supportive tissue in the male is a combination of all the ducts, glands, and other organs aside from the gonads. This is called STROMAL tissue.

Case Study Continued

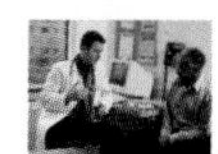

When Mr. Trudell confesses that he doesn't know much about the prostate, Adam sketches a rough drawing of the male urinary system on a notepad. "Here's the bladder where the urine is stored, and here's the urethra that carries it outside your body. This," he says, pointing at the bulge he'd drawn just below the bladder, "is a prostate. It's shaped like a donut surrounding the urethra. As many men age, parts of the prostate enlarge. If the prostate enlarges, it can close off the urethra. You can see how that would cause problems." Mr. Trudell grimaces and asks what can be done to correct the problem.

Adam explains that standard blood and urine laboratory tests are necessary, along with a digital rectal examination (DRE) and a prostate-specific antigen (PSA). Diagnostic imaging will probably include an intravenous urogram (IVU) or a renal ultrasound. Mr. Trudell is not overjoyed about the DRE but is anxious to get some relief. He jokes that he may have trouble providing the urine specimen. Adam smiles and tells him to do the best he can.

PATHOLOGY

Terms Related to Congenital Disorders

TERM	WORD ORIGIN	DEFINITION
Anorchism AN or kih zum	*an-* without *orch/o* testis *-ism* condition	Condition of being born without a testicle.
Cryptorchidism kript OR kid iz um	*crypt-* hidden *orchid/o* testis *-ism* condition	Condition in which the testicles fail to descend into the scrotum before birth. Also called **cryptorchism.**
Hyperspadias hye pur SPAY dee ahs	*hyper-* above *spadias* from Greek, meaning *rent* or *tear*	Urethral opening on the dorsum of the penis rather than on the tip. Also called **epispadias.**
Hypospadias hye poh SPAY dee ahs	*hypo-* below *spadias* from Greek, meaning *rent* or *tear*	Urethral opening on the ventral surface of the penis instead of on the tip (Fig. 7-2).
Phimosis fih MOH sis		Congenital condition of tightening of the prepuce around the glans penis so that the foreskin cannot be retracted.

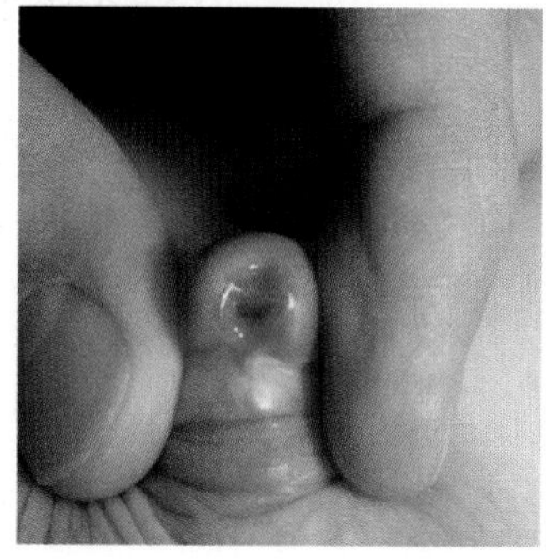

Fig. 7-2 Hypospadias.

Terms Related to Other Male Reproductive Disorders

TERM	WORD ORIGIN	DEFINITION
Aspermia a SPUR mee ah	*a-* without *sperm/o* sperm *-ia* condition	Condition in which no spermatozoa are present, nor any semen formed or ejaculated.
Azoospermia a zoh uh SPUR mee ah	*a-* without *zo/o* life *sperm/o* sperm *-ia* condition	Condition of no living sperm in the semen.
Balanitis bal en EYE tis	*balan/o* glans penis *-itis* inflammation	Inflammation of the glans penis.
Benign prostatic hyperplasia (BPH) beh NYNE pros TAT ick hye pur PLAY zsa	*prostat/o* prostate *-ic* pertaining to *hyper-* excessive *-plasia* formation	Abnormal enlargement of the prostate gland surrounding the urethra, leading to difficulty with urination (Fig. 7-3). Also known as **benign prostatic hypertrophy.**
Epididymitis ep ih did ih MYE tis	*epididym/o* epididymis *-itis* inflammation	Inflammation of the epididymis, usually as a result of an ascending infection through the genitourinary tract.
Erectile dysfunction		Inability to achieve or sustain a penile erection for sexual intercourse. Also known as **impotence** (IM poh tense).
Gynecomastia gye neh koh MASS tee ah	*gynec/o* female *mast/o* breast *-ia* condition	Enlargement of either unilateral or bilateral breast tissue in the male. The *gynec/o* is a reference to the appearance of the breast, not to a female.
Hydrocele HYE droh seel	*hydr/o* water, fluid *-cele* herniation, protrusion	Accumulation of fluid in the tunica vaginalis testis (Fig. 7-4).
Oligospermia oh lih goh SPUR mee ah	*oligo-* scanty *sperm/o* sperm *-ia* condition	Condition of temporary or permanent deficiency of sperm in the seminal fluid; related to azoospermia.
Orchitis or KYE tis	*orch/o* testis *-itis* inflammation	Inflammation of the testicles; may or may not be associated with the mumps virus. Also known as **testitis** (tess TYE tis).
Prostatitis pros tah TYE tis	*prostat/o* prostate *-itis* inflammation	Inflammation of the prostate gland.

Continued

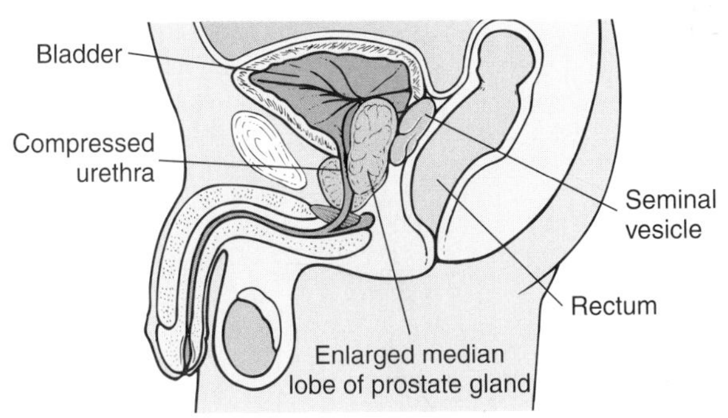

Fig. 7-3 BPH.

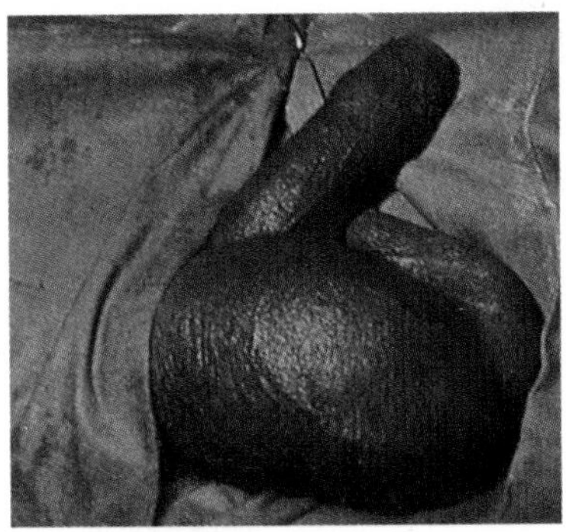

Fig. 7-4 Hydrocele.

DID YOU KNOW?

Azoospermia is expected in a man who has had a vasectomy but is a concern for a man who wants to father children.

Terms Related to Other Male Reproductive Disorders—cont'd

TERM	WORD ORIGIN	DEFINITION
Testicular torsion tes TICK kyoo lur	*testicul/o* testicle *-ar* pertaining to	Twisting of a testicle on its spermatic cord, usually due to trauma. May lead to ischemia of the testicle.
Varicocele VAIR ih koh seel	*varic/o* varices *-cele* herniation, protrusion	Abnormal dilation of the veins of the spermatic cord; can lead to infertility.
Vesiculitis veh sick yoo LYE tis	*vesicul/o* seminal vesicle *-itis* inflammation	Inflammation of a seminal vesicle, usually associated with prostatitis.

Exercise 2: MALE REPRODUCTIVE DISORDERS

Matching.

____ 1. lack of a testicle

____ 2. tightening of foreskin

____ 3. undescended testicles

____ 4. opening of urethra on ventral surface of penis

____ 5. procedure to correct phimosis

____ 6. opening of urethra on dorsal aspect of penis

A. epispadias
B. phimosis
C. hypospadias
D. cryptorchidism
E. circumcision
F. anorchism

Fill in the blanks with one of the following terms.

azoospermia, hydrocele, balanitis, epididymitis, testitis, gynecomastia, benign prostatic hyperplasia, erectile dysfunction, varicocele, testicular torsion

7. What is a synonym for orchitis? ____________
8. An abnormal growth of the prostate is called ____________.
9. A twisting of one or both testicles on the spermatic cord is called ____________.
10. An abnormal dilation of veins around the testicles is called a/an ____________.
11. What is a synonym for impotence? ____________
12. Enlarged breasts in a male is called ____________.
13. Inflammation of the glans penis is called ____________.
14. Accumulation of fluid in the scrotum is called ____________.
15. Inflammation of the sac that stores the spermatozoa is called ____________.
16. A condition of no spermatozoa in the seminal fluid is called ____________.

Terms Related to Sexually Transmitted Diseases (STDs)

The pathogens that cause STDs are various, but what they have in common is that they are all most efficiently transmitted by sexual contact.

TERM	WORD ORIGIN	DEFINITION
Gonorrhea gon uh REE ah	*gon/o* seed *-rrhea* flow, discharge	Disease caused by the gram-negative diplococcus *Neisseria gonorrhoeae* bacterium, which manifests itself as inflammation of the urethra, prostate, rectum, or pharynx. The cervix and fallopian tubes may also be involved in females, although they may appear to be **asymptomatic,** meaning without symptoms.
Herpes genitalis (herpes simplex virus, HSV-2) HER peez jen ih TAL is		Form of the herpesvirus transmitted through sexual contact, causing recurring painful vesicular eruptions (Fig. 7-5).
Human papilloma virus (HPV) pap ih LOH mah		Virus that causes common warts of the hands and feet, as well as lesions of the mucous membranes of the oral, anal, and genital cavities. A genital wart is referred to as a **condyloma** (kon dih LOH mah) (*pl.* condylomata).
Nongonococcal urethritis (NGU) non gon uh KOCK ul yoor ih THRY tis	*urethr/o* urethra *-itis* inflammation	Inflammation of the urethra caused by *Chlamydia trachomatis, Mycoplasma genitalium,* or *Ureaplasma urealyticum.*
Syphilis SIFF ill is		Multistage STD caused by the spirochete *Treponema pallidum.* A highly infectious **chancre** (SHAN kur), a painless, red pustule, appears in the first stage, usually on the genitals.

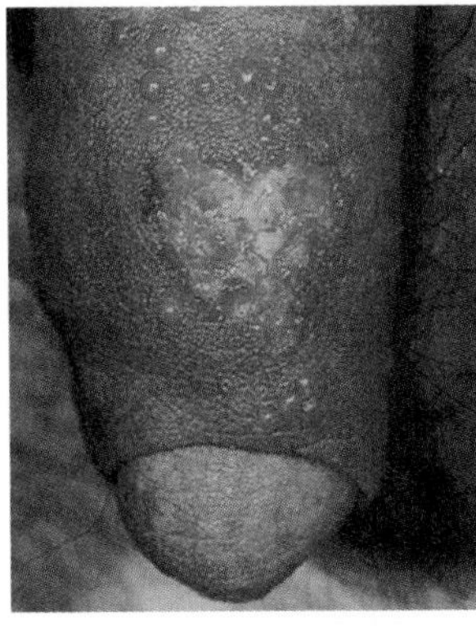

Fig. 7-5 Genital herpes.

DID YOU KNOW?

Nongonococcal urethritis accounts for the majority of cases of STDs in the population today.

Exercise 3: SEXUALLY TRANSMITTED DISEASES

Fill in the blanks with one of the following terms.

chlamydia, condylomata, asymptomatic, human papilloma virus, chancres, herpes simplex virus-2, nongonococcal urethritis, syphilis, gonorrhea

1. HPV causes genital warts that are referred to as Condylomata.
2. The majority of cases of STDs are caused by chlamydia.

3. Which STD has multiple stages? Syphilis

4. Inflammation of the urethra not caused by the gonorrhea bacterium is called nongonococcal urethritis.

5. An STD caused by a gram-negative bacteria is called gonorrhea.

6. Syphilitic lesions that are painless ulcers are called Chnncres.

7. When a patient has no symptoms, he is considered to be Asystomatic.

8. Genital warts are caused by the Human Papilloma Virw.

9. A viral infection resulting in painful, recurring vesicular eruptions is called Herpes Simplex Virw-2.

DIAGNOSTIC PROCEDURES

Terms Related to Diagnostic Procedures

TERM	WORD ORIGIN	DEFINITION
Digital rectal examination (DRE)	***digit/o*** digit (finger or toe) ***-al*** pertaining to ***rect/o*** rectum ***-al*** pertaining to	Insertion of a gloved finger into the rectum to palpate the prostate (Fig. 7-6).
Fluorescent treponemal antibody absorption test (FTA-ABS) floor ES unt trep uh NEE mul		Definitive test for diagnosing syphilis (Fig. 7-7).
Gram stain		Test that can be used to diagnose gonorrhea.
Prostate-specific antigen (PSA) AN tih jen		Blood test for prostatic hypertrophy.
Sperm analysis		Count and analysis of the number and health of the spermatozoa as a test for male fertility. Also called **sperm count** or **semen analysis.**
Ultrasonography	***ultra-*** beyond ***son/o*** sound ***-graphy*** process of recording	Use of high-frequency sound waves that can be used to examine the testicles for abnormalities.
Venereal Disease Research Laboratory (VDRL) test		Test used to screen for syphilis.

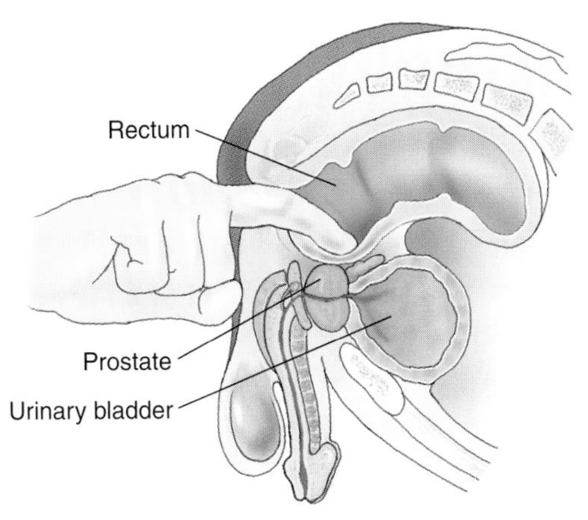

Fig. 7-6 DRE.

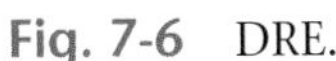

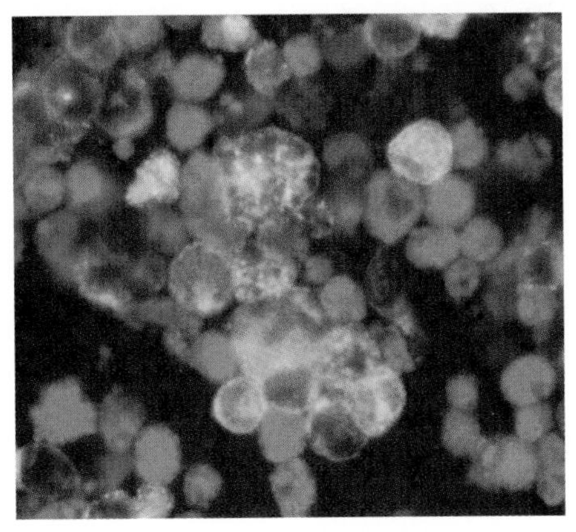

Fig. 7-7 Fluorescent antibody test.

> **BE CAREFUL!**
>
> Don't confuse *proct/o,* which means *rectum* and *anus,* and *prostat/o,* which means *prostate.*

Exercise 4: DIAGNOSTIC PROCEDURES

Fill in the blanks.

1. What is/are laboratory test(s) for the following?

   A. prostatic hypertrophy PSA (blood) DRE (manual)

   B. syphilis VDRL (screen) FTA-ABS (definitive)

   C. male fertility Sperm analysis

   D. gonorrhea gram stain

2. Palpation of the prostate using a finger is part of a D*igital* R*ectal* E*xamination*.

3. Use of high-frequency sound waves to image the sac that holds the testicles is called a scrotal *ultrasonography*.

THERAPEUTIC INTERVENTIONS

Terms Related to Therapeutic Interventions

TERM	WORD ORIGIN	DEFINITION
Ablation ah BLAY shun		Removal of tissue by surgery, chemical destruction, electrocautery, or radiofrequency energy.
Castration kas TRAY shun		Removal of both gonads in the male or the female.
Circumcision sur kum SIH zhun	*circum-* around *-cision* process of cutting	Surgical procedure in which the prepuce of the penis (or that of the clitoris of the female) is excised.
Orchidectomy or kih DECK tuh mee	*orchid/o* testis *-ectomy* excision	Removal of one or both testicles.

Continued

Terms Related to Therapeutic Interventions—cont'd

Term	Word Origin	Definition
Orchiopexy or kee oh PECK see	*orchi/o* testis *-pexy* fixation	Surgical procedure to mobilize an undescended testicle, attaching it to the scrotum.
Prostatectomy pros tuh TECK tuh mee	*prostat/o* prostate *-ectomy* excision	Removal of the prostate gland. If termed a **radical prostatectomy,** the seminal vesicles and area of vas ampullae are also removed.
Sterilization		Process of rendering a male or female barren.
Transurethral resection of the prostate (TUR, TURP) trans yoo REE thrul	*trans-* through *urethr/o* urethra *-al* pertaining to	Removal of the prostate in sections through a urethral approach (Fig. 7-8).
Transurethral incision of the prostate (TUIP)	*trans-* through *urethr/o* urethra *-al* pertaining to *in-* in *-cision* process of cutting	Form of prostate surgery involving tiny incisions of the prostate. The prostate is not removed.
Vasectomy vas SECK tuh mee	*vas/o* vas deferens *-ectomy* removal	Incision, ligation, and cauterization of both of the vas deferens for the purpose of male sterilization (Fig. 7-9).
Vasovasostomy vay zoh vuh SOS tuh mee	*vas/o* vas deferens *-stomy* new opening	Anastomosis of the ends of the vas deferens as a means of reconnecting them to reverse the sterilization procedure.

DID YOU KNOW?

Ritual circumcision is required by the religions of approximately one sixth of the world's population.

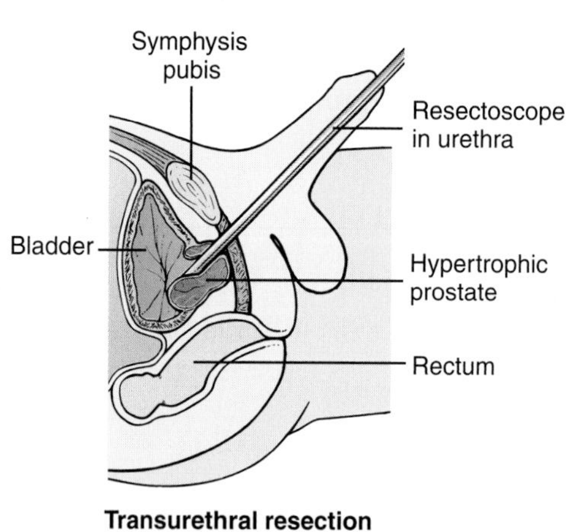

Fig. 7-8 TURP.

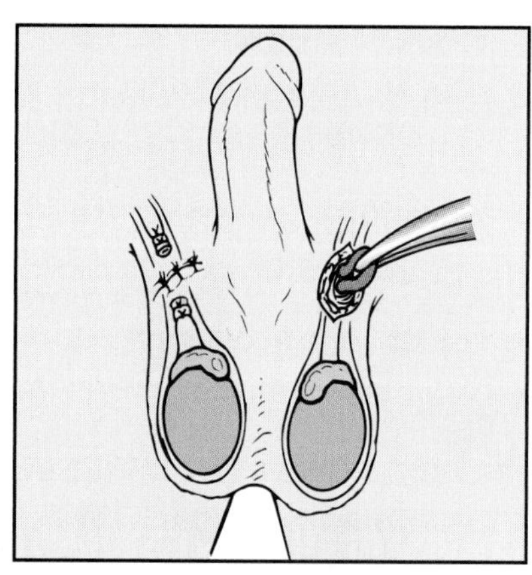

Fig. 7-9 Vasectomy.

Exercise 5: THERAPEUTIC INTERVENTIONS

Matching.

____ 1. removing both gonads
____ 2. destruction of tissue
____ 3. removal of prepuce
____ 4. removal of testicle
____ 5. fixation of testicle
____ 6. rendering barren
____ 7. resection of prostate
____ 8. reversal of vasectomy
____ 9. through the urethra
____ 10. ligation of ductus deferens

A. circumcision
B. orchiopexy
C. vasectomy
D. sterilization
E. vasovasostomy
F. castration
G. orchidectomy
H. transurethral
I. ablation
J. prostatectomy

Case Study Continued

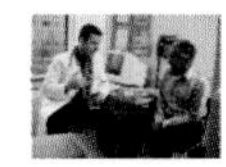

Mr. Trudell's tests come back positive for benign prostatic hyperplasia (BPH). Adam tells him that prostate surgery will be necessary. Mr. Trudell's physician comes in and further explains that the procedure he recommends—the TURP—will help alleviate his symptoms. He explains the surgery to Mr. Trudell. Adam adds more information to what the doctor has said by telling Mr. Trudell that he'll be in the hospital for a couple of days and that when he goes home, he will need to drink a lot of water, urinate often, and avoid strenuous exercise for a couple of weeks, until he comes in again for a checkup. "How soon can we schedule the surgery?" Mr. Trudell asks. "I'm ready right now to just get this over with."

PHARMACOLOGY

Antibiotics: Used to treat microbial infections. Penicillin, tetracycline, and doxycycline can all be used to treat syphilis.

Antiimpotence drugs: Used to alleviate erectile dysfunction. Sildenafil citrate (Viagra) is most commonly used.

Antivirals: Used to treat viral infections. For instance, acyclovir (Zovirax) is used to treat the genital herpesvirus.

Complementary medicine: Saw palmetto *(Serenoa repens),* which has been shown to be as effective as finasteride for treatment of symptoms of BPH.

Nonsurgical treatment of symptoms of BPH: Shrinkage of prostatic tissue and increase of urine flow through the use of finasteride (Proscar, Propecia).

Exercise 6: PHARMACOLOGY

Matching.

_____ 1. class of drug used to treat microbial infections

_____ 2. class of drug used to treat viral infections

_____ 3. class of drug used to treat erectile dysfunction

_____ 4. an example of a drug used to treat BPH

_____ 5. herbal, alternative medicine

A. antivirals
B. antiimpotence
C. complementary medicine
D. antibiotic
E. finasteride

Case Study Continued

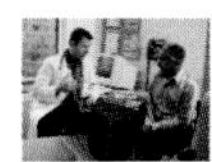

Adam smiles as he looks over the operative report from Mr. Trudell's recent surgery. Mr. Trudell had called to say that he was home from the hospital, drinking lots of water, and having no problems urinating. He went on to say, "I wanted to say thanks for all your help. And by the way, my daughter's a biology major and says she's interested in a medical career. Would you be willing to spend a few minutes talking to her about your career? I think she'd be a great PA, just like you!"

Abbreviations

Abbreviation	Definition	Abbreviation	Definition
BPH	Benign prostatic hyperplasia/ hypertrophy	NGU	Nongonococcal urethritis
		PSA	Prostate-specific antigen
Bx	Biopsy	STD	Sexually transmitted disease
DRE	Digital rectal exam	TUIP	Transurethral incision of the prostate
F	Female		
FTA-ABS	Fluorescent treponemal antibody test	TUR	Transurethral resection [of the prostate]
Gc	Gonococcus	TURP	Transurethral resection of the prostate
HPV	Human papilloma virus		
HSV-2	Herpes simplex virus-2, herpes genitalis	VD	Venereal disease
		VDRL	Venereal Disease Research Laboratory test (for syphilis)
M	Male		

BE CAREFUL!

Don't confuse the gastrointestinal (GI) system with the genitourinary (GU) system.

Exercise 7: ABBREVIATIONS

1. The patient had a TURP to relieve his ________________ (answer with another abbreviation).

2. Someone who has a Gc infection has a/an ________________ (answer with another abbreviation).

3. A patient tested with VDRL is suspected of having ________________.
4. What is a DRE, and for what is it used?

____

5. If condylomata are present, the patient may have ________________.

6. What is the GU system? ________________________________

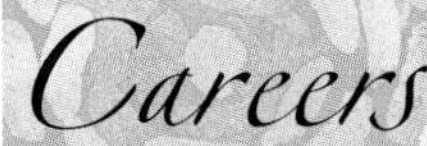

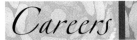

Careers

Physician Assistants

Employment opportunities for physician assistants (PAs) are expected to be plentiful through the year 2010 as a result of an increase in demand for healthcare services and an accompanying need for the cost-effectiveness that PAs provide.

Individual state laws and supervising physicians determine the exact nature of PAs' duties, but they are trained to diagnose, treat, and provide preventive care services to patients. In the majority of states, they may also prescribe medications.

All states require that PAs complete an accredited, formal education program and also pass the PA national certifying examination. As with most other healthcare professions, PAs must continually keep themselves abreast of changes in their field through formal continuing education programs. The training programs range from an associate's to a master's degree, and most last at least 2 years. Approximately two thirds of current applicants hold a bachelor's degree, and many have prior healthcare experience.

Although most PAs practice in general primary care settings, opportunities for specialization are available in emergency medicine, pediatrics, surgery, and other areas.

For more information on a career as a PA, contact the American Academy of Physician Assistants Information Center at http://www.aapa.org, or for a list of accredited programs, the Association of Physician Assistant Programs at http://www.apap.org.

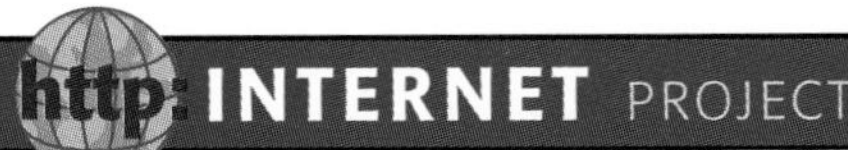

http: INTERNET PROJECT

The National Institutes of Health report that BPH is present in 50% of men aged 51 to 60 and in 90% of men over the age of 80. Although there are currently no effective preventive measures, treatments may be divided into healthcare and surgical options. For this Internet project, you will be searching for the current treatments, both medical and surgical, including alternative therapies, where appropriate.

For surgical treatments, list at least six different options, aside from those listed in the chapter. For pharmaceuticals, list the current drugs as well as those being tested in clinical trials.

Be sure to include your reference sites and define any terms not covered in the chapter but used in your report.

You may want to start your research at the following sites:

For an exhaustive listing of categories covering prostate health, try the government's MEDLINEplus at http://www.nlm.nih.gov/medlineplus/prostatediseases.html.

The National Cancer Institute has an interesting summary of BPH treatment options at http://www.pueblo.gsa.gov/cic_text/health/prost-change/prost-ch.htm.

For an explanation of the different types of surgeries, try the American College of Surgeons Website at http://www.medem.com/default.cfm.

Try http://clinicaltrials.gov for information on clinical research studies of investigational drugs and treatments. This site is made available through the National Library of Medicine.

Chapter Review

A. Functions of the Male Reproductive System

1. In your own words, explain the function(s) of the male reproductive system.

Continue Species

B. Anatomy and Physiology

Define the following terms.

2. copulation Sexual intercourse
3. ejaculation release of sperm & semen
4. conception = Fertilization
5. Label the illustration below with the anatomic structures and their combining forms.

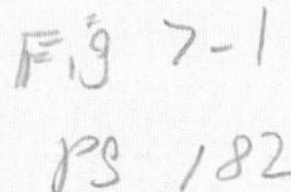

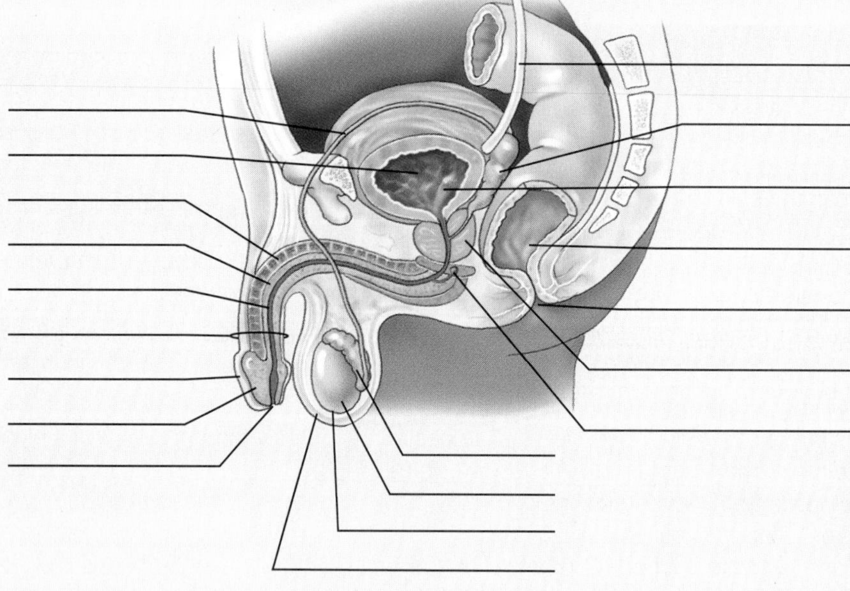

C. Pathology

Build a term.

6. What is the term for undescended (hidden) testicles? crypto orchidism
7. What is the term for an inflammation of the ducts that store spermatozoa?

epididymitis

8. What is the term for an absence of one testicle? Anorchism
9. What is a term for inflammation of the testes? orchitis
10. What is the term for swollen, twisted veins surrounding a testicle?

Decode the term.

11. balanitis ______________________________

12. nongonococcal urethritis ______________________________

13. oligospermia ______________________________

14. orchitis ______________________________

15. prostatic hypertrophy ______________________________

Name the disorder.

16. What is a term for the abnormal opening of the urethra on the underside of the penis?

____

17. What is a term for the tightening of the foreskin over the glans penis?

____

18. In what condition is one testicle twisted out of its normal position?

____

19. What is a nonmalignant enlargement of the prostate? ______________________________

20. What is another term for impotence? ______________________________

D. Diagnostic Procedures

21. John Walls has made an appointment with his physician to have a physical and blood test for a suspected prostate enlargement. What are these tests? ______________________________

22. When Paul realized that the sore on his penis could be the result of a STD, he went to his doctor, who called it a chancre and ordered a test called a/an ______________________________.

23. Roger went in to have an imaging procedure that uses high-frequency sound waves to examine a mass in his scrotum. It is called a/an ______________________________.

24. The Williams couple was having trouble conceiving. Fertility testing was started by their physician, who ordered a/an ______________________________ for Mr. Williams.

E. Therapeutic Interventions

Build a term.

25. surgical fixation of a testicle ______________________________

26. to cut around ______________________________

27. removal of the prostate ______________________________

Decode the term.

28. bilateral orchiectomy ______________________________

29. vasectomy ______________________________

30. vasovasostomy ______________________________

Recall the term.

31. removal of both gonads in either sex ______________________________

32. removal of a body part by electrocautery, chemical destruction, or radiofrequency

____

33. the treatment for phimosis ______________________________

34. a surgical procedure used to treat benign prostatic hyperplasia ______________________________

35. the term for "rendering barren" ______________________________

F. Pharmacology

Fill in the blanks.

36. Robert was given a prescription of doxycycline for his epididymitis. Doxycycline is an example of what class of drug? ______________________________

37. Andrew was behind Robert at the pharmacy, picking up a prescription of acyclovir for genital herpes. Acyclovir is an example of what class of drug? ______________________________

38. Saw palmetto has been used to treat the symptoms of which disorder?

____

39. Sildenafil citrate has been used to treat erectile dysfunction. What class of drug is it?

____

40. Urinary flow is increased through the use of finasteride, which acts to shrink the tissue of which male reproductive organ? ______________________________

G. Abbreviations

41. What is the abbreviation for the bacterium that causes gonorrhea?

____

42. A patient is being treated for HPV. What is the disorder? ______________________________

43. What is the abbreviation for the virus that causes genital herpes? ______________________________

44. What is the abbreviation for the technique of removing sections of the prostate through the urethra?

____

45. A patient with gonorrhea is being treated for what type of disease (the abbreviation)?

____

H. Singulars and Plurals

Change the following terms from singular to plural.

46. testis testes
47. epididymis - mides
48. scrotum scrota
49. penis penes
50. spermatozoon - zoa

I. Translations

Rewrite the following sentences, translating the underlined terms in your own words.

51. A semen analysis revealed oligospermia that caused the couple's infertility.

52. The patient's BPH was diagnosed after a DRE and PSA.

Benign prostatic hypertrophy
Digital Rectal Exam & Prostatic-Specific antigen

53. Sam's painful testicular swelling was diagnosed as epididymitis.

inflammation of epididymis

54. When the college student appeared at the clinic, he had been experiencing dysuria and mucopurulent discharge. He was asked to bring in his girlfriend, even though he said she was asymptomatic.

mucopurulent mucous & pus discharge

55. The physician suggested circumcision to treat the patient's phimosis.

J. Cumulative Exercises

Circle the correct answer.

56. When Mr. Jones had his left testicle removed he had a *(unilateral, bilateral)* orchiectomy.
57. The term *vasovasostomy* is an example of an *(anastomosis, ostomy)*.
58. The patient with BPH who complained of being unable to urinate was exhibiting *(urinary retention, urinary incontinence)*.
59. A patient examined while lying on his/her stomach is in a *(prone, supine)* position.

K. Be Careful

Explain the difference between the following combining forms.

60. vesic/o, vesicul/o vesic = bladder vesicul = Seminal vesicle

61. cry/o, crypt/o cry = cold crypt = hidden

62. phall/o, phalang/o Phall = penis phalang = Bone finger or Toe

63. urethr/o, ureter/o

64. proct/o, prostat/o proct = anus & Rectum prostat = prostrate

Cedar Lake Hospital
72 N. Main St.
Cedar Lake, IA 50672

OPERATIVE REPORT

Patient Name: Samuel Trudell MR#: 455 768
Physician: Hamid Ali, MD Date: 8/23/02
Preoperative Diagnosis: BPH, urinary retention
Postoperative Diagnosis: BPH, urinary retention
History of Present Illness: Patient is a 64-year-old African-American male with past medical history of hiatal hernia with gastritis, BPH, and UTI with h/o urinary retention. Patient denies dysuria, incontinence, hematuria, urgency, and urinary frequency. Urinary retention has been managed with a Foley catheter after a bout of UTI on past admission.
Operation: TURP
Anesthesia: Spinal
Procedure: The patient was brought to the operating room, properly identified, and, following adequate administration of spinal anesthesia, was placed in the dorsal lithotomy position, and the genitalia prepared with Betadine and draped in the sterile manner.

A #26 French scope was used to inspect the urethra and bladder. Trilobar hypertrophy of the prostate was easily identified.

A transurethral resection of the prostate was carried out in the usual fashion. Chips of prostatic tissue were evacuated from the bladder with a Toomey syringe. Hemostasis was achieved with a Bovie. On final inspection, the urethra was free of obstruction, and both the external sphincter and the ureteral orifices were intact. A Foley catheter was attached for drainage, and the patient was sent to the recovery room in satisfactory condition.

Zachary James, MD (surgeon)

L. Healthcare Report

65. The patient's past medical history included a hiatal hernia. Describe this condition.

Protrusion of part of stomach thru the diaphram

66. Explain what the patient does *not* complain of:

A. dysuria ______
B. incontinence ______
C. urgency ______
D. urinary frequency ______
E. hematuria ______

67. How many lobes of the prostate were enlarged? ______

68. What does the abbreviation for the patient's surgery, TURP, mean? Trans urethral resection of the prostate

69. If this patient had had periprostatic lesions, where would they have been?

Surrounding the prostate

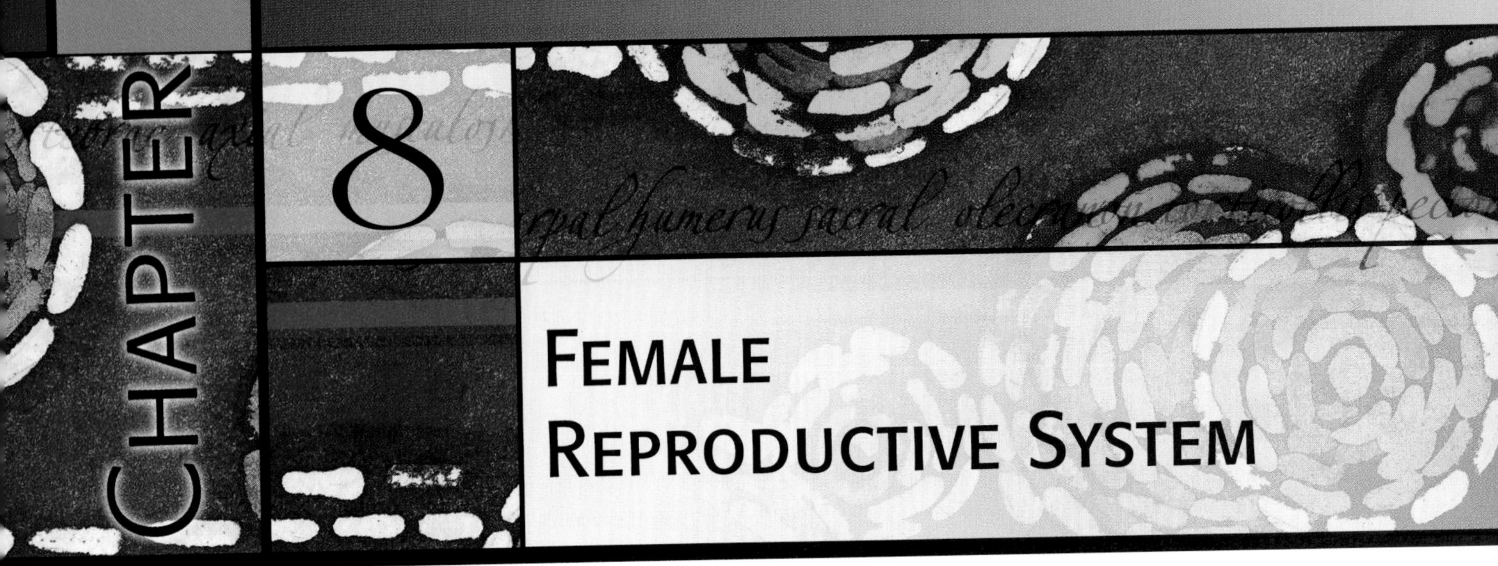

CHAPTER 8 FEMALE REPRODUCTIVE SYSTEM

"He not busy being born, is busy dying." ***—Bob Dylan***

Case Study

After years of working as an RN on an OB-GYN floor in one of the local hospitals, Linda Santos longed to have more autonomy. She decided to return to school to get her certification in nurse midwifery. Now certified as a nurse midwife, Linda has several patients who are in various stages of pregnancy. Today, she is going to meet with one of her patients, Susan Banfield, who is newly pregnant with her first child and anxious about her new role as a soon-to-be mother.

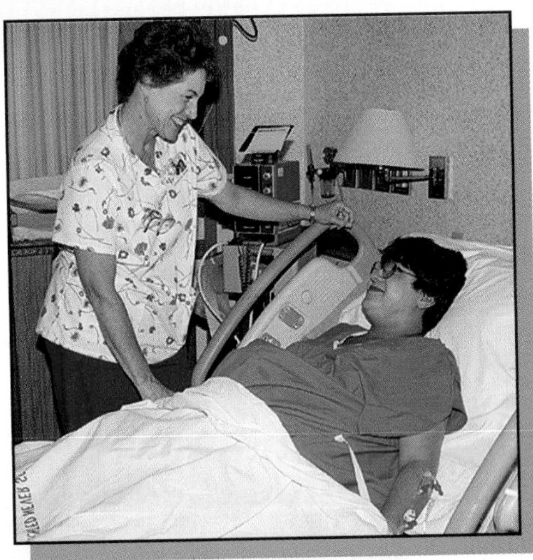

OBJECTIVES

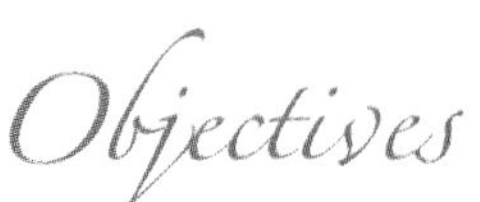

- In your own words, explain the functions of the female reproductive system.
- Recognize, recall, and apply healthcare terms related to the anatomy and physiology of the female reproductive system.
- Recognize, recall, and apply healthcare terms related to the pathology of the female reproductive system.
- Recognize, recall, and apply healthcare terms related to diagnostic procedures of the female reproductive system.
- Recognize, recall, and apply healthcare terms related to the therapeutic interventions of the female reproductive system.
- Recognize, recall, and apply the abbreviations introduced in this chapter.
- Recognize, recall, and apply word components used in this chapter to build and decode healthcare terms relevant to the female reproductive system.
- Recognize, recall, and apply material learned in previous chapters.

FUNCTIONS OF THE FEMALE REPRODUCTIVE SYSTEM

The role of the female reproductive system is to keep one's genetic material in the world's gene pool. Through sexual reproduction, the 23 pairs of chromosomes of the female must join with 23 pairs of chromosomes from a male to create new life. To do this, the system must produce the hormones necessary to provide a hospitable environment for the **ovum** (OH vum) (*pl.* **ova**), the female gamete, to connect with the **spermatozoon** (spur mah toh ZOH un), the male gamete, for fertilization to occur. Once an egg is fertilized, it is nurtured throughout its growth process until the delivery of the neonate (newborn).

Exercise 1: FUNCTIONS OF THE FEMALE REPRODUCTIVE SYSTEM

Matching.

__C__ 1. female gametes

__D__ 2. male gametes

__A__ 3. neonates

__E__ 4. genetic information is passed on through

__B__ 5. the system's reproductive functions are coordinated by

A. newborns
B. hormones
C. ova
D. spermatozoa
E. chromosomes

ANATOMY AND PHYSIOLOGY

Internal Anatomy

Because the primary function of the female reproductive system is to create new life through the successful fertilization of an ovum, discussion of this system begins with this very important germ cell.

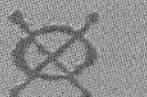

BE CAREFUL!

The term *germ* comes from the Latin word for *sprout* or *fetus,* here referring to its reproductive nature; however, it can also mean a type of *microorganism* that can cause disease.

Ova and Ovaries

From **menarche** (meh NAR kee), the first menstrual period, to **menopause** (MEN oh poz), the cessation of menstruation, mature ova are produced by the female gonads, the **ovaries** (OH vuh reez) (Fig. 8-1). The ovaries are small, almond-shaped, paired organs located on either side of the uterus in the female pelvic cavity. They are attached to the uterus by the ovarian ligaments and lie close to

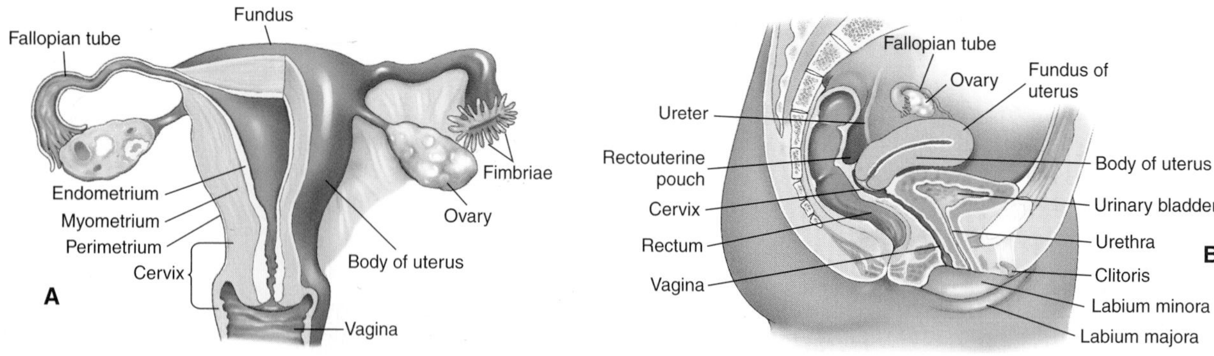

Fig. 8-1 Female reproductive organs. **A,** Frontal view. **B,** Sagittal view.

the opening of the **fallopian** (fuh LOH pee un) **tubes.** Approximately every 28 days, in response to hormonal stimulation, the ovaries alternate releasing one ovum. This egg matures in one of the **follicles** (FALL ih kuls), which are tiny secretory sacs within an ovary. The **pituitary** (pih TOO ih tair ee) **gland** secretes two hormones that influence the activity of the ovaries. **Follicle-stimulating hormone (FSH)** causes the ovarian follicles to begin to mature and secrete estrogen. Because of the increase of estrogen in the bloodstream, **luteinizing** (LOO tin eye zing) **hormone (LH)** is released by the anterior lobe of the pituitary gland. LH then stimulates the follicle to mature and release its ovum **(ovulation)** and aids in the development of the **corpus luteum** (KORE pus LOO tee um). The corpus luteum is then responsible for secreting **estrogen** (ES troh jen) and **progesterone** (proh JES teh roan), hormones responsible for female secondary sex characteristics and the cyclical maintenance of the uterus for pregnancy.

If two eggs are released and fertilized, the resulting twins will be termed **fraternal,** because they will be no more or less alike in appearance than brothers (or sisters) occurring in sequential pregnancies. If, however, one of the fertilized eggs divides and forms two infants, these are **identical** twins, who share the same appearance and genetic material.

Fallopian Tubes

Once the mature ovum has been released, it is drawn into the **fimbriae** (FIM bree ee) (*sing.* fimbria), the feathery ends of the fallopian tube (see Fig. 8-1). These tubes, about the width of a pencil, and about as long (10 to 12 cm), transport the ovum to the uterus. The fallopian tubes (also called *oviducts* or *uterine tubes*) and the ovaries make up what is called the **uterine adnexa** (YOO tuh rin add NECKS ah), or accessory organs of the uterus.

Uterus

Once the ovum has traversed the fallopian tube, it is secreted into the uterus, or womb, a pear-shaped organ that is designed to nurture a developing embryo/fetus (see Fig. 8-1). The uterus is composed of three layers: the outer layer, called the **perimetrium** (pair ih MEE tree um), or serosa; the **myometrium** (mye oh MEE tree um), or muscle layer; and the **endometrium** (en doh MEE tree um), the lining of the uterus. As a whole, it can be divided into several areas. The body or **corpus** (which means *body* in Latin) is the large central area; the **fundus** (FUN dus) is the raised area at the top of the uterus between the outlets for the fallopian tubes; and the **cervix** (SUR vicks) is the narrowed lower area, often referred to as the neck of the uterus.

Rectouterine Pouch

An area associated with the female reproductive system that does not play a direct role in its function, the **rectouterine pouch** (reck toh YOO tur in), is also

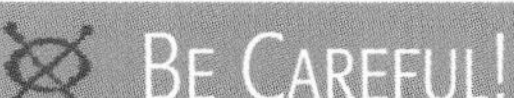

called *Douglas's cul-de-sac,* a space in the pelvic cavity between the uterus and the rectum.

BE CAREFUL!

Do not confuse *ureter/o,* which means the *ureter,* with *uter/o,* which means *uterus.*

Vagina

If the ovum does not become fertilized by a spermatozoon, the corpus luteum stops producing estrogen and progesterone, and the lining of the uterus is shed through the muscular, tubelike vagina by the process of **menstruation (menses).**

COMBINING FORMS FOR INTERNAL FEMALE GENITALIA

MEANING	COMBINING FORM	MEANING	COMBINING FORM
born	nat/o	ovary	ovari/o, oophor/o
cervix	cervic/o	rectouterine pouch	culd/o
egg, ovum	ov/i, ov/o	rectum	rect/o
fallopian tube	salping/o	uterus	uter/o, hyster/o, metri/o, metr/o
menses, menstruation	men/o		
muscle	my/o	vagina	vagin/o, colp/o

PREFIXES FOR INTERNAL FEMALE GENITALIA

PREFIX	MEANING
endo-	within
neo-	new
peri-	surrounding

BE CAREFUL!

Don't confuse *culd/o,* which means the *recto-uterine pouch,* with *colp/o,* which means *vagina.*

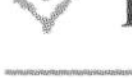

Exercise 2: INTERNAL FEMALE GENITALIA

Matching.

____ 1. hormones that stimulate production of the ova

____ 2. beginning of menstruation

____ 3. cessation of the menses

____ 4. inner lining of the uterus

____ 5. monthly shedding of uterine lining

____ 6. eponym for rectouterine pouch

____ 7. hormone that stimulates follicles to release ovum

____ 8. muscular layer of the uterus

____ 9. release of ovum

____ 10. neck of uterus

____ 11. outer layer of uterus

____ 12. gland that secretes hormones influencing ovaries

____ 13. accessory organs of uterus

____ 14. muscular tube, entrance to internal genitalia

A. menstruation
B. cervix
C. LH
D. uterine adnexa
E. pituitary
F. perimetrium
G. vagina
H. ovulation
I. FSH
J. menopause
K. endometrium
L. Douglas's cul-de-sac
M. menarche
N. myometrium

Exercise 3: Combining Forms for Internal Female Genitalia

Match the following. There may be more than one answer per question.

___ 1. culd/o
___ 2. oophor/o
___ 3. metr/o
___ 4. hyster/o
___ 5. colp/o
___ 6. ov/o
___ 7. salping/o
___ 8. cervic/o
___ 9. ovari/o
___ 10. uter/o
___ 11. vagin/o
___ 12. men/o

A. uterus
B. vagina
C. fallopian tube
D. cervix
E. rectouterine pouch
F. ovary
G. female germ cell
H. menstruation, menses

External Genitalia

The external female genitalia are collectively called the **vulva** (VUL vah) (Fig. 8-2). The vulva consists of the vaginal opening, or **orifice** (ORE ih fis); the membrane covering the opening, or **hymen** (HYE men); the two folds of skin surrounding the opening, or **labia majora** (LAY bee ah muh JOR ah) (the larger folds) and **labia minora** (LAY bee ah min NOR uh) (the smaller folds); the **clitoris** (KLIT uh ris), which is sensitive, erectile tissue; and the **perineum** (pair ih NEE um), the area between the opening of the vagina and the anus. The paired glands in the vulva that secrete a mucous lubricant for the vagina are the **Bartholin's** (BAR toh lin) **glands.** The **mons pubis** (mons PYOO bis) is a fatty cushion of tissue over the pubic bone.

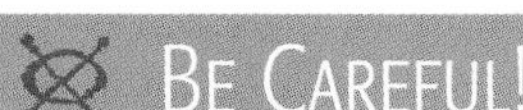

The combining form *cervic/o* has two meanings: the *neck* and the *cervix.*

The Breast

The breasts, or mammary glands, function to secrete milk. The breast tissue is composed of glandular, fatty, and fibrous tissue. The nipple of the breast is the **mammary papilla** (MAM uh ree puh PILL ah) (*pl.* **papillae**), and the darker colored skin surrounding the nipple is the **areola** (ah REE oh lah) (*pl.* **areolae**).

Combining Forms for External Genitalia

Meaning	Combining Form
Bartholin's glands	bartholin/o
hymen	hymen/o
labia	labi/o
perineum	perine/o
vulva	vulv/o, episi/o

Combining Forms for the Breast

Meaning	Combining Form
breast	mamm/o, mast/o
milk	lact/o, galact/o
nipple	papill/o, thel/o

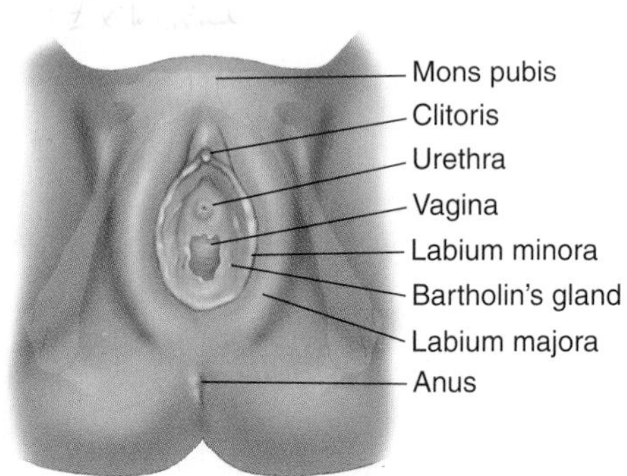

Fig. 8-2 Female external genitalia.

Exercise 4: EXTERNAL FEMALE GENITALIA AND THE BREAST

Matching.

_____ 1. membrane that covers the vaginal orifice

_____ 2. area between the opening of the vagina and the anus

_____ 3. healthcare term for the nipple

_____ 4. darker colored skin surrounding the nipple

_____ 5. paired glands that lubricate the vagina

A. areola
B. mammary papilla
C. perineum
D. Bartholin's glands
E. hymen

Match the following combining forms with their meanings. There may be more than one answer.

_____ 6. vulva
_____ 7. nipple
_____ 8. hymen
_____ 9. milk
_____ 10. labia
_____ 11. breast
_____ 12. perineum
_____ 13. Bartholin's glands

A. galact/o
B. episi/o
C. bartholin/o
D. papill/o
E. mamm/o
F. thel/o
G. hymen/o
H. perine/o
I. lact/o
J. vulv/o
K. mast/o
L. labi/o

Pregnancy and Delivery

Pregnancy begins with the fertilization of an ovum by a spermatozoon, often in the fallopian tube, as the ovum travels toward the uterus. Conception is usually the result of sexual intercourse (also termed *copulation* or *coitus*). However, other methods of conception are possible, if the couple has difficulty conceiving. These methods are discussed in the section on therapeutic interventions and may include artificial insemination and in vitro fertilization.

The fertilized egg, or **zygote** (ZYE gote), divides as it moves through the fallopian tube to the uterus, where it becomes implanted. From the third to the eighth week of life, it is called an **embryo** (EM bree oh). From the ninth through the thirty-eighth week of life (a normal length for **gestation** [jes TAY shun], or pregnancy), it is called a **fetus** (FEE tus). During implantation, the zygote functions as an endocrine gland by secreting **human chorionic gonadotropin (hCG)** (kore ee AH nick goh nad doh TROH pin). The function of the hormone is to prevent the corpus luteum from deteriorating, which allows the continued production of estrogen and progesterone to support the pregnancy and prevent menstruation.

At the same time that the embryo is developing, extraembryonic membranes are forming to sustain the pregnancy: Two of these, the **amnion** (AM nee on) and the **chorion** (KORE ee on), form the inner and outer sacs that contain the embryo (Fig. 8-3). The fluid that forms inside the amnion is the **amniotic** (am nee AH tick) **fluid.** It functions to cushion the embryo, protect it against temperature changes, and allow it to move. The **placenta** (plah SEN tah) is a highly vascular structure that acts as a physical communication between the mother and embryo. The **umbilical** (um BILL ih kul) **cord** is the tissue that connects the embryo to the placenta (and hence to the mother). When the baby is delivered, the umbilical cord is cut, and the baby is then dependent on his/her own body for all physiologic processes. The remaining "scar" is the **umbilicus** (um BILL il kus), or navel. The delivery of an infant is termed **parturition** (par tur RIH shun).

Babies born before 37 weeks are referred to as *premature infants*. Those weighing less than 2500 grams (5 lbs, 8 oz) are referred to as *low–birth-weight infants*.

DID YOU KNOW?

The abbreviation GPA is used in obstetric notation to indicate the *number of pregnancies* (G for gravida), *the number of deliveries* of either a live or stillborn infant over 20 weeks of gestation (P for para), and *the number of miscarriages/abortions* that occur before 20 weeks of gestation (A for abortion). A woman described as G4P3A1 has had 4 pregnancies, 3 deliveries, and 1 abortion.

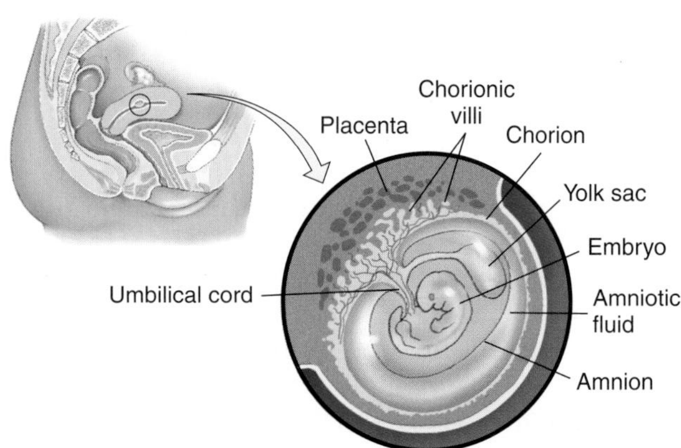

Fig. 8-3 The uterus of a pregnant woman.

COMBINING FORMS FOR PREGNANCY AND DELIVERY

MEANING	COMBINING FORM
amnion	amni/o
chorion	chori/o, chorion/o
fetus	fet/o
pregnancy	gravid/o
umbilicus	omphal/o, umbilic/o

SUFFIXES FOR PREGNANCY AND DELIVERY

SUFFIX	MEANING
-gravida, -cyesis	pregnancy
-tocia, -para	labor, delivery

Exercise 5: PREGNANCY

1. Trace the development of the fertilized egg to the thirty-eighth week of pregnancy with stages of development and time frames.

____

____

Matching.

____ 2. outer sac that encloses the embryo

____ 3. inner sac that encircles the embryo

____ 4. organ of communication between mother and baby

____ 5. navel

____ 6. another term for pregnancy

____ 7. childbirth

A. gestation
B. placenta
C. parturition
D. amnion
E. chorion
F. umbilicus

Match the word parts with their correct meanings. There may be more than one answer.

____ 8. pregnancy

____ 9. umbilicus

____ 10. labor, delivery

____ 11. amnion

____ 12. chorion

____ 13. fetus

A. -tocia
B. omphal/o
C. gravid/o
D. amni/o
E. umbilic/o
F. chori/o
G. -para
H. -cyesis
I. chorion/o
J. -gravida
K. fet/o

Case Study Continued

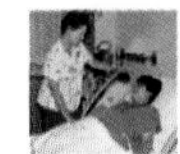

Susan, Linda Santos's patient, is a 36-year-old woman experiencing her first pregnancy. "Just because I'm older doesn't necessarily mean I know anything," she warns Linda with a smile. "We had such a hard time getting pregnant! We didn't have any miscarriages, any ectopics, any anything! Until now . . . I just didn't think that it would be an issue . . . Anyways! I've got so many questions for you!" Linda laughs and quickly gets down to business reviewing Susan's health record, including the date of her last menstrual period. "Well, the first thing I can tell you is your expected due date—it's St. Patrick's Day. Although, you know you'll need the cooperation of the baby for that."

PATHOLOGY

Terms Related to Disorders of the Ovaries

TERM	WORD ORIGIN	DEFINITION
Anovulation an ah vyoo LAY shun	*an-* without *ovul/o* ovulation *-ation* process	Failure of the ovary to release an ovum.
Ovarian cyst oh VAIR ee un sist	*ovari/o* ovary *-an* pertaining to	Benign, fluid-filled sac. Can be either a follicular cyst, which occurs when a follicle does not rupture at ovulation, or a cyst of the corpus luteum, caused when it does not continue its transformation (Fig. 8-4).
Polycystic ovary pall ee SIS tick	*poly-* many *cyst/o* sac *-ic* pertaining to	Bilateral presence of numerous cysts, caused by a hormonal abnormality leading to the secretion of androgens. Can cause acne, facial hair, and infertility.

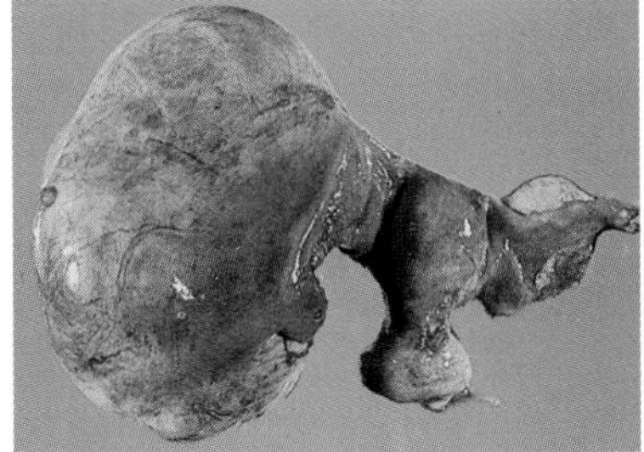

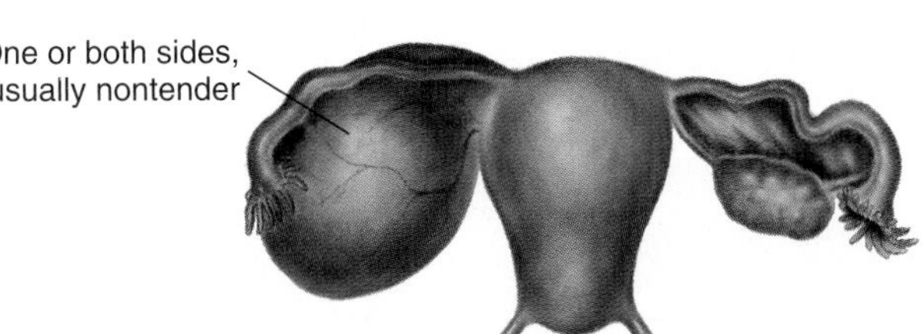

Fig. 8-4 Ovarian cyst.

Terms Related to Disorders of the Fallopian Tubes

TERM	WORD ORIGIN	DEFINITION
Adhesions, fallopian tubes add HEE zhuns		Scar tissue that binds surfaces together; a sequela of pelvic inflammatory disease (PID), in which, as a result of the inflammation, the tubes heal closed, causing infertility.
Hematosalpinx hee mah toh SAL pinks	*hemat/o* blood *-salpinx* fallopian tubes	Condition of blood in the fallopian tubes.

Continued

Terms Related to Disorders of the Fallopian Tubes—cont'd		
TERM	**WORD ORIGIN**	**DEFINITION**
Hydrosalpinx hye droh SAL pinks	*hydr/o* fluid *-salpinx* fallopian tubes	Condition of fluid in the fallopian tubes.
Pyosalpinx pye oh SAL pinks	*py/o* pus *-salpinx* fallopian tubes	Condition of pus in the fallopian tubes.
Salpingitis sal pin JYE tis	*salping/o* fallopian tubes *-itis* inflammation	Inflammation of the fallopian tubes. Also called PID.

Exercise 6: Ovarian and Fallopian Tube Disorders

Fill in the blanks with the terms provided.

polycystic ovary syndrome, anovulation, ovarian cyst, adhesions, hematosalpinx, salpingitis, hydrosalpinx, pyosalpinx

1. condition of pus in the fallopian tubes pyo salpinx
2. scar tissue that binds surfaces together ________________
3. inflammation of the fallopian tubes ________________
4. condition of blood in the fallopian tubes ________________
5. failure of the ovary to release an ovum ________________
6. benign fluid-filled sac in female gonads ________________
7. condition of fluid in fallopian tubes ________________
8. condition of multiple sacs on both ovaries leading to acne, facial hair, and infertility ________________

Terms Related to Disorders of the Uterus		
TERM	**WORD ORIGIN**	**DEFINITION**
Endometriosis en doh mee tree OH sis	*endometri/o* endometrium *-osis* abnormal condition	Condition in which the tissue that makes up the lining of the uterus, the endometrium, is found ectopically (outside the uterus); causes are unknown (Fig. 8-5).
Hysteroptosis hiss tur op TOH sis	*hyster/o* uterus *-ptosis* drooping, sagging	Falling or sliding of the uterus from its normal location in the body. Also called **uterine prolapse** (Fig. 8-6).
Leiomyoma (*pl.* leiomyomata, leiomyomas) lye oh mye OH mah	*lei/o* smooth *my/o* muscle *-oma* tumor, mass	Benign growths occurring in the muscle layer of the uterus. Also called **fibroids** (FYE broyds).
Retroflexion of uterus reh troh FLECK shun	*retro-* backward *flex/o* bend *-ion* process	Condition in which the body of the uterus is bent backwards, forming an angle with the cervix; often called a "tipped uterus."

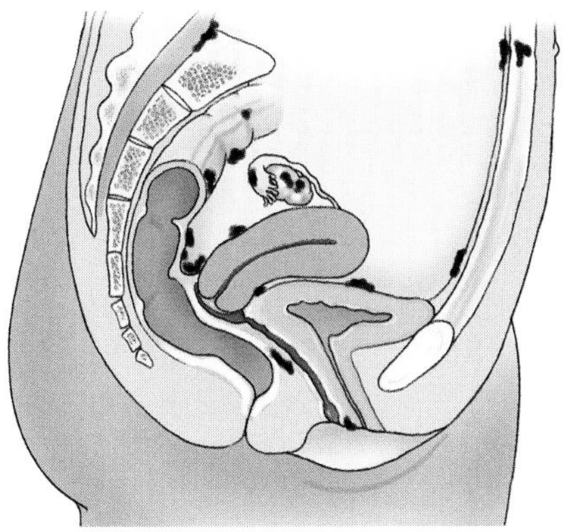

Fig. 8-5 Common sites of endometriosis.

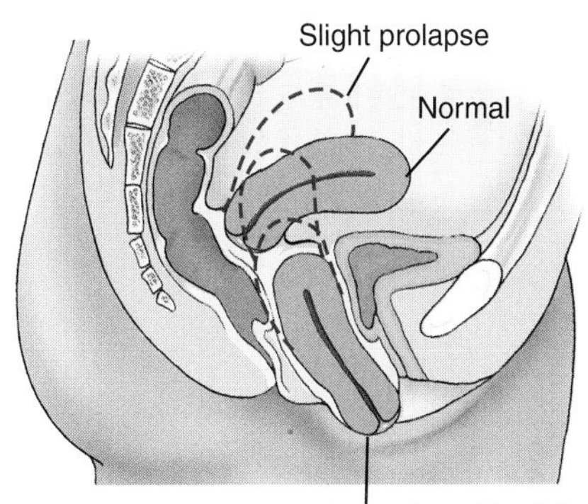

Fig. 8-6 Prolapse of uterus.

DID YOU KNOW?

Human papillomavirus (HPV) may be a cause of dysplastic cervical changes in women and has been implicated as a cause of cervical intraepithelial neoplasia (CIN) and cervical cancer.

Terms Related to Disorders of the Cervix

TERM	WORD ORIGIN	DEFINITION
Cervicitis sur vih SYE tis	*cervic/o* cervix *-itis* inflammation	Inflammation of the cervix.
Dysplasia, cervical dis PLAY zsa	*dys-* abnormal *-plasia* formation	Abnormal formation of the cells of the cervix, sometimes discovered as an abnormal laboratory finding from a Pap smear.
Leukorrhea loo kuh REE ah	*leuk/o* white *-rrhea* flow, discharge	Whitish discharge usually resulting from an inflammation of the cervix.

Exercise 7: DISORDERS OF THE UTERUS AND CERVIX

Fill in the blanks with the terms provided.

hysteroptosis, leukorrhea, cervicitis, leiomyoma, endometriosis, dysplasia, retroflexion of uterus

1. uterine prolapse ________________
2. white-colored cervical discharge ________________
3. uterus bent toward spine ________________
4. inflammation of cervix ________________
5. healthcare term for fibroids leiomyoma
6. abnormal formation (of cells of cervix) ________________
7. condition of ectopic endometrial tissue ________________

Terms Related to Disorders of the Vagina and Vulva		
TERM	**WORD ORIGIN**	**DEFINITION**
Vaginal prolapse PRO laps	*pro-* forward *-lapse* fall	Downward displacement of the vagina. Also called **colpoptosis** (kohl pop TOH sis).
Vaginitis vaj ih NYE tis	*vagin/o* vagina *-itis* inflammation	Inflammation of the vagina.
Vulvitis vul VYE tis	*vulv/o* vulva *-itis* inflammation	Inflammation of the external female genitalia.
Vulvodynia vul voh DIN ee ah	*vulv/o* vulva *-dynia* pain	Idiopathic syndrome of nonspecific complaints of pain of the vulva.
Vulvovaginitis vul voh vaj ih NYE tis	*vulv/o* vulva *vagin/o* vagina *-itis* inflammation	Inflammation of the vulva and the vagina.

Terms Related to Disorders of the Breast		
TERM	**WORD ORIGIN**	**DEFINITION**
Fibrocystic disease fye broh SIS tick	*fibr/o* fiber *cyst/o* sac *-ic* pertaining to	Normally benign condition of the palpable presence of single or multiple cysts in the breast.
Mastitis mass TYE tis	*mast/o* breast *-itis* inflammation	Inflammation of the breast.
Thelitis thee LYE tis	*thel/o* nipple *-itis* inflammation	Inflammation of the nipples; also referred to as **acromastitis** (ack kroh mass TYE tis), meaning an inflammation of the extremities of the breast.

Exercise 8: DISORDERS OF THE VAGINA, VULVA, AND BREASTS

Fill in the blanks with the terms provided.

vaginitis, vulvitis, thelitis, mastitis, vulvodynia, vaginal prolapse, vulvovaginitis, fibrocystic disease

1. also known as colpoptosis VAGINAL prolapse
2. inflammation of the external female genitalia vulvitis
3. inflammation of the vagina Vagin itis
4. pain of external female genitalia Vulvodynia
5. also known as acromastitis thelitis
   └ Extremities of the Breast

DID YOU KNOW?

Fibrocystic disease does have the potential for malignancy and must be monitored.

6. inflammation of the breast ____________

7. benign condition of multiple cysts in the breast ____________

8. inflammation of female external genitalia and vagina ____________

Terms Related to Menstrual Disorders

TERM	WORD ORIGIN	DEFINITION
Amenorrhea ah men uh REE ah	*a-* without *men/o* menses *-rrhea* flow	Lack of menstrual flow.
Dysfunctional uterine bleeding (DUB)		Abnormal uterine bleeding not caused by a tumor, inflammation, or pregnancy.
Dysmenorrhea diss men uh REE ah	*dys-* painful *men/o* menses *-rrhea* discharge	Painful menstrual flow, cramps.
Menometrorrhagia men oh met roh RAH zsa	*men/o* menses *metr/o* uterus *-rrhagia* burst forth	Excessive menstrual flow and uterine bleeding other than that caused by menstruation.
Menorrhagia men or RAH zsa	*men/o* menses *-rrhagia* burst forth	Abnormally heavy or prolonged menstrual period; may be an indication of fibroids.
Metrorrhagia met roh RAH zsa	*metr/o* uterus *-rrhagia* burst forth	Uterine bleeding other than that caused by menstruation. May be caused by uterine lesions.
Oligomenorrhea oh lig oh men oh REE ah	*oligo-* scanty *men/o* menses *-rrhea* discharge	Abnormally light menstrual flow; **menorrhea** refers to the normal discharge of blood and tissue from the uterus.
Premenstrual dysphoric disorder (PMDD)	*pre-* before *menstru/o* menses *-al* pertaining to *dys-* abnormal *phor/o* carry, bear *-ic* pertaining to	Mood disorder that includes depression, irritability, fatigue, changes in appetite or sleep, and difficulty in concentrating; occurs 1 to 2 weeks before the onset of the menstrual flow.
Premenstrual syndrome (PMS)	*pre-* before *menstru/o* menses *-al* pertaining to *syn-* together *-drome* run	Poorly understood group of symptoms that occur in some women on a cyclical basis: Breast pain, irritability, fluid retention, headache, and lack of coordination are some of the symptoms.
Polymenorrhea pol ee men or REE ah	*poly-* excessive *men/o* menses *-rrhea* discharge	Abnormally frequent menstrual flow.

 Exercise 9: MENSTRUAL DISORDERS

Fill in the blanks with the terms provided.

premenstrual syndrome, menometrorrhagia, dysmenorrhea, amenorrhea, polymenorrhea, dysfunctional uterine bleeding, oligomenorrhea, menorrhagia, premenstrual dysmorphic disorder

1. What is the term for the lack of menstruation? ______________________________
2. What is the term for an excessively heavy menstrual period? ______________________________
3. What is the term for menstrual cramps? ______________________________
4. What is the term for bleeding from the uterus that is not a result of menstruation? ______________________________
5. What is the term for scanty menstruation? ______________________________
6. What is the term for the group of symptoms occurring on a cyclical basis that include irritability, retention of fluid, lack of coordination, and so on? ______________________________
7. What is the term for excessive menstrual and dysfunctional bleeding? ______________________________
8. What mood disorder occurs before menstruation and includes depression, appetite loss, and sleep disorders? ______________________________
9. What is the term for frequent menstrual bleeding? ______________________________

Infertility

Couples who are infertile are unable to produce offspring. The causes of infertility in the female may be endometriosis, ovulation problems, poor egg quality, polycystic ovarian syndrome, or female tube blockages. In the male, the problems may be lack of sperm production or viability, or male tube blockages. His partner may even be allergic to his sperm. Treatments are dependent on the variety of causal factors and are discussed in the Therapeutic Interventions and Pharmacology sections.

DID YOU KNOW?

One out of 10 women diagnosed with eclampsia die from it.

Terms Related to Pregnancy Disorders

TERM	WORD ORIGIN	DEFINITION
Abruptio placentae ah BRUP she oh plah SEN tee		Premature separation of the placenta from the uterine wall; may result in a severe hemorrhage that can threaten both infant and maternal lives. Also called **ablatio placentae** (ah BLAY she oh).
Cephalopelvic disproportion seh fah loh PELL vick	*cephal/o* head *pelv/i* pelvis *-ic* pertaining to	Condition in which the infant's head is larger than the pelvic outlet it must pass through, thereby inhibiting normal labor and birth. It is one of the indications for a cesarean section.
Eclampsia eck LAMP see ah	See **Did You Know?** box	Extremely serious form of hypertension secondary to pregnancy. Patients are at risk for coma, convulsions, and death.

Terms Related to Pregnancy Disorders—cont'd

TERM	WORD ORIGIN	DEFINITION
Ectopic pregnancy eck TAH pick	*ec-* out of *top/o* place *-ic* pertaining to	Implantation of the embryo in any location but the uterus (Fig. 8-7).
Erythroblastosis fetalis eh RITH roh blas toh sis feh TAL is	*erythr/o* red (blood cell) *blast/o* immature *-osis* abnormal condition	Condition in which mother is Rh negative and her fetus is Rh positive, causing the mother to form antibodies to the Rh-positive factor. Subsequent Rh-positive pregnancies will be in jeopardy because the mother's anti-Rh antibodies will cross the placenta and destroy fetal blood cells (Fig. 8-8).
Miscarriage/abortion		Termination of a pregnancy before the fetus is viable. If spontaneous, it may be termed a **miscarriage** or a **spontaneous abortion.** If induced, it can be referred to as a **therapeutic abortion.**
Oligohydramnios oh lih goh hye DRAM nee ohs	*oligo-* scanty *hydr/o* fluid *-amnios* amnion	Condition of low or missing amniotic fluid.
Placenta previa plah SEN tah PREE vee ah	*previa* in front of	Placenta that is malpositioned in the uterus, so that it covers the opening of the cervix.
Polyhydramnios pah lee hye DRAM nee ohs	*poly-* excessive *hydr/o* fluid *-amnios* amnion	Condition of excessive amniotic fluid.
Preeclampsia pre eh KLAMP see ah	*pre-* before See **Did You Know?** box	Abnormal condition of pregnancy with unknown etiology, marked by hypertension, edema, and proteinuria. Also called **toxemia of pregnancy.**

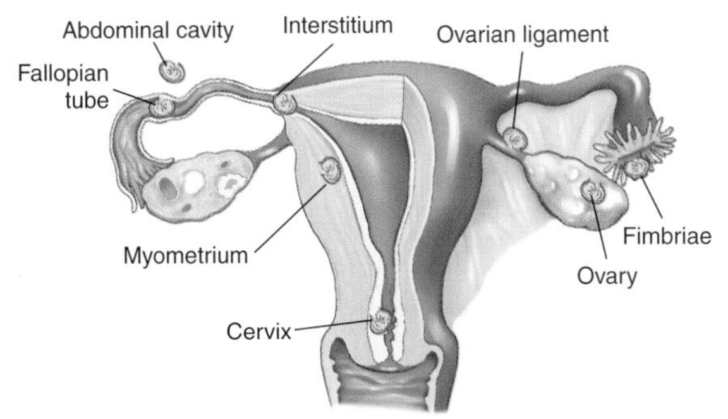

Fig. 8-7 Sites of ectopic pregnancy.

DID YOU KNOW?

Because 95% of ectopic pregnancies occur in the fallopian tubes, these are also called *tubal pregnancies.*

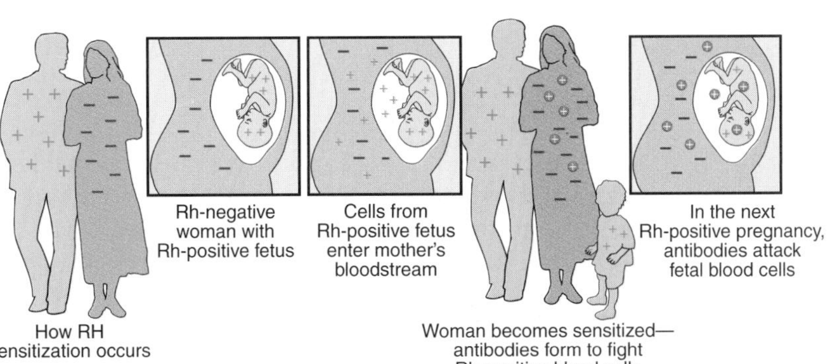

Fig. 8-8 Diagram illustrating the concept of Rh sensitization.

DID YOU KNOW?

The term *eclampsia* comes from a Greek word meaning *a flash of light,* referring to what a victim of convulsions may experience. Later, the term was restricted to mean a *disorder of pregnancy* that can result in convulsions.

Terms Related to Neonatal Disorders		
TERM	**WORD ORIGIN**	**DEFINITION**
Meconium staining meh KOH nee um	See **Did You Know?** box	Refers to fetal defecation while in utero and indicates fetal distress. **Meconium** is the first feces of the newborn.
Nuchal cord NOO kul	*nuch/o* neck *-al* pertaining to	Abnormal but common occurrence of the umbilical cord wrapped around the neck of the neonate.

Exercise 10: DISORDERS OF PREGNANCY AND THE NEWBORN

Fill in the blanks with the terms provided.

ectopic pregnancy, nuchal cord, abortion, oligohydramnios, eclampsia, placenta previa, meconium, erythroblastosis fetalis, preeclampsia, placenta abruptio, cephalopelvic disproportion

1. What are the first feces of the newborn called? ________________
2. What is the term for the cord wrapped around the neck of the neonate? ________________
3. What is the term for a placenta that separates prematurely from the wall of the uterus? ________________
4. What is the term for a baby's head being larger than the pelvic outlet? ________________
5. What is the term for a pregnancy that takes place anywhere but in the uterus? ________________
6. What is the term for the termination of a pregnancy, intentionally or not, before the fetus is viable? ________________
7. What is the term for a complication of pregnancy characterized by protein in the mother's urine, hypertension, and swelling? ________________
8. What is the term for a placenta that is attached to the opening of the cervix? ________________
9. What is the term for an abnormally small amount of amniotic fluid? ________________
10. What is the term for a severe form of toxemia that may result in convulsions, coma, and death? ________________
11. Incompatibility between Rh factors of mother and baby that leads to destruction of red blood cells in the fetus is called ________________

Case Study Continued

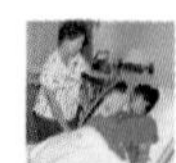

As Susan and Linda talk, Linda reviews the results from her blood work, urine tests, height, weight, and blood pressure measurements. Because of Susan's age, she discusses prenatal testing with her, and Susan agrees to discuss amniocentesis, chorionic villus sampling, and alpha-fetoprotein testing with her husband. "I will be able to keep working, won't I?" asks Susan. "We'll monitor you for possible abnormal prenatal conditions, but they really aren't that common," replies Linda. "Generally, I can say that you can work as long as you feel well." They conclude the appointment by discussing the expected schedule of visits for the next few months.

DIAGNOSTIC PROCEDURES

Terms Related to Imaging

TERM	WORD ORIGIN	DEFINITION
Cervicography sur vih KAH gruh fee	*cervic/o* cervix *-graphy* process of recording	Photographic procedure in which a specially designed 35-mm camera is used to image the entire cervix to produce a slide called a **cervigram.** It is used to detect early cervical intraepithelial neoplasia (CIN) or invasive cervical cancer. Can be combined with **colposcopy** or be done on its own.
Hysterosalpingography (HSG) his tur oh sal pin GAH gruh fee	*hyster/o* uterus *salping/o* fallopian tube *-graphy* process of recording	X-ray procedure using contrast medium to image the uterus and fallopian tubes (Fig. 8-9).
Mammography mam MOG gruh fee	*mamm/o* breast *-graphy* process of recording	Imaging technique for the early detection of breast cancer.
Pelvimetry pell VIH meh tree	*pelv/i* pelvis *-metry* process of measurement	Measurement of the birth canal. Types of pelvimetry include clinical and x-ray, although x-ray pelvimetry is not commonly done.
Ultrasonography	*ultra-* beyond *son/o* sound *-graphy* process of recording	Use of high-frequency sound waves to image the pelvic area **(pelvic ultrasounds)** and the uterus **(sonohysterography).** A **transvaginal ultrasound** of the pelvic cavity is obtained through the use of a probe introduced into the vagina (Fig. 8-10).

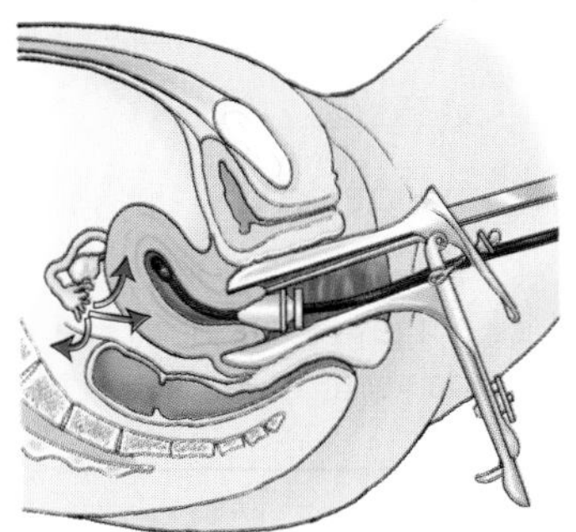

Fig. 8-9 Hysterosalpingography.

DID YOU KNOW?

Meconium derives its name from the Greek term for *poppy juice,* which is a purplish-black color.

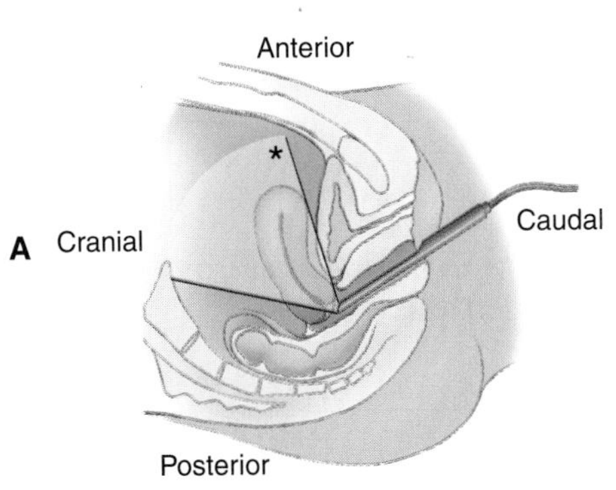

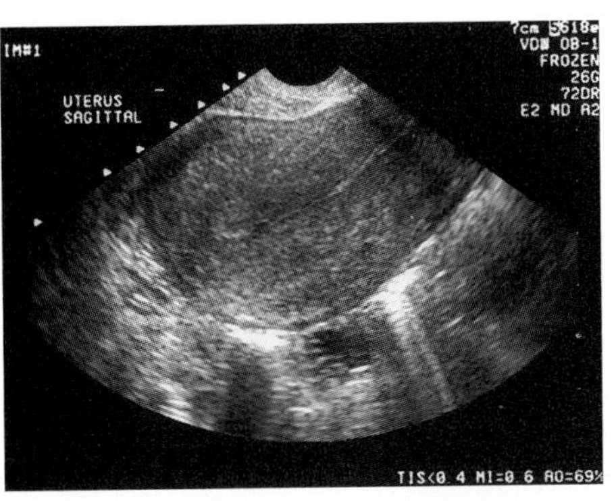

Fig. 8-10 **A,** Transvaginal sonography. **B,** Transvaginal sagittal view of the uterus.

BE CAREFUL!

Don't confuse the suffix *-metry,* which means the *process of measurement,* with *metr/o,* the combining form for the uterus.

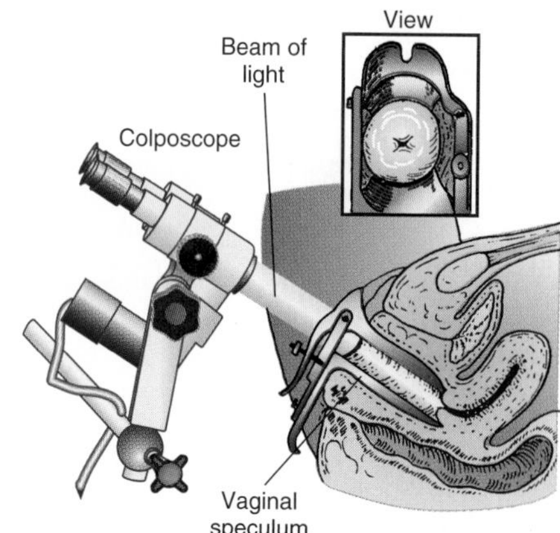

Fig. 8-11 Colposcopy.

Terms Related to Endoscopies

TERM	WORD ORIGIN	DEFINITION
Colposcopy kohl PAH skuh pee	*colp/o* vagina *-scopy* visual examination	Endoscopic procedure used for a cervical/vaginal biopsy. The instrument used is called a **colposcope** (Fig. 8-11).
Culdoscopy kull DAH skuh pee	*culd/o* cul-de-sac *-scopy* visual examination	Endoscopic procedure used for biopsy of Douglas's cul-de-sac. The instrument used is called a **culdoscope.**
Hysteroscopy hiss tuh RAH skuh pee	*hyster/o* uterus *-scopy* visual examination	Endoscopic procedure used for a myomectomy (fibroid removal) or polypectomy (polyp removal). The instrument used is called a **hysteroscope.**
Laparoscopy lap uh RAH skuh pee	*lapar/o* abdomen *-scopy* visual examination	Endoscopic procedure for removing lesions (lysis), a hysterectomy, or ovarian biopsy. The instrument used is called a **laparoscope.**

Terms Related to Laboratory Tests

TERM	WORD ORIGIN	DEFINITION
Culdocentesis kull doh sen TEE sis	*culd/o* cul-de-sac *-centesis* removal of fluid	Removal of fluid and cells from the rectouterine pouch to detect dysplasia.
Hormone levels		Lab specimens taken to test for hormone levels, indicating a range of conditions from pregnancy to menopause.
Pap smear		Exfoliative cytology procedure useful for the detection of vaginal and cervical cancer.

Exercise 11: FEMALE REPRODUCTIVE IMAGING TECHNIQUES, ENDOSCOPIES, AND LABORATORY TESTS

Fill in the blanks with the terms provided.

cervicography, culdoscopy, pelvimetry, hysterosalpingography, mammography, sonohysterography, colposcopy, hysteroscopy, laparoscopy, hormone levels, Pap smear, culdocentesis

1. process of imaging the uterus and fallopian tubes ____________________

2. removal of fluid from Douglas's cul-de-sac ____________________

3. measurement of the birth canal ______________

4. photographic recording of the cervix ______________
5. endoscopic procedure for fibroid/polyp removal ______________

6. endoscopic procedure for vaginal biopsy ______________

7. imaging of the breast ______________
8. high-frequency sound waves used to image the uterus ______________

9. endoscopic procedure for removing lesions ______________

10. endoscopic procedure for biopsy of Douglas's cul-de-sac ______________

11. lab test to detect a range of conditions from pregnancy to menopause ______________

12. removal of cells from cervix to detect abnormal cells ______________

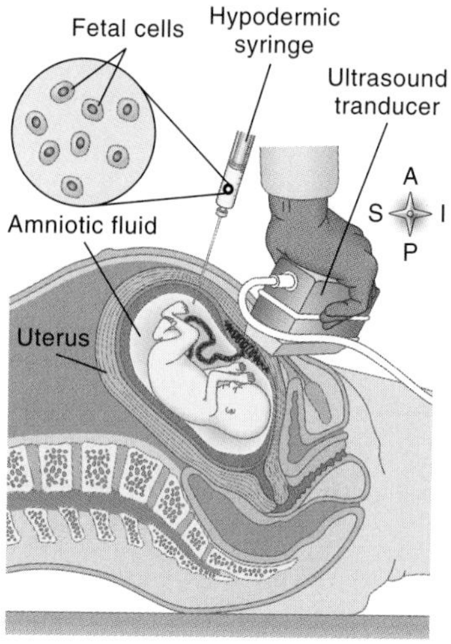

Fig. 8-12 Amniocentesis.

Terms Related to Prenatal Diagnosis

TERM	WORD ORIGIN	DEFINITION
Alpha-fetoprotein (AFP) test al fah fee toh PROH teen		Maternal serum (blood) alpha-fetoprotein test performed between 14 and 19 weeks of gestation; may indicate a variety of conditions such as neural tube defects (spina bifida is the most common finding) and multiple gestation.
Amniocentesis am nee oh sen TEE sis	*amni/o* amnion *-centesis* removal of fluid for diagnostic purposes	Removal and analysis of a sample of the amniotic fluid with the use of a guided needle through the abdomen of the mother into the amniotic sac to diagnose fetal abnormalities (Fig. 8-12).
Chorionic villus sampling (CVS) kore ee AH nick VILL us	*chorion/o* chorion *-ic* pertaining to	Removal of a small piece of the outer covering of the fetus, the chorion, either transvaginally or through a small incision in the abdomen, to test for chromosomal abnormalities.
Contraction stress test (CST)		Test to predict fetal outcome and risk of intrauterine asphyxia by measuring fetal heart rate throughout a minimum of 3 contractions within a 10-minute period.
Pregnancy test		Test available in two forms: a standard over-the-counter pregnancy test, which examines urine for the presence of hCG; or a serum (blood) pregnancy test performed in a physician's office or laboratory to get a quantitative hCG.
Nonstress test (NST)		Stimulation of the fetus to monitor for a normal, expected acceleration of the fetal heart rate (FHR). A nonreactive stress test should be followed by a CST and possible ultrasound studies.

Terms Related to Postnatal Diagnosis		
TERM	**WORD ORIGIN**	**DEFINITION**
Apgar score		Rates the physical health of the infant with a set of criteria 1 minute and 5 minutes after birth.
Congenital hypothyroidism	*hypo-* below *thyroid/o* thyroid *-ism* condition	Condition of deficient thyroid hormones. Undiscovered and untreated, it can lead to retarded growth and brain development. If caught at birth, oral doses of the missing thyroid hormone will allow normal development.
Phenylketonuria (PKU) fee null kee tone YOOR ee ah	*keton/o* ketones *-uria* urine condition	Test for deficiency of enzyme phenylalanine hydroxylase, which is responsible for converting phenylalanine, found in certain foods, into tyrosine. Failure to treat this condition will lead to brain damage and mental retardation.

Exercise 12: PRENATAL AND POSTNATAL DIAGNOSIS

Fill in the blanks with the terms provided.

alpha-fetoprotein, human chorionic gonadotropin, Apgar, nonstress test, phenylketonuria, amniocentesis, chorionic villus sampling, contraction stress test, congenital hypothyroidism

1. What hormone does a pregnancy test look for? ______________
2. What is the term for removal of fluid from the amniotic cavity? ______________
3. What is the name of the test done 1 and 5 minutes after birth that scores the physical health of the neonate? ______________
4. What is a measurement of fetal heart rate through contractions? ______________
5. What test determines fetal health by measuring the heart rate? ______________
6. What test of maternal blood between 14 and 19 weeks indicates neural tube defects and/or multiple gestation? ______________
7. What is a condition of deficient thyroid hormones that is present at birth? ______________
8. What is a test of neonates for a specific enzyme, the lack of which may lead to brain damage and mental retardation? ______________
9. What test of a sample from the outer covering of the fetus determines chromosomal abnormalities? ______________

THERAPEUTIC INTERVENTIONS

Terms Related to Nonpregnancy Procedures

TERM	WORD ORIGIN	DEFINITION
Cervicectomy sur vih SECK tuh mee	*cervic/o* cervix *-ectomy* removal	Resection (removal) of the uterine cervix.
Colpopexy KOHL poh peck see	*colp/o* vagina *-pexy* fixation, suspension	Fixation of the vagina to an adjacent structure to hold it in place.
Colpoplasty KOHL poh plas tee	*colp/o* vagina *-plasty* surgical repair	Surgical repair of the vagina.
Dilation and curettage (D&C) dye LAY shun KYOOR ih tahj		Procedure involving widening (dilation) of the cervix until a curette, a sharp scraping tool, can be inserted to remove the lining of the uterus (curettage). Used to treat and diagnose conditions such as heavy menstrual bleeding or to empty the uterus of the products of conception.
Hysterectomy hiss tur RECK tuh mee	*hyster/o* uterus *-ectomy* removal	Resection (removal) of the uterus; may be partial, pan- (all), or include other organs as well (e.g., *t*otal *a*bdominal *h*ysterectomy with a *b*ilateral *s*alpingo-*o*ophorectomy [TAH-BSO]). The surgical approach is usually stated: whether it is laparoscopic, vaginal, or abdominal.
Hysteropexy HISS tur roh peck see	*hyster/o* uterus *-pexy* fixation, suspension	Suspension and fixation of a prolapsed uterus.
Lumpectomy lum PECK tuh mee	*-ectomy* removal	Removal of a tumor from the breast.
Mammoplasty MAM oh plas tee	*mamm/o* breast *-plasty* surgical repair	Surgical or cosmetic repair of the breast. Options may include augmentation, to increase the size of the breasts, or reduction, to reduce the size of the breasts.
Mastectomy mass TECK tuh mee	*mast/o* breast *-ectomy* removal	Removal of the breast; may be unilateral or bilateral.
Mastopexy MASS toh peck see	*mast/o* breast *-pexy* fixation, suspension	Reconstructive procedure to lift and fixate the breasts.
Oophorectomy oo ah fore ECK tuh mee	*oophor/o* ovary *-ectomy* removal	Resection of an ovary; may be unilateral or bilateral.
Pelvic exenteration eck sen tuh RAY shun		Removal of the contents of the pelvic cavity. Pelvic exenteration is done usually in response to widespread cancer to remove the uterus, fallopian tubes, ovaries, bladder, vagina, rectum, and lymph nodes (Fig. 8-13).
Salpingectomy sal pin JECK tuh mee	*salping/o* fallopian tubes *-ectomy* removal	Resection of a fallopian tube; may be unilateral or bilateral.
Salpingolysis sal ping GALL ih sis	*salping/o* fallopian tubes *-lysis* destroy	Removal of the adhesions in the fallopian tubes to reestablish patency, with the goal of fertility.
Uterine artery embolization (UAE) em boh lye ZAY shun		Injection of particles to block a uterine artery supplying blood to a fibroid with resultant death of fibroid tissue.

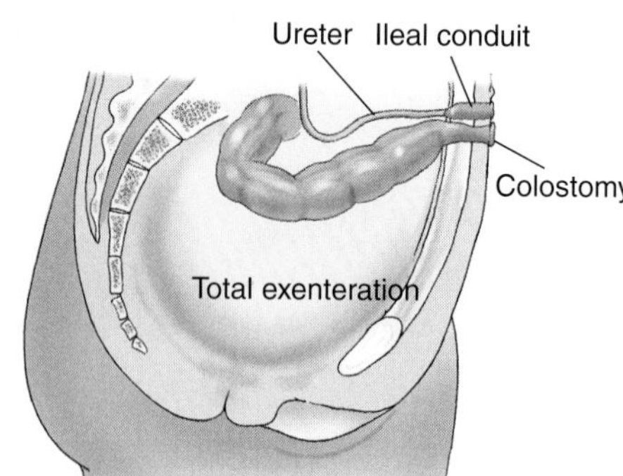

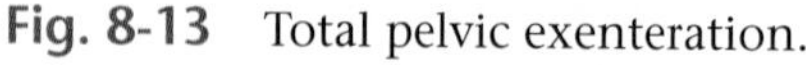
Fig. 8-13 Total pelvic exenteration.

Exercise 13: Therapeutic Interventions Not Related to Pregnancy

Fill in the blanks with the terms provided.

lumpectomy, dilation and curettage, salpingolysis, colpoplasty, hysteropexy, pelvic exenteration, uterine artery embolization, mastopexy, bilateral oophorectomy, TAH-BSO

1. What surgical procedure suspends the uterus? _______________
2. What surgical procedure removes adhesions from the fallopian tubes? _______________
3. What surgical procedure resects both ovaries? _______________
4. What surgical procedure resects the entire uterus, fallopian tubes, and ovaries through an incision in the abdomen? _______________
5. What is removal of a tumor from the breast called? _______________
6. What is the term for the removal of the contents of the pelvic cavity? _______________
7. What procedure treats fibroids without surgically removing them? _______________
8. What is the term for a procedure that widens the cervix in order to remove the lining of the uterus? _______________
9. What is surgical repair of the vagina called? _______________
10. What is the term for the lifting and fixation of sagging breasts? _______________

Case Study Continued

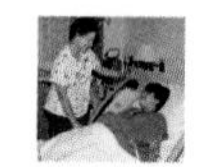

Susan comes in for a routine examination during her thirty-second week of pregnancy. Susan's eyes widen as she sees the scale reading as she is weighed. "Oh, no! Are you *sure* there's only one baby?" Linda reviews the urinalysis results and the blood pressure reading. "Well, the good news is that you're not preeclamptic, but the bad news is that we'll have to have a little diet discussion."

As Linda advises Susan to replace her cheese steak lunches with salad, she asks about Susan's scheduled Lamaze classes. "We really want to have a natural birth," says Susan. "I want this baby to have every advantage possible." Linda nods, "Of course, but please remember that we'll do what's best for the baby—whatever that may be. You should have a little information about a C-section, just in case."

Terms Related to Pregnancy and Delivery Procedures

TERM	WORD ORIGIN	DEFINITION
Cephalic version seh FAL ick	*cephal/o* head *-ic* pertaining to *version* process of turning	Process of turning the fetus so that the head is at the cervical outlet for a vaginal delivery.
Cerclage sur KLAHZH		Suturing the cervix closed to prevent a spontaneous abortion in a woman with an incompetent cervix. The suture is removed when the pregnancy is at full term to allow the delivery to proceed normally (Fig. 8-14).
Cesarean section (C-section, CS)	See **Did You Know?** box	Delivery of an infant through a surgical abdominal incision (Fig. 8-15).
Episiotomy eh pee zee AH tuh mee	*episi/o* vulva *-tomy* incision	Incision to widen the vaginal orifice to avoid tearing the tissue of the vulva during delivery.
Oxytocia ock see TOH sha	*oxy-* rapid *-tocia* labor, delivery	Rapid birth. **Dystocia** is a difficult labor.
Vaginal birth after C-section (VBAC) VAJ ih nul	*vagin/o* vagina *-al* pertaining to	Delivery of subsequent babies vaginally after a C-section. In the past, women were told "once a C-section, always a C-section." Currently, this is being changed by recent developments in technique.
Vaginal delivery	*vagin/o* vagina *-al* pertaining to	(Usually) cephalic presentation (head first) through the vagina. Feet or buttock presentation is a **breech** delivery.

DID YOU KNOW?

Cesarean section derives its name from one of the first individuals purported to be delivered in this manner: Julius Caesar.

DID YOU KNOW?

Contractions often continue after birth to deliver the placenta and its membranes, called *afterbirth*. Subsequent uterine contractions help the uterus return to its nongravid size and shape.

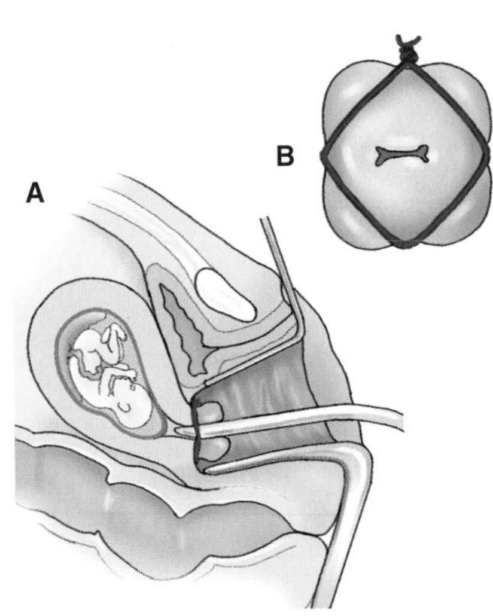

Fig. 8-14 **A,** Cerclage correction of premature dilation of the cervix. **B,** Cross-sectional view of closed cervix.

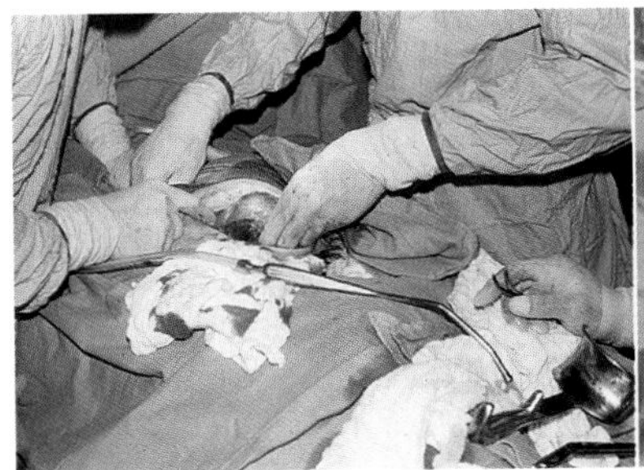
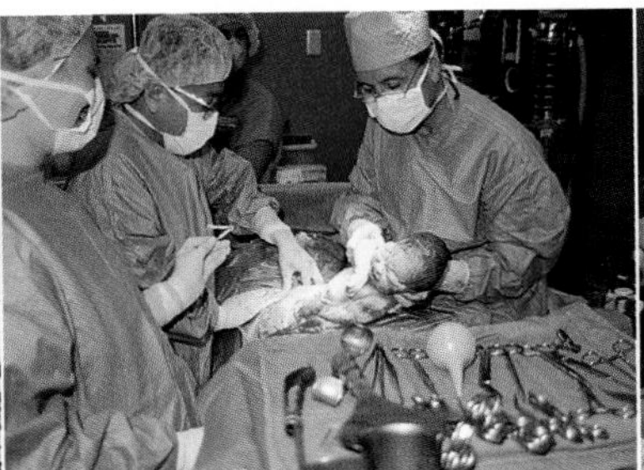
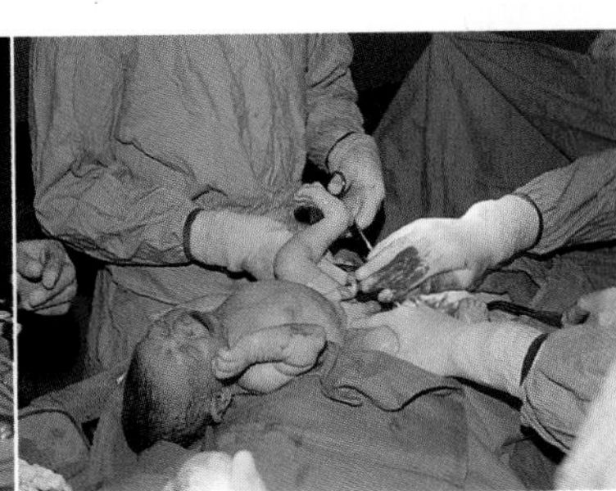

Fig. 8-15 Cesarean birth.

Terms Related to Infertility Procedures

Term	Word Origin	Definition
Artificial insemination (AI)	*in-* in *semin/i* semen *-ation* process of	Introduction of semen into the vagina by mechanical or instrumental means.
Gamete intrafallopian transfer (GIFT) GAM eet in trah fah LOH pee un	*intra-* within *fallopi/o* fallopian tube	Laboratory mixing and injection of the ova and sperm into the fallopian tubes so that fertilization occurs naturally within the body.
Intracytoplasmic sperm injection (ICSI)	*intra-* within *cyt/o* cell *plasm/o* formation *-ic* pertaining to	Injection of one sperm into the ovum and subsequent transplantation of the resulting zygote into the uterus.
In vitro fertilization (IVF) in VEE tro	*in* in *vitro* life	Procedure that allows the mother's ova to be fertilized outside the body and then implanted in the uterus of either the biologic mother or a surrogate to carry to term.
Zygote intrafallopian transfer (ZIFT)	*intra-* within *fallopi/o* fallopian tube	Mixing of the ova and sperm in the laboratory, with fertilization confirmed before the zygotes are returned to the fallopian tubes.

Terms Related to Sterilization

Term	Word Origin	Definition
Sterilization		Surgical procedure rendering a person unable to produce children; for women may involve hysterectomy, bilateral oophorectomy, or tubal ligation.
Tubal ligation TOO bul lye GAY shun		Sterilization procedure in which the fallopian tubes are cut, ligated (tied), and cauterized to prevent the ova released from being fertilized by spermatozoa (Fig. 8-16).

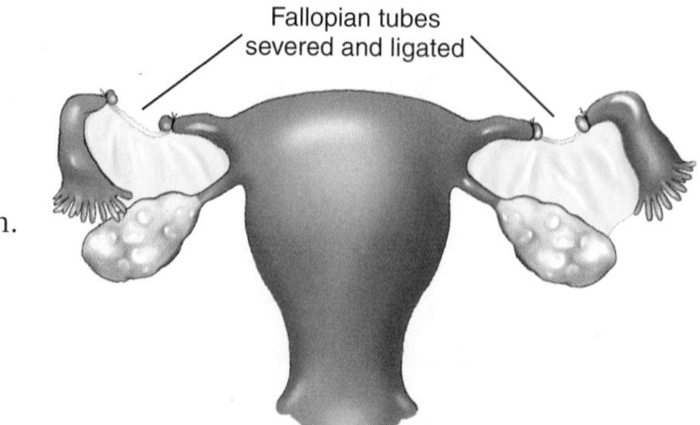

Fig. 8-16 Tubal ligation.

Exercise 14: INTERVENTIONS RELATED TO PROCREATION AND CONTRACEPTION

Fill in the blanks with the terms provided.

episiotomy, C-section, VBAC, tubal ligation, cerclage, cephalic version, sterilization, vaginal delivery

1. The fallopian tubes are cut, tied, and cauterized in which procedure? ______________
2. A patient who has a baby vaginally after having a cesarean section may have what abbreviation on her chart? ______________
3. A procedure performed to widen the vaginal opening during delivery is a/an ______________.
4. What is the term for a normal delivery? ______________
5. What is the procedure to turn the infant if its head is not down? ______________
6. What is the term for a delivery via an incision? ______________
7. A bilateral oophorectomy would effectively cause ______________.
8. A procedure to keep an incompetent cervix closed until the due date is called ______________.

Match the abbreviations with the type of fertilization technique.

__A__ 9. IVF

__C__ 10. ZIFT

__B__ 11. AI

__D__ 12. GIFT

__E__ 13. ICSI

A. ova fertilized outside of the body, then implanted in the uterus of biologic mother or surrogate.
B. semen introduced in vagina by means other than sexual intercourse.
C. ova and sperm mixed outside of the body; confirmed zygotes are implanted in uterus.
D. ova and sperm injected in oviducts; fertilization occurs within the body.
E. ovum injected with one sperm; confirmed zygote is implanted in uterus.

PHARMACOLOGY

Contraceptive Management

Abortifacient (ah bore tih FAY shee ent): Medication that terminates pregnancy.
Abstinence: Total avoidance of sexual intercourse as a contraceptive option that does not involve medications, surgery, or devices; 100% effective.
Barrier methods: See **diaphragm** and **cervical cap.**
Cervical cap: Small rubber cup that fits over the cervix to prevent sperm from entering.
Contraceptive sponge: Intravaginal barrier with a spermicidal additive.
Diaphragm: Soft, rubber hemisphere that fits over the cervix after being filled with a contraceptive cream or gel.
Emergency contraception pill (ECP): Pill that can prevent pregnancy after unprotected vaginal intercourse; does not affect existing pregnancies or cause abortions.
Female condom: Soft, flexible sheath that fits within the vagina and prevents sperm from entering the vagina.
Implant: Timed-release medication placed under the skin of the upper arm, providing long-term protection.

DID YOU KNOW?

Both male and female condoms also offer some protection against sexually transmitted diseases.

> **DID YOU KNOW?**
>
> Although adverse publicity surrounding one type of IUD years ago has deterred many women from considering it as a contraceptive option, the American Medical Association, the American College of Obstetricians and Gynecologists, and the World Health Organization recognize it as one of the safest and most effective forms of reversible birth control.

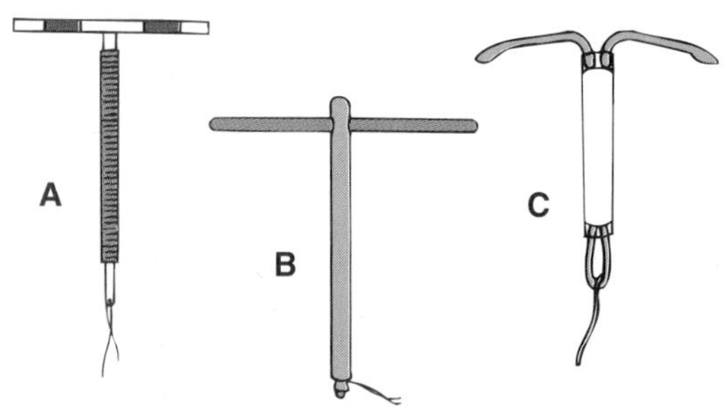

Fig. 8-17 IUDs. **A,** Copper T380A. **B,** Progesterone T. **C,** Levonorgestrel-releasing IUD.

Injection: Contraceptive such as Depo-Provera that may be given approximately four times a year to provide 99.7% reliability in preventing pregnancies.
Intrauterine device (IUD): Small, flexible device inserted into the uterus that prevents implantation of a zygote (Fig. 8-17).
Male condom: Soft, flexible sheath that covers the penis and prevents sperm from entering the vagina.
Mifepristone: Medication that—followed with a dose of misoprostol, a prostaglandin—induces spontaneous abortion. Previously known as RU-486.
Oral contraceptive pill (OCP): Pill containing estrogen and/or progesterone taken daily to fool the body into thinking that it is pregnant, so that ovulation is suppressed.
Procreative and contraceptive management: Term for a variety of medications and techniques that describe the options available for women's reproductive health.
Rhythm method: A natural family planning method that involves charting the menstrual cycle to recognize fertile and infertile periods.
Spermicides: Foam or gel inserted into the vagina before intercourse to kill sperm.
Transdermal patch: Timed-release contraceptive worn on the skin.

Exercise 15: CONTRACEPTIVE OPTIONS

Fill in the blanks with the terms provided.

abstinence, rhythm method, abortifacient, OCP, spermicides, IUDs, condoms, ECP, barrier methods

1. A contraceptive method that works by suppressing ovulation. ______________
2. Diaphragms and cervical caps are examples of what type of contraceptive method? ______________
3. Soft, flexible sheaths that prevent sperm from entering the vagina are called ______________.
4. Small flexible devices that fit within the uterus are called ______________.
5. A medication intended to terminate a pregnancy is a/an ______________.
6. A natural family planning method that has participants chart the woman's menstrual cycle to determine fertile and infertile periods. ______________
7. The only 100% effective contraceptive method. ______________
8. Foams and gels may be used as contraceptives in what type of birth control method? ______________
9. An emergency contraceptive measure that prevents pregnancy but does not affect an existing pregnancy is called a/an ______________.

Fertility Drugs

Bromocriptine: Oral or vaginal medication that reduces prolactin levels that suppress ovulation.

Clomiphene: Oral medication taken daily to stimulate the pituitary gland to produce the hormones that trigger ovulation.

Human menopausal gonadotropin (hMG): Fertility treatment that uses two different gonadotropins: one to stimulate the production of egg follicles, and the other to cause the eggs to be released once they are developed.

Drugs to Manage Delivery

Oxytocin: Medication given to induce labor.

Uterine relaxant: Medication given to slow down or stop labor.

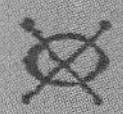

BE CAREFUL!

Do not confuse *oxytocin,* a labor-inducing drug, with *oxytocia,* which means *rapid birth.*

Hormone Replacements

Hormone replacement therapy (HRT), also called estrogen replacement therapy (ERT): The healthcare replacement of estrogen and progesterone perimenopausally in several forms (tablet, transdermal patch, injection, or vaginal suppository) to relieve symptoms of menopause and protect against osteoporosis.

Phytoestrogens: An alternative source of estrogen replacement through the ingestion of soy proteins.

Exercise 16: FERTILITY, DELIVERY, AND HORMONE REPLACEMENT DRUGS

Circle the correct answer in parentheses.

1. Bromocriptine, clomiphene, and hMG are all used to *(increase, decrease)* fertility.
2. Use of drugs to replace hormones missing as a result of menopause is called *(hormone replacement therapy, contraceptive management).*
3. A natural source of estrogen is found in *(carbohydrates, soy proteins).*
4. Oxytocin is used to *(inhibit, induce)* labor.
5. Medications given to slow down or stop labor are called *(uterine relaxants, phytoestrogens).*

Case Study Continued

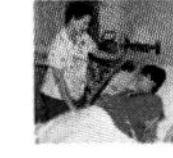

Linda's advice proved valuable, because as a result of a poor nonstress test and low amniotic volume, Susan's baby was delivered via a C-section before term. "I can't believe we spent all that time in Lamaze classes," Susan sighed as she gazed at her baby daughter in her husband's arms. "But, you know what?" she said as her eyes met Linda's, "the bottom line is that we have a beautiful healthy daughter, and I loved having you on my 'team' through the whole pregnancy. Thank you so much!"

Abbreviations

Abbreviation	Definition	Abbreviation	Definition
AFP	Alpha-fetoprotein test	ICSI	Intracytoplasmic sperm injection
AI	Artificial insemination	IUD	Intrauterine device
CIN	Cervical intraepithelial neoplasia	IVF	In vitro fertilization
CS	Cesarean section	LMP	Last menstrual period
CST	Contraction stress test	NST	Nonstress test
CVS	Chorionic villus sampling	Ob	Obstetrics
Cx	Cervix	OCP	Oral contraceptive pill
D&C	Dilation and curettage	PID	Pelvic inflammatory disease
DUB	Dysfunctional uterine bleeding	PKU	Phenylketonuria
ECP	Emergency contraceptive pills	PMDD	Premenstrual dysphoric disorder
EDD	Estimated delivery date	PMS	Premenstrual syndrome
ERT	Estrogen replacement therapy	Rh	Rhesus factor
FHR	Fetal heart rate	TAH-BSO	Total abdominal hysterectomy with a bilateral salpingo-oophorectomy
GIFT	Gamete intrafallopian transfer		
hCG	Human chorionic gonadotropin	UAE	Uterine artery embolization
hMG	Human menopausal gonadotropin	VBAC	Vaginal birth after cesarean section
HRT	Hormone replacement therapy	ZIFT	Zygote intrafallopian transfer

Exercise 17: ABBREVIATIONS

Matching.

____ 1. baby is due

____ 2. pregnancy hormone

____ 3. infertility treatment

____ 4. birth control medication

____ 5. salpingitis

____ 6. removal of uterine lining

____ 7. test for cervical/vaginal cancer

____ 8. removal of uterus, oviducts, and ovaries

A. TAH-BSO
B. OCP
C. Pap smear
D. hCG
E. D&C
F. AI
G. PID
H. EDD

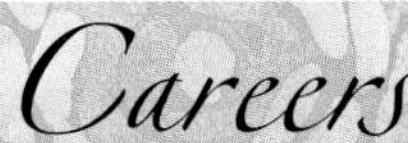

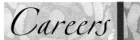

Careers

Midwives and Doulas

Midwives are healthcare providers who assist women through labor and birth. Statistics for expected job growth through the year 2010 are not available through the Bureau of Labor Statistics, but the profession of nursing is expected to grow faster than average. Credentialed midwives in the United States are either Certified Nurse Midwives (CNMs) or Certified Midwives (CM) and are accredited by the American College of Nurse-Midwives. Although most midwives are Registered Nurses before pursuing a specialized credential in midwifery, CMs are individuals credentialed in another healthcare field (e.g., physical therapy) and sit for the same examination as the CNMs. Licensing requirements vary from state to state. For programs and licensing requirements in your area, inquire at http://www.midwife.org.

The term *doula* originates from the Greek term, in ancient times, for the woman servant of the household whose job it was to care for the woman of the house through pregnancy, labor, and delivery. Currently, there are two types of doulas. A birth doula aids a pregnant mother through labor and delivery, providing emotional and psychosocial support as a member of her healthcare team. A birth doula may also provide physical comfort for the laboring mother through the use of massage. A postpartum doula provides support after the delivery of the baby and is instrumental in caring for the mother and the baby, giving breastfeeding advice, cooking, and doing light household chores. Certification may be obtained through a variety of organizations with different requirements and training options. Visit the following Websites for more information:

Doulas of North America: http://www.dona.org
International Childbirth Education Association: http://www.icea.org
Association of Labor Assistants and Childbirth Educators: http://www.alace.org

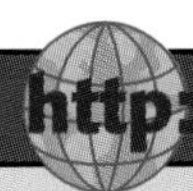

INTERNET PROJECT

Newborn Screening

Many birth defects are not visible, especially those problems due to body chemistry. Early detection and treatment can often help prevent subsequent physical problems and/or mental retardation caused by many of the disorders. Screening newborns for disorders of body chemistry, however, is *not* uniform throughout the United States. Visit http://www.aap.org/policy and review the table of Newborn Screening by States and Jurisdictions to see which disorders hospitals are required to screen for where you live. Choose one of the disorders that your area is not required to screen for and submit a brief description of it. How do you think the decision should be made as to which disorders should be screened?

Chapter Review

A. Functions of the Female Reproductive System

1. In your own words, describe the overall function of the female reproductive system and the three activities the system must accomplish to meet this goal.

____

____

____

B. Anatomy and Physiology

2. Label the diagram of the internal female reproductive system with the correct terms and their corresponding combining forms.

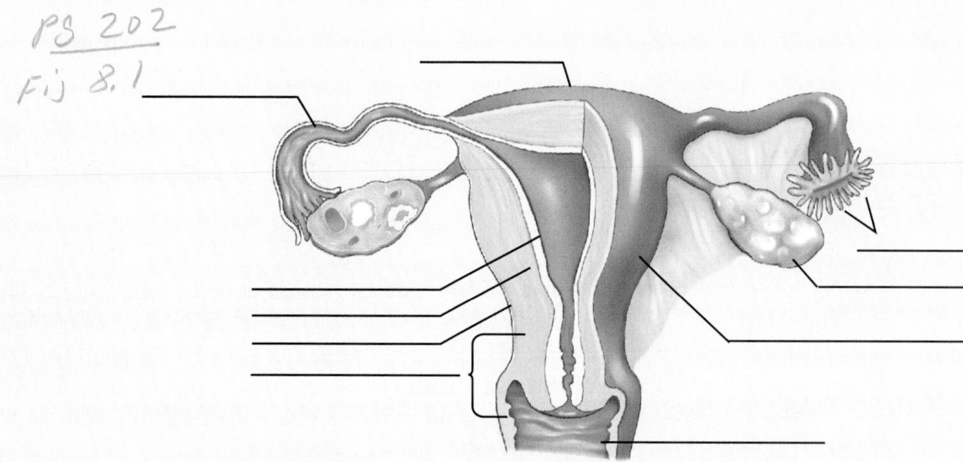

3. Name the term and combining forms for the female gonad. ________________

4. Name the term and combining forms for the female gamete. ________________

5. The release of an egg is called ________________.

6. The release of an egg is influenced by which hormones? ________________

7. The cyclical shedding of the lining of the uterus is called ________________.

8. The beginning of a woman's fertile period is termed ________________, whereas the cessation of fertility is termed ________________.

9. The ovaries are influenced by two hormones secreted by the pituitary: FSH, which causes ________________, and LH, which stimulates the follicle to ________________.

10. The corpus luteum produces which two hormones, and for what are they responsible?

Estrogen & progesterone
Female sex characteristics & cyclical maintenace

11. Name the parts of the external female genitalia, including their combining forms.

labia labi; clitoris, vaginal orifice, hymen
perineum, Bartholin's glands

12. Name the parts of the breast, being sure to include all relevant combining forms.

nipple (thel papill)
areola

13. What is the term that means the production of milk, and what are its combining forms?

lactation lact, galact

14. What are the terms for sexual intercourse?

Copulation Coitus

15. What is the term for pregnancy, and what are its component word parts?

Gestation gravid - gravida - cyesis

16. Label the following drawing of the uterus of a pregnant woman.

PG 206
Fig 8-3

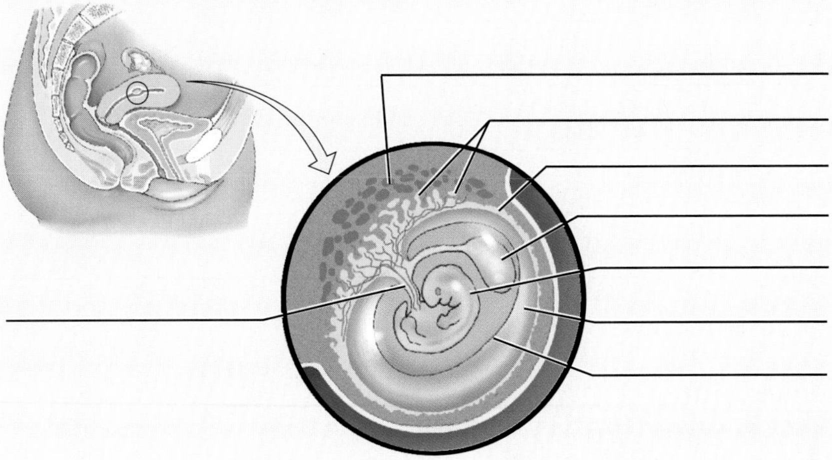

17. What hormone does the fertilized egg secrete, and what is its function?

Human chorionic gonadotropin hCG   Helps the Corpus luteum From Deteriorating

18. What two sacs enclose the embryo, and what are their combining forms?

Chorion (chorion) & Amnion (Amnio)

19. What is the highly vascular structure that acts as communication between the mother and the embryo?

Placenta

20. What are the combining forms for the umbilical cord? omphal umbilic

21. What is the healthcare term for delivery? ParTurition

22. A. How many weeks is a normal pregnancy? 38

B. Neonates born at <37 weeks are termed Pre- .

C. Neonates weighing less than 2500 grams at birth are termed Low .

23. What are the suffixes for labor and delivery? -tocia ; -para

C. Pathology
Build a term.

24. What is the term for too little amniotic fluid? oligohydramnios

25. What is the term for a lack of menstruation? Amenorrhea

26. What is the term for a lack of ovulation? anovulation

27. What is the term for prolapse of the uterus? hysteroptosis

28. What is the term for a whitish discharge due to cervicitis? leukorrhea

Decode the term.

29. thelitis inflammation of nipple

30. ectopic pregnancy preg out of Place

31. endometriosis abnormal condition lining of the uterus

32. retroflexion process of turning backwards

33. vulvovaginitis inflam vulva & vagina

34. pyosalpinx Pus in The fallopian tube

Name the term.

35. What is the term for first feces of the newborn? meconium

36. Ms. Ross was diagnosed with what disorder characterized by multiple sacs on both ovaries? She had symptoms of facial hair, acne, and infertility. Polycystic ovary Syndrome

37. What is the term for an induced termination of a pregnancy before the fetus is viable?
ABortion

38. What is another term for fibroids? leiomyomata

39. What was the term used on the healthcare chart to indicate that Ms. Wright's first son was born with the cord wrapped around his neck? nuchal cord

40. The young mother was diagnosed with what condition that is a complication of pregnancy characterized by hypertension, edema, and protein in the urine? Pre-eclampsia

41. What is the term for the presence of benign cysts in the breasts that have the potential for malignancy?

Fibrocystic disease

42. The patient complained of both abnormally heavy menstrual periods and dysfunctional uterine bleeding. What would the healthcare term be? menorrhagia

Define the underlined terms.

43. A vaginal delivery was not an option for the patient who presented with placenta previa.

____

44. Ms. Gross was a candidate for a cesarean section because of cephalopelvic disproportion.

Head too Big for Pelvis

D. Diagnostic Procedures
Build a term.

45. an x-ray image of the breast ______________________________
46. the process of imaging the uterus and fallopian tubes using x-rays and a contrast medium

hysterosalpingography

47. the process of visually examining Douglas's cul-de-sac Culdoscopy

Decode the term.

48. cervicography record the neck of the uterus

49. colposcope Instrument to Examine The Vagina

50. sonohysterography uterus w/ ultrasound

What is the function of the following tests and procedures?

51. Pap smear Cancer ck

52. AFP multi gestation & neural tube disorder

53. hysteroscopy ______________________________

54. CVS detect chromosomal abnormalities

55. CST Contraction Stress Test

56. NST Non-Stress Test

57. Apgar Physical Health of new born
58. Decode the term *amniocentesis* and explain its purpose.

____

____

59. Screening for PKU and congenital hypothyroidism are done at birth. Why?

____

____

E. Therapeutic Interventions

Build a term.

60. What is the term for the removal of both ovaries? ________________

61. What is the term for removal of one breast (one side)? ________________

62. What is a surgical repair of the vagina called? ________________

63. What is the term for removal of adhesions from the fallopian tubes? ________________

64. What is the term for an incision of the vulva to prevent laceration during delivery?

____

Name the term.

65. What is the term for the removal of the entire contents of the pelvic cavity?

____

66. What is the term for a procedure used in pregnancy to treat an incompetent cervix?

____

67. What is the term for turning the baby in utero so that the head is delivered first?

____

68. The healthcare term for "tying" is ________________.

69. Procedure for widening the cervix and removing the lining of the uterus.

____

70. Fertilization of the ovum takes place outside the body in which procedures?

____

71. What hormones secreted by the corpus luteum are responsible for female secondary sex characteristics and the maintenance of the uterus for pregnancy? ________________

72. If a woman desires permanent protection from conception, a surgical option is a tying, cutting, and burning of the fallopian tubes. This is called a ________________.

Decode the term.

73. hysteropexy ________________

74. salpingolysis ________________

75. episiotomy ________________

76. bilateral oophorectomy ________________

77. colpoplasty ________________

F. Pharmacology

78. Procreative and contraceptive management describes

    ____

    ____

79. A woman has a doctor's order in her chart for OCPs. You know that she has been prescribed

    ____________________________.

80. If a term ends in the suffix *-cide,* you know that whatever precedes the term is meant to be

    ____________________________.

81. An IUD is a/an ____________________________.
82. What is an example of a contraceptive method that also provides protection from sexually transmitted

    diseases? ____________________________

83. Abortifacients are intended to ____________________________.
84. A woman taking clomiphene, bromocriptine, or hMG is probably doing so because she has been having

    difficulty with ____________________________.

85. The purpose of HRT is to ____________________________.

86. Oxytocin is given because ____________________________.

87. Decode the term *oxytocia.* ____________________________

G. Abbreviations

Define the following abbreviations.

88. Ms. Smith made an appointment with her gynecologist because of persistent symptoms of PMS.

    ____

89. When Ms. Jones went in for her first prenatal visit, she was asked the date of her LMP.

    ____

90. Ms. Brown was described as being G2P1A0. ____________________________

91. hCG, LH, and FSH are all abbreviations for what? ____________________________

92. Marquita's chart said her baby's FHT had dropped. ____________________________

93. Ms. Chou's EDD is October 13 of next year. ____________________________

94. An IUD was prescribed for Ms. Donner. ____________________________

95. Maria had a D&C after suffering a miscarriage. ____________________________

96. Ms. Swift is having a biopsy of her Cx. ____________________________
97. After difficulty with conceiving for a year, Ms. Kennedy and her husband are considering IVF.

    ____

H. Singulars and Plurals

Define and change the following terms from singular to plural.

98. papilla ______________________________

99. areola ______________________________

100. ovum ______________________________

101. cervix ______________________________

102. uterus ______________________________

103. fimbria ______________________________

104. placenta ______________________________

105. chorionic villus ______________________________

I. Translations

Translate the following sentences into your own words.

106. Ms. Costello made an appointment to visit her gynecologist because of intense dysmenorrhea, DUB, and questions about the possibility that she might be experiencing PMS.

____

____

107. Anna Walker is a 37-year-old G2P1A0 who is visiting her obstetrician for an amniocentesis.

____

____

108. The neonate was born with a nuchal cord and was recorded as a low–birth-weight baby.

____

____

109. Maria Olmos presented with leukorrhea that was a symptom of cervicitis.

____

____

110. Ms. Robinson was treated for fallopian adhesions with salpingolysis.

____

____

J. Cumulative Review

Circle the correct answer.

111. The outer layer of the uterus is the *(peri-, endo-, myo-)* metrium.
112. The female reproductive organs are contained in the *(pelvic, abdominal, thoracic)* cavity.
113. The ovaries are *(bilateral, unilateral)* organs.
114. The fimbriae are at the *(distal, proximal)* end of the fallopian tubes.
115. The 5-year-old patient was admitted with a broken tibia that was partially bent and partially broken. This is considered a *(comminuted, greenstick)* fracture.
116. A patient with reddened swollen skin covered with blisters was treated for *(first-, second-, third-, fourth-)* degree burns.
117. A patient with Crohn's disease had his entire ileum removed and an anastomosis of the remaining intestine called a/an *(ileostomy, jejunocecostomy).*
118. Mr. Wofford presented with painful urination, which was recorded in his patient record as *(dysuria, dyurea).*
119. A patient presented with adhesions in the tube that led from the bladder to the outside of the body. The surgery performed on him was *(urethrolysis, ureterolysis, uterolysis).*

K. Be Careful

Define the following similar groupings of word parts.

120. -metry ______________________ metr/o ______________________

121. ureter/o ______________________ uter/o ______________________

122. culd/o ______________________ colp/o ______________________

Give two meanings for each of the following.

123. cervic/o ______________________

124. germ ______________________

Define the following tricky term.

125. gynecomastia ______________________

St. Gerard's Hospital
123 Hope St.
Philadelphia, PA 19128

OPERATIVE REPORT

Patient Name: Susan Banfield MR#: 23 76 00
Physician/Surgeon: Louis Macharia, MD Date: 12/17/01
Preoperative Diagnosis: Pregnancy at 34 weeks, poor nonstress test, oligohydramnios
Postoperative Diagnosis: Pregnancy at 34 weeks, poor nonstress test, oligohydramnios
Procedure: Low transverse cervical cesarean section
Estimated Blood Loss: 300 cc
Anesthesia: Epidural anesthesia
Description of Procedure: Routine preparation and draping of the abdomen. Abdominal cavity was opened with a Pfannenstiel skin incision. Bladder flap of peritoneum was incised and bluntly stripped downward over the lower uterine segment.

A transverse incision was made in the lower uterine segment, and a normal, living girl child weighing 6 pounds 1 ounce was delivered with an Apgar of 5 and 9. Cord blood was taken. Placenta removed complete with membranes.

Edge of uterine incision was then closed with two layers of a continuous #1 chromic catgut, with the second layer placed in a running type Lembert suture. All bleeding was controlled. Bladder flap of peritoneum was replaced.

Sponge and pack counts were correct before and after closing the abdomen. Routine closure of the abdomen. Staples were used for the skin.

Immediate postoperative condition of mother and baby was good. Amniotic fluid was noted to be meconium stained.

Louis Macharia, MD

L. Operative Report

126. An infant born at 34 weeks' gestation would be considered what type of infant?

____

127. What does the term *meconium* mean? _______________

128. What is a nuchal cord? _______________

129. What does an Apgar score measure? _______________

130. The nonstress test was probably done because there was concern about

____

____

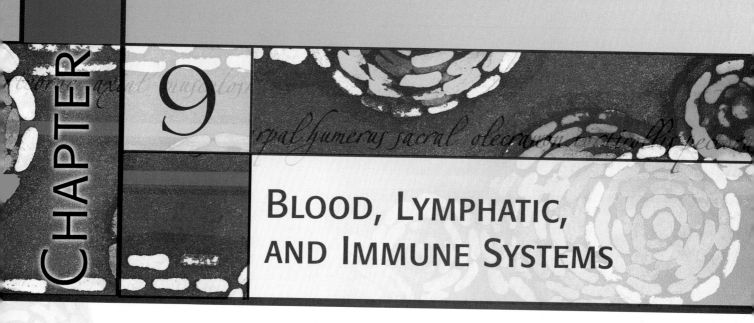

CHAPTER 9

BLOOD, LYMPHATIC, AND IMMUNE SYSTEMS

"The family you come from isn't as important as the family you are going to have." **—Ring Lardner**

Quote

Case Study

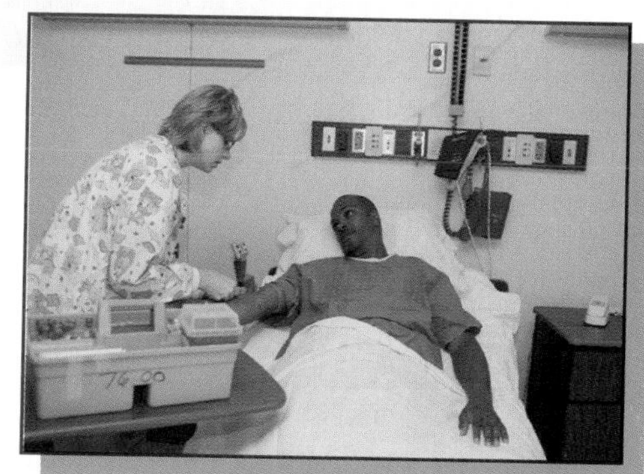

Ozzie Samuelson is a 42-year-old African-American with a history of sickle-cell disease. Diagnosed as a child, he has been treated for the disease and its complications numerous times at the hospital. On this day, Ozzie is admitted for a probable sickle-cell crisis accompanied by acute bronchitis. Marta Erickson, a clinical lab technologist at the hospital, has been assigned to draw Ozzie's blood for tests.

OBJECTIVES

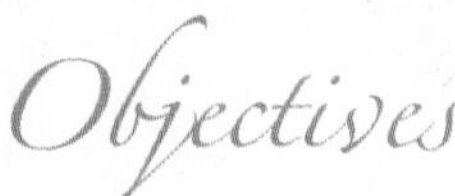

- In your own words, explain the functions of the blood, lymphatic, and immune systems.
- Recognize, recall, and apply healthcare terms related to the anatomy and physiology of the blood, lymphatic, and immune systems.
- Recognize, recall, and apply healthcare terms related to the pathology of the blood, lymphatic, and immune systems.
- Recognize, recall, and apply healthcare terms related to diagnostic procedures of the blood, lymphatic, and immune systems.
- Recognize, recall, and apply healthcare terms related to the therapeutic interventions of the blood, lymphatic, and immune systems.
- Recognize, recall, and apply the abbreviations introduced in this chapter.
- Recognize, recall, and apply word components used in this chapter to build and decode healthcare terms relevant to the blood, lymphatic, and immune systems.
- Recognize, recall, and apply material learned in previous chapters.

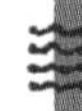

FUNCTIONS OF THE BLOOD, LYMPHATIC, AND IMMUNE SYSTEMS

Homeostasis (hoh mee oh STAY sis), or a "steady state," is a continual balancing act of the body systems to provide an internal environment that is compatible with life. The two liquid tissues of the body, the **blood** and **lymph** (limf), have separate but interrelated functions in maintaining this balance. They combine with a third system, the **immune** (ih MYOON) system, to protect the body against **pathogens** (PATH oh jenz) that could threaten the organism's viability. The **blood** is responsible for the following:

- Transportation of gases (oxygen [O_2] and carbon dioxide [CO_2]), chemical substances (hormones, nutrients, salts), and cells that defend the body.
- Regulation of the body's fluid and electrolyte balance, acid-base balance, and body temperature.
- Protection of the body from infection.
- Protection of the body from loss of blood by the action of clotting.

The **lymph system** is responsible for the following:

- Cleansing the cellular environment.
- Returning proteins and tissue fluids to the blood (drainage).
- Providing a pathway for the absorption of fats and fat-soluble vitamins into the bloodstream.
- Defending the body against disease.

The **immune system** is responsible for the following:

- Defending the body against disease via the immune response.

Fig. 9-1 is a Venn diagram of the interrelationship between the three systems, with the shared goals of homeostasis and protection at the intersection of the three circles.

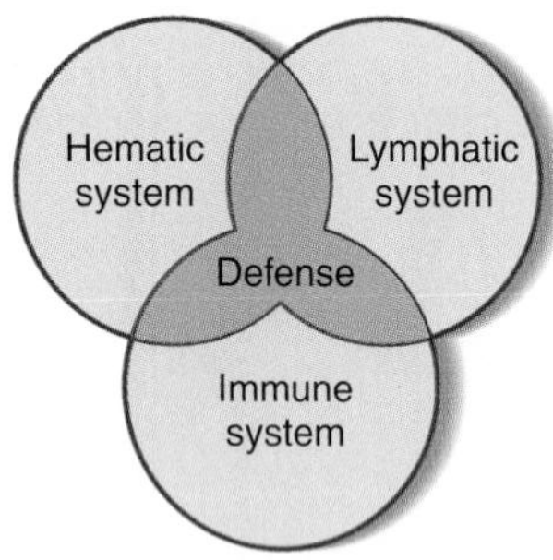

Fig. 9-1 Diagram of interrelationship between the hematic, lymphatic, and immune systems.

Exercise 1: FUNCTIONS OF THE BLOOD, LYMPHATIC, AND IMMUNE SYSTEMS

1. What is the term for the process of maintaining a "steady state" within the body?

____

2. Sort the following functions into their respective systems by writing the name of the system *(blood, lymphatic, or immune)* responsible for each.

_______________ A. cleansing the cellular environment

_______________ B. defending the body via the immune response

_______________ C. protection of the body from infection

_______________ D. transportation of substances throughout the body

_______________ E. providing a pathway for absorption of substances into the bloodstream

_______________ F. regulation of body temperature, fluids, and acid-base balance

_______________ G. returning proteins and tissue fluids to the blood

_______________ H. protecting the body from blood loss by clotting

_______________ I. defending the body against disease

ANATOMY AND PHYSIOLOGY

The **hematic** (hem AT ick) and **lymphatic** (lihm FAT ick) systems flow through separate yet interconnected and interdependent channels. Both are systems composed of vessels and the liquids that flow through them. The **immune** system, a very complex set of levels of protection for the body, includes blood and lymph cells.

Fig. 9-2 shows the relationship of the lymphatic vessels to the circulatory system. Note the close relationship between the distribution of the lymphatic vessels and the venous blood vessels. Tissue fluid is drained by the lymphatic capillaries and transported by a series of larger lymphatic vessels toward the heart.

The clearest path to understanding the interconnected roles of these three systems is to look at the hematic system first.

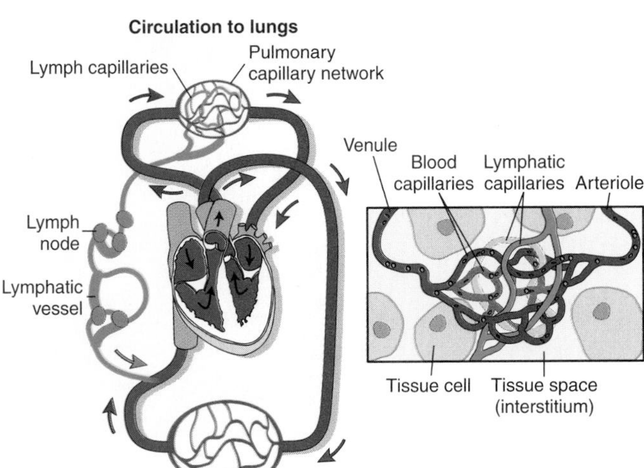

Fig. 9-2 Relationship of the lymphatic vessels to the circulatory system.

Hematic System

The hematic system is composed of blood and the vessels that carry the blood throughout the body. Because blood can be an extremely important part of the diagnostic process, students need to understand its normal composition. Blood is composed of a solid portion that consists of formed elements, or **cells**, and a liquid portion called **plasma** (PLAZ muh). Blood cells make up 45% of the total blood volume, and plasma makes up the other 55% (Fig. 9-3).

(Whole) Blood = Blood Cells (45%) + Plasma (55%)

The solid portion of blood is composed of three different types of cells:

1. **Erythrocytes** (eh RITH roh sites), also called red blood cells **(RBCs).**
2. **Leukocytes** (LOO koh sites), also called white blood cells **(WBCs).**
3. **Thrombocytes** (THROM boh sites), also called clotting cells, cell fragments, or **platelets** (PLATE lets).

BE CAREFUL!

Hgb, HB, Hb, and HG are all abbreviations for hemoglobin. Hg is the abbreviation for mercury.

In a milliliter of blood, there are 4.2 to 5.8 million RBCs, 250,000 to 400,000 platelets, and 5000 to 9000 WBCs. These cells together account for approximately 8% of body volume. Converted to more familiar liquid measure, there are about 10.5 pints (5 liters) of blood in a 150-pound (68-kilogram) person.

Components of Blood

Erythrocytes (Red Blood Cells)

The erythrocytes (which are normally present in the millions) have the important function of transporting O_2 and CO_2 throughout the body (Fig. 9-4). The vehicle for this transportation is a protein-iron pigment called **hemoglobin** (HEE moh gloh bin).

The formation of RBCs in the bone marrow is stimulated by a hormone from the kidneys called **erythropoietin** (eh rith roh POY uh tin). RBCs have a lifespan of approximately 120 days, after which they decompose into **hemosiderin** (hee moh SID uh rin), an iron pigment resulting from **hemolysis** (heh MALL uh sis), and bilirubin. The iron is stored in the liver to be recycled into new RBCs, and the bile pigments are excreted via the liver.

Abnormal RBCs can be named by their **morphology** (more FALL uh jee), the study of shape or form. RBCs normally have a biconcave, disklike shape (although the center is depressed, there is not an actual hole). Those that are shaped differently often have difficulty in carrying out their function.

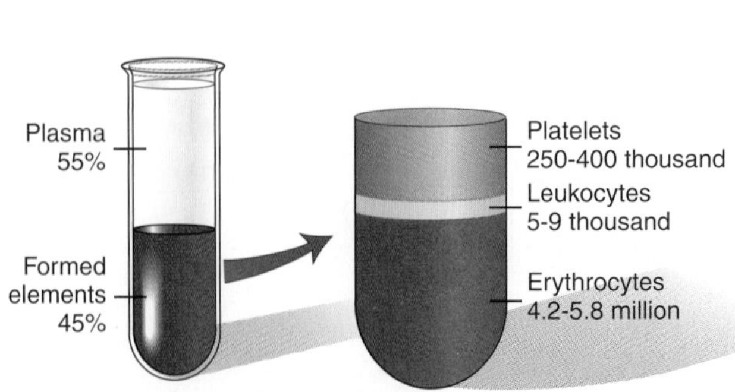

Fig. 9-3 Composition of blood.

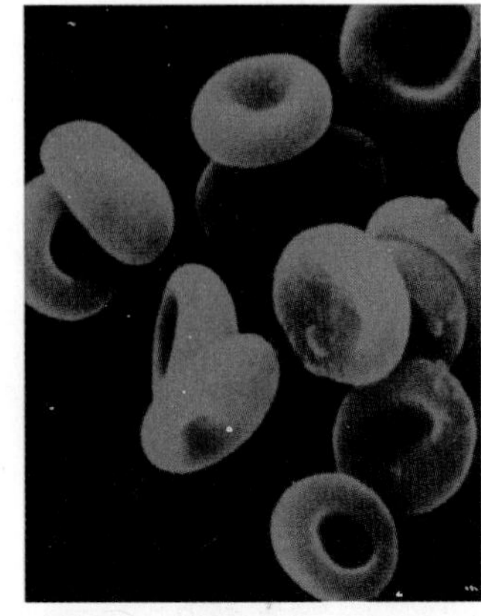

Fig. 9-4 Erythrocytes, or red blood cells.

For example, sickle-cell anemia is a hereditary condition characterized by erythrocytes (RBCs) that are abnormally shaped. They resemble a crescent or sickle. An abnormal hemoglobin found inside these erythrocytes causes sickle-cell anemia in a number of Africans and African-Americans.

Leukocytes (White Blood Cells)

Although there are fewer leukocytes (thousands, not millions), there are different types with different functions. In general, WBCs protect the body from invasion by pathogens. The different types of cells provide this defense in a number of different ways. There are two main types of WBCs: granulocytes and agranulocytes.

GRANULOCYTES (POLYMORPHONUCLEOCYTES)

Named for their appearance, **granulocytes** (GRAN yoo loh sites), also called **polymorphonucleocytes** (pah lee morf oh NOO klee oh sites), have small grains within the cytoplasm and multilobed nuclei. Both names are used interchangeably.

There are three types of granulocytes, each with its own function. Each of them is named for the type of dye that it attracts.

1. **Eosinophils** (ee ah SIN oh fils) are cells that absorb an acidic dye, causing them to appear reddish. An increase in eosinophils is a response to their function in defending the body against allergens and parasites.
2. **Neutrophils** (NOO troh fils) are cells that do not absorb either an acidic or basic dye and consequently are a purplish color. They are also called **phagocytes** (FAG oh sites) because they specialize in **phagocytosis** (fag oh sye TOH sis) and generally combat bacteria in pyogenic infections. This means that these cells are drawn to the site of a pathogenic "invasion," where they consume the enemy and remove the debris resulting from the battle.
3. **Basophils** (BAY soh fils) are cells that absorb a basic (or alkaline) dye and stain a bluish color. Especially effective in combatting parasites, they release histamine (a substance that initiates an inflammatory response) and heparin (an **anticoagulant** [an tee koh AGG yoo lunt]), both of which are instrumental in healing damaged tissue.

AGRANULOCYTES (MONONUCLEAR LEUKOCYTES)

Agranulocytes (a GRAN yoo loh sites) are cells named for their lack of granules. The alternative name, **mononuclear leukocytes,** is so given because they have one nucleus. Both names are used interchangeably. Although these cells originate in the bone marrow, they mature after entering the lymphatic system. There are two types of these WBCs:

1. **Monocytes** (MON oh sites): These cells, named for their single, large nucleus, transform into **macrophages** (MACK roh fay jehs), which eat pathogens (phagocytosis) and are effective against severe infections.
2. **Lymphocytes** (LIM foh sites): These cells are key in what is called the **immune response,** which involves the "recognition" of dangerous, foreign (viral) substances and the manufacture of their neutralizers. The foreign substances are called **antigens** (AN tih juns), and the neutralizers are called **antibodies** (AN tih bod ees).

Thrombocytes (Platelets)

Platelets (also known as *thrombocytes*) have a round or oval shape and are so named because they look like small plates. Their function is to clot blood, also called **coagulation** (koh agg yoo LAY shun), after an injury. When blood cells escape their normal vessels, they **agglutinate** (ah GLOO tih nate), or clump together, by the following process: First, they release **factor X** (formerly called *thrombokinase*), which, in the presence of calcium, reacts with the blood protein

DID YOU KNOW?

Sickle-cell anemia is the most common hereditary disorder among African-Americans. Approximately 8% of African-Americans carry the gene, and 1 in 400 are affected with the disease.

BE CAREFUL!

Whereas granulocytes are also known as *polymorphonucleocytes,* abbreviated *PMNs* or *polys,* the matter is further confused in that neutrophils are commonly referred to as *polymorphs (PMNs, polys),* because they have the greatest degree of nuclear polymorphism, in addition to being the most common type of leukocyte.

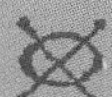

BE CAREFUL!

Don't confuse *cyt/o,* meaning *cell,* with *cyst/o,* meaning *a bladder or a sac.*

DID YOU KNOW?

The process of blood formation is called **hematopoiesis** (hee muh toh poy EE sis). All blood cells originate from a single type of cell called a **stem cell.** Hematopoietic stem cell research is currently an exciting area of healthcare investigation. The National Institutes of Health has a Website that keeps an updated list of news links titled "NIH Stem Cell Information" at http://www.nih.gov/news/stemcell/.

prothrombin (proh THROM bin) to form **thrombin.** Thrombin then converts another blood protein, **fibrinogen** (fye BRIN ah jen), to **fibrin** (FYE brin), which eventually forms a meshlike fibrin clot (blood clot), achieving **hemostasis** (hee moh STAY sis) (control of blood flow; that is, stopping the bleeding). See Fig. 9-5 for a visual explanation of the clotting process.

Plasma

Plasma, the liquid portion of blood, is composed of the following:

1. Water, or H_2O (90%)
2. Inorganic substances (calcium, potassium, sodium)
3. Organic substances (glucose, amino acids, fats, cholesterol, hormones)
4. Waste products (urea, uric acid, ammonia, creatinine)
5. Plasma proteins (serum albumin, serum globulin, and two clotting proteins: fibrinogen and prothrombin)

Serum (SEER um) (*pl.* sera) is plasma minus the clotting proteins. Serology is the branch of laboratory medicine that studies blood serum for evidence of infection by evaluating antigen-antibody reactions in vitro.

$$\text{Serum} = \text{Plasma} - (\text{Prothrombin} + \text{Fibrinogen})$$

COMBINING FORMS FOR THE HEMATIC SYSTEM

MEANING	COMBINING FORM	MEANING	COMBINING FORM
alkaline, basic	bas/o	neutral	neutr/o
blood	hem/o, hemat/o	nucleus	nucle/o
cell	cyt/o	red	erythr/o
clotting	thromb/o	rosy, acidic	eosin/o
clumping	agglutin/o	safety, protection	immun/o
eat, swallow	phag/o	serum	ser/o
fiber	fibr/o	shape	morph/o
fibrin	fibrin/o	small grain	granul/o
iron	sider/o	white	leuk/o
lymph	lymph/o, lymphat/o		

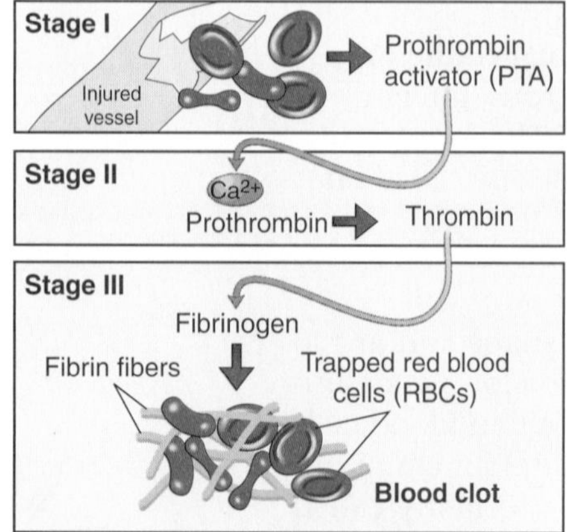

Fig. 9-5 The clotting process.

PREFIXES AND SUFFIXES FOR HEMATIC ANATOMY AND PHYSIOLOGY

PREFIX, SUFFIX	MEANING
a-	without
-gen	producing, produced by
macro-	large
mono-	one, singular
pro-	before, in front of
-stasis	stopping, controlling

 Exercise 2: HEMATIC SYSTEM

Circle the correct answer.

1. Whole blood is composed of *(blood cells and lymph, blood cells and plasma).*
2. An average-sized person has about *(25, 11)* pints of blood in his/her body.
3. RBCs are called *(leukocytes, erythrocytes)* and are responsible for transporting *(O_2 and CO_2, Ca and K)* through the use of *(hemosiderin, hemoglobin).*
4. A normal RBC count should be in the *(thousands, millions, billions).*
5. RBCs decompose in a process called *(hemostasis, hemolysis).*
6. WBCs are called *(leukocytes, leukemia)* and generally *(defend the body against disease, regulate the body's fluid balance).*
7. A normal WBC count should be in the *(thousands, millions, billions).*
8. *(Agranulocytes, Granulocytes)* are so named because they have grains within their cytoplasm. The alternative name is *(mononuclear leukocytes, polymorphonucleocytes).*
9. One type of WBC is named for its one-lobed nucleus *(mononuclear leukocyte, polymorphonucleocyte)* and its alternate name *(agranulocyte, granulocyte),* for its lack of tiny grains in its nucleus.

Fill in the blank with the correct term from the following list.

neutrophils, eosinophils, basophils

10. Cells that absorb an acidic dye and defend against allergens and parasites. ______________
11. Cells that absorb an alkaline dye, combat parasites, and release histamine and heparin.

    ____

12. Cells that absorb a neutral dye and specialize in phagocytosis. ______________

Match the types of plasma components with examples of each.

_____ 13. plasma protein

_____ 14. inorganic substance

_____ 15. organic substance

_____ 16. waste product

A. urea
B. cholesterol
C. serum albumin
D. calcium

Fill in the blanks.

17. Plasma is the ______________ part of blood.

18. What is the principal component of plasma? ______________

19. Plasma becomes serum when which two substances are removed? ______________

20. Clotting cells are called ______________cytes or platelets. They are responsible for the process of *(phagocytosis, coagulation)* (circle one).

21. Cut → ______________ → release of Ca^+ and prothrombin → ______________ → fibrinogen →

    ______________ → hemostasis.

Match the following combining forms, prefixes, and suffixes with their meanings.

_____ 22. hem/o, hemat/o

_____ 23. erythr/o

_____ 24. leuk/o

_____ 25. thromb/o

_____ 26. lymph/o, lymphat/o

_____ 27. immun/o

_____ 28. morph/o

_____ 29. cyt/o

_____ 30. sider/o

_____ 31. bas/o

_____ 32. eosin/o

_____ 33. neutr/o

_____ 34. phag/o

_____ 35. mon/o

_____ 36. -stasis

_____ 37. nucle/o

_____ 38. fibr/o

_____ 39. pro-

_____ 40. ser/o

_____ 41. granul/o

_____ 42. -gen

_____ 43. agglutin/o

_____ 44. macro-

_____ 45. fibrin/o

_____ 46. a-

A. safety, protection
B. rosy, acidic
C. stopping, controlling
D. iron
E. before, in front of
F. producing, produced by
G. blood
H. small grain
I. eat, swallow
J. nucleus
K. fiber
L. red
M. large
N. serum
O. lymph
P. without
Q. clotting
R. neutral
S. fibrin
T. cell
U. clumping
V. alkaline, basic
W. white
X. one, singular
Y. shape

Blood Groups

Human blood is divided into four major different types: A, B, AB, and O. See Fig. 9-6 for a table of blood types, agglutinogens, and agglutinins. The differences are due to antigens present on the surface of the red blood cells. **Antigens** (ANN tih jens) are substances that produce an immune reaction by their nature of being perceived as foreign to the body. In response, the body produces substances called **antibodies** that nullify or neutralize the antigens. In blood, these antigens are called **agglutinogens** (ah gloo TIN oh jens) because their presence can cause the blood to clot. The antibody is termed an **agglutinin** (ah GLOO tin nin). For example, type A blood has A antigen, type B has B antigen, type AB has both A and B antigens, and type O has neither A nor B antigens. If an individual with type A blood is transfused with type B blood, the A antigens will form anti-B antibodies because they perceive B blood as being foreign. Following the logic of each of these antigen-antibody reactions, an individual with type AB blood is a **universal recipient,** and an individual with type O blood is a **universal donor.**

Another antigen, the **Rh factor,** is important in pregnancy because a mismatch between the fetus and the mother can cause erythroblastosis fetalis, or **hemolytic** (hee moh LIT ick) disease of the newborn (HDN). In this disorder, a mother with a negative Rh factor will develop antibodies to an Rh+ fetus during the first pregnancy. If another pregnancy occurs with an Rh+ fetus, the antibodies will destroy the fetal blood cells.

Blood Type	Antigen (RBC membrane)	Antibody (plasma)	Can receive blood from	Can donate blood to
A (40%)	A antigen	Anti-B antibodies	A, O	A, AB
B (10%)	B antigen	Anti-A antibodies	B, O	B, AB
AB (4%)	A antigen, B antigen	No antibodies	A, B, AB, O	AB
O (46%)	No antigen	Both Anti-A and Anti-B antibodies	O	O, A, B, AB

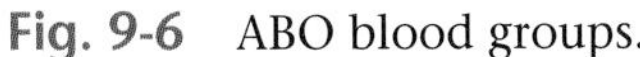
Fig. 9-6 ABO blood groups.

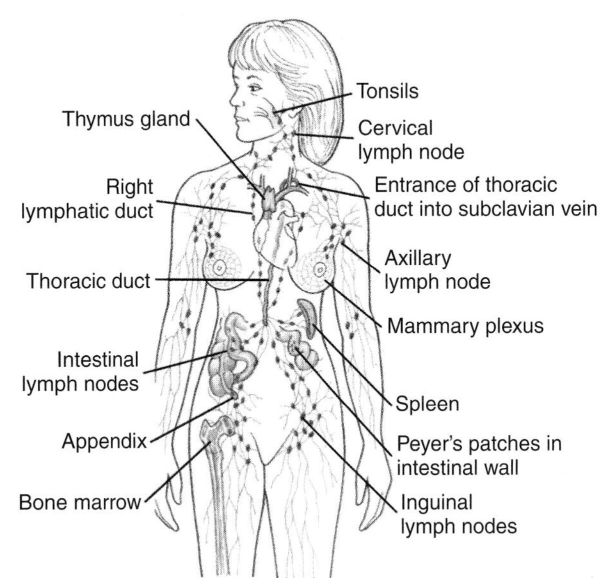

Fig. 9-7 The lymphatic system.

Exercise 3: BLOOD GROUPS

1. The four blood types are ______________________________.
2. Not all blood types are interchangeable because of ____.
3. A person with type A blood can donate blood to people with which blood type? ______________________________
4. Type O blood type is the *(universal donor, universal recipient)*, whereas type AB is the *(universal donor, universal recipient)* (circle one).
5. HDN is an example of an antigen-antibody reaction of what blood factor? Rh ______________________________

Lymphatic System

The lymphatic system is responsible for the following:

- Cleansing the cellular environment
- Returning proteins and tissue fluids to the blood
- Providing a pathway for the absorption of fats into the bloodstream
- Defending the body against disease.

The lymphatic system (Fig. 9-7) is composed of **lymph** (or **interstitial fluid**), **lymph vessels, lymph nodes**, lymph organs (e.g., tonsils, adenoids, appendix, spleen, thymus gland, and patches of tissue in the intestines called *Peyer's patches*), and lymphoid tissue. Monocytes and lymphocytes pass from the bloodstream through the blood capillary walls into the spaces between the cells in body tissue. When they pass into this lymph or interstitial fluid that surrounds cells, they perform their protective functions. Monocytes change into **macrophages** (MACK roh fay jehs), destroy pathogens, and collect debris from damaged cells. Lymphocytes are much more complicated and are essential to the immune response, so they are discussed in the next section. Once monocytes and lymphocytes pass into the lymphatic capillaries, the fluid is termed *lymph* or *lymphatic fluid.*

Lymph moves in one direction to prevent pathogens from flowing through the entire body. The system filters out the microorganisms as the lymph passes through its various capillaries, vessels, and nodes. Lymph travels in the following sequence:

1. From the interstitial spaces between the cells, then
2. Toward the heart through lymphatic capillaries.
3. To lymphatic vessels that carry lymph using a valvular system.
4. To the lymphatic nodes, which are also called **lymph glands,** that filter the debris that has been collected through the use of macrophages. These nodes can become enlarged when pathogens are present. Note the major lymph nodes in Fig. 9-7, including the cervical, axillary, inguinal, and mediastinal nodes.
5. Then to either the **right lymphatic duct** or the **thoracic duct,** both of which empty into the large subclavian veins in the neck.
6. Once in the venous blood, the lymph is then recycled through the body through the circulatory system.

BE CAREFUL!

Don't confuse *thym/o,* which means *thymus,* with *thyr/o,* which means *thyroid.*

The organs in the lymphatic system are the spleen, the thymus gland, the tonsils, the appendix, and Peyer's patches. The spleen is located in the upper left quadrant and serves to filter, store, and produce blood cells; remove RBCs; and activate B lymphocytes. The thymus gland is located in the mediastinum and is instrumental in the development of T lymphocytes (T cells). The tonsils are lymphatic tissue (lingual, pharyngeal, and palatine) that help protect the entrance to the respiratory and digestive systems. The vermiform appendix and Peyer's patches are lymphoid tissue in the intestines.

COMBINING FORMS FOR THE LYMPHATIC SYSTEM

MEANING	COMBINING FORM	MEANING	COMBINING FORM
armpit	axill/o	neck	cervic/o
groin	inguin/o	space between	interstit/o
lymph gland	lymphaden/o	spleen	splen/o
lymph vessel	lymphangi/o	thymus	thym/o
mediastinum	mediastin/o		

Exercise 4: LYMPHATIC SYSTEM

Fill in the blanks.

1. What are the two types of cells found in lymph? ______________________
2. How do these cells become part of lymphatic fluid?

____

3. What are the names of the two ducts that drain lymph back into the circulatory system?

RT Lymphatic Duct, Thoracic Duct

Circle the correct answer.

4. The *(thymus, spleen)* changes lymphocytes into T lymphocytes.
5. The *(thymus, spleen)* activates B lymphocytes.
6. Macrophages develop from *(monocytes, lymphocytes).*
7. The *(tonsils, spleen, appendix)* protect(s) the entrances to the digestive and respiratory systems.

Match the following combining forms with their meanings.

_____ 8. spleen

_____ 9. lymph vessel

_____ 10. armpit

_____ 11. neck

_____ 12. groin

_____ 13. space between

_____ 14. lymph gland

_____ 15. mediastinum

_____ 16. thymus

A. lymphangi/o
B. thym/o
C. interstit/o
D. splen/o
E. inguin/o
F. cervic/o
G. mediastin/o
H. lymphaden/o
I. axill/o

Immune System

The immune system is composed of organs, tissues, cells, and chemical messengers that interact to protect the body from external invaders and its own internally altered cells. The chemical messengers are **cytokines** (SYE toh kynes), which are secreted by cells of the immune system that direct immune cellular interactions. Lymphocytes (leukocytes that are categorized as either **B cells** or **T cells**) secrete **lymphokines** (LIM foh kynes). Monocytes and macrophages secrete **monokines** (MAH noh kynes). **Interleukins** (in tur LOO kins) are a type of cytokine that sends messages among leukocytes to direct protective action.

The best way to understand this system is through the body's various levels of defense. The goal of pathogens is to breach these levels to enter the body, reproduce, and, subsequently, exploit healthy tissue, causing harm. The immune system's task is to stop them.

Fig. 9-8 illustrates the levels of defense. The two outside circles represent **nonspecific immunity** and its two levels of defense. The inner circle represents the various mechanisms of **specific immunity**, which can be **natural (genetic)** or **acquired** in four different ways. Most pathogens can be contained by the first two lines of nonspecific defense. However, some pathogens deserve a "special" means of protection, which is discussed under "Specific Immunity."

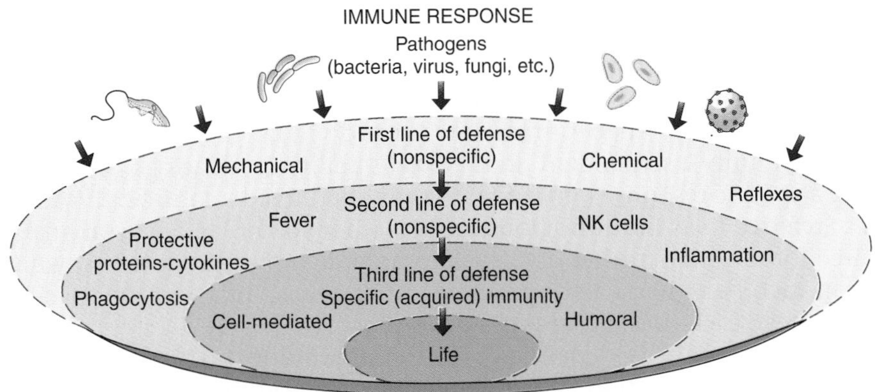

Fig. 9-8 The levels of defense.

Nonspecific Immunity

This term refers to the various ways that the body protects itself from many types of pathogens, without having to "recognize" them. The *first line of defense* in a nonspecific immunity (the outermost layer) consists of the following methods of protection:

- **Mechanical**—Examples include the skin, which acts as a barrier, and the sticky mucus on mucous membranes, which serves to trap pathogens.
- **Physical**—Examples include coughing, sneezing, vomiting, and diarrhea. Although not pleasant, these serve to expel pathogens that have gotten past the initial barriers.
- **Chemical**—Examples include tears, saliva, and perspiration. These have a slightly acidic nature that deters pathogens from entering the body while also washing them away. In addition, stomach acids and enzymes serve to kill germs.

The *second line of defense* in nonspecific immunity comes into play if the pathogens make it past the first line. Defensive measures include certain processes, proteins, and specialized cells.

Defensive processes include the following:

- **Phagocytosis** (fag oh sye TOH sis)—Pathogens that make it past the first line of defense and enter into the bloodstream may be consumed by neutrophils and monocytes.
- **Inflammation**—Acquiring its name from its properties, this is a protective response to irritation or injury. The characteristics (heat, swelling, redness, and pain) arise in response to an immediate vasoconstriction, followed by an increase in vascular permeability. These provide a good environment for healing. If caused by a pathogen, the inflammation is called an **infection.**
- **Pyrexia** (pye RECK see uh)—When infection is present, fever may serve a protective function by increasing the action of phagocytes and decreasing the viability of certain pathogens.

The **protective proteins** are part of the second line of defense. These include **interferons** (in tur FEER ons), which get their name from their ability to "interfere" with viral replication and limit a virus's ability to damage the body. A second protein type, the **complement proteins,** exist as inactive forms in blood circulation that become activated in the presence of bacteria, enabling them to lyse (destroy) the organisms.

Finally, the last of the "team" in the second line of defense are the **natural killer (NK) cells.** This special kind of lymphocyte acts nonspecifically to kill cells that have been infected by certain viruses and cancer cells.

Specific Immunity

Specific immunity may be either **genetic**—an inherited ability to resist certain diseases due to one's species, race, sex, or individual genetics—or **acquired.** Specific immunity is dependent on the body's ability to identify a pathogen and prepare a specific response (antibody) to only that invader (antigen). Antibodies are also referred to as **immunoglobulins (Ig)** (ih myoo noh GLOB you lins). The acquired form can be further divided into natural and artificial forms, which in turn can each be either active or passive. After a description of the specific immune process, each of the four types is discussed.

Specific immunity is dependent on the agranulocytes (lymphocytes and monocytes) for its function. The monocytes metamorphose into macrophages, which dispose of foreign substances. The lymphocytes differentiate into either T lymphocytes (they mature in the thymus) or B lymphocytes (they mature in the bone marrow or fetal liver). Although both types of lymphocytes take part in specific immunity, they do it in different ways.

The T cells neutralize their enemies through a process of **cell-mediated immunity.** This means that they attack antigens directly. They are effective against fungi, cancer cells, protozoa, and, unfortunately, organ transplants. B cells use a process of **humoral immunity** (also called **antibody-mediated immunity**). This means that they secrete antibodies to "poison" their enemies.

DID YOU KNOW?

The word *humoral* in the term *humoral immunity* gets its name from the medieval term for body fluids—humors.

Types of Acquired Immunity

Acquired immunity is categorized as *active* or *passive* and then is further subcategorized as *natural* or *artificial.* All describe ways that the body has acquired antibodies to specific diseases.

Active acquired immunity can take either of the following two forms:

1. **Natural:** Development of memory cells to protect the individual from a second exposure.
2. **Artificial:** Vaccination (immunization) that uses a greatly weakened form of the antigen, thus enabling the body to develop antibodies in response to this intentional exposure. Examples are the DPT and MMR vaccines.

Passive acquired immunity can take either of the following two forms:

1. **Natural:** Passage of antibodies through the placenta or breast milk.
2. **Artificial:** Use of immunoglobulins harvested from a donor who developed resistance against specific antigens.

COMBINING FORMS FOR THE IMMUNE SYSTEM

MEANING	COMBINING FORM
eat	phag/o
fever	pyr/o
flame	flamm/o
liquid	humor/o
white	leuk/o

PREFIXES AND SUFFIXES FOR THE IMMUNE SYSTEM

PREFIX, SUFFIX	MEANING
inter-	between
non-	not
-kine	movement

Exercise 5: IMMUNE SYSTEM

1. How do nonspecific and specific immunity differ?

general
____

2. Name examples of first-line defenses.

____

3. Name examples of second-line defenses.

____

4. What pathogens are neutralized by the following:

   A. interferons ______________________

   B. complement proteins ______________________

   C. NK cells ______________________

5. B cells get their name because they mature in the ______________________.
6. T cells are responsible for what type of immunity? ______________________
7. B cells are responsible for what type of immunity? ______________________
8. Monocytes change into ______________________.

Circle the correct answer.

9. *(Granulocyte, Agranulocyte)* cells participate in specific immunity.
10. T cells get their name because they mature in the *(thymus, thyroid).*
11. If a patient has resistance to a disease because of heredity, this is called *(genetic, artificial)* immunity.

Choose from the following types of acquired immunity to fill in the blanks.

active natural, active artificial, passive natural, passive artificial

12. If a child has an immunization against measles, he/she has what type of immunity? ______________
13. If an individual receives maternal antibodies, then this is a type of ______________ immunity.
14. If an individual receives a mixture of antibodies from a donor, he/she has received ______________ immunity.
15. Acquiring a disease and producing memory cells for that disease is a type of ______________ immunity.

Match the following word parts with their meanings.

_____ 16. fever

_____ 17. eat

_____ 18. flame

_____ 19. between

_____ 20. white

_____ 21. liquid

_____ 22. not

_____ 23. movement

A. humor/o
B. pyr/o
C. leuk/o
D. flamm/o
E. inter-
F. phag/o
G. non-
H. -kine

PATHOLOGY

Dyscrasia (dis KRAY zsa), a term that means *disease,* is used more specifically to describe only diseases of the blood or bone marrow. Many disorders of the blood have to do with too many or too few of certain types of blood cells. Many others have to do with an abnormality of their morphology or shape.

Terms Related to Blood Dyscrasias

TERM	WORD ORIGIN	DEFINITION
Acute posthemorrhagic anemia	*post-* after *hem/o* blood *-rrhagia* burst forth *-ic* pertaining to *an-* no, not *-emia* blood condition	RBC deficiency due to blood loss.
Anemia ah NEE mee ah	*an-* no, not *-emia* blood condition	Condition of lacking an adequate level of red blood cells for any of a variety of reasons.
B_{12} deficiency		Anemia characterized by the absence of **intrinsic factor** (a substance in the GI system that assists in B_{12} absorption) or by a strict vegetarian diet.
Chronic blood loss		Long-term internal bleeding. May cause anemia.
Folate deficiency FOH late		Anemia due to a lack of folate from dietary, drug-induced, congenital, or other etiologies.
Iron-deficiency anemia	*an-* no, not *-emia* blood condition	Condition of having reduced numbers of RBCs due to chronic blood loss, inadequate iron intake, or unspecified causes. **Sideropenia** (sih dur roh PEE nee ah) is a type of iron-deficiency anemia.
Pernicious anemia pur NIH shush	*an-* no, not *-emia* blood condition	Progressive anemia that results from a lack of intrinsic factor essential for the absorption of vitamin B_{12}.

Terms Related to Hemolytic Anemias

TERM	WORD ORIGIN	DEFINITION
Aplastic anemia a PLAS tick	*a-* no, not *plast/o* formation *-ic* pertaining to *an-* no, not *-emia* blood condition	Suppression of bone marrow function leading to a reduction of RBC production. Although etiologies of this often fatal type of anemia may be hepatitis, radiation, or cytotoxic agents, most causes are idiopathic. Also called **hypoplastic anemia.**
Autoimmune acquired hemolytic anemia hee moh LIT ick	*auto-* self *immune* safety, protection *hem/o* blood *-lytic* destruction *an-* no, not *-emia* blood condition	Anemia caused by the body's destruction of its own RBCs by serum antibodies.
Nonautoimmune acquired hemolytic anemia	*non-* not *hem/o* blood *-lytic* destruction *an-* no, not *-emia* blood condition	Anemia that may be drug-induced or caused by an infectious disease.
Pancytopenia pan sye toh PEE nee ah	*pan-* all *cyt/o* cell *-penia* deficiency	Deficiency of all blood cells due to dysfunctional stem cells.

Continued

Terms Related to Hemolytic Anemias—cont'd		
TERM	**WORD ORIGIN**	**DEFINITION**
Sickle-cell anemia	*an-* no, not *-emia* blood condition	Inherited anemia characterized by crescent-shaped RBCs. This abnormality in morphology causes RBCs to block small-diameter capillaries, thereby decreasing the oxygen supply to the cells (Fig. 9-9).
Thalassemia thal ah SEE mee ah	See **Did You Know?** box	Group of inherited disorders of people of Mediterranean, African, and Southeast Asian descent, in which the anemia is the result of a decrease in the synthesis of hemoglobin, resulting in the decreased production and increased destruction of RBCs.

DID YOU KNOW?

Sickle-cell anemia is expressed only in individuals who inherit the gene from both parents. If only one gene is present, the patient is said to have the sickle-cell trait but not the disease.

DID YOU KNOW?

The term *thalassemia* comes from the Greek word *thalassa,* meaning *sea,* especially the Mediterranean. Many people with thalassemia are of Mediterranean descent.

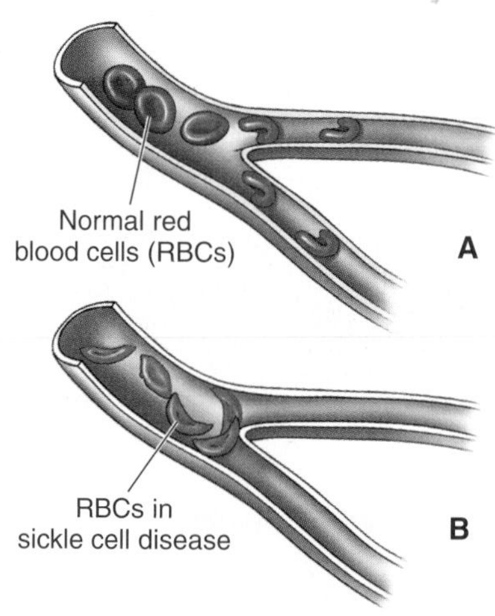

Fig. 9-9 **A,** Normal, donut-shaped red blood cells bend to fit through capillaries. **B,** Sickled red blood cells cannot bend and therefore block the flow of blood through the vessel.

Exercise 6: DYSCRASIAS AND ANEMIAS

Matching.

____ 1. -penia
____ 2. megal/o
____ 3. sider/o
____ 4. -lytic
____ 5. a, an-
____ 6. post-
____ 7. -emia
____ 8. plast/o
____ 9. hypo-
____ 10. pan-

A. after
B. all
C. iron
D. deficiency (prefix)
E. pertaining to destruction
F. no, not, without
G. blood condition
H. formation
I. decrease (suffix)
J. large

Fill in the blank with one of the following terms.

pancytopenia, thalassemia, aplastic anemia, sickle-cell anemia, autoimmune acquired hemolytic anemia, pernicious anemia, acute hemorrhagic anemia

11. What type of inherited anemia has misshapen blood cells that block blood vessels, causing oxygen deprivation to the cells? ________________
12. What type of anemia is caused by the body destroying its own blood cells? ________________
13. What type of inherited anemia may affect people of Mediterranean, African, and Southeast Asian descent? ________________
14. What type of anemia is caused by bone marrow suppression? ________________
15. Deficiency of all types of blood cells due to dysfunctional stem cells is called ________________.
16. Lack of intrinsic factor causes this type of progressive anemia. ________________
17. Anemia due to sudden blood loss is called ________________.

Terms Related to Coagulation Disorders

TERM	WORD ORIGIN	DEFINITION
Hemophilia hee moh FEE lee ah	*hem/o* blood *-philia* tendency	Group of inherited bleeding disorders characterized by a deficiency of one of the factors necessary for the coagulation of the blood.
Polycythemia vera pah lee sye THEE mee ah VARE ah	*poly-* many *cyt/o* cell *-emia* blood condition *vera* true	Chronic increase in the number of RBCs and the concentration of hemoglobin. "Vera" signifies that this is not a sequela of another condition.
Purpura PURR purr uh	See **Did You Know?** box	Bleeding disorder characterized by hemorrhage into the tissues (Fig. 9-10).
Thrombocytopenia throm boh sye toh PEE nee ah	*thromb/o* clot *cyt/o* cell *-penia* deficiency	Deficiency of platelets causing an inability of the blood to clot. The most common cause of bleeding disorders.

DID YOU KNOW?

In the term *hemophilia,* the *-philia* suffix means a *tendency;* in this case, to bleed.

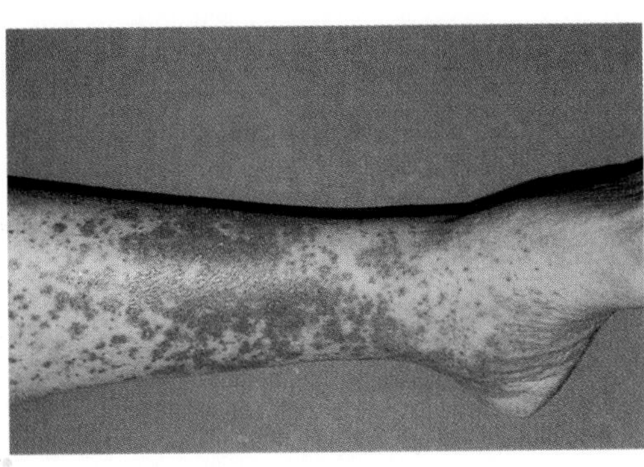

Fig. 9-10 Purpura.

DID YOU KNOW?

Purpura comes from the Latin word for *purple.*

Terms Related to Leukocytic Disorders

Term	Word Origin	Definition
Leukemia loo KEE mee ah	*leuk/o* white (blood cell) *-emia* blood condition	Any of a group of hematologic malignancies that manifest with the increase of immature WBCs at the expense of normal blood cells.
Leukocytosis loo koh sye TOH sis	*leuk/o* white (blood cell) *-cytosis* abnormal increase of cells	Abnormal increase in WBCs. Abnormal increases in each type of granulocyte are termed **eosinophilia, basophilia,** or **neutrophilia,** where the suffix *-philia* denotes *a slight increase.* Abnormal increases in the number of each type of agranulocyte are termed **lymphocytosis** or **monocytosis.**
Leukopenia loo koh PEE nee ah	*leuk/o* white (blood cell) *-penia* deficiency	Abnormal decrease in WBCs. Specific deficiencies are termed **neutropenia, eosinopenia, monocytopenia,** and **lymphocytopenia.**

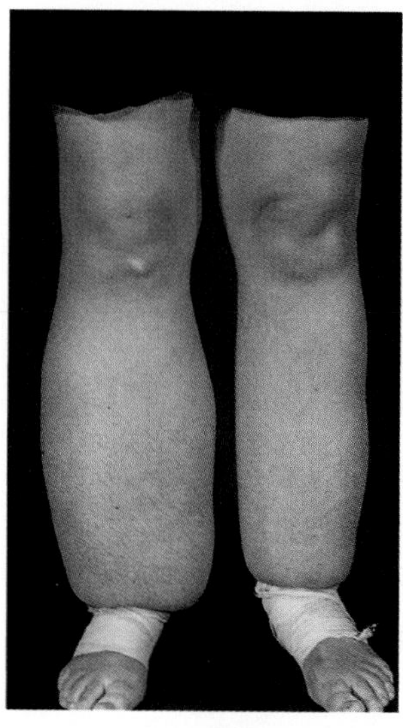

Fig. 9-11 Lymphedema. The patient had to bind her feet so that she could wear shoes.

Exercise 7: Coagulation and WBC Disorders

Matching.

____ 1. leukemia

____ 2. hemophilia

____ 3. purpura

____ 4. polycythemia

____ 5. leukopenia

____ 6. leukocytosis

____ 7. thrombocytopenia

A. platelet deficiency
B. slight increase of WBCs
C. hereditary bleeding disorder
D. deficiency of WBCs
E. excessive RBCs
F. hematologic malignancy
G. hemorrhagic bleeding disorder of tissues

Terms Related to Lymphatic Disorders

Term	Word Origin	Definition
Edema eh DEE muh		Abnormal accumulation of fluid in the interstitial spaces of tissues.
Hypersplenism hye purr SPLEE niz um	*hyper-* excessive *splen/o* spleen *-ism* condition	Increased function of the spleen, resulting in hemolysis.
Lymphedema lim fuh DEE muh	*lymph/o* lymph *-edema* swelling	Accumulation of lymphatic fluid and resultant swelling due to obstruction, removal, or hypoplasia of lymph vessels (Fig. 9-11).

Terms Related to Lymphatic Disorders—cont'd

TERM	WORD ORIGIN	DEFINITION
Lymphadenitis lim fad uh NYE tis	*lymphaden/o* lymph gland *-itis* inflammation	Inflammation of a lymph node.
Lymphadenopathy lim fad uh NOP puh thee	*lymphaden/o* lymph gland *-pathy* disease	Disease of the lymph nodes or vessels that may be localized or generalized.
Lymphangitis lim fan JYE tis	*lymphangi/o* lymph vessel *-itis* inflammation	Inflammation of lymph vessels.
Lymphocytopenia lim foh sye toh PEE nee ah	*lymphocyt/o* lymphocyte *-penia* deficiency	Deficiency of lymphocytes due to infectious mononucleosis, malignancy, nutritional deficiency, or a hematologic disorder.
Lymphocytosis lim foh sye TOH sis	*lymph/o* lymph *-cytosis* increase of cells	Abnormal increase in lymphocytes.
Mononucleosis mah noh noo klee OH sis	*mono-* single, one *nucle/o* nucleus *-osis* abnormal condition	Increase in the number of mononuclear cells (monocytes and lymphocytes) in the blood caused by the Epstein-Barr virus. Can result in **splenomegaly** (enlarged spleen).

Terms Related to Immune Disorders

TERM	WORD ORIGIN	DEFINITION
Acquired immunodeficiency syndrome (AIDS)		Syndrome caused by the human immunodeficiency virus (HIV) and transmitted through body fluids via sexual contact or intravenous exposure. HIV attacks the helper T cells, which diminishes the immune response (Fig. 9-12).
Allergy		Immune system's overreaction to irritants that are perceived as antigens. The substance that causes the irritation is called an **allergen.** Also called **hypersensitivity.**

Continued

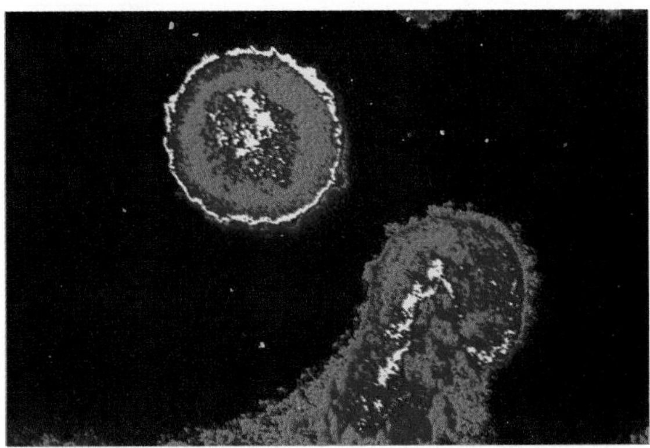

Fig. 9-12 HIV virus.

DID YOU KNOW?

Although **organ rejection** may not be viewed as an abnormal response, it is certainly an undesired one. The immune system recognizes any foreign tissue as such and responds to it with its characteristic search-and-destroy techniques. In order to inhibit this reaction to an organ transplant, immunosuppressant drugs are used.

Terms Related to Immune Disorders—cont'd

TERM	WORD ORIGIN	DEFINITION
Anaphylaxis an uh fuh LACK sis	*an-* without *-phylaxis* protection	Extreme form of allergic response in which the patient suffers severely decreased blood pressure and constriction of the airways.
Autoimmunity	*auto-* self *immunity* protection	Condition in which a person's T cells attack his/her own cells, causing extensive tissue damage and organ dysfunction. Examples of resultant **autoimmune diseases** include myasthenia gravis, rheumatoid arthritis, systemic lupus erythematosus, and multiple sclerosis.
Delayed-reaction allergy		Immune system hypersensitivity caused by activated T cells that respond to an exposure of the skin to a chemical irritant up to 2 days later. Examples are poison ivy and nickel. The resulting rash is called *contact dermatitis.*
Immediate-reaction allergy		Hypersensitivity of the immune system caused by IgE. Examples are insect bites and tree or grass pollens.

DID YOU KNOW?

The term *anaphylaxis* is a misnomer. Early physiologists thought that the phenomenon was a lack of protection, not, as we know now, an exaggerated allergic response.

Fighting Future Diseases

The National Institute of Allergy and Infectious Diseases (NIAID) is one of the branches of the National Institutes of Health (NIH). Because its mission is to conduct and support research on immunologic and infectious diseases, students may be interested in visiting its Website and reading about its plans to combat emerging infectious diseases in the twenty-first century at http://www.niaid.nih.gov/strategicplan2000/emerge.htm.

For those interested in a more global view, another site that may be of interest is that of the World Health Organization at http://www.who.int/home-page/. Links include "Disease Outbreaks," "Traveller's Health," a "Press Media Centre," and "Information Resources."

Exercise 8: ABNORMAL IMMUNE RESPONSES

Fill in the blank with one of the following terms.

anaphylaxis, lymphadenitis, autoimmune, allergy, immunosuppressant, lymphocytopenia, mononucleosis, hypersplenism, lymphocytosis

1. Hypersensitivity to a substance that would not otherwise threaten the life of an organism is called a/an ________________.
2. If a person's immune system attacks its own cells, he has a/an ________________ disease.
3. What type of drugs are used to inhibit the rejection of transplanted organs? ________________
4. What is the healthcare term for an extremely severe allergic reaction resulting in restricted airways and decreased blood pressure? ________________

5. An abnormal increase in cells caused by the Epstein-Barr virus is called ________________.

6. A lack of lymphocytes is called ________________.

7. Inflammation of a lymph gland is called ________________.

8. Increased splenic function is called ________________.

9. An abnormal increase in lymphatic cells is called ________________.

Fill in the blanks.

10. AIDS is caused by ________________, which attacks ________________ cells, resulting in diminished ________________ response.

Exercise 9: LYMPHATIC AND IMMUNE DISORDERS

Match the word part with the correct term.

_____ 1. -pathy

_____ 2. lymphaden/o

_____ 3. lymphangi/o

_____ 4. edema

_____ 5. -megaly

A. disease
B. lymph vessel
C. enlargement
D. lymph gland
E. swelling

Case Study Continued

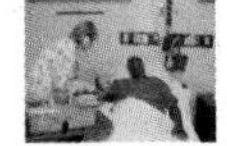

Sickle-cell anemia causes RBCs to become sickle-shaped, which causes them to block up small blood vessels and stop the flow of blood. Pain is the main symptom, but respiratory infections are common, and severe anemia sometimes occurs, necessitating blood transfusions.

Ozzie is exhausted by this most recent, painful, sickle-cell crisis episode, which this time has been accompanied by bronchitis. **Sickle-cell crisis** is an acute exacerbation of sickle-cell anemia. Ozzie is also worried about his unborn daughter, who is being tested for the trait.

DIAGNOSTIC PROCEDURES

Terms Related to Imaging

TERM	WORD ORIGIN	DEFINITION
Lymphadenography lim fad uh NAH gruh fee	*lymphaden/o* lymph gland *-graphy* process of recording	Radiographic visualization of the lymph gland after injection of a radiopaque substance. Also called **lymphography.**
Lymphangiography lim FAN jee ah gruh fee	*lymphangi/o* lymph vessel *-graphy* process of recording	Radiographic visualization of a part of the lymphatic system after injection with a radiopaque substance (Fig. 9-13).
Splenic arteriography	*splen/o* spleen	Radiographic visualization of the spleen with the use of a contrast medium.

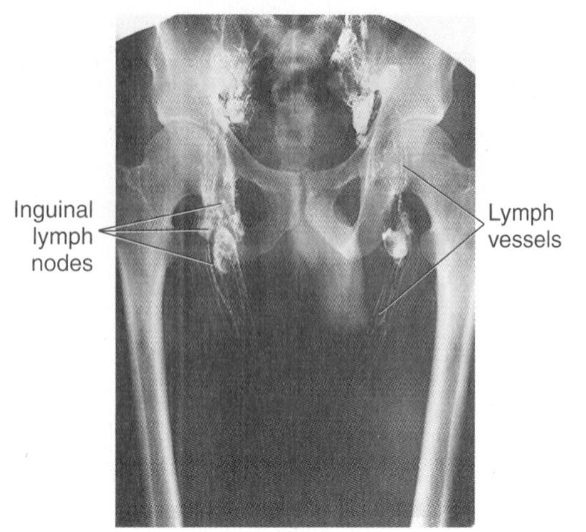

Fig. 9-13 Lymphangiogram of inguinal region and upper thighs.

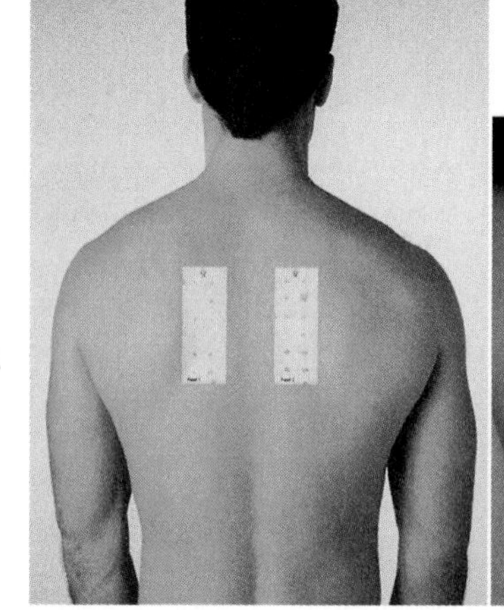

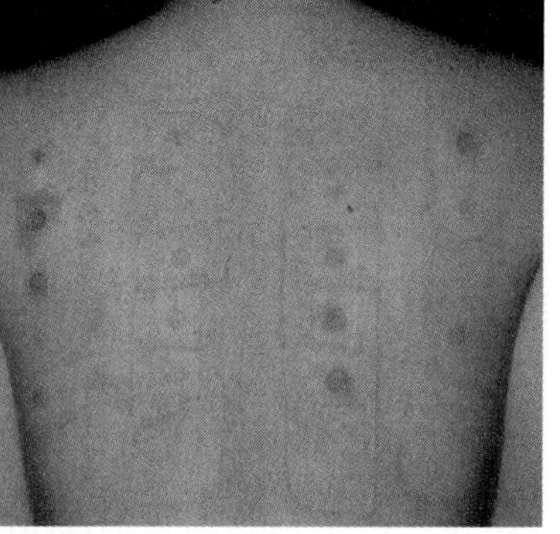

Fig. 9-14 **A,** Allergen patch test impregnated with individual allergens is applied to the back of the patient. **B,** Positive allergy reactions of varying intensity.

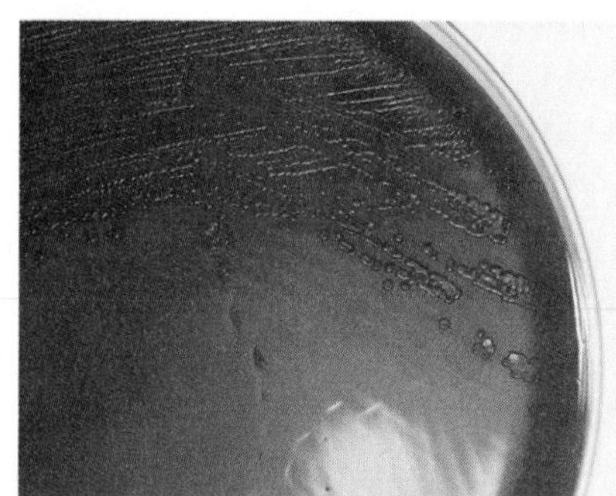

Fig. 9-15 Blood culture.

Terms Related to Laboratory Tests

TERM	WORD ORIGIN	DEFINITION
AIDS tests—ELISA, Western blot		Tests to detect the presence of HIV types 1 and 2.
Allergy testing		Series of tests involving a patch, scratch, or intradermal injection of an attenuated amount of an allergen to test for hypersensitivity (Fig. 9-14).
Blood cultures		Blood samples are submitted to propagate microorganisms that may be present. Cultures may be indicated for bacteremia or septicemia, or to discover other pathogens (fungi, viruses, or parasites) (Fig. 9-15).
Complete blood cell count (CBC)		Twelve tests, including RBC (red blood cell count), WBC (white blood cell count), Hg (hemoglobin), Hct/PCV (hematocrit/packed cell volume), and diff (WBC differential).

Terms Related to Laboratory Tests—cont'd

TERM	WORD ORIGIN	DEFINITION
Coombs' antiglobulin test koomz an tee GLOB yoo lin		Blood test to diagnose hemolytic disease of the newborn (HDN), acquired hemolytic anemia, or a transfusion reaction.
Diff count		Measure of the numbers of the different types of WBCs.
Erythrocyte sedimentation rate (ESR) eh RITH roh syte seh dih men TAY shun		Measurement of time for mature RBCs to settle out of a blood sample after an anticoagulant is added. An increased ESR indicates inflammation.
Hematocrit (Hct), Packed cell volume (PCV) hee MAT oh krit		Measure of the percentage of RBCs in the blood.
Hemoglobin (Hgb, Hb) HEE moh gloh bin		Iron-containing pigment of RBCs that carries oxygen to tissues.
Mean corpuscular hemoglobin (MCH) kor PUS kyoo lur		Test to measure the average weight of hemoglobin per RBC. Useful in diagnosing anemia.
Mean corpuscular hemoglobin concentration (MCHC)		Test to measure the concentration of hemoglobin in RBCs. This test is useful for measuring a patient's response to treatment for anemia.
Monospot MAH noh spot		Test for infectious mononucleosis.
Prothrombin time (PT) proh THROM bin		Test that measures the amount of time taken for clot formation. It is used to determine the cause of unexplained bleeding, to assess levels of anticoagulation in patients taking warfarin, or with vitamin K deficiency, and to assess the ability of the liver to synthesize blood-clotting proteins.
Partial thromboplastin time (PTT) THROM boh plas tin		Test of blood plasma to detect coagulation defects of the intrinsic system; used to detect hemophilias.
Schilling test SHILL ing		Nuclear medicine test used to diagnose pernicious anemia and other metabolic disorders.
White blood cell count (WBC)		Measurement of the number of leukocytes in the blood. An increase may indicate the presence of an infection; a decrease may be caused by radiation or chemotherapy.

Exercise 10: Diagnostic Procedures

Matching. Some answers may be used more than once.

____ 1. Coombs' antiglobulin
____ 2. Schilling test
____ 3. PTT
____ 4. PCV
____ 5. Monospot
____ 6. ESR
____ 7. blood culture
____ 8. WBC
____ 9. Western blot
____ 10. Hct
____ 11. ELISA
____ 12. MCH
____ 13. MCHC
____ 14. allergy test
____ 15. PT

A. % RBCs
B. if increased, inflammation indicated
C. anemia
D. HIV
E. response to anemia treatment
F. determines cause of bleeding
G. hemophilia
H. pernicious anemia
I. infectious mononucleosis
J. hypersensitivity
K. HDN, transfusion reaction
L. microorganisms
M. prothrombin time

Circle the correct answer.

16. Splenic arteriography is an x-ray *(record, process of recording)* of the spleen.
17. A lymphangiogram is a *(record, process of recording)* of a lymph *(gland, vessel)*.
18. Lymphadenography is an x-ray *(record, process of recording)* of a lymph *(gland, vessel)*.

THERAPEUTIC INTERVENTIONS

Case Study Continued

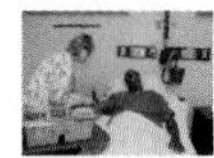

Marta processes Ozzie's bloodwork, noting the low hematocrit and the high WBC that accompanies a sickle-cell crisis. Ozzie is given intravenous pain medication, along with antibiotics for his bronchitis. Luckily, the RBC is not low enough to necessitate a blood transfusion.

Terms Related to Blood and Bone Marrow Interventions

Term	Word Origin	Definition
Apheresis aff ur EE sis	*-pheresis* removal	Temporary removal of blood from a donor, in which one or more components are removed and the rest of the blood is reinfused into the donor. Examples include **leukapheresis,** removal of WBCs; **plasmapheresis,** removal of plasma; and **plateletpheresis,** removal of thrombocytes.
Autologous transfusion ah TALL uh gus	*auto-* self *log/o* study *-ous* pertaining to *trans-* across *-fusion* pouring	Process in which the donor's own blood is removed and stored in anticipation of a future need (Fig. 9-16).

Terms Related to Blood and Bone Marrow Interventions—cont'd

Term	Word Origin	Definition
Autologous bone transplant	*auto-* self *log/o* study *-ous* pertaining to	Harvesting of patient's own healthy bone marrow before treatment, for reintroduction later.
Autotransfusion	*auto-* self *trans-* across *-fusion* pouring	Process in which the donor is transfused with his/her own blood, after anticoagulation and filtration, from an active bleeding site in cases of major surgery or trauma.
Blood transfusion	*trans-* across *-fusion* pouring	Intravenous transfer of blood from a donor to a recipient, giving either whole blood or its components.
Homologous bone marrow transplant (BMT) hoh MALL uh gus	*homo-* same (species) *log/o* study *-ous* pertaining to	Transplantation of healthy bone marrow from a donor to a recipient to stimulate formation of new blood cells.

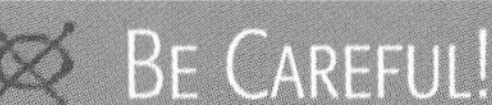

BE CAREFUL!

Do not confuse *apheresis,* meaning *removal of blood,* with *poiesis,* which means *formation.*

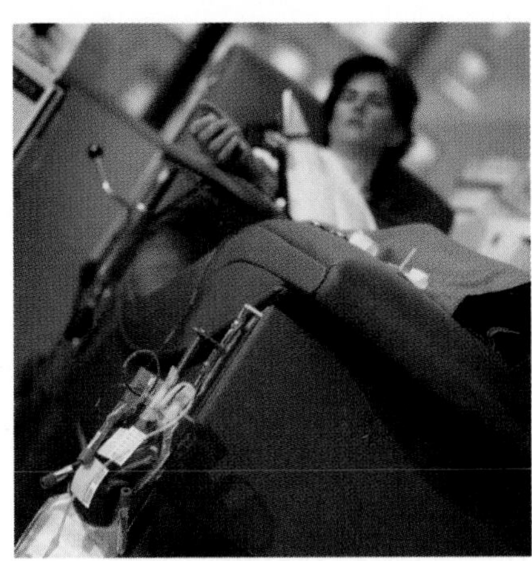

Fig. 9-16 Autologous blood transfusion.

DID YOU KNOW?

Apheresis is from a Greek word meaning *removal.* It may also be used as a suffix to create a term that means *to remove blood constituents* such as *leukapheresis,* the removal of WBCs.

Terms Related to Lymphatic and Immune System Interventions

Term	Word Origin	Definition
Adenoidectomy ad eh noyd ECK tuh mee	*adenoid/o* adenoid *-ectomy* removal	Removal of the adenoids. Also called the *pharyngeal tonsils.*
Biopsy of lymphatic structures	*bi/o* living *-opsy* viewing *lymphat/o* lymph *-ic* pertaining to	Removal of the lymph nodes or lymphoid tissue to be examined for disease.
Lymphadenectomy lim fad uh NECK tuh mee	*lymphaden/o* lymph gland *-ectomy* removal	Removal of a lymph node.
Splenectomy spleh NECK tuh mee	*splen/o* spleen *-ectomy* removal	Removal of the spleen.

Exercise 11: THERAPEUTIC INTERVENTIONS

Fill in the blanks with one of the following terms.

adenoidectomy, plasmapheresis, splenectomy, leukapheresis, autologous, homologous

1. Someone who has a transfusion of his/her own blood that has been stored in advance has what type of transfusion? ________________
2. A patient who receives a bone marrow transplant from a donor has a/an ________________ bone marrow transplant.
3. A resection of the pharyngeal tonsils is called ________________.
4. A separation of the white blood cells from the rest of the blood is called ________________.
5. If plasma is separated from the rest of a unit of donated blood, the process is called ________________.
6. Removal of the lymphoid tissue in the upper left quadrant of the body is a/an ________________.

PHARMACOLOGY

Hematic Drugs

Anticoagulants: Drugs that prevent or delay the coagulation of the blood. Examples: anisindione (Miradon), dicumarol, and warfarin (Coumadin and generic).

Antiplatelets: Drugs that inhibit the function of platelets or destroy them. Examples: aspirin, clopidogrel (Plavix), dipyridamole (Persantine), sulfinpyrazone (Anturane), ticlopidine (Ticlid), and tirofiban (Aggrastat).

Blood-flow agents: Drugs that promote blood flow by keeping platelets from clumping. Examples: ginkgo biloba, cilostazol (Pletal), and pentoxifylline (Trental).

Epoetin alfa: Drug that increases products of RBCs.

Hematinic (hee muh TIN ick) **agents:** Drugs that increase the number of erythrocytes and/or hemoglobin concentration in the erythrocytes. Examples: iron and B-complex vitamins.

Hematopoietic (hem uh toh poy EH tick) **agents:** Drugs that help to increase WBC counts. Example: filgrastim (Neupogen).

Hemostatics (coagulants): Drugs that stop the flow of blood. Example: hydroxyurea (Droxia, Hydrea).

Thrombolytics (throm boh LIT icks): Drugs that cause the destruction of blood clots; used to decrease the severity and frequency of sickle-cell crises.

Lymphatic and Immune Drugs

Antihistamines: Drugs that reduce the effects of histamine, part of the allergic inflammatory response. Examples: diphenhydramine (Benadryl), clemastine (Tavist), dimenhydrinate (Dramamine), cetirizine (Zyrtec), fexofenadine (Allegra), and loratadine (Claritin).

Anti-IgE: Investigational agent currently being researched for use as injectable anti-IgE monoclonal antibodies against asthma and allergic rhinitis. It appears to work in both adults and children without major side effects.

Antineoplastic drug: Drug used to treat cancer by preventing growth of neoplastic (tumor) cells.
Azidothymidine (AZT) (also called *zidovudine*): Classed as an antiviral and anti-HIV drug, this drug interferes with the virus's replication by disrupting the function of essential enzymes. Examples: Retrovir and Combivir.
Corticosteroids or "steroids": Drugs used as antiinflammatories and immunosuppressants.
Cytotoxic drug: Drug used as an immunosuppressant or antineoplastic for its ability to damage or destroy cells.
Immunosuppressants: Drugs that have the effect of lessening the immune response. Examples: azathioprine (Imuran), chlorambucil (Leukeran), cyclophosphamide (Cytoxan), cyclosporine (Sandimmune), hydroxychloroquine (Plaquenil), leflunomide (Arava), sirolimus (Rapamune), and tacrolimus (Prograf).
Protease (PRO tee aze) **inhibitors:** Also classed as antivirals and anti-AIDS drugs. By blocking the production of an essential enzyme called *protease,* these drugs keep the virus from replicating. Examples are Amprenavir, Indinavir, Nelfinavir, Ritonavir, and Saquinavir.
Trizivir: A combination of three potent anti-AIDS drugs (zidovudine or AZT, lamivudine [3TC], and abacavir or Ziagen) in one pill.
Vaccines (immunizations): Substances administered to induce immunity or reduce the pathologic effects of a disease. Examples are measles, mumps, and chicken pox vaccines.

Exercise 12: PHARMACOLOGY

Match each drug group with its action.

_____ 1. thrombolytics
_____ 2. antiplatelets
_____ 3. hematopoietic agents
_____ 4. hematinics
_____ 5. anticoagulants
_____ 6. antihistamines
_____ 7. immunosuppressants
_____ 8. diuretics
_____ 9. hemostatics
_____ 10. vaccines

A. treat allergic reactions
B. delay clotting of blood
C. inhibit clotting, destroy thrombocytes
D. help induce immunity
E. increase WBCs
F. stop the flow of blood
G. decrease fluid retention
H. lessen the immune response
I. increase RBC or Hgb concentration
J. destroy clots

Case Study *Continued*

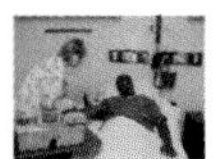

On Ozzie's last day in the hospital, Marta comes to his room to draw blood for one last test. She is glad to see that he is feeling much better. She asks him how the tests on his daughter came out. Ozzie grins and says that the amniocentesis was negative for the sickle-cell trait, and she is not a carrier. At least one member of his family has escaped the agony of sickle-cell anemia.

Abbreviations

Abbreviation	Definition	Abbreviation	Definition
A, B, AB, O	Blood types	HIV	Human immunodeficiency virus
AIDS	Acquired immunodeficiency syndrome	Ig	Immunoglobin
ANA	Antinuclear antibody	Lymphs	Lymphocytes
Baso	Basophils	MCH	Mean corpuscular hemoglobin
BMT	Bone marrow transplant	MCHC	Mean corpuscular hemoglobin concentration
CBC	Complete blood cell count	Neut	Neutrophils
CO_2	Carbon dioxide	NK	Natural killer cells
Diff	Differential WBC count	O_2	Oxygen
EBL	Estimated blood loss	PCV	Packed cell volume, hematocrit
EBV	Epstein-Barr virus	Plats	Platelets, thrombocytes
Eosins	Eosinophils	PMNs, polys	Polymorphonucleocytes
ESR	Erythrocyte sedimentation rate	PT	Prothrombin time
Hb	Hemoglobin	PTT	Partial thromboplastin time
Hct	Hematocrit, packed cell volume	RBC	Red blood cell (count)
HDN	Hemolytic disease of the newborn	Rh	Rhesus
Hgb	Hemoglobin	WBC	White blood cell (count)

Exercise 13: ABBREVIATIONS

Write out the term for the following abbreviations.

1. Karl was admitted with a Dx of EBV.

____

2. The patient's blood sample was tested for Hct and Hb.

____

3. The AIDS patient was HIV positive.

____

4. The patient left surgery with a EBL of 300 cc.

____

5. The patient was admitted for a BMT with his twin as the donor.

____

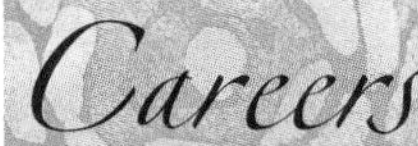

Careers

Clinical Laboratory Technologists and Technicians

Clinical laboratory technologists and technicians are instrumental in the diagnosis of diseases by preparing, examining, and analyzing samples of cells, tissues, and bodily fluids. Although about half of the clinical laboratory technologists and technicians work in hospitals, the other half work in physician clinics and stand-alone healthcare laboratories. The Occupational Outlook Handbook of the Bureau of Labor Statistics describes the attributes necessary to work in the field: "good analytical judgment . . . ability to work under pressure . . . close attention to detail . . . manual dexterity . . . computer skills are important . . . expected to be good at problem solving."

Healthcare and clinical laboratory technologists usually have a bachelor's degree with a major in healthcare technology, whereas clinical laboratory technicians have an associate's degree or a certificate. The field is expected to have average growth, although competition for jobs has increased because of organizational consolidation and restructuring and laboratory automation.

The professional organizations for these careers are as follows:

American Society of Clinical Pathologists, Board of Registry at http://www.ascp.org/bor
American Medical Technologists at http://www.amt1.com
American Society of Cytopathology at http://www.cytopathology.org
International Society for Clinical Laboratory Technology, 917 Locust St., Suite 1100, St. Louis, MO 63101-1413.

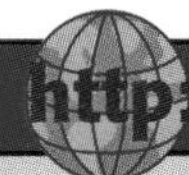

http: INTERNET PROJECT

Fifteen million units of blood are needed each year for emergency and scheduled transfusions. Currently, the only method to obtain this blood is through donations. Although most people are amenable to accepting a transfusion, fewer are willing to donate. Starting with the following sites, research the question of who donates blood in our society and why. Or stated another way—why are some people unwilling to donate blood? You should examine at least two of the following parameters: sex, age, ethnicity, and religious belief. Present your findings in a 3-page, double-spaced paper, with at least three cited sources.

Use the following sites:

American Red Cross: http://www.redcross.org/services/biomed/blood
American Association of Blood Banks: http://www.aabb.org/All about Blood/
Johns Hopkins Medical Institutions: Article titled "Mistrust, Religious Beliefs Hinder Blood and Organ Donation": http://www.hopkinsmedicine.org
National Institutes of Health MEDLINEplus: Blood/Blood Transfusion: http://www.nlm.nih.gov/medlineplus/bloodbloodtransfusion.html

Chapter Review

A. Functions of the Blood, Lymphatic, and Immune Systems

1. What functions do the blood, lymphatic, and immune systems share?

defense

2. Give an example of how one of these systems maintains homeostasis.

3. Explain how the three systems are different.

B. Anatomy and Physiology

4. Write the formula for the composition of blood (solid and liquid elements) with percentages.

Blood 45% formed elements + 55% plasma

5. What is the term for a red blood cell and what is its function?

erythrocyte O_2 & CO_2 transport

6. If someone has a low red blood cell count, what functions are being compromised? What other body systems may be involved?

x-port of gases & nutrients; All other Body Systems Are involved

7. How are the terms hemoglobin, hemosiderin, and hemolysis related?

Hemoglobin = protein iron pigment; Decomposes → hemosiderin (iron pigment) Formed result of Hemolysis

8. Name the two main kinds of leukocytes (be sure to include their alternative names also).

granulocyte (PMN) & Agranulocyte

9. Name all three types of granulocytes.

10. Name the two types of agranulocytes.

11. What do thrombocytes do and what is their other name?

Clot Platelets

12. Fill in the steps to complete the process of blood clotting.

Cut → ________ → ________ → ________ → ________ →

________ → Hemostasis

13. Of what is plasma composed?

H_2O Inorg. substance, Org. substance; waste prod.; plasma protein

14. What is the relationship of serum to plasma?

Serum = plasma − clotting proteins

15. What is the term for the formation of blood? ____________________
16. Name the four blood types, specifying which is the universal donor and which is the universal recipient.

____

17. The differences between the blood types are due to a/an ____________ present on the surface of the blood cells, called a/an ____________, and the body produces antibodies called ____________.
18. Name the parts of the lymphatic system with their combining forms.

____

19. What type of cell is responsible for phagocytosis? ____________________
20. Explain the path of lymph from the interstitial spaces to the blood capillaries.

____

21. Chemical messengers of the immune system are called ____________________. The three different types are called ____________.
22. What is the difference between cell-mediated and antibody-related immunity?

____

23. What are the levels of defense in the immune system?

____

24. What is the difference between specific and nonspecific immunity?

____

C. Pathology

25. What is the general term for blood disorders? ____________________
26. Why is anemia a problem? What functions are diminished?

____

Decode the term.

27. leukopenia ____

28. lymphocytosis ____

29. sideropenia ____

30. splenomegaly ____

31. lymphadenitis ____

Build a term.

32. deficiency of all cells ______________________________

33. increase of WBCs ______________________________

34. disease of a lymph gland ______________________________

35. inflammation of a lymph vessel ______________________________

36. pertaining to destruction of blood Hemolytic

Fill in the blank.

37. What is a type of anemia that is inherited by African American, Mediterranean, and Southeast Asian people? Thalassemia

38. What type of anemia is an inherited malformation of the red blood cells?

____

39. Which group of disorders has an inherited lack of a factor necessary for blood to clot?

Hemophilia

40. What is the term for a disease caused by the Epstein-Barr virus? ______________________________

41. What is the term for accumulation of lymphatic fluid? ______________________________

42. What is the term for blood disorders? Dyscrasia

43. What is the term for a hypersensitivity to a normally nonpathogenic substance?

____

44. An extreme allergic response is called ANAphylAxis.

45. What is a chronic increase in the number of red blood cells and concentration of hemoglobin?

Polycythemia vera

D. Diagnostic Procedures

Fill in the blank with one of the following terms.

ESR, blood cultures, monospot, Coombs' test, PTT, MCH, diff, ELISA, hematocrit, Schilling test

46. number of varieties of white blood cells diff

47. recognition of HIV antibodies Elisa

48. percentage of solid elements in blood Hematocrit

49. test for mononucleosis ______________

50. increase may indicate infection ESR

51. transfusion reaction Coombs Test

52. anemia MCH

53. clotting problems ______________

54. pernicious anemia ______________

55. septicemia ______________

Decode the term.

56. lymphangiogram ______________

57. lymphadenography ______________

58. splenic arteriography ______________

E. Therapeutic Interventions

59. Build the terms for the following resections:

   A. lymph vessels ______________

   B. spleen ______________

   C. thymus gland ______________

   D. lymph nodes ______________

60. What is the term for the separation of blood into component parts? ______________

61. A. What is the term for taking blood from one donor and introducing it into a recipient?

   ____

   B. If the transfusion takes place immediately because of major trauma or surgery, it is called

   ______________.

   C. If the transfusion is done in advance for an event in the future, it is called ______________.

62. What is the term for removal of tissue from the lymph nodes for examination?

   ____

F. Pharmacology

63. A patient is prescribed a/an ______________ for an allergic reaction.

64. ______________ are used to prevent the formation of blood clots.

65. ______________ are administered to dissolve blood clots.

66. Substances that induce immunity are ______________.

67. Classed also as an antiviral drug, this drug is used to combat AIDS. ______________

68. Drugs used as antineoplastics or immunosuppressants with cell-damaging properties are called

   ______________.

G. Abbreviations

Spell out the abbreviations in the following sentences.

69. The patient with posthemorrhagic anemia needed a transfusion to raise her Hct.

    ____

70. An elevated ESR indicated that Jasper had some type of infection. ____________________
71. Because the patient's PCV was so low, she was unable to donate blood.

    ____

72. Upon admission, Sally had a CBC and a diff. ____________________

73. The patient and her fetus had different Rh factors. ____________________

H. Singulars and Plurals

Change the following terms from singular to plural.

74. nucleus ____________________

75. serum ____________________

I. Cumulative Review

76. In what quadrant is the spleen located? ____________________

77. In what quadrant is the appendix located? ____________________

78. The thymus is located in the mediastinum. Where is that? ____________________
79. Define the locations of the following lymph nodes:

    A. cervical ____________________

    B. axillary ____________________

    C. inguinal ____________________

80. Emesis means ____________________. If in response to a pathogen, it may illustrate

    which line of defense? ____________________

J. Translations

Translate the following into your own words.

81. Ms. Cooper was seen by her physician for complaints of fatigue and weakness accompanied by a tendency to bruise easily. On physical examination, her physician observed hepatosplenomegaly, lymphadenopathy, and purpura. Laboratory findings indicated pancytopenia. She was diagnosed with aplastic anemia and treated with RBCs and platelet transfusions.

    ____

    ____

82. Dr. Douglas was seen for chills, fever, loss of appetite and an inflamed cut on his upper arm. Laboratory testing revealed leukocytosis, and a blood culture was positive for staphylococci. His physician diagnosed lymphadenitis.

    ____

    ____

83. Tyra Wilson worried that her weight loss, diarrhea, night sweats, and occasional pyrexia might be symptoms of an HIV infection. After anonymous testing with ELISA, she was relieved to find that she was not HIV positive.

    ____

    ____

K. Be Careful

84. What is the difference between *apheresis* and *poiesis?*

    ____

85. What is the difference between *Hgb* and *Hg?*

    ____

86. What is the difference between *thym/o* and *thyr/o?*

    ____

87. What is the difference between *cyt/o* and *cyst/o?*

    ____

River City Hospital
7777 S. Shore Dr.
Mason City, IA 50428

DISCHARGE SUMMARY

Patient Name: Ozzie Samuelson
Med Rec #: 935634
Adm Date: 3/1/2001
Discharge Date: 3/5/2001
Principal Diagnosis: Sickle-Cell Crisis
Secondary Diagnosis: Acute Bronchitis
Surgical Procedure: None
History of Present Illness: On the above date, the patient was admitted to River City Hospital via the Emergency Room, with a chief complaint of pain all over his body since the night before.

The patient, a 42-year-old African-American male with a history of sickle-cell anemia, stated that he started having pain all over his body, especially at the back of the legs. He also notes having chills, but denies sweats.

Medical History: The patient has a medical history of sickle-cell anemia and pneumonia in 1998.
Surgical History: Surgical history includes a total hip replacement and an appendectomy.
Allergies: The patient has no history of allergies.
Medications: Motrin and Darvon.
Occupation: The patient is unemployed, on disability. The patient is a nonsmoker and nondrinker.
Family History: The patient's family history is positive for mother and father with sickle-cell trait; otherwise unremarkable.
Review of Systems: Unremarkable except for global body pain.
Physical Examination: Temperature was 98.1 degrees, blood pressure was 155/90, heart rate of 75, respiratory rate of 23.
Consultations: The consultations included Dr. Smith for sickle-cell disease.
Pertinent Laboratory Studies: Reticulocyte count of 13.8; white blood cell count of 12.9; hemoglobin and hematocrit of 12.0 and 29.4, respectively; albumin of 2.1.
Hospital Course: The patient was admitted on 3/1/2001, and progressed steadily with intravenous analgesic support until discharge on 3/5/2001, when the patient was deemed stable.
Condition on Discharge: Stable.
Discharge Instructions: The patient is to limit activity and follow up with Dr. Rohr in his office in 1 week.
Medications on Discharge: Biaxin, Suprax, Trental, folic acid, Toradol, and vitamin E.

____
Marvin Kinley, MD

L. Healthcare Report

88. What statement in the discharge summary indicates that the patient was in sickle-cell crisis?

____

89. What medications were used to treat the patient's symptoms?

____

90. The patient's past healthcare history mentions a resection of his ____________________.

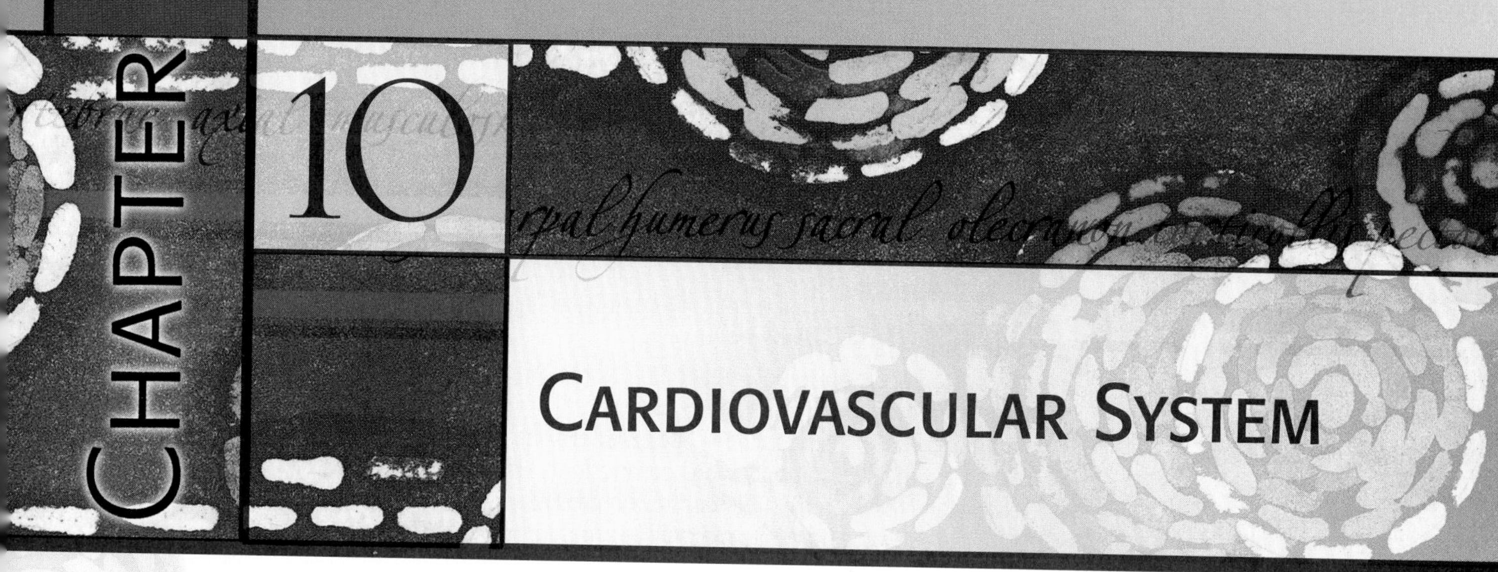

CHAPTER 10 CARDIOVASCULAR SYSTEM

"The patient must combat the disease along with the physician." ***—Hippocrates***

Quote

Case Study

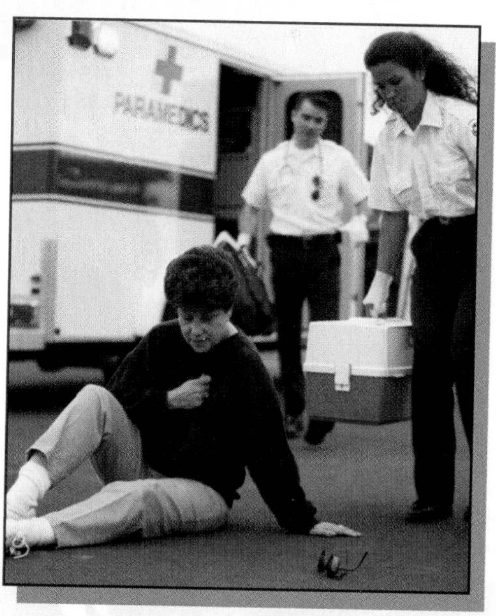

Cheryl Miller has been shopping all day and is tired. She stops for a quick burger and fries at the food court and then heads out of the mall. As Cheryl walks toward her car, she begins to experience symptoms of sweating, nausea, and extreme pain and pressure in her chest. She wants nothing more than to get home and lie down, but the pain is so bad that she sinks down in the parking lot, grabbing her chest. A passerby calls 911.

OBJECTIVES

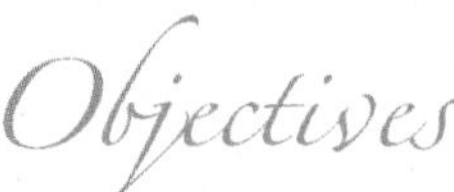

- In your own words, explain the functions of the cardiovascular system.
- Recognize, recall, and apply healthcare terms related to the anatomy and physiology of the cardiovascular system.
- Recognize, recall, and apply healthcare terms related to the pathology of the cardiovascular system.
- Recognize, recall, and apply healthcare terms related to diagnostic procedures of the cardiovascular system.
- Recognize, recall, and apply healthcare terms related to the therapeutic interventions of the cardiovascular system.
- Recognize, recall, and apply the abbreviations introduced in this chapter.
- Recognize, recall, and apply word components used in this chapter to build and decode healthcare terms relevant to the cardiovascular system.
- Recognize, recall, and apply material learned in previous chapters.

DID YOU KNOW?

Since 1900, cardiovascular disease (CVD) has been the number-one killer in the United States every year but 1918. CVD claims almost 10,500 more lives each year than the next six leading causes of death combined.

FUNCTIONS OF THE CARDIOVASCULAR SYSTEM

The primary function of the **cardiovascular** (kar dee oh VAS kyoo lur) **system** (CV), also called the **circulatory system**, is to provide transportation of oxygen, nutrients, water, body salts, hormones, and other substances to every cell in the body. It also acts to carry waste products, such as carbon dioxide (CO_2), away from the cells, eventually to be excreted. The heart functions as a pump; the blood vessels act as "pipes"; and the blood is the transportation medium. If the system does not function properly, causing oxygen or the other critical substances to be withheld from the cells, dysfunction results, and the cells (and the person) may be injured or die.

Exercise 1: FUNCTIONS OF THE CARDIOVASCULAR SYSTEM

Fill in the blanks.

1. The function of the CV system is to carry substances to and from every cell in the body.
2. The CV system is composed of a pump, which is the heart; pipes, which are the Vessels; and a transportation medium that flows through the pipes, which is the blood.

ANATOMY AND PHYSIOLOGY

Pulmonary and Systemic Circulation

To accomplish its task of pumping substances to and from the cells of the body, the heart is involved in two overlapping cycles of circulation: **pulmonary** and **systemic.**

Pulmonary Circulation

Pulmonary circulation begins with the right side of the heart sending blood to the lungs to absorb oxygen (O_2) and release carbon dioxide (CO_2). Note in Fig.

10-1 that the vessels that carry blood to the lungs from the heart are blue—to show the blood as being **deoxygenated** (dee OCK sih juh nay tid), or oxygen deficient. Once the oxygen is absorbed, the blood is considered **oxygenated**, or oxygen rich. Note in Fig. 10-1 that the vessels traveling away from the lungs are red—to show oxygenation. The blood then progresses back to the left side of the heart, where it is pumped out to begin its route through the systemic circulatory system. The systemic circulation carries blood to the cells of the body, where nutrient and waste exchange takes place; the wastes, such as CO_2, are carried back to the heart on the return trip. This blood is then pumped out of the right side of the heart to the lungs to dispose of its CO_2, absorb O_2, and repeat the cycle.

Systemic Circulation

Fig. 10-2 shows the oxygenated/deoxygenated status of blood. In systemic circulation, the blood traveling away from the heart first passes through the largest artery in the body called the aorta (a ORE tuh). From the aorta, the vessels branch into conducting **arteries** (AR tur reez), then smaller **arterioles** (ar TEER ee oles), and finally to the **capillaries** (CAP ih lair eez). Note in Fig. 10-2 that the color has changed from the red of oxygenated blood to a purple color at the capillaries. This is the site of exchange between the cells' fluids and the plasma of the circulatory system. Oxygen and other substances are supplied, and carbon dioxide collected, along with a number of other wastes. Once the blood begins its journey

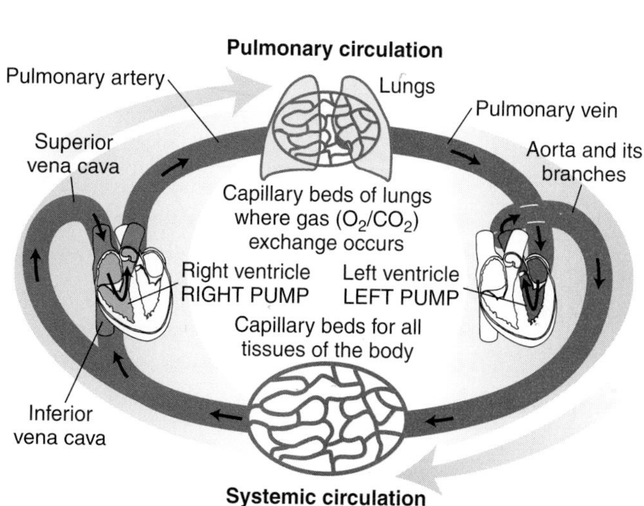

Fig. 10-1 Pulmonary and systemic circulation.

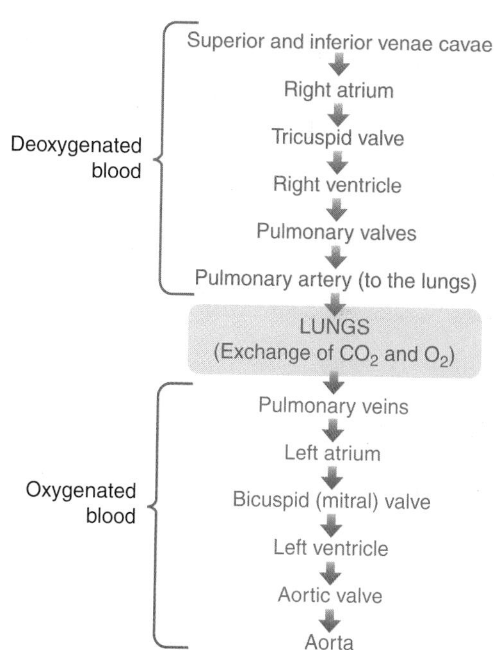

Fig. 10-2 Oxygenated/deoxygenated status of blood.

back to the heart, it first goes through **venules** (VEEN yools), then **veins** (vayns), and finally into one of the two largest veins, the **superior** and **inferior venae cavae** (VEE nuh KAY vuh). Fig. 10-3 illustrates the muscular, thick nature of arteries; the valvular, thinner nature of veins; and the delicate exchange function of capillaries. Arteries are generally thicker than veins, because they must withstand the force of the heart's pumping action.Veins do not have the thick muscle coat of the arteries to propel the blood on its journey through the circulatory system but instead rely on one-way valves that prevent the backflow of blood. In addition, skeletal muscle contraction provides pumping action. The capillaries' diameters are so tiny that only one blood cell at a time can pass through them.

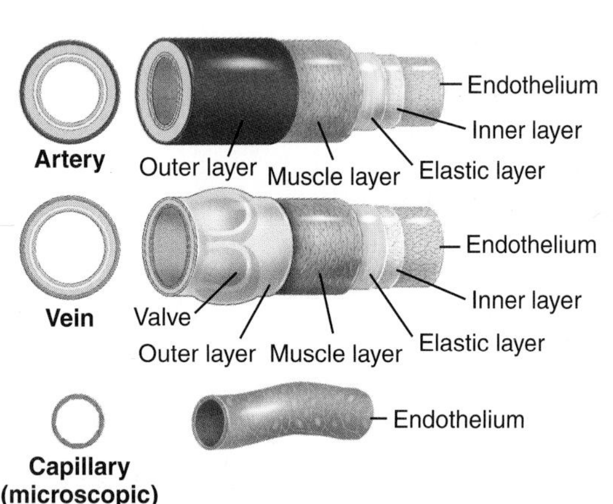

Fig. 10-3 Differences among arteries, veins, and capillaries.

COMBINING FORMS FOR THE CARDIOVASCULAR SYSTEM

MEANING	COMBINING FORM
aorta	aort/o
arteriole	arteriol/o
artery	arteri/o
capillary	capillar/o
heart	cardi/o, coron/o
lung	pulmon/o
system	system/o
vein	ven/o, phleb/o
venule	venul/o
vessel	vascul/o, angi/o, vas/o

Exercise 2: PULMONARY AND SYSTEMIC CIRCULATION

Fill in the blanks.

1. The heart is the center of which two types of circulation? ____________________
2. Which type of circulation takes blood to and from the cells of the lungs?

   ____
3. Which type of circulation begins with blood being pumped out of the left side of the heart?

   ____
4. What waste product is excreted by the lungs? ____________________

Circle the correct answer.

5. Blood traveling to the lungs from the heart is *(deoxygenated, oxygenated)*.
6. Arteries carry blood *(to, away from)* the heart.
7. Veins carry blood *(to, away from)* the heart.
8. Using red and blue pencils, write, in order, the names of the vessels that travel, first, *away from* the heart to the capillaries (in red), and *then back* to the heart (in blue). Begin with the word "heart."

   ____

   ____

Match the following combining forms with their meanings. More than one answer may be correct.

____ 9. vein
____ 10. artery
____ 11. heart
____ 12. venule
____ 13. capillary
____ 14. lung
____ 15. aorta
____ 16. arteriole
____ 17. vessel

A. vas/o
B. coron/o
C. pulmon/o
D. angi/o
E. phleb/o
F. arteri/o
G. ven/o
H. cardi/o
I. capillar/o
J. vascul/o
K. arteriol/o
L. aort/o
M. venul/o

Anatomy of the Heart

The human heart is about the size of a fist. It is located in the mediastinum of the thoracic cavity, slightly left of the midline. Its pointed tip, the apex, rests just above the diaphragm. The area of the chest wall anterior to the heart and lower thorax is referred to as the **precordium** (pree KORE dee um). The heart muscle has its own dedicated system of blood supply, the **coronary** (KORE ih nair ee) **arteries** (Fig. 10-4, *A*). The two main coronary arteries are called the left and right coronary arteries. They supply a constant, uninterrupted blood flow to the heart. The areas of the heart wall that they feed are designated as *inferior, lateral, anterior,* and *posterior.*

The heart has four chambers (Fig. 10-4, *B*). The upper chambers are called **atria** (A tree uh) (*sing.* atrium). The lower chambers are called **ventricles** (VEN trih kuls). Between the atria and ventricles, and between the ventricles and vessels, are valves that allow blood to flow through in one direction. The tissue walls between the chambers are called **septa** (SEP tuh) (*sing.* septum). The heart wall is constructed of three layers. The **endocardium** (en doh KAR dee um) is the thin tissue that acts as a lining of each of the chambers and valves. The **myocardium** (mye oh KAR dee um) is the cardiac muscle surrounding each of these chambers. The **pericardium** (pare ee KAR dee um) is the double-folded layer of connective tissue that surrounds the heart. The inner surface of this double fold is called the **visceral** (VIS uh rul) **pericardium**, and the outer membrane, closest to the body wall, is the **parietal** (puh RYE uh tul) **pericardium.** Another name for the visceral pericardium is the **epicardium** (eh pee KAR dee um), because it is the structure on top of the heart.

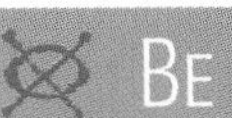

BE CAREFUL!

Do not confuse *aort/o,* meaning *aorta; atri/o,* meaning *atrium; arteri/o,* meaning *artery;* and *arteriol/o,* meaning *arteriole.*

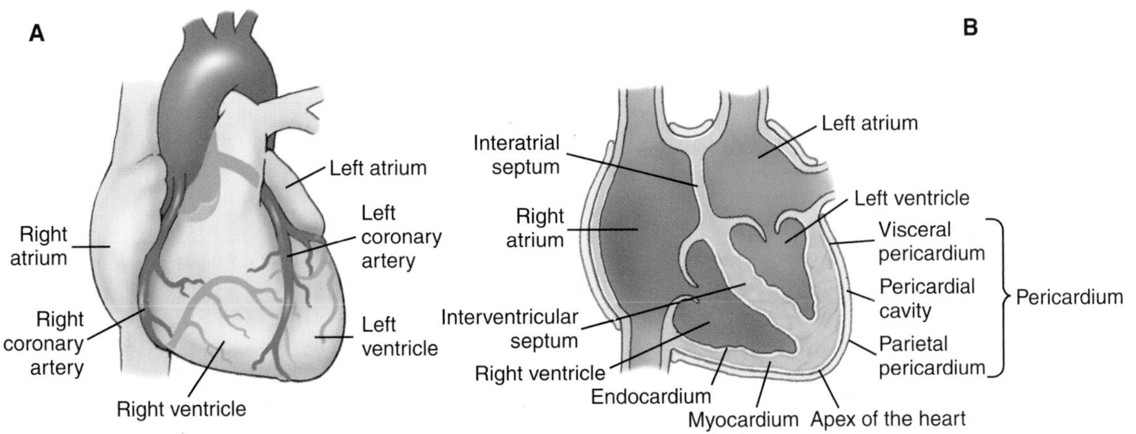

Fig. 10-4 **A,** Location of the coronary arteries. **B,** Chambers of the heart.

Combining Forms for the Anatomy of the Heart

Meaning	Combining Form	Meaning	Combining Form
apex	apic/o	myocardium	myocardi/o
endocardium	endocardi/o	pericardium	pericardi/o
heart	cardi/o, cordi/o, coron/o	septum	sept/o
muscle	my/o	ventricle	ventricul/o

Exercise 3: Anatomy of the Heart

Match the combining form with the correct body part.

______ 1. sept/o
______ 2. valv/o
______ 3. atri/o
______ 4. ventricul/o
______ 5. aort/o
______ 6. cardi/o, cordi/o, coron/o
______ 7. apic/o
______ 8. endocardi/o
______ 9. myocardi/o
______ 10. pericardi/o
______ 11. pulmon/o
______ 12. arteri/o

A. upper chamber of the heart
B. lower chamber of the heart
C. heart
D. largest artery
E. inner lining of chambers of heart
F. outer sac surrounding the heart
G. lung
H. muscle layer of the heart
I. valve
J. vessel that carries blood away from the heart
K. wall between chambers
L. the top, end, or tip of a structure

Did You Know?

A good way to remember how the blood flows through the heart valves is to memorize the phrase "Try (tri) before you buy (bi)." In the heart, blood flows through the tricuspid valve and then through the bicuspid (mitral) valve.

Blood Flow Through the Heart

Using Fig. 10-5 as a guide, follow the route of the blood through the heart. The pictures and words in this diagram are shaded red and blue to represent oxygenated and deoxygenated blood. Blood is squeezed from the **right atrium** to the **right ventricle** through the **tricuspid** (try KUSS pid) **valve.** Valves are considered to be competent if they open and close properly, letting through

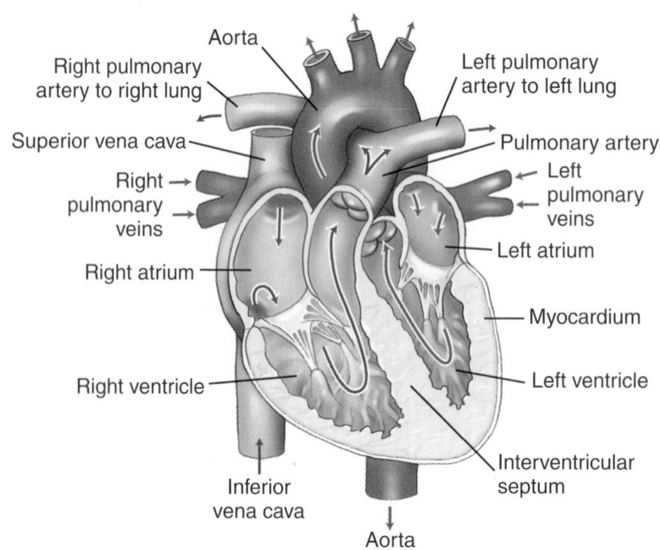

Fig. 10-5 Route of the blood through the heart.

or holding back an expected amount of blood. Once in the right ventricle, the blood is squeezed out through the **pulmonary semilunar valve** into the **pulmonary arteries,** which carry blood to the lungs and are the only arteries that carry deoxygenated blood. In the capillaries of the lungs, the CO_2 is passed out of the blood and O_2 is taken in. The now-oxygenated blood continues its journey back to the left side of the heart through the **pulmonary veins.** These are the only veins that carry oxygenated blood. The blood then enters the heart through the **left atrium** and has to pass the **mitral** (MYE trul) **valve,** also termed the **bicuspid valve,** to enter the **left ventricle.** When the left ventricle contracts, the blood is finally pushed out through the **aortic semilunar valve** into the **aorta** and begins yet another cycle through the body.

The amount of blood expelled from the left ventricle compared with the total volume of blood filling the ventricle is referred to as the stroke volume and is a measure of the **ejection fraction** of cardiac output. Typically around 65%, this amount is reduced in certain types of heart disease.

If a woman's heart rate is 80 beats per minute (bpm), then that means her heart contracts almost 5000 times per hour and over 100,000 beats per day, every day, for a lifetime. Truly an amazing amount of work is accomplished by an individual's body without a bit of conscious thought!

Exercise 4: BLOOD FLOW THROUGH THE HEART

Circle the correct answer.

1. *(Pulmonary arteries, Coronary arteries)* are the only arteries that carry deoxygenated blood.
2. The *(mitral, tricuspid)* valve is between the right atrium and right ventricle.
3. The *(mitral, tricuspid)* valve is between the left atrium and left ventricle.
4. *(Patent, Competent)* valves open and close properly.
5. The amount of blood expelled from the left ventricle compared to total heart volume is a measure of the *(ejection fraction, cardiac contraction).*

Case Study Continued

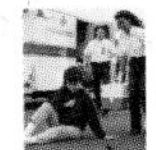

When paramedics, Cyn and David, arrive at the mall to take care of Cheryl Miller, one of the first things they assess is whether she is breathing freely. When they see that she is, they check her blood pressure with an instrument called a sphygmomanometer and listen to her heart rate with a stethoscope. Cheryl's blood pressure is very high, and her heart rate is irregular and faster than normal. Cyn tells Cheryl that she should be taken to the hospital for an electrocardiogram (ECG). Cheryl says that she thinks it is just stress or maybe a virus, but she agrees to go to the emergency department (ED).

The Cardiac Cycle

Systemic and pulmonary circulations occur as a result of a series of coordinated, rhythmic pulsations, called contractions and relaxations, of the heart muscle. The normal *rate* of these pulsations in humans is 60 to 100 bpm and is noted as a patient's **heart rate.** Fig. 10-6 illustrates various pulse points, places where heart rate can be measured in the body. **Blood pressure (BP)** is the resulting *force* of blood against the arteries. The contractive phase is **systole** (SIS toh lee), and the relaxation phase is **diastole** (dye AS toh lee). When blood pressure is measured with a **sphygmomanometer** (sfig moh muh NOM uh tur), it is recorded in millimeters of mercury (Hg) as a fraction representing the systolic pressure over the

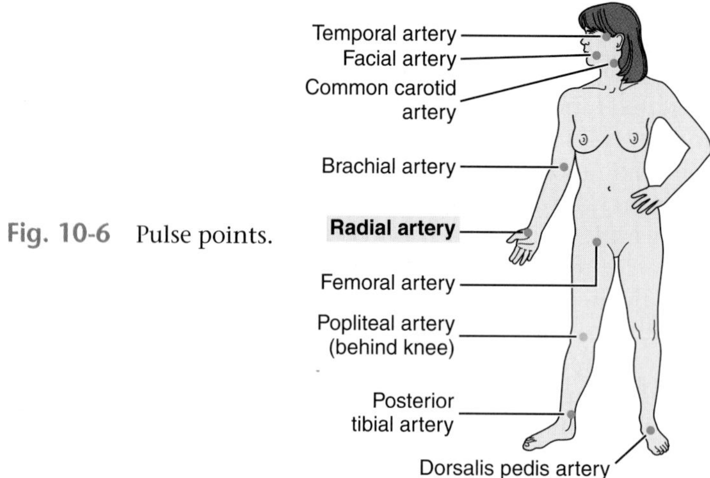

Fig. 10-6 Pulse points.

diastolic pressure. Optimal blood pressure is a systolic reading <120 and a diastolic reading <80. This is written as 120/80. Normal blood pressure is represented by a range. See the table below for blood pressure guidelines.

Blood Pressure Guidelines

	SYSTOLIC	DIASTOLIC
Optimal	Under 120 and	Under 80
Normal	120-139 or	80-84
High-normal	130-139 or	85-89

If the systolic and diastolic readings are in different categories, the higher of the two is used. Hypertension is defined as ≥140 systolic or ≥90 diastolic.

The cues for the timing of the heartbeat come from the electrical pathways in the muscle tissue of the heart (Fig. 10-7). The heartbeat begins in the right atrium at the **sinoatrial** (sin oh A tree ul) **(SA) node,** called the natural pacemaker of the heart. The initial electrical signal causes the atria to undergo electrical changes that signal contraction. This electrical signal is sent to the **atrioventricular** (a tree oh ven TRICK yoo lur) **(AV) node,** which is located at the base of the right atrium proximal to the interatrial septum. From the AV node, the signal travels next to the **bundle of His** (also called the **atrioventricular bundle**). This bundle is in the interatrial septum, and its right and left bundle branches transmit the impulse to the **Purkinje** (poor KIN jee) **fibers** in the right and left ventricles. Once the Purkinje fibers receive stimulation, they cause the ventricles to undergo electrical changes that signal contraction to force blood out to the pulmonary arteries and the aorta. If the electrical activity is normal, it is referred to as a **normal sinus rhythm** or **heart rate.** Any deviation of this electronic signaling may lead to an **arrhythmia** (ah RITH mee ah), an abnormal heart rhythm that compromises an individual's cardiovascular functioning by pumping too much or too little blood during that segment of the cardiac cycle. Normal or abnormal, the electronic impulses may be recorded as **wave deflections** of a needle on an instrument called an **electrocardiograph (ECG).**

One can hear the heart (also lung and bowel) sounds through a **stethoscope,** an instrument used to listen to sounds within the body.

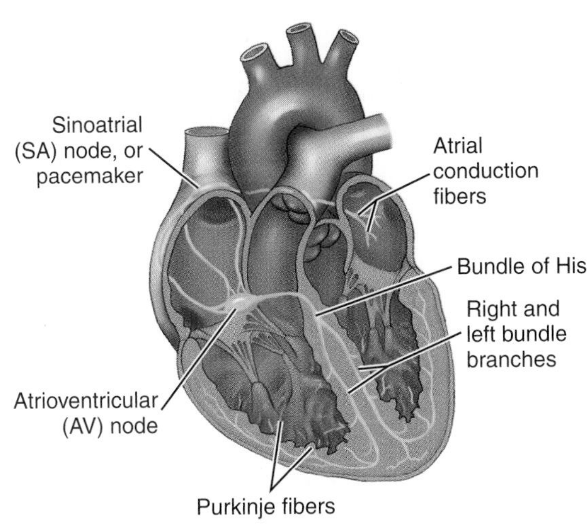

Fig. 10-7 Electrical conduction pathways of the heart.

Exercise 5: THE CARDIAC CYCLE

Circle the correct answer.

1. The contractive phase of the heart beat is *(systole, diastole)* and the relaxation phase is *(systole, diastole)*.
2. A normal heart rhythm is described as *(sinus rhythm, coronary rhythm)*.
3. List in order the structures that make up the normal pathway of electrical stimulation through the heart.

    ________________ → ________________ → ________________ → ________________ → ________________

4. Electrical impulses of the heart may be recorded graphically on an instrument called an

    ________________. The recording would be termed an ________________, and the process of recording the electrical activity of the heart would be called ________________. The abbreviation for these is ________________.

PATHOLOGY

Case Study Continued

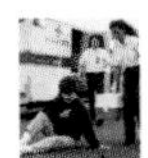

The paramedics, Cyn and David, give the ED staff their report on Cheryl Miller. They report that she complained of shortness of breath and nausea while shopping. On their arrival, they noticed that she was experiencing diaphoresis and was very pale. When questioned, she reported intense chest pain and palpitations but no syncope. She reports that she knows she has "high cholesterol" but has had difficulty changing her lifestyle of high-fat diets and minimal exercise.

Terms Related to Cardiac Signs and Symptoms

Term	Word Origin	Definition
Bradycardia bray dee KAR dee ah	*brady-* slow *-cardia* heart condition	Slow heartbeat, with ventricular contractions less than 60 bpm (Fig 10-8, *B*).
Bruit BROO ee		Abnormal sound heard when auscultating an artery. Usually a blowing or swishing sound, higher pitched than a murmur.
Cardiac pain		**Atypical pain** is a stabbing or burning pain that is variable in location and intensity and unrelated to exertion. **Ischemic pain** is a pressing, squeezing, or weightlike cardiac pain caused by decreased blood supply and usually lasts only minutes. **Pericardial pain** is stabbing, burning, or cutting cardiac pain.
Cardiomegaly kar dee oh MEG uh lee	*cardi/o* heart *-megaly* enlargement	Enlargement of the heart.
Cyanosis sye uh NOH sis	*cyan/o* blue *-osis* abnormal condition	Lack of oxygen in blood, seen as a bluish or grayish discoloration of skin, nail beds, and/or lips.
Diaphoresis dye uh foh REE sis		Profuse secretion of sweat.
Dyspnea; dyspnea on exertion (DOE) DISP nee uh	*dys-* difficult *-pnea* breathing	Difficult and/or painful breathing; if DOE, it is experienced when effort is expended.
Edema eh DEE muh		Abnormal accumulation of fluid in interstitial spaces of tissues.
Emesis EM uh sis	*emesis* to vomit	Expelling the contents of the stomach through the esophagus and mouth; vomiting.
Fatigue fuh TEEG		Sense of exhaustion, regardless of adequacy of sleep.
Murmur		Abnormal heart sound heard during systole, diastole, or both, which may be described as a gentle blowing, fluttering, or humming sound.
Nausea NAH zsa		Sensation of the urge to vomit.
Pallor PAL ur		Paleness of skin and/or mucous membranes. On darker pigmented skin, it may be noted on the inner surfaces of the lower eyelids or the nail beds.
Palpitations pal pih TAY shuns		Pounding or racing of the heart, such that the patient is aware of his/her heartbeat.
Pulmonary congestion	*pulmon/o* lung *-ary* pertaining to	Excessive amount of blood in the pulmonary vessels. Usually associated with heart failure.
Shortness of breath (SOB)		Breathlessness, air hunger.

Terms Related to Cardiac Signs and Symptoms—cont'd

TERM	WORD ORIGIN	DEFINITION
Syncope SING kuh pee		Fainting, loss of consciousness.
Tachycardia tack ee KAR dee ah	*tachy-* rapid *-cardia* heart condition	Rapid heartbeat, over 100 bpm (Fig. 10-8, *C*).
Thrill		Fine vibration felt by the examiner on palpation.
Venous distension	*ven/o* vein *-ous* pertaining to	Enlarged or swollen veins.

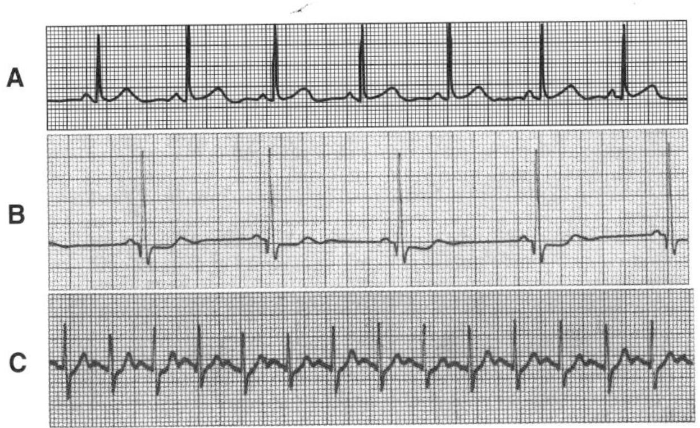

Fig. 10-8 ECGs. **A,** Normal; **B,** bradycardia; **C,** tachycardia.

> **BE CAREFUL!**
> Do not confuse *palpation,* which means *examination by touch,* and *palpitation,* which means *a pounding or racing of the heart.*

Exercise 6: CARDIAC SIGNS AND SYMPTOMS

Fill in the blanks.

1. Mr. Braun arrives at the ED complaining of feeling sick to his stomach, with an intense sensation of pressure in his chest and profuse sweating. These symptoms will be recorded as ______________, ______________, and ______________.
2. Another patient describes his problem of being out of breath whenever he tries to walk upstairs. This symptom may be described in healthcare terminology as one of two abbreviations: ______________ or ______________.
3. On examination, Ms. Fermetti's heart rate is 121 bpm. This can be described as ______________.
4. William Anson's family brings him to the ED because he fainted. Which symptom is this? ______________
5. On examination, the physician hears a gentle fluttering on systole. This is described as a/an ______________.

Matching.

_____ 6. bradycardia

_____ 7. tachycardia

_____ 8. syncope

_____ 9. diaphoresis

_____ 10. bruit

_____ 11. murmur

_____ 12. thrill

_____ 13. emesis

_____ 14. ischemia

_____ 15. fatigue

_____ 16. nausea

_____ 17. pallor

_____ 18. palpitations

_____ 19. dyspnea

_____ 20. cyanosis

_____ 21. SOB

A. fainting
B. paleness of skin
C. air hunger
D. exhaustion
E. fine vibration felt on palpation
F. difficult breathing
G. abnormal sound heard upon auscultation of an artery
H. rapid heartbeat
I. abnormal heart sound
J. lack of oxygen
K. urge to vomit
L. vomiting
M. decreased blood supply
N. slow heartbeat
O. profuse sweating
P. pounding of the heart

Terms Related to Congenital Disorders of the Heart

TERM	WORD ORIGIN	DEFINITION
Coarctation of the aorta koh ark TAY shun		Congenital cardiac anomaly characterized by a localized narrowing of the aorta. **Coarctation** is another term for a narrowing (Fig. 10-9).
Patent ductus arteriosus (PDA) PAY tent DUCK tus ar teer ee OH sis		Abnormal opening between the pulmonary artery and the aorta, caused by failure of the fetal ductus arteriosus to close after birth, most often in premature infants. **Patent** means *open*.
Septal defect SEP tul	***sept/o*** partition ***-al*** pertaining to	Any congenital abnormality to the walls between the heart chambers. **Atrial septal defect** is a hole in the wall between the top chambers of the heart. **Ventricular septal defect** is a hole in the wall between the bottom two chambers of the heart.
Tetralogy of Fallot teh TROL uh jee fah LOH	***tetra-*** four ***-logy*** study of	Congenital cardiac anomaly that consists of four defects: pulmonic stenosis; ventricular septal defect; malposition of the aorta, so that it arises from the septal defect or the right ventricle; and right ventricular hypertrophy.

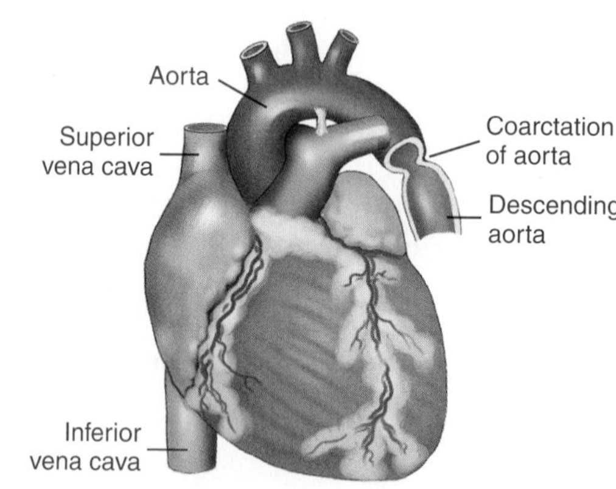

Fig. 10-9 Coarctation of the aorta.

Exercise 7: CONGENITAL DISORDERS

Matching.

_____ 1. sept/o

_____ 2. atri/o

_____ 3. ventricul/o

_____ 4. -trophy

_____ 5. hyper-

_____ 6. patent

_____ 7. stenosis

_____ 8. tetra-

_____ 9. pulmon/o

A. lower chamber of the heart
B. open
C. four
D. lung
E. development
F. wall, partition
G. excessive
H. narrowing
I. upper chamber of the heart

Terms Related to Valvular Heart Disease

The following valvular heart diseases (VHDs) present as incompetent or insufficient valvular function as a result of stenosis (narrowing), regurgitation (backflow), or prolapse (drooping). The causes are either congenital or acquired.

TERM	WORD ORIGIN	DEFINITION
Aortic stenosis (AS) a OR tick sten OH sis	***aort/o*** aorta ***-ic*** pertaining to ***stenosis*** narrowing	Narrowing of the aortic valve, which may be acquired or congenital (Fig. 10-10).
Mitral regurgitation (MR) MYE trul ree gur jih TAY shun		Backflow of blood from the left ventricle into the left atrium in systole across a diseased valve. It may be the result of congenital valve abnormalities, rheumatic fever, or MVP.
Mitral stenosis (MS) MYE trul sten OH sis	***stenosis*** narrowing	Narrowing of the valve between the left atrium and left ventricle, caused by adhesions on the leaflets of the valve, usually the result of recurrent episodes of rheumatic endocarditis. Left atrial hypertrophy develops and may be followed by right-sided heart failure and pulmonary edema (cor pulmonale) (see Fig. 10-10).

Continued

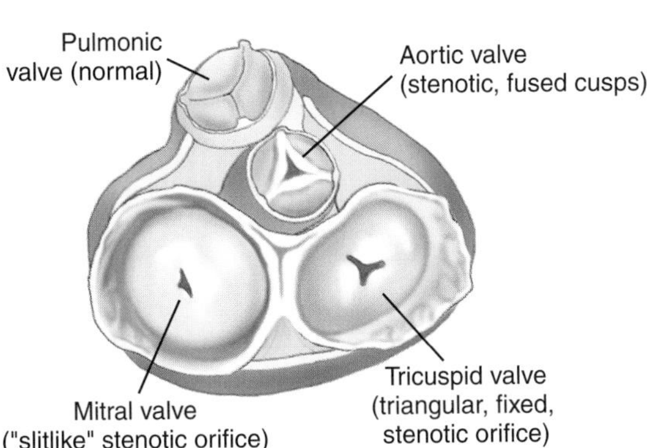

Fig. 10-10 Valvular heart disease: disorders of the aortic, mitral, and tricuspid valves.

DID YOU KNOW?

The term *mitral* is derived from the appearance of the valve and its similarity to a bishop's miter, or hat.

BE CAREFUL!

Do not confuse *stenosis,* which means *a narrowing,* with *sclerosis,* which means *a hardening.*

Terms Related to Valvular Heart Disease—cont'd

TERM	WORD ORIGIN	DEFINITION
Mitral valve prolapse (MVP) MYE trul valv PRO laps		Protrusion of one or both cusps of the mitral valve back into the left atrium during ventricular systole (Fig. 10-11).
Orthopnea or THOP nee uh	***orth/o*** straight, upright ***-pnea*** breathing	Condition seen in mitral stenosis in which a person must sit or stand to breathe comfortably.
Tricuspid stenosis (TS) try KUSS pid sten OH sis	***stenosis*** narrowing	Relatively uncommon narrowing of the tricuspid valve associated with lesions of other valves, caused by rheumatic fever. Symptoms include jugular vein distention and pulmonary congestion (see Fig. 10-10).
Valvulitis val vyoo LYE tis	***valvul/o*** valve ***-itis*** inflammation	Inflammatory condition of a valve, especially a cardiac valve, caused most commonly by rheumatic fever, and less frequently by bacterial endocarditis or syphilis. Results are stenoses and obstructed blood flow.

DID YOU KNOW?

Excessive alcohol ingestion is associated with atrial fibrillation.

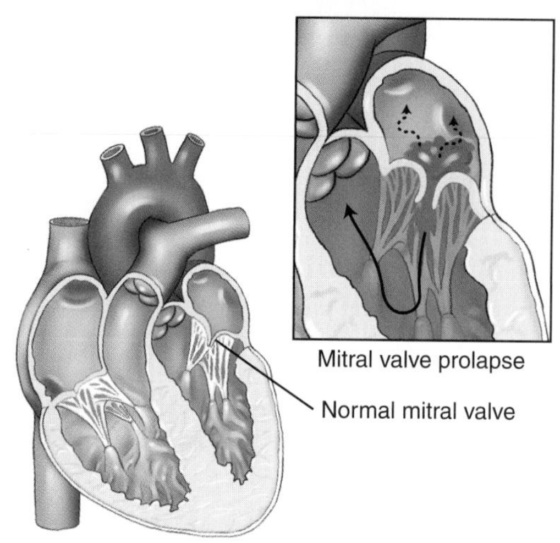

Fig. 10-11 Mitral valve prolapse.

Exercise 8: VALVULAR HEART DISORDERS

Matching.

_____ 1. stenosis

_____ 2. regurgitation

_____ 3. prolapse

_____ 4. orthopnea

A. breathing in an upright position
B. drooping
C. narrowing
D. backflow

Circle the correct answer.

5. The mitral valve is on the *(right, left)* side of the heart, whereas the tricuspid is on the *(right, left)* side of the heart.

Terms Related to Cardiac Dysrhythmias (Arrhythmias)

Term	Word Origin	Definition
Arrhythmia ah RITH mee ah	*a-* without *rrhythm/o* rhythm *-ia* condition	Abnormal variation from the normal heartbeat rhythm. Also called **dysrhythmia.**
Atrial ectopic beats A tree ul eck TOP ick	*atri/o* atrium *-al* pertaining to *ec-* out of *top/o* place *-ic* pertaining to	Premature atrial contractions (PACs).
Atrial fibrillation (AF) A tree ul fih brih LAY shun	*atri/o* atrium *-al* pertaining to	Most common type of cardiac arrhythmia; a series of extremely rapid and irregular atrial contractions (300-600 per minute) occurring with or without an underlying cardiovascular disorder, such as coronary artery disease or hypertension.
Atrial flutter	*atri/o* atrium *-al* pertaining to	Rapid regular atrial rhythm (250-350 bpm).
Atrial tachycardia A tree ul tack ee KAR dee ah	*atri/o* atrium *-al* pertaining to *tachy-* rapid *-cardia* heart condition	Abnormally rapid atrial contractions.
Atrioventricular block a tree oh ven TRICK yoo lur	*atri/o* atrium *ventricul/o* ventricle *-ar* pertaining to	Partial or complete heart block that is the result of a lack of electrical communication between the atria and the ventricles.
Bundle branch block (BBB)		Incomplete electrical conduction in the bundle branches, either right or left.
Paroxysmal atrial fibrillation par ock SIZ mul A tree ul fih brih LAY shun	*paroxysmal* marked episodic increase in symptoms	Atrial fibrillation occurring as a marked episode.
Sick sinus syndrome (SSS)		Any abnormality of the sinus node, which may include the necessity of an implantable pacemaker.
Ventricular ectopic beats (VEB) ven TRICK yoo lur eck TOP ick	*ventricul/o* ventricle *-ar* pertaining to *ec-* out of *top/o* place *-ic* pertaining to	Premature ventricular contractions (PVCs). Not always pathologic.
Ventricular fibrillation ven TRICK yoo lur fih brih LAY shun	*ventricul/o* ventricle *-ar* pertaining to	Rapid, irregular ventricular contractions; may be fatal unless reversed.
Ventricular tachycardia (VT) ven TRICK yoo lur tack ee KAR dee uh	*ventricul/o* ventricle *-ar* pertaining to *tachy-* rapid *-cardia* heart condition	Ventricular contractions at rates >120 bpm.

Exercise 9: CARDIAC DYSRHYTHMIAS

1. In your own words, what is a cardiac arrhythmia?

____

Circle the correct answer.

2. Extremely rapid and irregular cardiac contractions are called *(flutters, fibrillations).*
3. Rapid regular rhythms are called *(flutters, fibrillations).*
4. Premature atrial contractions are the same as *(atrial tachycardia, atrial ectopic beats).*
5. No electrical communication between the atria and the ventricles is called *(bundle branch block, atrioventricular block).*

Terms Related to Other Disorders of Coronary Circulation

TERM	WORD ORIGIN	DEFINITION
Angina pectoris an JYE nuh peck TORE us	***pector/o*** chest	Paroxysmal chest pain that is often accompanied by shortness of breath and a sensation of impending doom (Fig. 10-12).
Coronary artery disease (CAD) KORE uh nare ee	***coron/o*** heart ***-ary*** pertaining to	Accumulation and hardening of plaque in the coronary arteries that eventually can deprive the heart muscle of oxygen, leading to **angina.**
Myocardial infarction (MI) mye oh KAR dee ul in FARCK shun	***myocardi/o*** heart muscle ***-al*** pertaining to	Cardiac tissue death that occurs when the coronary arteries are occluded (blocked) by an **atheroma** (ath uh ROH mah), a mass of fat or lipids on the wall of an artery, or a blood clot caused by an atheroma, and are thus unable to carry enough oxygenated blood to the heart muscle. Depending on the area affected, the patient may die if enough of the heart muscle is destroyed (Fig. 10-13).

DID YOU KNOW?

CAD is the leading cause of death in both sexes in the United States, accounting for one third of all deaths each year.

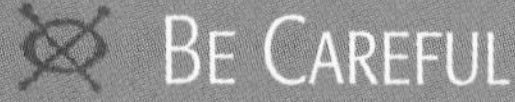

BE CAREFUL!

Infarction refers to tissue death. An *infraction* refers to a breaking, as in an incomplete bone fracture.

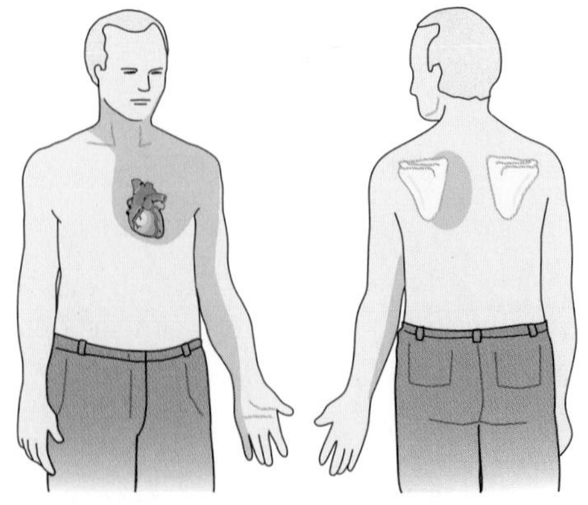

Fig. 10-12 Common sites of pain in angina pectoris.

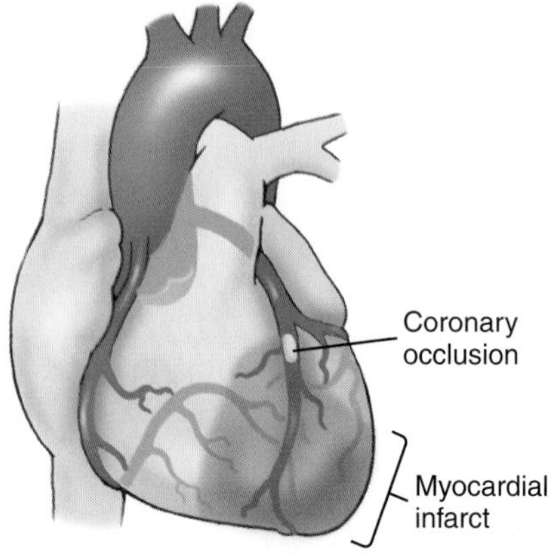

Fig. 10-13 Myocardial infarction.

 Exercise 10: OTHER DISORDERS OF CORONARY CIRCULATION

Circle the correct answer.

1. Coronary artery disease is a blockage of the arteries supplying blood to the *(heart, lungs)*.
2. The blockage is caused by fatty plaque called a/an *(atheroma, lipid)*.
3. If the blockage is enough to deprive the myocardium of oxygen, chest pain called *(angina pectoris, pleurodynia)* results.
4. If the blockage is complete, due to either the plaque or a blood clot, heart tissue will die in an event called a myocardial *(stenosis, infarction)*.

DID YOU KNOW?

Although the number of cases of endocarditis have not changed over the last few decades, twice as many men as women are diagnosed with this condition.

Fill in the blanks.

5. What are some of the symptoms of angina pectoris?

____

6. What is the leading cause of death in the United States? ____________________

7. What is the difference between an infarction and an infraction? ____________________

____

Inflammation and Heart Disease

Recent research has uncovered a link between higher levels of a protein present in the blood when blood vessels are inflamed and cardiovascular disease risk. Elevated C-reactive protein (CRP) levels are associated with a dramatically increased risk for heart attack and stroke, independent of an individual's cholesterol levels, obesity, smoking history, or blood pressure.

Although the research indicates that diagnosis and treatment of the inflammation may reduce one's risk of heart disease, the American Heart Association continues to recommend that individuals stop smoking, eat a healthy diet, exercise, maintain a healthy blood pressure, and manage diabetes if present for optimal cardiovascular health.

Terms Related to Other Cardiac Conditions

TERM	WORD ORIGIN	DEFINITION
Cardiac tamponade TAM pon ade		Compression of the heart caused by fluid in the pericardial sac.
Cardiomyopathy kar dee oh mye AH puh thee	*cardiomy/o* heart muscle *-pathy* disease	Progressive disorder of the ventricles of the heart.
Congestive heart failure (CHF)		Inability of the heart muscle to pump blood efficiently, so that it becomes overloaded. The heart enlarges with unpumped blood and the lungs fill with fluid.
Endocarditis en doh kar DYE tis	*endocardi/o* endocardium *-itis* inflammation	Inflammation of the endocardium and heart valves, characterized by lesions and caused by a number of different microbes (Fig. 10-14).
Pericarditis pair ee kar DYE tis	*pericardi/o* pericardium *-itis* inflammation	Inflammation of the sac surrounding the heart, with the possibility of pericardial effusion.

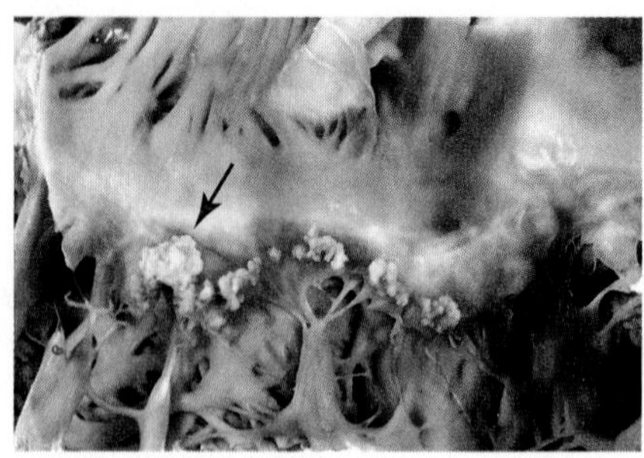

Fig. 10-14 Acute bacterial endocarditis. The valve is covered with large irregular vegetations.

A

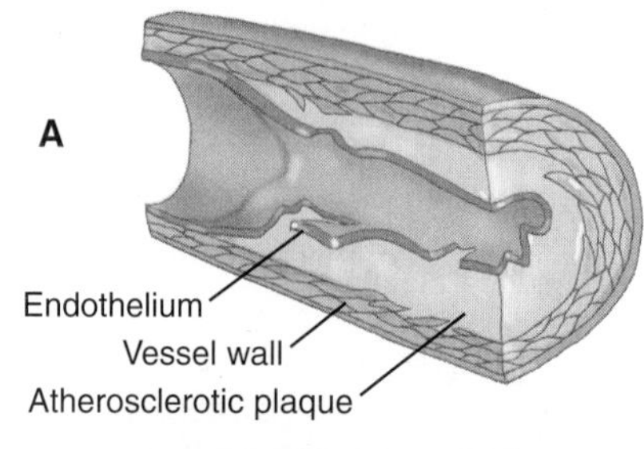

B

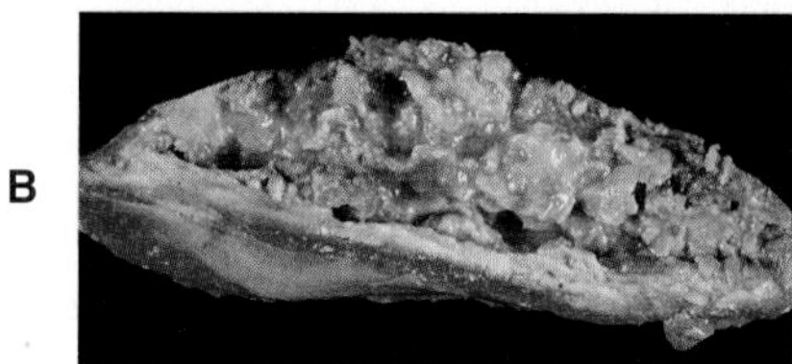

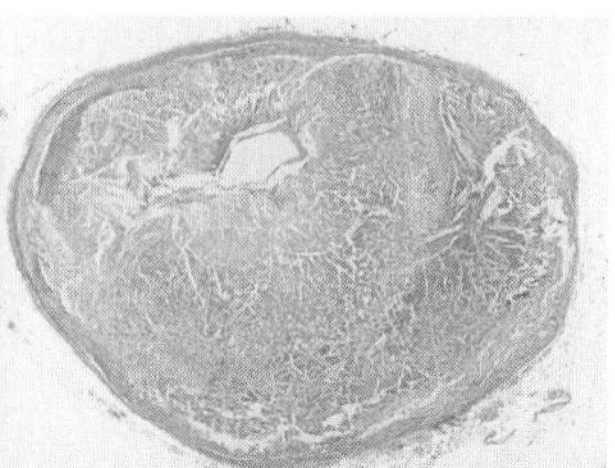

C

Fig. 10-15 Atherosclerosis. **A,** Artery is blocked by an atheroma. **B,** Fatty deposits on wall of artery. **C,** Image of the resultant narrowed coronary artery.

Terms Related to Vascular Disorders

Term	Word Origin	Definition
Arteriosclerosis ar teer ee oh sklah ROH sis	*arteri/o* artery *-sclerosis* abnormal condition of hardening	Disease in which the arterial walls become thickened and lose their elasticity, without the presence of atheromas (Fig. 10-15).
Atherosclerosis ath uh roh sklah ROH sis	*ather/o* fat, plaque *-sclerosis* abnormal condition of hardening	Form of arteriosclerosis in which the arteries present with atheromas of medium and large arteries, which can reduce or obstruct blood flow. Patients with peripheral atherosclerosis complain of intermittent claudication.
Aneurysm AN yoo rizz um	See **Did You Know?** Box	Localized dilation of an artery due to a congenital or acquired weakness in the wall of the vessel. The acquired causes may be arteriosclerosis, trauma, infection, and/or inflammation.
Claudication klah dih KAY shun		Cramplike pains in the calves due to poor circulation in the leg muscles.
Esophageal varices eh sof uh JEE ul VARE ih seez	*esophag/o* esophagus *-eal* pertaining to *varic/o* dilated vein	Varicose veins that appear at the lower end of the esophagus as a result of portal hypertension; they are superficial and may cause ulceration and bleeding.
Hemorrhoid HEM uh royd		Varicose condition of the external or internal rectal veins that causes painful swellings at the anus.
Hypertension hye pur TEN shun	*hyper-* excessive *-tension* pressure	Condition of high or elevated blood pressure, also known as **arterial hypertension;** occurs in two forms—**primary** (or **essential**) **hypertension,** which has no identifiable cause; and **secondary hypertension,** which occurs in response to another disorder.
Peripheral arterial occlusion puh RIFF uh rul ar TEER ree ul oh KLOO zhun	*arteri/o* artery *-al* pertaining to	Blockage of blood flow to the extremities. Acute or chronic conditions may be present, but both types of patients are likely to have underlying atherosclerosis.
Peripheral vascular disorder puh RIFF uh rul VAS kyoo lur	*vascul/o* vessel *-ar* pertaining to	Any vascular disorder limited to the extremities; may affect not only the arteries and veins but also the lymphatics.

Terms Related to Vascular Disorders—cont'd

TERM	WORD ORIGIN	DEFINITION
Raynaud's disease ray NOZE		**Idiopathic** disease—that is, of unknown cause—of the peripheral vascular system that causes intermittent cyanosis/erythema of the distal ends of the fingers and toes, sometimes accompanied by numbness; occurs almost exclusively in young women. Presentation is bilateral. **Raynaud's phenomenon** is secondary to rheumatoid arthritis, scleroderma, or trauma. Presentation is unilateral.
Thrombophlebitis throm boh fluh BYE tis		Inflammation of either deep (**deep vein thrombosis,** or **DVT**) or superficial veins, with the formation of one or more blood clots (Fig. 10-16).
Varicose veins VARE ih kose	***varic/o*** dilated vein ***-ose*** pertaining to	Elongated, dilated superficial veins with incompetent valves that permit reverse blood flow. These veins may appear in various parts of the anatomy, but the term varicose vein(s) has been reserved for those in the lower extremities.

Exercise 11: OTHER CARDIAC CONDITIONS

Fill in the blanks with one of the following terms.

endocarditis, atherosclerosis, pericarditis, arteriosclerosis, congestive heart failure

1. An inflammation of the lining of the heart is called ________.
2. The inability of the heart muscle to pump blood efficiently is called ________.
3. An inflammation of the sac surrounding the heart is termed ________.
4. Hardening of the arteries without fatty plaque is called ________.
5. Hardening of the arteries with fatty plaque is called ________.

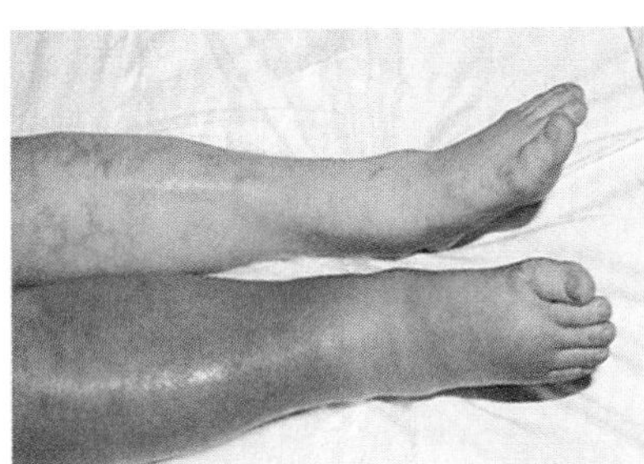

Fig. 10-16 Deep vein thrombophlebitis.

DID YOU KNOW?

Arteriosclerosis is the leading cause of morbidity and mortality in the United States today.

DID YOU KNOW?

Aneurysms are dilations of **a**rteries, and **v**aricosities are dilations of **v**eins.

DID YOU KNOW?

Almost 1 out of 5 Americans have been diagnosed with hypertension. The highest incidences are in African Americans (approximately 1 out of 3), followed by Caucasians and Mexican Americans (approximately 1 out of 4).

DID YOU KNOW?

The term *varicose vein* is redundant, in that a varix itself is a dilated vein.

Exercise 12: VASCULAR DISORDERS

Fill in the blanks with one of the following terms.

essential, primary, secondary, varicose veins, thrombophlebitis, claudication, hemorrhoids, esophageal varices, aneurysm, peripheral artery occlusion, Raynaud's disease

1. A localized dilation of an artery due to a weakness in the vessel wall is a/an ______________.
2. Cramplike pains in the calves due to poor circulation are called ______________.
3. If hypertension is idiopathic, it is called ______________ or ______________ hypertension.
4. ______________ hypertension is due to another disorder.
5. An inflammation of veins with the formation of one or more blood clots is called ______________.
6. Swollen, twisted veins in the region of the anus are called ______________.
7. Varicose veins of the lower end of the tube from the throat to the stomach are called ______________.
8. A blockage of blood flow to the extremities is called ______________.
9. An idiopathic disease of the peripheral vascular system is called ______________.
10. Elongated superficial dilated veins are called ______________.

Match the combining form with the correct term.

____ 11. vessel	____ 15. vein	A.	phleb/o
		B.	arteri/o
____ 12. clot	____ 16. dilation	C.	varic/o
		D.	vascul/o
____ 13. esophagus	____ 17. dilated vein	E.	aneurysm/o
		F.	esophag/o
____ 14. artery		G.	thromb/o

Heart Disease in Women

Heart disease is the number-one killer of women in the United States, killing more women every year than men. The Office of Research on Women's Health at the National Institutes of Health is charged with understanding how biologic and physiologic differences between the sexes affect their health. As a result of this research, hormonal fluctuations are now believed to vary the results of a number of diagnostic tests and the optimal time for certain types of treatments. Visit http://www.4woman.gov to view the latest results of studies that examine the differences gender makes on cardiovascular and other diseases.

DIAGNOSTIC PROCEDURES

Terms Related to Noninvasive Imaging		
TERM	**WORD ORIGIN**	**DEFINITION**
Echocardiography eck oh kar dee AH gruh fee	*echo-* sound *cardi/o* heart *-graphy* process of recording	Use of ultrasonic waves directed through the heart to study the structure and motion of the heart. **Transesophageal echocardiography (TEE)** images the heart through a transducer introduced into the esophagus (Fig. 10-17).
Exercise stress test (EST)		Imaging of the heart during exercise on a treadmill, with the use of radioactive thallium or technetium Tc 99m sestamibi.
Magnetic resonance imaging (MRI)		Computerized imaging that uses radiofrequency radiation in a magnetic field to detect areas of myocardial infarction, stenoses, and areas of blood flow.
Myocardial perfusion imaging mye oh KAR dee ul pur FYOO zhun	*myocardi/o* myocardium *-al* pertaining to	Use of radionuclide to diagnose CAD, valvular or congenital heart disease, and cardiomyopathy.
Positron emission tomography (PET) POZ ih tron ee MIH shun toh MAH gruh fee	*e-* out *-mission* sending *tom/o* slice *-graphy* process of recording	Computerized nuclear medicine procedure that uses inhaled or injected radioactive substances to help identify how much a patient will benefit from revascularization procedures.
Radiography	*radi/o* rays *-graphy* process of recording	Posteroanterior and lateral chest x-rays may be used to evaluate the size and shape of the heart.

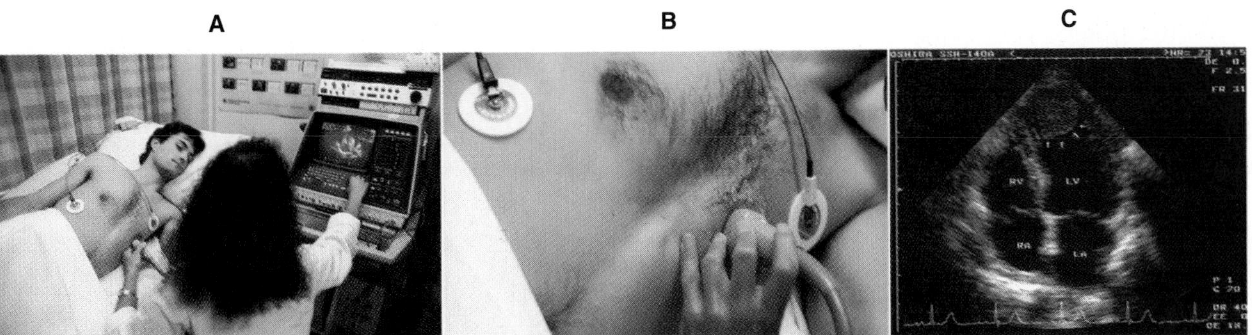

Fig. 10-17 **A** and **B**, Echocardiography. **C**, Resultant image showing large apical thrombus. *RV,* Right ventricle; *LV,* left ventricle; *RA,* right atrium; *LA,* left atrium.

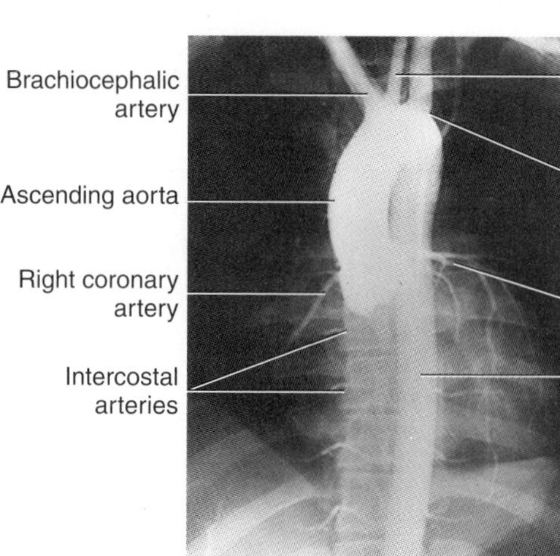

Fig. 10-18 Angiocardiography. Aorta and right and left coronary arteries are shown.

Terms Related to Invasive Imaging

Term	Word Origin	Definition
Angiocardiography an jee oh kar dee AH gruh fee	*angi/o* vessel *cardi/o* heart *-graphy* process of recording	Injection of a radiopaque substance during cardiac catheterization for the purpose of imaging the heart and related structures (Fig. 10-18).
Cardiac catheterization KAR dee ack kath ih tur ih ZAY shun	*cardi/o* heart *-ac* pertaining to	Threading of a catheter (thin tube) into the heart to collect diagnostic information about structures in the heart, coronary arteries, and great vessels; also used to aid in treatment of CAD, congenital abnormalities, and heart failure.
Digital subtraction angiography (DSA) an jee AH gruh fee	*angi/o* vessel *-graphy* process of recording	Digital imaging process wherein contrast images are used to "subtract" the noncontrast image of surrounding structures, leaving only a clear image of blood vessels.
Electrocardiography (ECG)	*electr/o* electricity *cardi/o* heart *-graphy* process of recording	Process of graphing the electrical activity of the heart muscle.
Holter monitor		Portable electrocardiograph that is worn to record the reaction of the heart to daily activities.
Swan-Ganz catheter		Long, thin cardiac catheter with a tiny balloon at the tip that is fed into the femoral artery near the groin and extended up to the left ventricle. This instrument is then used to determine left ventricular function by measuring pulmonary capillary wedge pressure.

Terms Related to Laboratory Tests

Term	Word Origin	Definition
Cardiac enzymes test		Blood test that measures the amount of cardiac enzymes characteristically released during a myocardial infarction; examines the amount of lactate dehydrogenase (LDH) and creatine phosphokinase (CPK) in the blood.
Lipid profile		Blood test to measure the lipids (cholesterol and triglycerides) in the circulating blood.

 Exercise 13: DIAGNOSTIC PROCEDURES

Fill in the blanks with one of the following terms.

cardiac enzymes test, cardiac catheterization, lipid profiles, radiography, transesophageal echocardiography, PET scan, exercise stress test, electrocardiography, digital subtraction angiography

1. What test measures the electrical activity of the heart? ____________
2. What test measures cholesterol and triglycerides? ____________
3. What test measures the enzymes released during a heart attack? ____________
4. What technique "subtracts" background structures to image vessels? ____________
5. What ultrasound technique images the heart through the esophagus? ____________
6. Heart size and shape can be evaluated with ____________.
7. The reaction of the heart to exercise is measured through what type of test? ____________
8. An invasive technique that is commonly used either to help diagnose or to treat disorders of the heart is called ____________.
9. A computerized nuclear medicine procedure to help identify the extent to which a patient will benefit from a vessel repair procedure is called ____________.

Case Study Continued

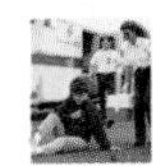

Cheryl Miller was admitted through the ED. During her admission she had an ECG, an echocardiogram, a stress test, a lipid profile, and a cardiac catheterization. The results indicated extensive coronary artery disease, an inferolateral wall myocardial infarction, hypercholesterolemia, and hypertension. When surgery was recommended, she was surprised and frightened. She had not thought of herself as someone who could have serious heart disease. She was scheduled for a coronary artery bypass graft.

THERAPEUTIC INTERVENTIONS

Terms Related to Cardiac Procedures

TERM	WORD ORIGIN	DEFINITION
Atherectomy ath uh RECK tuh mee	*ather/o* fat, plaque *-ectomy* removal	Removal of plaque from the coronary artery (or other arteries) through a catheter with a rotating shaver or a laser. If a laser is used, the procedure is termed **laser angioplasty** and the plaque is vaporized by pulsating beams of light through a catheter introduced into the coronary artery to the site of the blockage. May be used alone or with balloon angioplasty.

Continued

Terms Related to Cardiac Procedures—cont'd

TERM	WORD ORIGIN	DEFINITION
Cardiac defibrillator dee FIB ruh lay tur		Either external or implantable device that provides an electronic shock to the heart to restore a normal rhythm.
Cardiac pacemaker		Small, battery-operated device that helps the heart beat in a regular rhythm; can be either internal (permanent) or external (temporary) (Fig. 10-19).
Cardiopulmonary resuscitation (CPR) kar dee oh PULL muh nare ee	*cardi/o* heart *pulmon/o* lung *-ary* pertaining to	Manual external cardiac massage and artificial respiration used to restart the heartbeat and breathing of a patient.
Commissurotomy kom ih shur AH tuh mee	*commissur/o* connection *-tomy* incision	Surgical division of a fibrous band or ring connecting corresponding parts of a body structure. Commonly performed to separate the thickened, adherent leaves of a stenosed mitral valve.
Coronary artery bypass graft (CABG)		Open-heart surgery in which a piece of a blood vessel from another location is grafted onto one of the coronary arteries to reroute blood around a blockage (Fig. 10-20).
Extracorporeal circulation (ECC) ecks truh kore PORE ee ul	*extra-* outside *corpor/o* body *-eal* pertaining to	Use of a cardiopulmonary machine to do the work of the heart during open-heart procedures.
Heart transplantation		Removal of a diseased heart and transplantation of a donor heart when cardiac disease can no longer be treated by any other means.
Left ventricular assist device (LVAD)		Mechanical pump device that assists a patient's weakened heart by pulling blood from the left ventricle into the pump and then ejecting it out into the aorta. LVADs may be used on those patients awaiting a transplant.

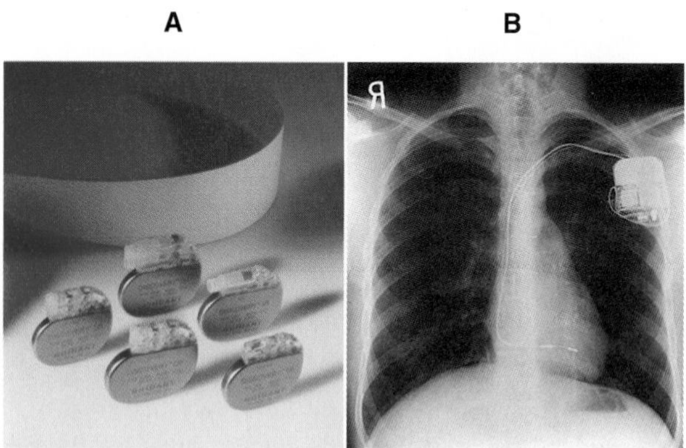

Fig. 10-19 **A,** Pacemakers. **B,** Chest radiograph of patient with permanent pacemaker implanted.

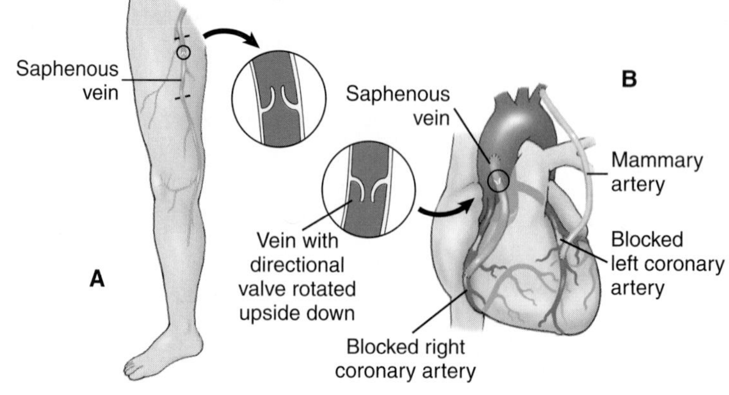

Fig. 10-20 CABG. **A,** A section of vein is harvested from the left leg and anastomosed to a coronary artery to bypass an occlusion of the right coronary artery. **B,** Bypass of the left coronary artery with a mammary artery.

Terms Related to Cardiac Procedures—cont'd

TERM	WORD ORIGIN	DEFINITION
Minimally invasive coronary artery bypass (MIDCAB)		Surgical procedure in which the heart is still beating while a minimal incision is made over the blocked coronary artery and an artery from the chest wall is used as the bypass.
Percutaneous transluminal coronary angioplasty (PTCA) pur kyoo TAY nee us trans LOO mih nul kor in NARE ee AN jee oh plas tee	***per-*** through ***cutane/o*** skin ***-ous*** pertaining to ***trans-*** across ***lumin/o*** lumen ***-al*** pertaining to ***coron/o*** heart ***-ary*** pertaining to ***angi/o*** vessel ***-plasty*** surgical repair	Surgical procedure in which a catheter is threaded into the coronary artery affected by atherosclerotic heart disease. The balloon at the tip of the catheter is inflated and deflated to compress the plaque against the wall of the artery and increase blood flow. **Stents,** wire mesh tubes, are placed in the arteries and used to prop them open after the angioplasty (Fig. 10-21).
Pericardiocentesis pair ee kar dee oh sen TEE sis	***peri-*** around ***cardi/o*** heart ***-centesis*** surgical puncture	Aspiration of fluid from the pericardium to diagnose and treat cardiac tamponade.
Port-access coronary artery bypass (PACAB)		Procedure in which the heart is stopped and surgery is accomplished through small incisions in the chest.
Radiofrequency catheter ablation ray dee oh FREE kwen see uh BLAY shun		Destruction of abnormal cardiac electrical pathways causing arrhythmias.
Transmyocardial revascularization (TMR) trans mye oh KAR dee ul ree vas kyoo lair ih ZAY shun	***trans-*** through ***myocardi/o*** myocardium ***-al*** pertaining to ***re-*** again ***vascul/o*** vessel ***-ization*** process	Procedure used to relieve severe angina in a patient who cannot tolerate a CABG or PTCA. With a laser, a series of holes are made in the heart tissue in the hope of increasing blood flow by stimulating new blood vessels to grow **(angiogenesis).**
Valvuloplasty VAL vyoo loh plas tee	***valvul/o*** valve ***-plasty*** surgical repair	Repair of a stenosed heart valve with the use of a balloon-tipped catheter.

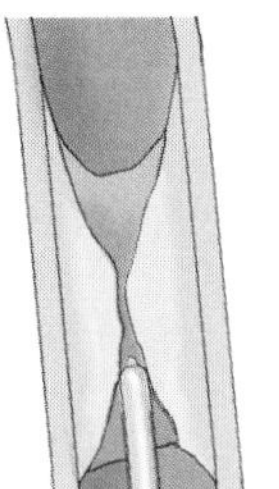
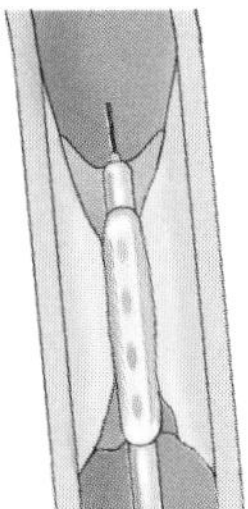
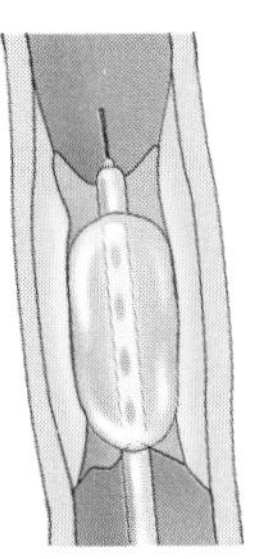
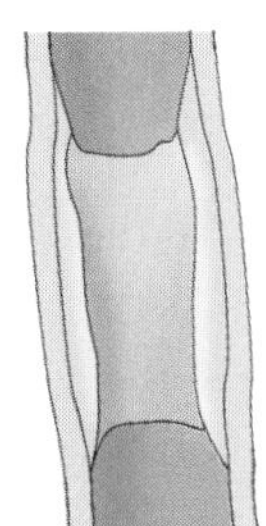

Fig. 10-21 PTCA.

DID YOU KNOW?

Heart transplantation is a reality for over 2000 Americans every year. Many more of these candidates die each year for lack of donor organs. Research continues in the development of an artificial heart.

Terms Related to Varicose Vein Surgical Treatment		
TERM	**WORD ORIGIN**	**DEFINITION**
Hemorrhoidectomy hem uh royd ECK tuh mee	*hemorrhoid/o* hemorrhoids *-ectomy* removal	Excision of hemorrhoids.
Ligation and stripping lye GAY shun		Tying (ligating) of varicose veins and their removal in severe cases.
Sclerotherapy sklih roh THER uh pee	*scler/o* hard *-therapy* treatment	Injection of chemical solution into varicosities to cause inflammation, resulting in an obliteration of the lining of the vein; blood flow is then rerouted through adjoining vessels.

Exercise 14: THERAPEUTIC INTERVENTIONS

Fill in the blanks with one of the following terms.

radiofrequency catheter ablation, CABG, hemorrhoidectomy, stripping, PTCA, pericardiocentesis, commissurotomy, atherectomy, CPR, LVAD, ligation, sclerotherapy

1. What procedure removes an atheroma from an artery? ________________
2. What procedure detours a blockage in a coronary artery to reestablish blood flow around the blockage? ________________
3. What emergency procedure restarts the heartbeat and breathing? ________________
4. What is removal of swollen, twisted veins around the rectum and anus? ________________
5. What is the procedure to correct mitral stenosis? ________________
6. What procedure introduces a balloon into a coronary artery via a catheter to reestablish patency? ________________
7. Varicose veins may be treated surgically by tying and removing them in a procedure called ________________ and ________________, or by injecting chemicals to destroy the lining of the veins, which is called ________________.
8. Destruction of abnormal cardiac electrical pathways is called ________________.
9. A mechanical pump device implanted in the lower left chamber of the heart to lessen the work of the heart is called a/an ________________.
10. Aspiration of fluid from the sac surrounding the heart to diagnose and treat cardiac tamponade is called ________________.

Match the term with its combining form, prefix, or suffix.

____ 11. vessel
____ 12. body
____ 13. resection
____ 14. space
____ 15. treatment
____ 16. hardening
____ 17. outside
____ 18. skin
____ 19. surgical puncture
____ 20. through, across
____ 21. ventricle
____ 22. a connection
____ 23. surgical repair
____ 24. plaque
____ 25. through
____ 26. lung
____ 27. again
____ 28. heart
____ 29. pericardium
____ 30. incision

A. ather/o
B. -tomy
C. extra-
D. cutane/o
E. -centesis
F. pulmon/o
G. coron/o
H. pericardi/o
I. corpor/o
J. commissur/o
K. -therapy
L. angi/o
M. per-
N. trans-
O. -ectomy
P. lumin/o
Q. re-
R. ventricul/o
S. -plasty
T. scler/o

PHARMACOLOGY

As in other body systems, medications may be described as over the counter (OTC) or prescribed (Rx). An example of an OTC drug used in this system is chewable baby (81 mg) aspirin, sometimes given to patients suspected of having a myocardial infarction. Rx drugs used to treat the cardiovascular system may be grouped as follows:

Angiotensin-converting enzyme (ACE) inhibitors: Drugs that relax blood vessels by preventing the formation of a vasoconstrictor, angiotensin II, causing a decrease in water retention and blood pressure, and an improvement in cardiac output. Used to treat hypertension and heart failure. Examples are captopril (Capoten), enalapril (Vasotec), and quinapril (Accupril).

Antiadrenergics (an tee ad ruh NUR jicks) **(beta blockers or beta-adrenergic blocking agents):** Drugs that lessen the heart rate and force of heart contractions by decreasing the effectiveness of the nerve impulses to the cardiovascular system; prescribed to treat angina pectoris, hypertension, and cardiac arrhythmias. Examples are propranolol (Inderal) and metoprolol (Lopressor).

Antiarrhythmic drugs: Medications, such as digitalis, that strengthen the heartbeat; may also be referred to as **cardiotonics** because they improve the tone of the heart muscle. Examples are digoxin (Lanoxin), amiodarone (Cordarone), or dofetilide (Tikosyn).

Anticoagulants: Drugs used to prevent the formation of blood clots, such as warfarin (Coumadin) and heparin.

Calcium channel blockers (CCBs): Drugs that effect a lessened myocardial oxygen demand by slowing the flow of calcium to smooth muscle cells, causing arterial relaxation. Used to treat angina, hypertension, and congestive heart failure. Examples are diltiazem (Cardizem), bepridil (Vascor), and nifedipine (Procardia).

DID YOU KNOW?

Patients taking nitrates must avoid alcohol because of its added blood vessel–relaxing effect, which may result in episodes of dangerous hypotension.

Diuretics (dye ur REH tiks): Drugs that help the body form and excrete urine, and are used in the treatment of hypertension and congestive heart failure. Examples of diuretics are furosemide (Lasix), hydrochlorothiazide (Hydrodiuril), and triamterene (Dyazide).

HMG-CoA reductase inhibitors (statins): Drugs that reduce the rate of LDL; used to lower cholesterol and consequently reduce the risk of heart attack or stroke. Examples are atorvastatin (Lipitor), pravastatin (Pravachol), and simvastatin (Zocor).

Nitrates (antianginals): Drugs that relax blood vessels and reduce the myocardial oxygen consumption to lessen the pain of angina pectoris; also used to treat hypertension and congestive heart failure. Examples include isosorbide dinitrate (Isordil) and nitroglycerin (Nitro, Nitro-dur, and Transderm-Nitro). Nitroglycerine (NTG) has two main routes of administration: **sublingual** and as a **transdermal (TDNTG or TDN)** patch.

Thrombolytics: Drugs that act on plasminogen, converting it to plasmin, which breaks up the fibrin in the clot, causing the clot to disintegrate. "Clot busters" are used on patients who have intracoronary thromboses (clots). Examples are tissue plasminogen activator (tPA), streptokinase, alteplase, reteplase, and tenecteplase.

Exercise 15: CARDIOVASCULAR MEDICATIONS

Match the type of drug with the disease(s) it treats. There may be more than one answer.

_____ 1. antiarrhythmic

_____ 2. antiadrenergic

_____ 3. ACE inhibitor

_____ 4. antianginal

_____ 5. calcium channel blocker

_____ 6. diuretic

_____ 7. thrombolytic

_____ 8. anticoagulant

_____ 9. HMG-CoA reductase inhibitors

A. hypertension
B. existing thrombosis
C. dysrhythmia
D. angina
E. congestive heart failure
F. formation of thromboses
G. high LDL cholesterol

Case Study Continued

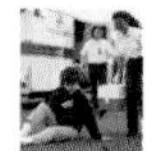

Four weeks after being discharged, Cheryl has recovered from her coronary artery bypass. She makes her first return visit to the mall, this time to buy a new pair of walking shoes and a comfortable set of sweats. She has given her husband a list for the supermarket. It includes lots of her favorite fruits, vegetables, and low-fat alternatives for the high-cholesterol foods she had been eating. When she looks back at how poorly she had taken care of herself, Cheryl can't help but be excited about looking forward to a happy, healthier lifestyle.

Abbreviations (Anatomic)

Abbreviations	Definition	Abbreviations	Definition
AV	Atrioventricular	MV	Mitral valve
CV	Cardiovascular	PA	Pulmonary artery
LA	Left atrium	PV	Pulmonary vein
LAD	Left anterior descending (coronary artery)	RA	Right atrium
		RCA	Right coronary artery
LCA	Left circumflex artery, left coronary artery	RV	Right ventricle
		SA	Sinoatrial
LMCA	Left main coronary artery	TV	Tricuspid valve
LV	Left ventricle		

Abbreviations (Pathology)

Abbreviations	Definitions	Abbreviations	Definitions
AEB	Atrial ectopic beat	MR	Mitral regurgitation
AF	Atrial fibrillation	MS	Mitral stenosis
AMI	Acute myocardial infarction	MVP	Mitral valve prolapse
AS	Aortic stenosis	NSR	Normal sinus rhythm
ASD	Atrial septal defect	PAC	Premature atrial contraction
ASHD	Arteriosclerotic heart disease	PDA	Patent ductus arteriosus
BBB	Bundle branch block	PVC	Premature ventricular contraction
CAD	Coronary artery disease	SOB	Shortness of breath
CCF	Congestive cardiac failure	SSS	Sick sinus syndrome
CHF	Congestive heart failure	TS	Tricuspid stenosis
DOE	Dyspnea on exertion	VEB	Ventricular ectopic beat
DVT	Deep vein thrombosis	VSD	Ventricular septal defect
MI	Myocardial infarction	VT	Ventricular tachycardia

Abbreviations (Diagnostic)

Abbreviations	Definition	Abbreviations	Definition
BP	Blood pressure	HDL	High-density lipids
BPM	Beats per minute	Hg	Mercury
Cath	(Cardiac) catheterization	LDH	Lactic dehydrogenase
CK	Creatine kinase	LDL	Low-density lipids
CO_2	Carbon dioxide	O_2	Oxygen
CPK	Creatine phosphokinase	SGOT	Serum glutamic oxaloacetate transaminase
DSA	Digital subtraction angiography		
ECG, EKG	Electrocardiogram	TEE	Transesophageal echocardiogram
ECHO	Echocardiography	VLDL	Very-low-density lipid(s)
EST	Exercise stress test		

Abbreviations (Therapeutic Interventions)

Abbreviations	*Definitions*	*Abbreviations*	*Definitions*
CABG	Coronary artery bypass graft	ICD	Implantable cardiac defibrillator
CCB	Calcium channel blocker(s)	RFA	Radiofrequency catheter ablation
CPR	Cardiopulmonary resuscitation	Rx	Prescription (drug)
ECC	Extracorporeal circulation	SK	Streptokinase
IU	International unit	TDN	Transdermal nitroglycerin
NTG	Nitroglycerin	TDNTG	Transdermal nitroglycerin
OTC	Over the counter (drug)	TEA	Thromboendarterectomy
PTCA	Percutaneous transluminal coronary angioplasty	TMR	Transmyocardial revascularization
		VAD	Ventricular assist device

Abbreviations

Other Cardiovascular Abbreviations	*Definitions*
CC	Cardiac care
CCU	Coronary care unit

Exercise 16: ABBREVIATIONS

Matching.

_____ 1. top right chamber of the heart

_____ 2. pertaining to top and bottom chambers of the heart

_____ 3. valve on right side of heart

_____ 4. valve on left side of heart

_____ 5. ultrasound procedure to examine the heart through the esophagus

_____ 6. heart attack

_____ 7. narrowing of largest artery in body

_____ 8. hole between top chambers of the heart

_____ 9. circulation of blood outside body during surgery

_____ 10. procedure to detour a blocked coronary artery

A. TEE
B. MI
C. ASD
D. TV
E. ECC
F. MV
G. CABG
H. RA
I. AS
J. AV

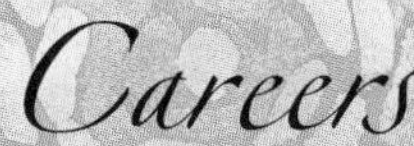

Emergency Medical Technicians (EMTs)

On the job, EMTs are expected to assess the nature and extent of the patient's condition, give appropriate medical care, and transport the patient to a medical facility. They may administer drugs orally and intravenously, interpret ECGs, and perform endotracheal intubations, among other duties. Hazards can include exposure to hepatitis B, AIDS, violence from disturbed patients, and physically strenuous conditions.

The *Occupational Outlook Handbook* of the Bureau of Labor Statistics reports a faster than average growth in this particular field. EMTs are required to have formal training and certification in all 50 states. Certification is in levels from the lowest level, EMT-Basic, to the highest level, EMT-Paramedics, who provide the most extensive prehospital care. To maintain certification, they must reregister, work as EMTs, and meet continuing education requirements.

Associations for EMTs include the following:

National Association of Emergency Medical Technicians
http://www.naemt.org
National Registry of Emergency Medical Technicians
http://www.nremt.org

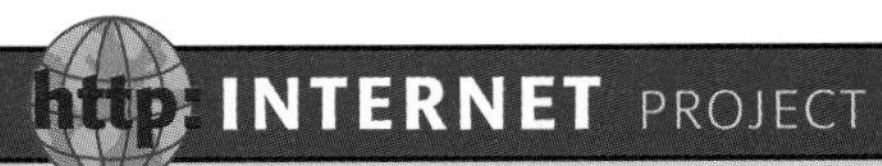

It is important to remember that treatments (including medicines) are recommended when their benefits outweigh their side effects. As mentioned in an earlier chapter, the United States Food and Drug Administration (FDA) regulates the use of drugs within the country. At the U.S. FDA's Center for Drug Evaluation and Research Website, http://www.fda.gov/cder/drug/default.html, information can be found on new and generic drug approvals, drug warnings, and the National Drug Code (NDC) Directory, which is a universal product identifier for human drugs.

Using this Website, choose either of the following assignments:

1. Find the approval date, trade name, dosage form, OTC/Rx status, and indications for the newest cardiovascular system drugs approved in the last 3 months.
2. Find the most recent posting of a warning regarding a drug currently on the market. Note its trade and generic names, OTC/Rx status, and the reason(s) for the warning.

Chapter Review

A. Functions of the Cardiovascular System

1. In your own words, explain the functions of the cardiovascular system.

____

____

____

B. Anatomy and Physiology

2. Explain the differences between systemic and pulmonary circulation.

____

____

____

3. Take a few minutes to think about the necessity of healthy, unblocked arteries, competent veins, and a strong heart. Choose one structure and explain what happens if it is not healthy.

____

____

____

4. Fill in the missing words for the figure below.

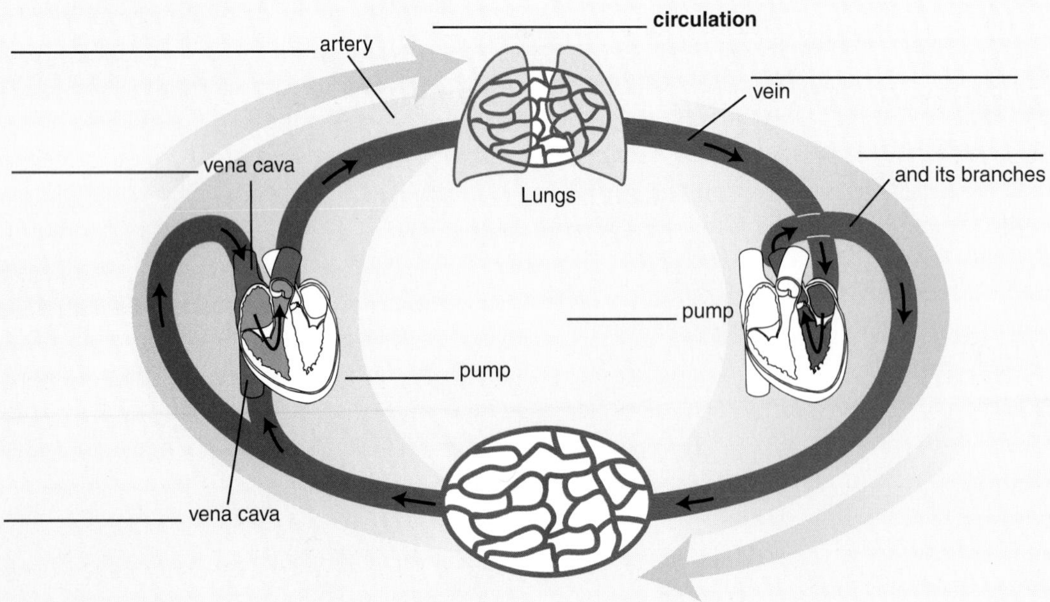

5. How is blood propelled through the arteries as opposed to the veins?

____

____

6. Vascul/o, vas/o, and angi/o are all combining forms for ______________.

7. Coronary arteries supply blood to ______________.

8. Oxygen/carbon dioxide exchange takes place in the ______________.

9. Arteries carry blood *away from/toward* (circle one) the heart.

10. Label the diagram with the structures and their combining forms.

11. The heart is located in the region of the chest called the ______________.

12. The combining form for the pointed tip of the heart is ______________.

13. The region over the heart and lower part of the thorax is the ______________.

14. The wall between the upper chambers of the heart is the ______________.

15. The thin tissue that acts as the lining of the chambers of the heart is the ______________.

16. The muscle layer of the heart is the ______________.

17. The double-folded membrane that surrounds the heart is the ______________, and the layer that is closest to the heart is the ______________ or ______________.

18. Indicate the flow of blood through the various structures of the heart, starting with the inferior and superior venae cavae and ending with the aorta.

____

____

19. Describe the pathway of the electrical impulse in the heartbeat, starting with the sinoatrial node.

____

____

20. What is the contractive phase of the heartbeat? ___Systole___

21. What instrument is used to measure blood pressure? ___Sphygmomanometer___

22. What is the range for a normal pulse rate? ___60-80 bpm___

23. What is the natural pacemaker of the heart? ___SA node___

24. What are the ranges of normal blood pressure? ___120/80 to 139/84___

25. Name an instrument used to listen to sounds in the chest. ______________

26. Name the instrument that measures the electrical activity of the heart.

____

27. What is the healthcare term for a normal heart rhythm? ___Sinus Rhythm___

28. An abnormal sound heard while listening to the heart is a/an ______________.

C. Pathology

Fill in the blanks with the correct term given below.

fatigue, dyspnea, shortness of breath, venous distension, thrill, murmur, bruit, bradycardia, tachycardia, syncope, cyanosis, edema, palpitations, pallor, diaphoresis, pulmonary congestion

29. What is the term for an abnormal accumulation of fluid in interstitial spaces of tissues?

____

30. What is the term for breathlessness? ______________

31. What is a fine vibration felt by the examiner called? ______________

32. What is a pounding or racing of the heart called? ______________

33. What is the term for fainting? ______________

34. What is the term for an excessive amount of blood in the lung tissue? ___Pulmonary Congestion___

35. What is the term for an absence of color or paleness of skin on the inner surfaces of the lower eyelids?

____

36. What is profuse secretion of sweat called? ______________

37. What is the term for a heartbeat below 60 bpm? ______________

38. What is difficult breathing called? ______________

39. What is the condition involving enlarged, swollen veins? ______________

40. What is the term for a gentle blowing, fluttering, or humming sound? ______________

41. What is the term for a heart rate over 100 bpm? ______________

42. What is an abnormal sound heard when auscultating an internal structure? ______________

43. What is the term for a sense of exhaustion, regardless of adequate sleep? ______________

44. What is lack of oxygen in the blood, seen as a bluish discoloration of skin/mucous membranes, nail beds, and/or lips? ______________

Fill in the blank.

45. Individuals born with ventricular septal defects have ______________________________.

46. A person with tetralogy of Fallot has how many defects? ______________________________

47. In patent ductus arteriosus, the fetal ductus arteriosus fails to do what after birth?

____

48. Coarctation of the aorta is characterized by a/an ______________ of the aorta.

Decode the term.

49. atrial septal defect ____

50. ventricular hypertrophy ____

51. aortic stenosis ____

52. valvulitis ____

53. cyanosis ____

54. orthopnea ____

Fill in the blank.

55. Explain the difference among mitral stenosis, mitral regurgitation, and mitral valve prolapse.

____

____

56. What is a normal heart rate called? ______________________________

57. What is a rapid (250 to 350 bpm) but regular type of arrhythmia? ______________________________

58. What is an extremely rapid and irregular type of arrhythmia? ______________________________

59. Atrial ectopic beats are the same as ______________.

60. Premature ventricular contractions are the same as ______________.

61. Ventricular fibrillation may be corrected with an ICD. What is that?

____

62. Ablation refers to ______________.

63. SSS is the abbreviation for ______________, which may be corrected with an ______________.

64. If a patient has RBBB, it means that there is an impairment of the electrical conductivity to the

______________.

Decode the terms.

65. ventricular tachycardia ______________________________

66. arrhythmia ______________________________

67. atrial ectopic beats ______________________________

Fill in the blank.

68. The leading cause of death in both sexes in the United States is ______________.

69. A decreased supply of oxygenated blood to tissues is ______________.

70. Paroxysmal chest pain that results from ischemic myocardial tissue is called ______________.

71. A medication to treat the symptom described in the previous question is ______________.

72. If an artery becomes blocked and a part of the heart muscle dies, the result is ______________.

73. The immediate pharmacologic treatment for the disorder in the previous question is ______________.

74. What are the similarities between esophageal varices and hemorrhoids?

____

75. In peripheral arterial occlusion, patients are likely to have underlying ______________.

Build a term.

76. mass of fat ______________________

77. hardening of fatty plaque in the arteries ______________________

78. inflammation of the lining of the heart ______________________

Decode the term.

79. coronary artery disease ______________________________

80. arteriosclerosis ______________________________

81. myocardial infarction ______________________________

Fill in the blank.

82. An aneurysm can be either ______________ or acquired.

83. Dilated superficial veins with incompetent valves are termed ______________ veins.

84. If dilated superficial veins are present in the rectum or anus, they are called ______________.

85. What are the cramplike pains in the lower extremities due to poor circulation called? ______________

Decode the term.

86. thrombophlebitis ______________________________

87. hypertension ______________________________

D. Laboratory Procedures

88. What is the instrument used to gather information about the electrical activity of the heart during daily activities? ______________________________

89. What is measured in a lipid profile? ______________________________

90. CPK and LDH are enzymes characteristically released during what type of cardiac disorder? ______________________________

91. What technique "subtracts" background structures to image vessels? ______________________________

92. What ultrasound technique creates an image of the heart? ______________________________

93. Posteroanterior and lateral chest x-rays are useful in determining what about the heart? ______________________________

94. The reaction of the heart to exercise is measured through what type of test? ______________________________

95. What type of catheter is used to visualize left ventricular function? ______________________________

E. Therapeutic Interventions

96. What device provides a shock to the heart to restore its normal rhythm? ______________________________

97. What device assists the heart to maintain a normal rhythm? ______________________________

98. What is a manual procedure to restart the breathing and heartbeat of a patient? ______________________________

99. What cardiac revascularization procedure bypasses a blockage in a coronary artery without stopping the heart? ______________________________

100. What is a CABG? ______________________________

101. What is CPR? ______________________________

102. What does a commissurotomy correct? ______________________________

103. What mechanical device, when inserted in a lower chamber, helps a patient's weakened heart? ______________________________

104. What does ligation mean? ______________________________

105. What procedure destroys abnormal electrical pathways in the heart? ______________________________

106. Sclerotherapy is done to correct ______________.

107. What is the difference between a MIDCAB and a PACAB? ______________________________

Decode the term.

108. atherectomy ______________________________

109. percutaneous transluminal coronary angioplasty ______________________________

110. pericardiocentesis ______________________________

Build a term.

111. surgical repair of a valve ______________________________

112. incision of a connection ______________________________

113. removal of hemorrhoids ______________________________

F. Pharmacology

114. Drugs that are purchased without a prescription are known by what abbreviation (and what is its meaning)? ______________________________

115. Drugs that lessen the heart rate and force of the heartbeat by decreasing the effectiveness of the nerve impulses to the cardiovascular system are what type of drugs? ______________________________

116. Drugs that prevent the formation of blood clots are called ________________.

117. Drugs that slow the flow of calcium to smooth muscle cells, causing arterial relaxation, are called ________________.

118. Drugs that relax blood vessels by preventing the formation of the vasoconstrictor, angiotensin II, are called ________________.

119. Drugs that strengthen the heartbeat are called ________________.

120. Drugs that the reduce the rate of LDL are called ________________.

121. Drugs that dissolve clots are called ________________.

122. Drugs that relax blood vessels and reduce the myocardial oxygen consumption to lessen the pain of angina pectoris are called ________________.

123. Drugs that help the body form and excrete urine and are used in the treatment of hypertension and CHF are called ________________.

Decode the term.

124. thrombolytic ______________________________

125. transdermal ______________________________

126. antiarrhythmic ______________________________

G. Abbreviations

Define the following abbreviations.

127. Mrs. Stephens was prescribed TDNTG for her angina pectoris.

____

128. Francis was admitted to the CCU with a massive MI.

____

129. The patient was treated for CAD with PTCA.

____

130. When a cath revealed a 90% blockage in John's LCA, he was scheduled for a CABG.

____

131. A patient with ASD was scheduled for septoplasty.

____

H. Singulars and Plurals

Define and change the following terms from singular to plural.

132. atrium ____

133. lumen ____

134. apex ____

135. septum ____

136. stenosis ____

137. thrombus ____

I. Translations

Rewrite the following sentences in your own words.

138. Laquita Washington was born with PDA that was originally detected by her doctor, who noted the presence of a continuous murmur and thrills. A left ventricular hypertrophy was noted on echocardiography. She was counseled as to the possibility of developing CHF later in life as a result of this disorder.

____

____

139. The 72-year-old man presented with advanced CAD. He had a history of cigarette smoking, hypertension, and blood lipid abnormalities.

____

____

140. The patient was treated with radiofrequency ablation for his paroxysmal atrial tachycardia.

____

____

141. Ms. Chong presented with dyspnea, substernal pain, leukocytosis, pyrexia, and ECG abnormalities. A diagnosis of pericarditis was made after a chest x-ray and echocardiogram.

____

____

142. A patient with hemorrhoids was scheduled for injection sclerotherapy.

____

J. Be Careful

What are the differences among the following?

143. arteri/o, atri/o, aort/o, arteriol/o, ather/o, arthr/o

____

____

144. palpation, palpitation

____

145. mitral regurgitation, digestive regurgitation

____

146. stenosis, sclerosis

____

147. infarction, infraction

____

K. Cumulative Review

Fill in the blank.

148. What is the tip of the heart called? _______________________

149. What is the term for the space between the lungs where the heart is located?

____

150. Blood vessels leading toward an organ are referred to as ________________, whereas those leading away from the organ are called ________________.

151. The heart is located (use the appropriate directional term) ________________ to the diaphragm.

152. Which vena cava returns blood to the right atrium from below the heart?

____

153. Which plane would image all four chambers of the heart? _______________________

154. The naming system for the layers of the heart is the same as the system for naming the layers of the ________________.

155. What is the term for a narrowing of a vessel? _______________________.

156. What are the three types of muscle and their combining forms? _______________________

157. What is the term for the cutting, tying, and burning of vessels in the male reproductive system for the purpose of sterilization? _______________________

Valleyview Hospital
90077 Santa Rosa Blvd.
Santa Rosa, CA 95011

DISCHARGE SUMMARY

Patient Name: Cheryl Miller
Age: 54

Admitted: 08/10/02
Discharged: 08/15/02

Principal Diagnosis: Inferolateral myocardial infarction
Secondary Diagnoses: Coronary artery disease; hypertension; hypercholesterolemia
Procedure: Coronary artery bypass graft
History of Present Illness: The patient, a 54-year-old Caucasian female, presents with a history of substernal chest pain, nausea, dyspnea, and diaphoresis for 1½ hours before being seen in the ED.
Medical History: Significant for hypertension and hypercholesterolemia.
Social History: Positive for social alcohol use, and patient has smoked 1 pack per day for the last 30 years.
Medications: The patient is not currently taking any medication.
Allergies: No known drug allergies.
Physical Examination: On physical examination, the patient's vital signs showed a blood pressure of 165/105, a pulse rate of 88, and a temperature of 98.6 degrees. The patient was a well-developed, well-nourished, Caucasian female in mild distress. The patient's head, eyes, ears, nose, and throat were unremarkable. The neck was supple, with no jugular venous distension. Heart showed irregularly regular rhythm. The lungs were clear to auscultation and percussion. The abdominal examination was soft and nontender. Extremities had no cyanosis, clubbing, or edema. The neurologic examination was nonfocal.
Laboratory Studies: White blood cell count 19, hematocrit 39.9, platelets 385. Differential included 89 neutrophils, 2 bands, 5 lymphocytes, and 1 mono. Sodium 142, potassium 4.3, BUN 11, creatinine 1.0, glucose 229, calcium 7.8, magnesium 1.9, phosphorus 8.4, CPK 375. Urinalysis revealed no abnormal findings. ECG revealed normal sinus rhythm at 85 bpm.
Hospital Course: The patient was admitted and started on intravenous nitroglycerin, heparin, aspirin, and Lopressor. Cardiac catheterization demonstrated significant occlusion of the right coronary artery. Echocardiogram showed an ejection fraction of 29%. A stress thallium demonstrated anterior ischemia after 6 minutes of exercise.

Patient underwent the bypass without incident and has progressed at a moderate pace through postoperative physical rehabilitation. At the time of discharge, she was ambulating well and demonstrated a good understanding of necessary lifestyle changes to maintain her health.
Medications on Discharge: Ascriptin, 325 mg po qd; Atenolol, 25 mg po qd.

Abegail Truskowski, MD, Resident Physician

L. Healthcare Report

158. Define the following symptoms presented by Ms. Miller:

    A. dyspnea ______________________________

    B. diaphoresis ______________________________

    C. hypertension ______________________________

159. Where was the chest pain perceived? ______________________________

160. How do you know that Ms. Miller had high cholesterol? ______________________________

161. What was the name of the ultrasound procedure to assess her cardiac function?

    ____

162. What procedure was done to treat her CAD? ______________________________

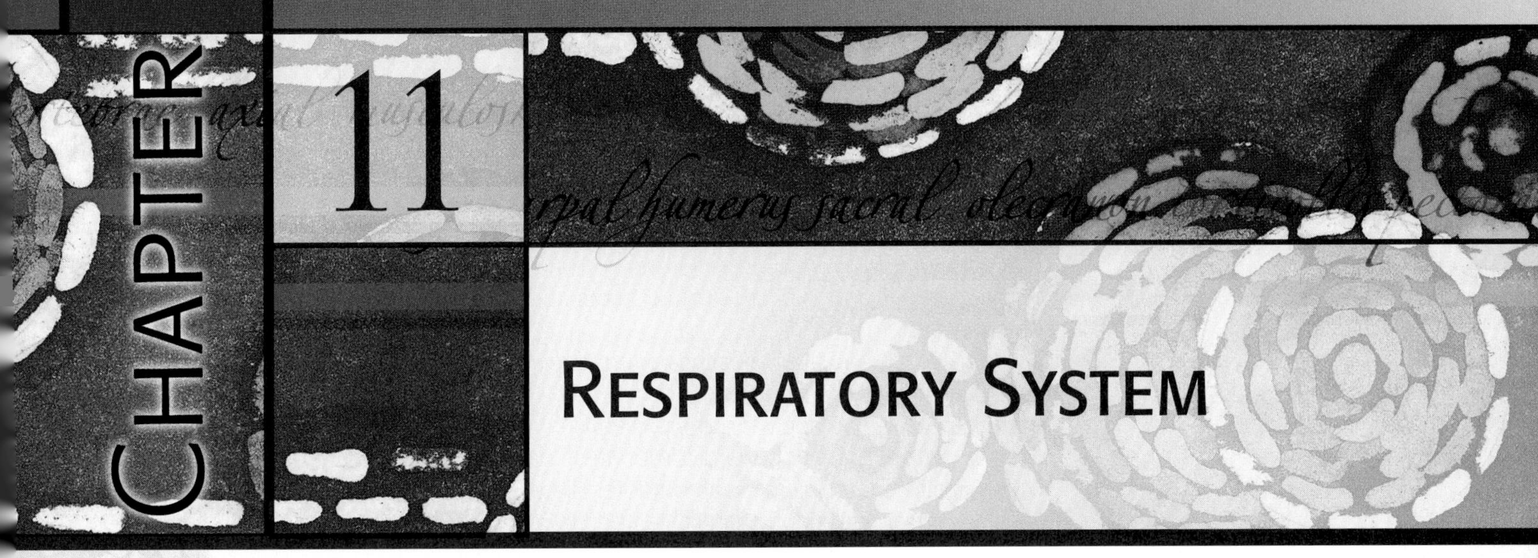

CHAPTER 11 RESPIRATORY SYSTEM

Roses are red,
Violets are blue,
Without your lungs,
Your blood would be too. —**Susan Ott**

Quote

Case Study

Casey Sandoval is a pitcher for her Little League softball team this year, but today on the field, she has so much difficulty catching her breath that now she can barely speak. Her mother has brought her to the emergency department (ED) for help. The respiratory therapist, Will Hamilton, speaks to the pair, asking whether Casey has hay fever (she does not) or allergies (none that she knows of). He also wants to know how hard she had been running during the game. Casey is pretty proud of her answer, in spite of her physical discomfort.

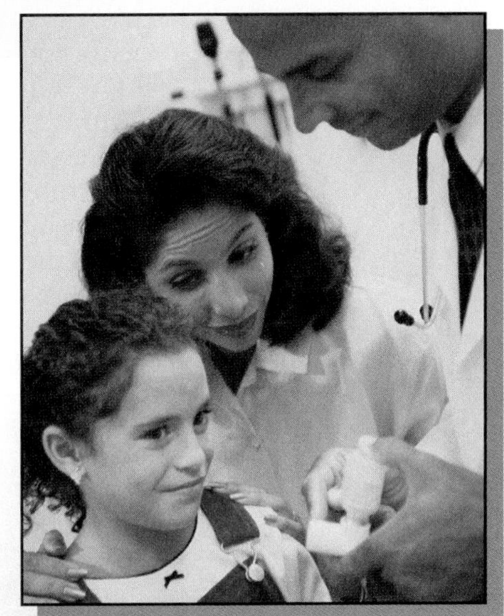

OBJECTIVES

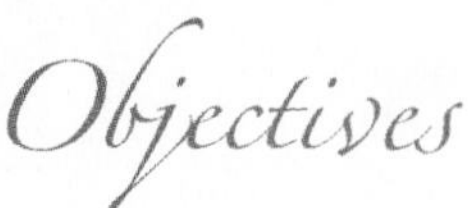

- In your own words, explain the functions of the respiratory system.
- Recognize, recall, and apply healthcare terms related to the anatomy and physiology of the respiratory system.
- Recognize, recall, and apply healthcare terms related to the pathology of the respiratory system.
- Recognize, recall, and apply healthcare terms related to diagnostic procedures of the respiratory system.
- Recognize, recall, and apply healthcare terms related to the therapeutic interventions of the respiratory system.
- Recognize, recall, and apply the abbreviations introduced in this chapter.
- Recognize, recall, and apply word components used in this chapter to build and decode healthcare terms relevant to the respiratory system.
- Recognize, recall, and apply material learned in previous chapters.

FUNCTIONS OF THE RESPIRATORY SYSTEM

The respiratory system handles the following functions for the body:

- Delivering oxygen (O_2) to the blood for transport to cells in the body.
- Excreting the waste product of cellular respiration, carbon dioxide (CO_2).
- Filtering, cleansing, warming, and humidifying air taken into the lungs.
- Helping to regulate blood pH.
- Helping the production of sound for speech and singing.
- Providing the tissue that receives the stimulus for the sense of smell, olfaction.

Analyzing the name for this system gives a clue as to its first two functions. The word **respiratory** (RES pur uh tore ee) comes from the combining form **spir/o,** which means *to breathe.* As a matter of fact, to breathe in is to **inspire,** and to breathe out is to **expire.** When one dies, one breathes out and no longer breathes in again—hence the expression is that the patient has "expired." **Inhalation** (in hull LAY shun) and **exhalation** (ex hull LAY shun) are alternative terms for **inspiration** and **expiration.**

The next two functions—filtering air and regulating blood pH—take place during breathing. The function of producing sound for speech and singing is accomplished by the interaction of air and the structures of the voice box, the larynx, and the hollow cavities, the sinuses, connected to the nasal passages.

Although the sense of smell, **olfaction** (ohl FACK shun), is not strictly a function of respiration, it is accomplished by the tissue in the nasal cavity, which receives the stimulus for smell and routes it to the brain through the nervous system.

Exercise 1: FUNCTIONS OF THE RESPIRATORY SYSTEM

1. The functions of the respiratory system are as follows:

   A. the delivery of ________________ to cells.

   B. the removal of ________________ from the body.

   C. to assist in regulating the blood's ________________.

   D. to condition and prepare air for the ________________.

   E. to assist in the production of ________________ for speech and singing.

   F. to provide tissue for receiving stimuli for the sense of smell, called ________________.

ANATOMY AND PHYSIOLOGY

The respiratory system is anatomically divided into the upper respiratory tract—the nose, pharynx, and larynx—and the lower respiratory tract—the trachea, bronchial tree, and lungs (Fig. 11-1). Physiologically, it is divided into conduction passageways and gas exchange surfaces.

There are two forms of respiration: **external respiration** and **internal respiration. External respiration** is the process of exchanging O_2 and CO_2 between the external environment and the lungs. **Internal respiration** is the exchange of gases between the lungs and the blood.

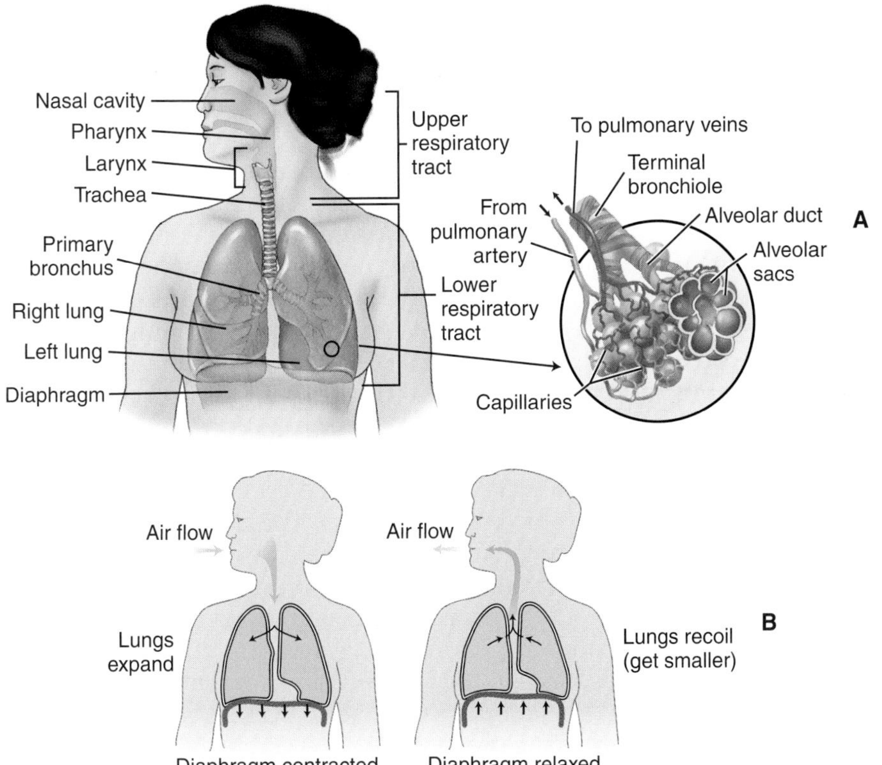

Fig. 11-1 **A,** The respiratory system showing a bronchial tree (inset). **B,** Inspiration and expiration.

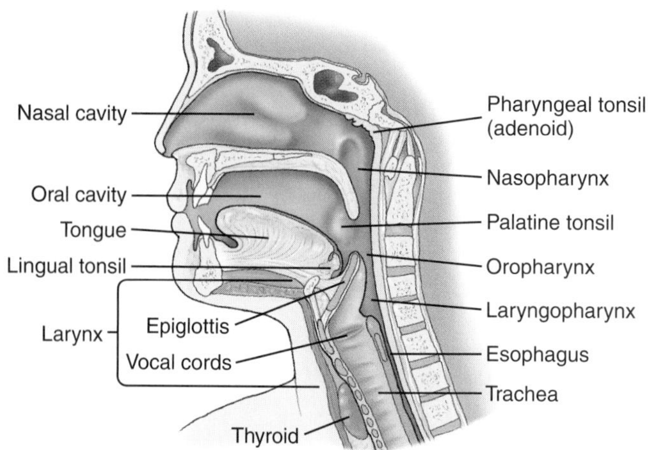

Fig. 11-2 The upper respiratory system.

BE CAREFUL!

The plural of sinus is not *sini*, but *sinuses*.

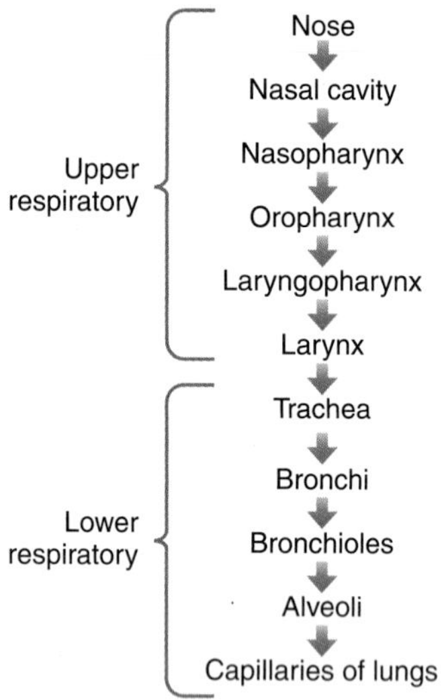

Fig. 11-3 Schematic of the order in which air passes through the upper respiratory system and into the lower respiratory system.

DID YOU KNOW?

An individual can survive the loss of a lobe of a lung, or even the removal of an entire lung.

Upper Respiratory Tract

The upper respiratory system encompasses the area from the nose to the larynx (Fig. 11-2). Air can enter the body through the mouth, but for the most part, it enters the body through the two **nares** (NAIR eez) (nostrils) of the **nose** that are separated by the **nasal septum** (NAY zul SEP tum). The hairs in the nose serve to filter out large particulate matter, and the mucus membrane and **cilia** (SEE lee uh) (small hairs) of the respiratory tract provide a further means of keeping air clean, warm, and moist as it travels to the lungs. The cilia continually move in a wavelike motion to push mucus and debris out of the respiratory tract. The air then travels up and backward, where it is filtered, warmed, and humidified by the environment in the upper portion of the nasal cavity. Fig. 11-3 illustrates the route of air into the body. The receptors for olfaction are located in the nasal cavity. The nasal cavity is connected to the **paranasal sinuses** (pair uh NAY zul SYE nus suhs).

The function of sinus cavities in the skull is to warm and filter the air taken in and to assist in the production of sound. These sinuses, divided into the frontal, maxillary, sphenoid, and ethmoid cavities, acquire their names from the bones in which they are located. They are lined with a mucous membrane that drains into the nasal cavity and can be the site of painful inflammation.

Air continues to travel past into the **nasopharynx** (NAY zoh fair inks), which is the part of the throat **(pharynx)** behind the nasal cavity. The **eustachian** (yoo STAY shun) **tubes** from the ears connect with the throat at this point to equalize pressure between the ears and the throat. This is the site of lymphatic tissue, the **pharyngeal tonsils** (fur IN jee ul TAHN suls), which are also termed the **adenoids** (AD uh noyds). These pharyngeal tonsils help to protect against pathogens. The next structure, the **oropharynx** (or oh FAIR inks), is the part of the throat posterior to the oral cavity and also the location of more lymphatic tissue, the **palatine tonsils** (PAL ah tyne TAHN suls), so named because they are continuous with the roof of the mouth (the palate). These tonsils, just like the adenoids, are made up of protective lymphatic tissue. The oropharynx is also part of the digestive system; food, as well as air, passes through it. Below the oropharynx is the part of the throat referred to as the **laryngopharynx** (luh ring goh FAIR inks), because of its proximity to the adjoining structure, the **larynx** (LAIR inks), or voice box. As air passes through the opening of the larynx, the **vocal cords** vibrate to produce speech. The **epiglottis** (eh pee GLOT is) is a flap of cartilage at the opening to the larynx that closes access to the **trachea** (TRAY kee uh) during swallowing, so that food is routed into the esophagus and is kept from entering the trachea. Though this is an effective protection most of the time, it can be overridden accidentally if the individual tries to talk and eat at the same time. When this happens, food can be pulled into the trachea, with possible serious consequences.

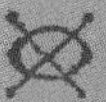

BE CAREFUL!

Salping/o means both *eustachian tubes* and *fallopian tubes.*

Lower Respiratory Tract

The lower respiratory tract begins with the **trachea** (or windpipe) that extends from the larynx into the thoracic cavity. The space between the lungs is called the **mediastinum** (mee dee uh STY num). Air travels into the lungs as the trachea bifurcates (branches) at the **carina** (kuh RIH nuh), where the right and left **bronchi** (BRONG kee) (*sing.* bronchus) divide into smaller branches, called **bronchioles** (BRONG kee ohls). These bronchioles end in microscopic ducts capped by air sacs called **alveoli** (al VEE oh lye) (*sing.* alveolus). Each alveolus is in contact with a blood capillary to provide a means of exchange of gases. It is at this point that O_2 is diffused across cell membranes into the blood cells, and CO_2 is diffused out to be expired. Each alveolus is coated with a substance called **surfactant** (sur FACK tunt) that keeps it from collapsing.

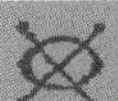

BE CAREFUL!

Don't confuse the combining form *ox/i,* which means *oxygen,* with the prefix *oxy-,* which means *rapid.*

Each lung is composed of sections, called **lobes.** The right lung is made up of three sections, whereas the left has only two. The abbreviations for the lobes of the lungs are RUL (right upper lobe), RML (right middle lobe), RLL (right lower lobe), LUL (left upper lobe), and LLL (left lower lobe).

Each lung is also enclosed by a double-folded, serous membrane called the **pleura** (PLOOR uh) (*pl.* pleurae). The side of the membrane that coats the lungs is the **visceral pleura** (VIH sur ul PLOOR ah); the side that lines the inner surface of the rib cage is the **parietal pleura** (puh RYE uh tul PLOOR ah). The two sides of the pleural membrane contain fluid that facilitates the expansion and contraction of the lungs with each breath.

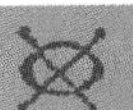

BE CAREFUL!

Don't confuse *bronchi/o,* which means the *bronchial tubes,* with *brachi/o,* which means the *arm.*

The muscles responsible for normal, quiet respiration are the **diaphragm** (DYE uh fram) and the **intercostal** (in tur KOS tul) **muscles.** On inspiration, the diaphragm is pulled down as it contracts and the intercostals muscles expand, pulling air into the lungs (see Fig 11-1, *B*).

COMBINING FORMS FOR THE RESPIRATORY SYSTEM

MEANING	COMBINING FORM	MEANING	COMBINING FORM
adenoids	adenoid/o	lung	pulmon/o, pneum/o, pneumon/o
air	pneum/o	mediastinum	mediastin/o
alveolus	alveol/o	mouth	or/o, stom/o, stomat/o
breathe	spir/o	mucus	muc/o
bronchiole	bronchiol/o	nose	nas/o, rhin/o
bronchus	bronch/o, bronchi/o	oxygen	ox/o
carbon dioxide	capn/o	pharynx	pharyng/o
chest	steth/o, thorac/o	pleura	pleur/o
diaphragm	diaphragm/o, diaphragmat/o, phren/o	rib	cost/o
eustachian tube	salping/o	sinus	sin/o, sinus/o
larynx	laryng/o	tonsil	tonsill/o
lobe	lob/o	trachea	trache/o

PREFIXES FOR THE RESPIRATORY SYSTEM			
PREFIX	**MEANING**	**PREFIX**	**MEANING**
ex-	out	para-	near
in-	in	re-	again
inter-	between		

Exercise 2: ANATOMY AND PHYSIOLOGY OF THE RESPIRATORY SYSTEM

Fill in the missing structures below to describe the route of the air through the upper respiratory system.

1. Nose →_______________→ nasopharynx →_______________→ laryngopharynx →_______________→ trachea (lower respiratory tract).
2. What mechanisms protect the respiratory system from pathogens?

____

3. What is the name of the substance that coats each alveolus? _______________

4. The pleura closest to the lungs is the _______________ pleura, whereas the pleura closest to the body wall is the _______________ pleura.

Match the respiratory structure with its combining form or prefix. More than one letter may be correct.

_____ 5. pleura
_____ 6. lobe
_____ 7. tonsil
_____ 8. mucus
_____ 9. diaphragm
_____ 10. windpipe
_____ 11. adenoids
_____ 12. eustachian tube
_____ 13. bronchiole
_____ 14. rib
_____ 15. breathe
_____ 16. pharynx
_____ 17. alveolus
_____ 18. lung
_____ 19. sinus
_____ 20. bronchus
_____ 21. voice box
_____ 22. mouth
_____ 23. nose
_____ 24. mediastinum

A. ox/o
B. bronch/o, bronchi/o
C. salping/o
D. pneum/o, pneumon/o
E. phren/o
F. stom/o, stomat/o
G. pharyng/o
H. adenoid/o
I. para-
J. rhin/o
K. re-
L. pulmon/o
M. capn/o
N. lob/o
O. diaphragm/o, diaphragmat/o
P. nas/o
Q. trache/o
R. alveol/o
S. tonsill/o
T. pleur/o
U. sin/o, sinus/o

_____ 25. in

_____ 26. near

_____ 27. out

_____ 28. between

_____ 29. again

_____ 30. carbon dioxide

_____ 31. oxygen

V. muc/o
W. inter-
X. laryng/o
Y. in-
Z. bronchiol/o
AA. cost/o
BB. mediastin/o
CC. ex-
DD. or/o
EE. spir/o

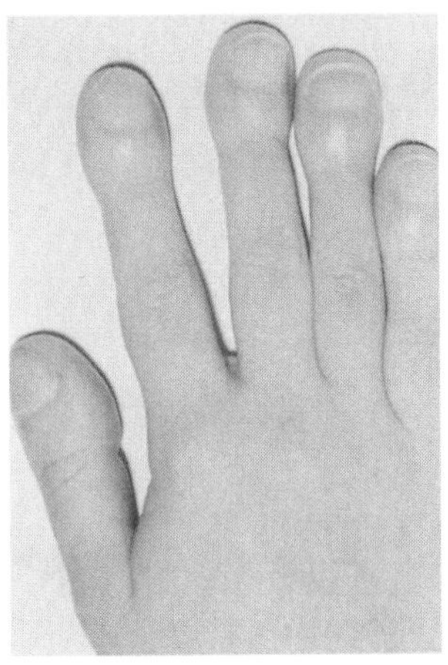

Fig. 11-4 Clubbing.

PATHOLOGY

Terms Related to Respiratory Symptoms

TERM	WORD ORIGIN	DEFINITION
Aphonia ah FOH nee ah	*a-* without *phon/o* sound *-ia* condition	Loss of ability to produce sounds.
Apnea AP nee ah	*a-* without *-pnea* breathing	Abnormal, periodic cessation of breathing.
Bradypnea brad IP nee ah	*brady-* slow *-pnea* breathing	Abnormally slow breathing.
Cheyne-Stokes respiration chayne stokes		Deep, rapid breathing followed by a period of apnea.
Clubbing		Abnormal enlargement of the distal phalanges as a result of diminished O_2 in the blood (Fig. 11-4).
Cough kof		Sudden, audible expulsion of air from the lungs.
Cyanosis sye uh NOH sis	*cyan/o* blue *-osis* abnormal condition	Discoloration of the skin and mucus membranes caused by insufficient oxygenation of the blood. The color of the skin, nailbeds, and/or mucous membranes may be blue, gray, slate, or dark purple.
Dysphonia dis FOH nee ah	*dys-* abnormal *phon/o* sound *-ia* condition	Impairment of speaking, hoarseness.
Dyspnea DISP nee ah	*dys-* difficult *-pnea* breathing	Any abnormal, difficult, or uncomfortable breathing.
Epistaxis ep ih STACK sis		Nosebleed.
Eupnea YOOP nee ah	*eu-* good, well *-pnea* breathing	Good, normal breathing.
Fatigue fuh TEEG		Overwhelming sense of exhaustion.

Continued

Terms Related to Respiratory Symptoms—cont'd

Term	Word Origin	Definition
Hemoptysis heh MOP tih sis	*hem/o* blood *-ptysis* spitting	Coughing up blood or blood-stained sputum.
Hypercapnia hye pur KAP nee ah	*hyper-* excessive *capn/o* carbon dioxide *-ia* condition	Condition of excessive CO_2 in the blood.
Hyperventilation hye pur ven tih LAY shun	*hyper-* excessive	Abnormally increased breathing.
Hypoxemia hye pock SEE mee ah	*hypo-* deficient *ox/o* oxygen *-emia* blood condition	Condition of deficient O_2 in the blood.
Orthopnea or THOP nee ah	*ortho-* straight *-pnea* breathing	Condition of difficult breathing unless in an upright position.
Pleurodynia ploor oh DIN ee ah	*pleur/o* pleura *-dynia* pain	Pain in the chest caused by inflammation of the intercostal muscles and their points of attachment of the diaphragm to the chest wall.
Precordial pain pre KORE dee ul	*pre-* before, in front of *-cordial* pertaining to the heart	Chest pain over the heart and lower thorax.
Pyrexia pye RECK see ah	*pyr/o* fire	Fever.
Rhinorrhea rye noh REE ah	*rhino-* nose *-rrhea* discharge	Discharge from the nose.
Shortness of breath (SOB)		Breathlessness; inability to fill the lungs adequately.
Sputum SPYOO tum		Mucus coughed up from the lungs and expectorated through the mouth. If abnormal, may be described as to its amount, color, or odor.
Stridor STRY dur		High-pitched inspiratory sound from the larynx; a sign of upper airway obstruction.
Tachypnea tack IP nee ah	*tachy-* fast *-pnea* breathing	Rapid, shallow breathing.
Thoracodynia thor uh koh DIN ee ah	*thorac/o* chest *-dynia* pain	Chest pain.
Wheezing		Whistling sound made during breathing.

Case Study Continued

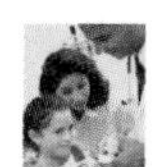

Casey has occasionally been short of breath when playing sports before, but not as severely as today. Even in the air-conditioned hospital she is sweaty, pale, and slightly cyanotic. Her inability to catch her breath is making her panicky, and Will can see that Casey's mother is worried too. Will speaks soothingly to them both, telling them that he can help Casey's breathing.

Terms Related to Abnormal Chest Sounds		
TERM	**WORD ORIGIN**	**DEFINITION**
Friction sounds		Sounds made by dry surfaces rubbing together.
Hiccup HICK up		Sound produced by the involuntary contraction of the diaphragm, followed by rapid closure of the glottis. Also called **hiccough, singultus.**
Rales rayls		Also called **crackles,** an abnormal lung sound heard on auscultation, characterized by discontinuous bubbling noises.
Rhonchi RONG kye		Abnormal rumbling sound heard on auscultation, caused by airways blocked by secretions or muscle contractions.
Tympany, chest TIM puh nee	*tympan/o* drum	Low-pitched resonant sound from the chest.

Exercise 3: SYMPTOMS OF RESPIRATORY DISEASE

Circle the correct answer.

1. Ms. Sims visits her physician's office and presents with hemoptysis. She has been *(vomiting blood, coughing up blood).*
2. Jeffrey Andar has been having persistent bouts of epistaxis, which is *(rhinorrhea, nosebleed).*
3. Singultus is another name for *(cough, hiccup).*
4. Hannah Moore exhibits rapid, shallow breathing. This is termed *(bradypnea, tachypnea).*
5. When Samuel Wrightson had laryngitis, he experienced aphonia. He cannot *(swallow, make sounds).*
6. A temporary lack of breathing is called *(dyspnea, apnea).*
7. Thoracodynia is *(pain, discharge)* in the chest.
8. Another name for rales is *(crackles, friction sounds).*
9. Pain caused by inflamed intercostal muscles and their points of attachment to the diaphragm is referred to as *(pleurodynia, singultus).*
10. A whistling sound made during inhalation is called *(rales, wheezing).*
11. The distal phalanges are abnormally enlarged in which symptom of advanced chronic pulmonary disease? *(cyanosis, clubbing)*

Match the term with its combining form or suffix. More than one letter may be correct.

_____ 12. spitting

_____ 13. blue

_____ 14. sound

_____ 15. nose

_____ 16. discharge

_____ 17. pleura

_____ 18. drum

_____ 19. breathing

_____ 20. straight

_____ 21. blood

_____ 22. chest

_____ 23. pain

A. phon/o
B. rhin/o
C. spir/o
D. -ptysis
E. orth/o
F. hem/o
G. -rrhea
H. thorac/o
I. tympan/o
J. -dynia
K. pleur/o
L. nas/o
M. cyan/o

Terms Related to Disorders of the Upper Respiratory Tract

TERM	WORD ORIGIN	DEFINITION
Croup croop		Acute viral infection of early childhood, marked by stridor caused by spasms of the larynx, trachea, and bronchi.
Deviated septum DEE vee a tid SEP tum	*sept/o* wall, partition *-um* noun ending	Deflection of the nasal septum that may obstruct the nasal passages, resulting in infection, sinusitis, shortness of breath, headache, or recurring epistaxis.
Epiglottitis eh pee glah TYE tis	*epiglott/o* epiglottis *-itis* inflammation	Inflammation of the epiglottis (Fig. 11-5).
Laryngitis lair in JYE tis	*laryng/o* voice box, larynx *-itis* inflammation	Inflammation of the voice box.
Pharyngitis fair in JYE tis	*pharyng/o* throat, pharynx *-itis* inflammation	Inflammation or infection of the pharynx, usually causing symptoms of a sore throat.
Polyps, nasal and vocal cord PALL ups		Small, tumorlike growth that projects from a mucous membrane surface, including the inside of the nose, paranasal sinuses, and the vocal cords (Fig. 11-6).
Rhinitis rye NYE tis	*rhin/o* nose *-itis* inflammation	Inflammation of the mucous membrane of the nose.
Rhinomycosis rye noh mye KOH sis	*rhin/o* nose *myc/o* fungus *-osis* abnormal condition	Abnormal condition of fungus in the nose.
Rhinosalpingitis rye noh sal pin JYE tis	*rhin/o* nose *salping/o* eustachian tube *-itis* inflammation	Inflammation of the mucous membranes of the nose and eustachian tubes.
Sinusitis sye nuh SYE tis	*sinus/o* sinus *-itis* inflammation	Inflammation of one or more of the paranasal sinuses.
Upper respiratory infection (URI)		Inflammation and/or infection of structures of the upper respiratory tract; sometimes referred to as **coryza** (kore EYE zuh), a head cold.

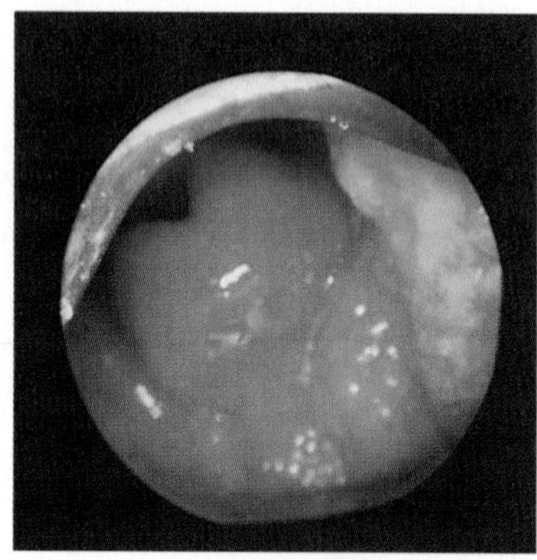

Fig. 11-5 Epiglottitis. The epiglottis is red and swollen.

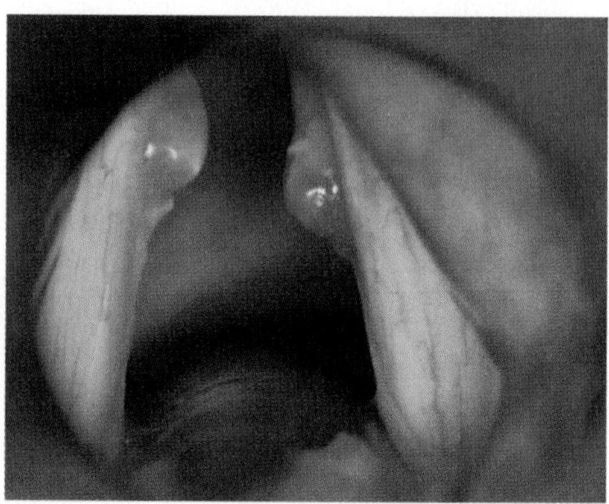

Fig. 11-6 Polypoid nodules of the vocal cords.

Terms Related to Disorders of the Lower Respiratory Tract

TERM	WORD ORIGIN	DEFINITION
Asthma AZ muh		Respiratory disorder characterized by recurring episodes of **paroxysmal** (sudden, episodic) dyspnea. Patients present with coughing, wheezing, and shortness of breath. If the attack becomes continuous (termed **status asthmaticus**), it may be fatal (Fig. 11-7).
Atelectasis at ih LECK tuh sis	*a-* not *tel/o* complete *-ectasis* dilation	Collapse of lung tissue or entire lung.
Bronchiectasis brong kee ECK tuh sis	*bronchi/o* bronchi *-ectasis* dilation	Chronic dilation of the bronchi. Symptoms include dyspnea, expectoration of foul-smelling sputum, and coughing.
Bronchiolitis brong kee oh LYE tis	*bronchiol/o* bronchiole *-itis* inflammation	Viral inflammation of the bronchioles; more common in children younger than 18 months.
Bronchitis brong KYE tis	*bronchi/o* bronchi *-itis* inflammation	Inflammation of the bronchi. May be acute or chronic.
Chronic obstructive pulmonary disease (COPD)	*pulmon/o* lung *-ary* pertaining to	Respiratory disorder characterized by a progressive and irreversible diminishment in inspiratory and expiratory capacity of the lungs. Patient experiences **dyspnea on exertion (DOE),** difficulty inhaling or exhaling, and a chronic cough.
Cystic fibrosis SIS tick fye BROH sis		Inherited disorder of the exocrine glands resulting in abnormal, thick secretions of mucus that cause COPD.
Emphysema em fah SEE mah		Abnormal condition of the pulmonary system characterized by distention and destructive changes of the alveoli. The most common cause is tobacco smoking, but exposure to environmental particulate matter may also cause the disease.
Flail chest		Thorax in which multiple rib fractures cause instability in part of the chest wall, in which the lung under the injured area contracts on inspiration and bulges out on expiration (Fig. 11-8).

Continued

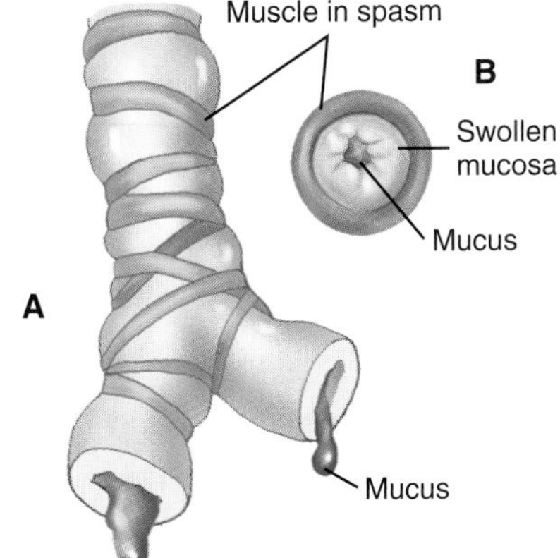

Fig. 11-7 Factors causing expiratory obstruction in asthma. **A,** Cross-section of a bronchiole occluded by muscle spasm, swollen mucosa, and mucus. **B,** Longitudinal section of a bronchiole.

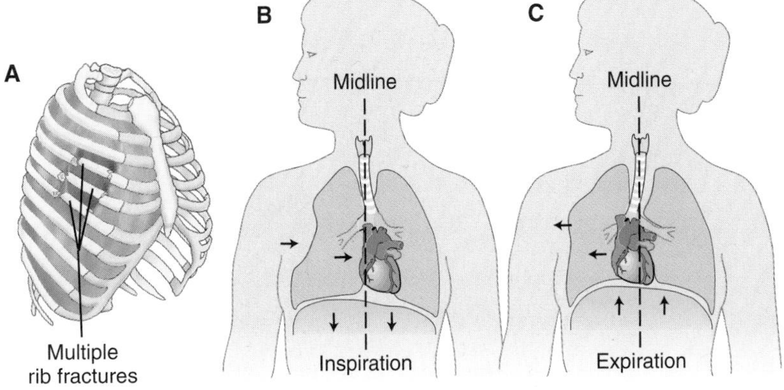

Fig. 11-8 Flail chest. **A,** Fractured rib sections are unattached to the rest of the chest wall. **B,** On inspiration, the flail segment of ribs is sucked inward, causing the lung to shift inward. **C,** On expiration, the flail segment of ribs bellows outward, causing the lung to shift outward. Air moves back and forth between the lungs instead of through the upper airway.

Terms Related to Disorders of the Lower Respiratory Tract—cont'd		
TERM	**WORD ORIGIN**	**DEFINITION**
Hemothorax hee moh THOR acks	*hem/o* blood *-thorax* pleural cavity	Blood in the pleural cavity (Fig. 11-9).
Influenza in floo EN zah		Also known as the **flu.** Acute infectious disease of the respiratory tract caused by a virus.
Pleural effusion PLOOR ul eh FYOO zhun	*pleur/o* pleura *-al* pertaining to	Abnormal accumulation of fluid in the intrapleural space.
Pleurisy PLOOR ih see	*pleur/o* pleura	Inflammation of the parietal pleura of the lungs. May be caused by cancer, pneumonia, or tuberculosis.
Pneumoconiosis noo moh koh nee OH sis	*pneum/o* lung *coni/o* dust *-osis* abnormal condition	Loss of lung capacity due to an accumulation of dust in the lungs. Types may include **asbestosis** (abnormal condition of asbestos in the lungs), **silicosis** (sil ih KOH sis) (abnormal accumulation of glass dust in the lungs), and **anthracosis** (abnormal accumulation of coal dust in the lungs—also known as **black lung disease** or **coal worker's pneumoconiosis [CWP]**) (Fig. 11-10).
Pneumonia noo MOH nya	*pneumon/o* lungs *-ia* condition	Inflammation of the lungs due to a variety of pathogens. If infectious, it is termed pneumonia; if noninfectious, **pneumonitis.** The name(s) of the lobes are used to describe the extent of the disease (e.g., **RML pneumonia** is pneumonia of the right middle lobe). If both lungs are affected, it is termed **double pneumonia.**
Pneumothorax noo moh THOR acks	*pneum/o* air *-thorax* pleural space	Air or gas in the pleural space causing the lung to collapse (Fig. 11-11).

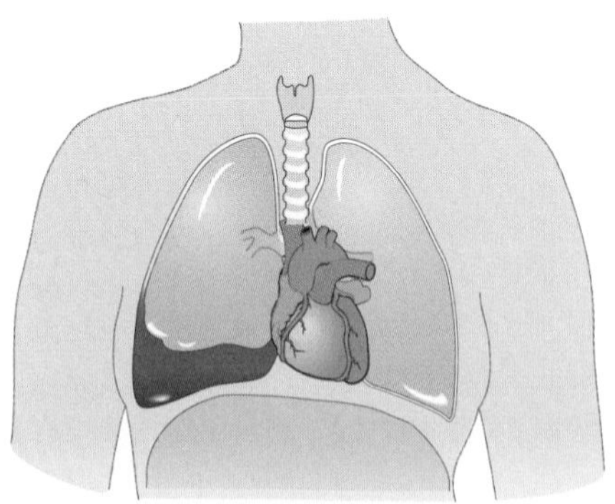

Fig. 11-9 Hemothorax. Blood below the left lung causes the lung to collapse.

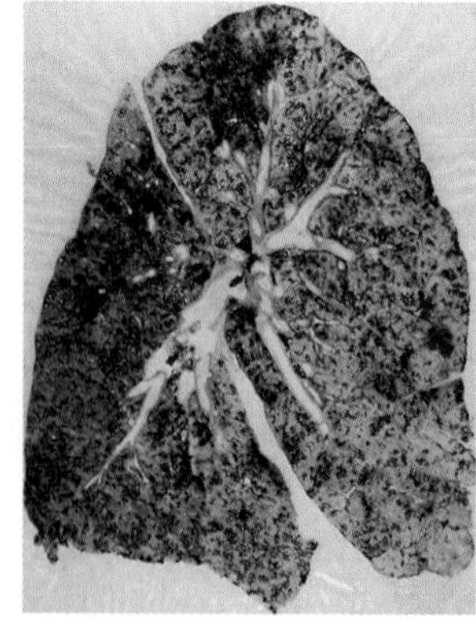

Fig. 11-10 Coal worker's pneumoconiosis. The lungs show increased black pigmentation.

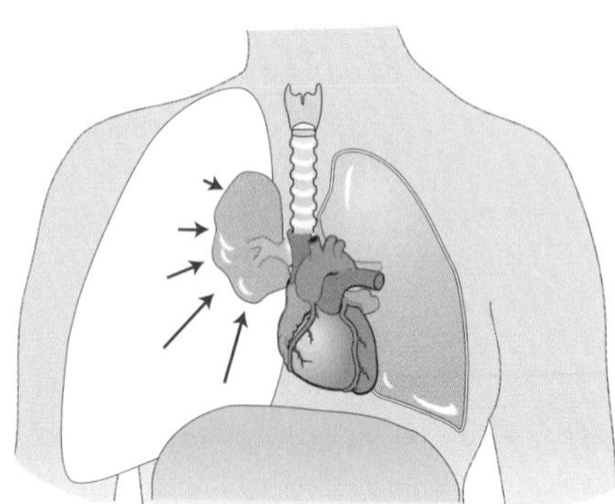

Fig. 11-11 Pneumothorax. The lung collapses as air gathers in the pleural space.

Terms Related to Disorders of the Lower Respiratory Tract—cont'd

TERM	WORD ORIGIN	DEFINITION
Pulmonary abscess PULL mun nair ee AB ses	*pulmon/o* lung *-ary* pertaining to	Localized accumulation of pus in the lung.
Pulmonary edema PULL mun nair ee eh DEE mah	*pulmon/o* lung *-ary* pertaining to	Accumulation of fluid in the lung tissue. Often present in congestive heart failure, it is caused by the inability of the heart to pump blood.
Pyothorax pye oh THOR acks	*py/o* pus *-thorax* pleural cavity	Pus in the pleural cavity. Also called **empyema.**
Tuberculosis (TB) too bur kyoo LOH sis		Chronic infectious disorder caused by an acid-fast bacillus, *Mycobacterium tuberculosis.* Transmission is normally by inhalation or ingestion of infected droplets. **Multidrug-resistant tuberculosis (MDR TB)** is fatal in 80% of cases.

Case Study Continued

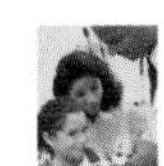

Will and the physician on staff suspect that Casey has exercise-induced asthma. Will gives her oxygen through a face mask and connects her to a cardiac monitor. He records Casey's heart and respiratory rates and notes the wheezing and bilateral rhonchi. Casey's eyes are wide and frightened as she watches Will work.

Exercise 4: DISORDERS OF THE UPPER AND LOWER RESPIRATORY TRACT

Circle the correct answer.

1. An inflammation of the voice box is called *(pharyngitis, laryngitis).*
2. A patient with an inflammation of the mucus membranes of the nose and eustachian tubes has *(rhinomycosis, rhinosalpingitis).*
3. A patient with an inflamed flap of tissue that covers the opening of the larynx has *(epiglottitis, sinusitis).*
4. A healthcare term for the common cold is *(chorea, coryza).*
5. An inflammation and/or infection of the structures of the upper respiratory tract is called a/an *(URI, SOB).*
6. A *(rhinorrhea, deviated septum)* is a deflection of the nasal wall that may result in nosebleeds, shortness of breath, infection, and/or headaches.
7. Growths that occur on the mucus membranes of the larynx are referred to as *(nasal polyps, vocal polyps).*
8. *(Pleurisy, Pleurodynia)* is an inflammation of the parietal pleura.
9. *(Croup, Asthma)* is an acute, infectious viral disease of the respiratory tract.
10. *(Atelectasis, Pneumoconiosis)* is the term for collapse of a lung.
11. *(Emphysema, Pneumoconiosis)* is a chronic pulmonary disease marked by distention of the alveoli.
12. *(Asthma, Tuberculosis)* is a respiratory disorder characterized by episodes of paroxysmal dyspnea.
13. Localized accumulation of pus in the lung is called a *(pulmonary abscess, pulmonary effusion).*
14. A chronic dilation of the bronchi is called *(bronchiectasis, bronchitis).*
15. Loss of lung capacity due to dust in the lung is called *(pleural effusion, pneumoconiosis).*
16. *(Tuberculosis, Cystic fibrosis)* is an inherited disorder of the exocrine glands that causes COPD.

17. The term that refers to abnormally slow breathing is *(bradypnea, tachypnea).*
18. The term that refers to good, easy breathing is *(eupnea, orthopnea).*
19. Patients with chest trauma who experience breathing in which the lung contracts on inspiration and expands on expiration have *(flail chest, atelectasis).*

Match the combining forms and suffixes with their meanings.

_____ 20. nas/o, rhin/o
_____ 21. -ectasis
_____ 22. pneum/o, pneumon/o
_____ 23. hem/o
_____ 24. laryng/o
_____ 25. epiglott/o
_____ 26. coni/o
_____ 27. sinus/o

_____ 28. sept/o
_____ 29. pharyng/o
_____ 30. bronchiol/o
_____ 31. py/o, purul/o
_____ 32. eustachian tube
_____ 33. -thorax
_____ 34. myc/o
_____ 35. tel/o

A. pleural cavity
B. complete
C. wall, partition
D. pus
E. nose
F. salping/o
G. bronchiole
H. fungus
I. dust
J. sinus
K. air, lung
L. epiglottis
M. throat
N. dilation
O. voice box
P. blood

DIAGNOSTIC PROCEDURES

BE CAREFUL!

The definition for a *scope* here is *to listen,* not *to look.*

The physical examination includes listening to the patient's chest by the process of **auscultation** (os kull TAY shun) (listening) and **percussion** (pur KUH shun) (tapping). If the patient's chest is free of fluid or exudates, it is considered *clear to auscultation* (CTA). Further examination of chest sounds may be accomplished through the use of a **stethoscope** (STETH oh scope).

Terms Related to Diagnostic Procedures

TERM	WORD ORIGIN	DEFINITION
Arterial blood gases (ABG)	*arteri/o* artery *-al* pertaining to	Blood test that measures the amount of O_2 and CO_2 in the blood.
Bronchoscopy brong KOS skuh pee	*bronch/o* bronchi *-scopy* visual examination	Endoscopic procedure used to examine the bronchial tubes visually (Fig. 11-12).
Chest x-ray (CXR)		One of the most common imaging techniques for the respiratory system; used to visualize abnormalities of the respiratory system. X-rays may also include the use of a contrast medium, as in a **pulmonary angiography,** which uses a dye injected into the blood vessels of the lung, followed by subsequent x-ray imaging to demonstrate the flow of blood through these vessels (Fig. 11-13).
Computed tomography (CT)	*tom/o* slice *-graphy* process of recording	Imaging technique that can image the respiratory system and associated structures by creating cross-sections or "slices" of tissue.

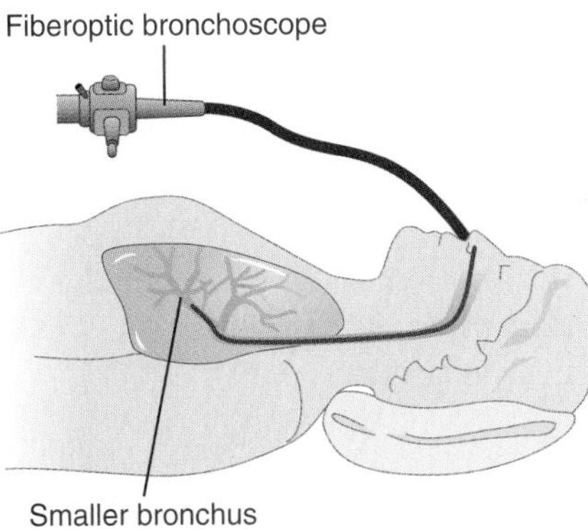

Fig. 11-12 Bronchoscopy.

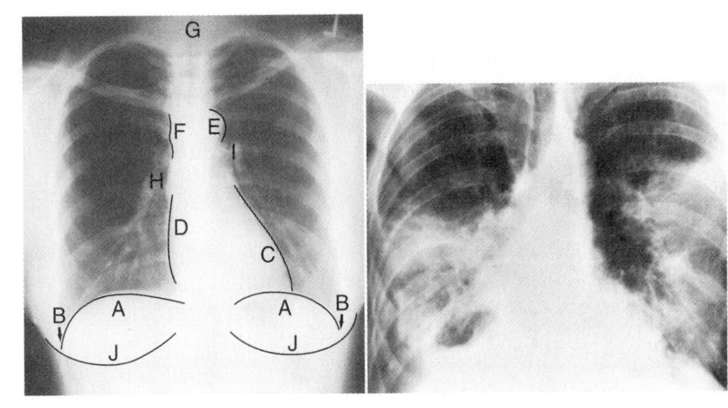

Fig. 11-13 **A,** Normal PA chest x-ray. The backward "L" in the upper right corner is placed on the film to indicate the left side of the client's chest. *A,* Diaphragm. *B,* Costophrenic angle. *C,* Left ventricle. *D,* Right atrium. *E,* Aortic arch. *F,* Superior vena cava. *G,* Trachea. *H,* Right bronchus. *I,* Left bronchus. *J,* Breast shadows. **B,** X-ray of lung with pneumonia.

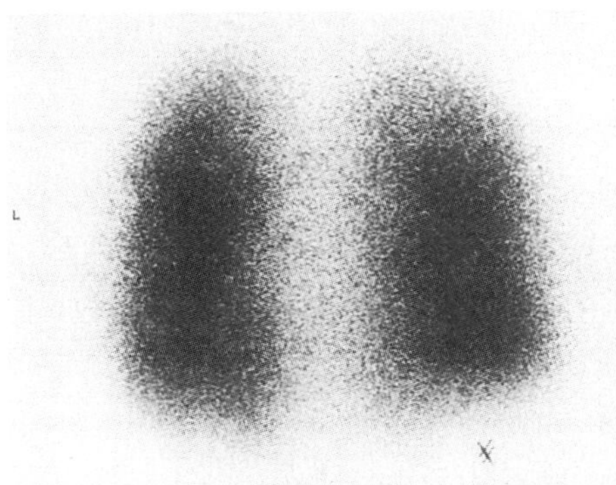

Fig. 11-14 Lung ventilation image of normal lungs.

Terms Related to Diagnostic Procedures—cont'd

TERM	WORD ORIGIN	DEFINITION
Laryngoscopy lair ing GOS skuh pee	*laryng/o* larynx, voice box *-scopy* visual examination	Endoscopic procedure used to visualize the interior of the larynx.
Lung perfusion scan		Nuclear medicine test that produces an image of blood flow to the lungs; used to detect pulmonary embolism.
Lung ventilation scan		Test using radiopharmaceuticals to produce a picture of how air is distributed in the lungs; measures the ability of the lungs to take in air (Fig. 11-14).
Magnetic resonance imaging (MRI)		Computerized imaging that uses radiofrequency radiation to detect lung tumors, embolisms, and chest trauma.
Mantoux skin test mon TOO		Intradermal injection of purified protein derivative (PPD) used to detect the presence of tuberculosis antibodies.
Mediastinoscopy mee dee as tih NAH skuh pee		Endoscopic procedure used for visual examination of the structures contained within the space between the lungs.

Continued

Terms Related to Diagnostic Procedures—cont'd		
TERM	**WORD ORIGIN**	**DEFINITION**
Peak flow meter		Instrument used in a PFT to measure breathing capacity.
Pulmonary function test (PFT)	*pulmon/o* lung *-ary* pertaining to	Procedure for determining the capacity of the lungs to exchange O_2 and CO_2 efficiently.
Pulse oximetry ock SIM uh tree	*ox/i* oxygen *-metry* process of measurement	Test to measure oxygen in arterial blood, in which a noninvasive, cliplike device is attached to either the earlobe or the fingertip (Fig. 11-15).
Spirometry spy ROM uh tree	*spir/o* breathing *-metry* process of measurement	Test to measure the air capacity of the lungs with a **spirometer.**
Sputum culture SPYOO tum		Cultivation of microorganisms from sputum that has been collected from expectoration.
Sweat test		Method of evaluating sodium and chloride concentration in sweat as a means of diagnosing cystic fibrosis.
Throat culture		Cultivation of microorganisms from a throat swab to determine the type of organism causing a disorder.
Ultrasonography	*ultra-* beyond *son/o* sound *-graphy* process of recording	Use of high-frequency sound waves to image structures within the body.

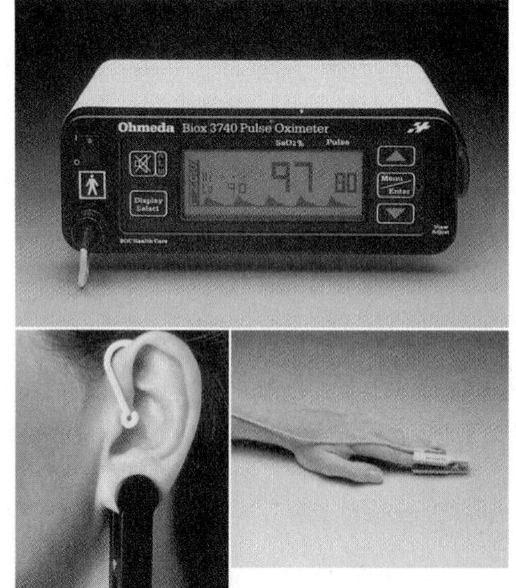

Fig. 11-15 Pulse oximetry.

Exercise 5: DIAGNOSTIC PROCEDURES

Circle the correct answer.

1. The test for tuberculosis is called *(spirometry, Mantoux skin test).*
2. A blood test that measures O_2 and CO_2 is a/an *(ABG, PFT).*
3. A *(Mantoux skin test, sweat test)* is used to diagnose cystic fibrosis.
4. A *(lung perfusion scan, lung ventilation scan)* is a test of how air is distributed in the lung.
5. An imaging technique that shows the flow of blood through the vessels of the lungs is called *(pulmonary angiography, ABG).*
6. *(Pulse oximetry, Spirometry)* is a noninvasive method of measuring oxygen saturation levels in arterial blood.

Match the combining forms and suffixes with their meanings.

_____ 7. -meter	_____ 12. -metry	A.	space between the lungs
		B.	bronchi
_____ 8. spir/o	_____ 13. steth/o	C.	voice box
		D.	chest
_____ 9. mediastin/o	_____ 14. pulmon/o	E.	lungs
		F.	breath
_____ 10. derm/o	_____ 15. laryng/o	G.	instrument to measure
		H.	vessel
_____ 11. angi/o	_____ 16. bronch/o	I.	skin
		J.	process of measurement

THERAPEUTIC INTERVENTIONS

Therapeutic interventions for the respiratory system involve removal (-ectomy), repair (-plasty), a new opening (-stomy), a surgical puncture to remove fluid (-centesis), or intubation. See examples in the following table.

Patients who need assistance in attaining adequate O_2 levels may need a mechanical device called a **ventilator** to provide positive-pressure breathing. The device delivers the O_2 in different ways. If a low level of O_2 is required, a nasal **cannula** (KAN you lah) (tube) may be adequate. Face masks are another option. The amount of O_2 may be monitored more accurately with a **Venturi mask.** If high O_2 concentrations are necessary, a nonrebreathing or partial **rebreathing mask** may be used.

Positive-pressure breathing (PPB) is a respiratory therapy technique designed to deliver air at greater than atmospheric pressure to the lungs. **Continuous positive airway pressure (CPAP)** may be delivered through a ventilator and endotracheal tube or a nasal cannula, face mask, or a hood over the patient's head. See Fig. 11-16 for several examples of oxygenation therapy.

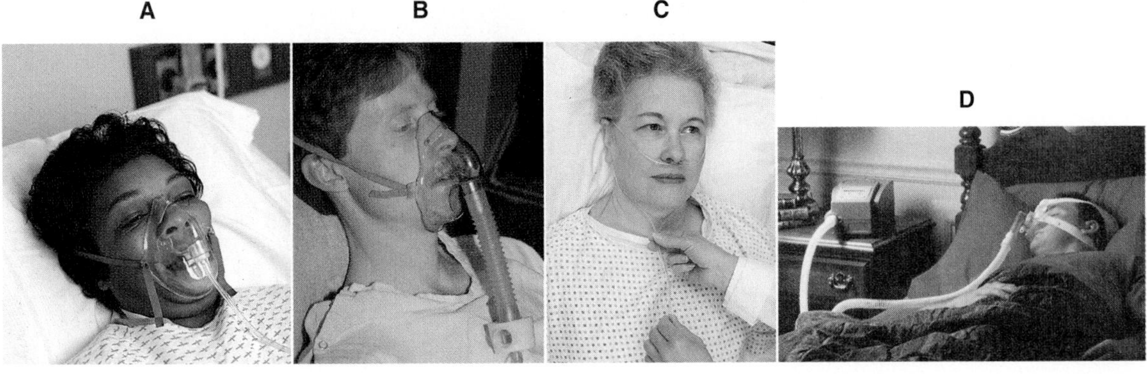

Fig. 11-16 Routes of oxygen therapy. **A,** Simple face mask. **B,** Venturi mask. **C,** Nasal cannula. **D,** CPAP.

Terms Related to Therapeutic Interventions

TERM	WORD ORIGIN	DEFINITION
Adenoidectomy ad uh noyd ECK tuh mee	***adenoid/o*** adenoid ***-ectomy*** excision, removal	Excision of the pharyngeal tonsils, or adenoids.
Bronchoplasty BRONG koh plas tee	***bronch/o*** bronchi ***-plasty*** surgical repair	Surgical repair of a bronchial defect.
Endotracheal intubation en doh TRAY kee ul in too BAY shun	***endo-*** within ***trache/o*** windpipe ***-al*** pertaining to	Passage of a tube through the mouth (or sometimes the nose) into the trachea to ensure a patent (open) airway.
Laryngectomy lair in JECK tuh mee	***laryng/o*** voice box ***-ectomy*** removal	Excision of the voice box.
Pulmonary resection		Excision of a portion or a lobe of the lung or the entire lung. Called a **lobectomy** when an entire lobe is excised, and a **pneumonectomy** when the entire lung is excised (Fig. 11-17).
Rhinoplasty RYE noh plas tee	***rhin/o*** nose ***-plasty*** surgical repair	Surgical repair of the nose for either healthcare or cosmetic reasons.
Septoplasty sep toh PLAS tee	***sept/o*** wall, partition ***-plasty*** surgical repair	Surgical repair of the wall between the nares.
Sinusotomy sye nuh SOT tuh mee	***sinus/o*** sinus ***-tomy*** incision	Incision of a sinus.
Thoracentesis thor oh sen TEE sis	***pleur/o*** pleura ***-centesis*** surgical puncture	Aspiration of a fluid from the pleural space. Also called **pleurocentesis.**
Tonsillectomy ton sih LECK tuh mee	***tonsill/o*** tonsil ***-ectomy*** removal	Excision of the palatine tonsils.
Tracheostomy tray kee OS tuh mee	***trache/o*** trachea, windpipe ***-stomy*** new opening	Opening through the neck into the trachea, through which an indwelling tube may be inserted either temporarily or permanently (Fig. 11-18).
Tracheotomy tray kee AH tuh mee	***trache/o*** trachea, windpipe ***-tomy*** incision	Incision made into the trachea below the larynx to gain access to the airway; usually as an emergency procedure.

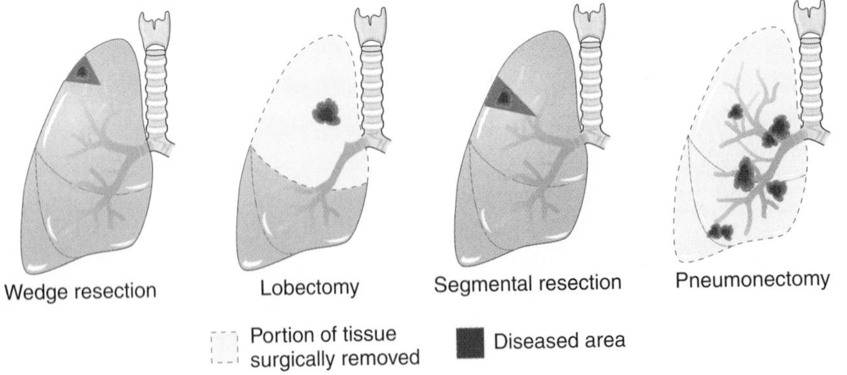

Fig. 11-17 Pulmonary resections.

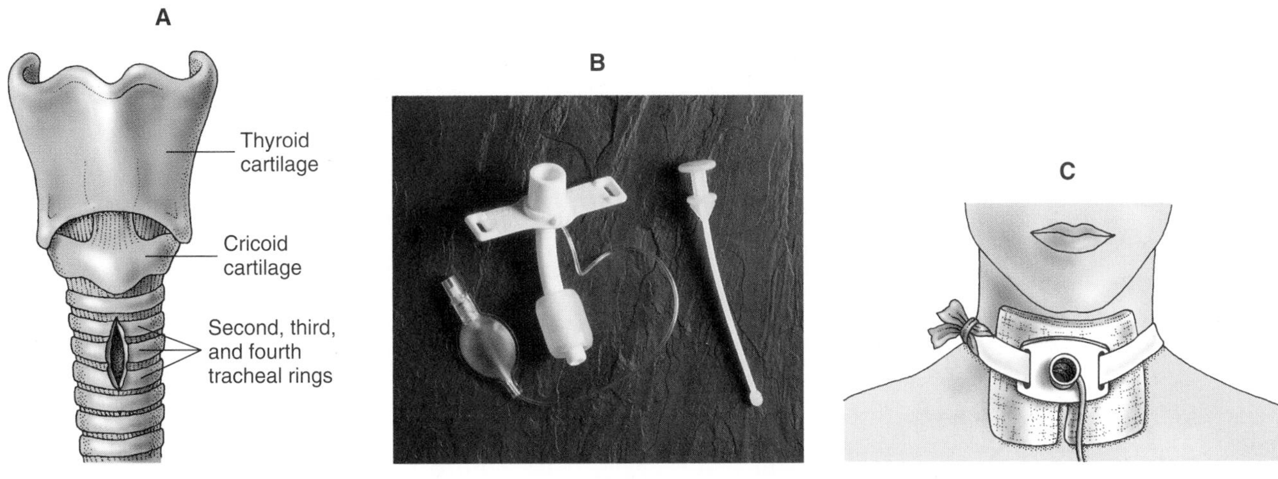

Fig. 11-18 **A,** Vertical tracheal incision for a tracheostomy. **B,** Tracheostomy tube. **C,** Placement of gauze and tie around a tracheostomy tube.

Exercise 6: THERAPEUTIC INTERVENTIONS

1. Name the term that means removal of the following:

   A. a lobe of the lung ______________

   B. part or all of the voice box ______________

   C. the palatine tonsils ______________

   D. the pharyngeal tonsils ______________

2. Name the term that means surgical repair of the following:

   A. the nose ______________

   B. the wall between the nostrils ______________

   C. the bronchi ______________

3. What is the term that means placement of a tube in the mouth or nose to the trachea to ensure an airway? ______________

4. A nasal cannula, Venturi mask, or endotracheal tube are means of delivering ______________ to patients with hypoxia.

Match the combining forms and suffixes with their meanings.

_____ 5. -centesis

_____ 6. tonsill/o

_____ 7. -ectomy

_____ 8. laryng/o

_____ 9. sinus/o

_____ 10. -plasty

_____ 11. bronch/o

_____ 12. sept/o

_____ 13. -tomy

_____ 14. trache/o

_____ 15. lob/o

_____ 16. pleur/o

_____ 17. -stomy

_____ 18. adenoid/o

_____ 19. rhin/o

A. windpipe
B. removal
C. voice box
D. wall, partition
E. pleura
F. nose
G. new opening
H. pharyngeal tonsils
I. incision
J. bronchus
K. surgical puncture
L. sinus
M. surgical repair
N. lobe
O. palatine tonsil

PHARMACOLOGY

Routes of administration for respiratory pharmaceuticals include the use of **ventilators**, devices that serve to assist respiration and intensive positive-pressure breathing. A hand-held **nebulizer** (HHN) is a device that produces a fine spray, such as for inhaled medications. An **inhaler** is a device for administering medications that are inhaled, such as vapors or fine powders. A spacer, a device connected to the inhaler that contains the mist expelled from the inhaler until the user can breathe it, is usually used for children.

Antihistamines: Block histamine receptors to manage allergies. Examples are clemastine (Tavist) and diphenhydramine (Benadryl).

Antitussives: Suppress the cough reflex. Examples include promethazine (Phenergan) and dextromethorphan (Hold DM).

Bronchodilators and antiasthmatics: Relax bronchi to improve ventilation to the lungs. Examples include theophylline (Bronkodyl), ipratropium (Atrovent), and albuterol (Proventil).

Decongestants: Reduce congestion or swelling of mucous membranes. An example is pseudoephedrine (Sudafed).

Expectorants: Promote the expulsion of mucus from the respiratory tract. An example is guaifenesin (Robitussin).

Exercise 7: PHARMACOLOGY

Matching.

_____ 1. drug that relaxes the bronchi

_____ 2. drug that expels mucus

_____ 3. drug that reduces congestion

_____ 4. drug that helps manage allergies

_____ 5. drug that suppresses coughs

A. antihistamine
B. antitussive
C. antiasthmatic
D. decongestant
E. expectorant

6. What type of device is used to produce a fine spray for inhaled medications?

nebulizer ________________

7. What type of device is used to administer medications that are inhaled, such as fine powders or vapors? ________________

8. A/An ________________ is a device to assist in respiration and intensive positive-pressure breathing.

Case Study Continued

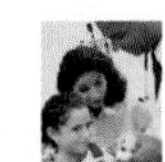

Will counsels Casey and her mother on how to manage Casey's asthma. She is prescribed a bronchodilator to relax the smooth muscle of the airways from the trachea to the bronchioles and an inhaled steroid to prevent mucus buildup in the bronchioles. She receives instructions in how to use an inhaler with a spacer, a tube that keeps the inhaler mist from scattering in the air. After a couple of tries, Casey is able to manage the inhaler.

Within a couple of days, Casey is back playing with her softball team. She occasionally experiences asthmatic symptoms but is able to treat them quickly with her inhalers.

Abbreviations

Abbreviation	Definition	Abbreviation	Definition
AP	Anteroposterior	LUL	Left upper lobe
COPD	Chronic obstructive pulmonary disease	MDI	Metered dose inhaler
CPAP	Continuous positive airway pressure	PA	Posteroanterior
CRT	Certified respiratory therapist	PPB	Positive-pressure breathing
CTA	Clear to auscultation	PPD	Purified protein derivative
CWP	Coal worker's pneumoconiosis	RAD	Reactive airway disease
CXR	Chest x-ray	RLL	Right lower lobe
DOE	Dyspnea on exertion	RML	Right middle lobe
ENT	Ear, nose, and throat	RRT	Registered respiratory therapist
HHN	Hand-held nebulizer	RUL	Right upper lobe
LLL	Left lower lobe	SOB	Shortness of breath
		TB	Tuberculosis
		URI	Upper respiratory infection

Exercise 8: ABBREVIATIONS

Write out the following abbreviations.

1. A CXR revealed RML pneumonia in the 43-year-old teacher. ________________
2. The patient was tested with PPD for suspected TB. ________________
3. Solange had rhinorrhea and a productive cough, and she was diagnosed with a URI.

____

4. The patient with COPD presented with dyspnea, DOE, and a chronic cough.

____

5. Years of work in the mines resulted in the patient's diagnosis of CWP.

____

Careers

Respiratory Therapists

Respiratory therapists assess, treat, and care for patients with respiratory disorders. They are qualified to treat all ages of patients, but, according to the *Occupational Outlook Handbook,* job opportunities will be greatest for those therapists with cardiopulmonary care skills and those who treat newborns and infants. Most therapists will work in a hospital setting and, as with many healthcare occupations, will risk catching infectious diseases.

Training for this field is offered in a variety of settings (e.g., hospitals, medical schools, trade schools), but the majority of programs are either 2-year programs leading to an associate degree or 4-year programs leading to a bachelor's degree. Coursework includes anatomy and physiology, chemistry, physics, microbiology, and mathematics.

Licensing is required by over 40 states. The National Board for Respiratory Care offers voluntary certification and registration. Individuals who complete coursework in a respiratory therapy program may sit for an exam to earn the credential of a Certified Respiratory Therapist (CRT). A Registered Respiratory Therapist (RRT) credential may be pursued after 2 years of experience.

Employment in respiratory therapy is expected to increase much faster than the average for all occupations through the year 2010 because of the aging population.

Information concerning respiratory therapy careers may be obtained from the American Association for Respiratory Care at http://www.aarc.org and the National Board for Respiratory Care, Inc. at http://www.nbrc.org. Information on CoARC-accredited educational programs for respiratory therapy occupations can be acquired from the Committee on Accreditation for Respiratory Care at http://www.coarc.com.

http: INTERNET PROJECT

Asthma is a condition that accounts for almost 500,000 hospital admissions each year. It affects both sexes and all ages, although the mortality rates are highest for African Americans between the ages of 15 and 24 years. Using the following Websites, write a 4-page report addressing the causes, signs and symptoms, treatments, and demographic statistics regarding asthma:

American Academy of Allergy, Asthma, and Immunology Online: http://www.aaaai.org
American Lung Association: http://www.lungusa.org
National Library of Medicine–Asthma: http://www.nlm.nih.gov/medlineplus/asthma.html

Chapter Review

A. Functions of the Respiratory System

Give four examples of functions you would lose if you were unable to use your respiratory system.

1. ______________________ 3. ______________________

2. ______________________ 4. ______________________

B. Anatomy and Physiology

5. Trace the route of air from the tip of the nose to the cells of the body. Include accessory structures and combining forms where appropriate (see Fig. 11-1, *A*).

____

____

____

6. What is the difference between internal and external respiration?

____

____

____

7. What are two terms for breathing in? ______________________

8. What are two terms for breathing out? ______________________

9. What is the structure that protects the airway from ingestion of food?

Epiglottis

10. What structure is equipped with vocal cords to produce speech? Larynx

11. Label the diagram provided with the terms for the structures of the respiratory system and their combining forms.

12. Label the diagram provided with the terms for the structures of the upper respiratory system and their combining forms.

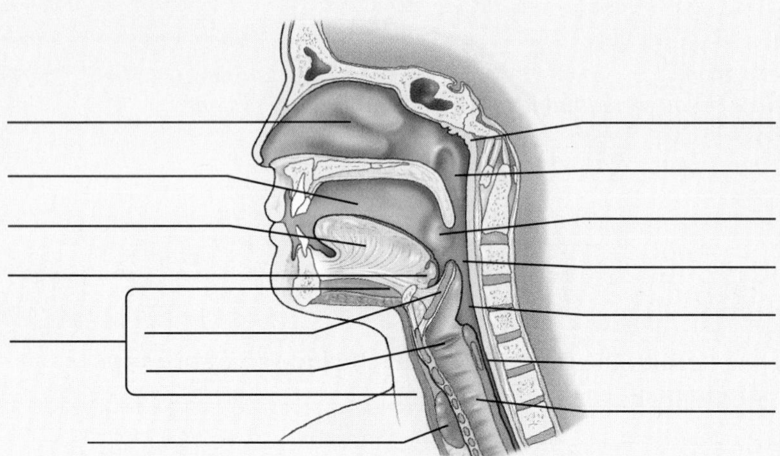

C. Pathology

13. What is the term for a runny nose? ______________________

14. What is the term for a bloody nose? ______________________

15. What is the term for an overwhelming sense of exhaustion? ______________________

16. What is the term for fever? ______________________

17. SOB stands for ______________________.
18. A condition of abnormal breathing marked by apnea and deep, rapid breathing is called

    ______________________.
19. What is an abnormal appearance of blueness, due to lack of oxygen?

    ____

20. What is a whistling sound heard during breathing? ______________________
21. What is material coughed up from the lungs and expectorated through the mouth?

    ____

22. What is a high-pitched inspiratory sound from the larynx? ______________________
23. What is a blunting of the distal phalanges seen in advanced chronic pulmonary disease?

    ____
24. What is a deflection of the nasal septum that may obstruct the nasal passages, possibly resulting in

    infection? ______________________

25. What is deficient O_2 in the tissues? ______________________
26. What is a rumbling sound heard on auscultation, usually caused by thick secretions or contractions of

    airways? ______________________

27. What is an abnormal condition of fungus in the nose? ____________

28. What type of chronic bacterial lung infection is resistant to drugs? ____________

29. What acute viral infection of early childhood is marked by stridor?

____

30. What is an accumulation of fluid in the lung? ____________

31. What is an accumulation of air in the pleural space? ____________

32. What is an infectious inflammation of the lungs? Pneumonia

33. What infection of the respiratory system is caused by an acid-fast bacillus?

TB

34. What is an inflammation of the parietal pleura that surrounds the lungs?

Pleurisy

35. What is the term for a collapsed lung or lung segment? ____________

Decode the term.

36. hypoxia ____________

37. hemoptysis ____________

38. dysphonia ____________

39. laryngitis ____________

40. pneumoconiosis ____________

41. pyothorax Pus pleural Cavity

Build a term.

42. excessive CO_2 in the blood ____________

43. discharge from the nose ____________

44. rapid breathing ____________

45. inflammation of the bronchi ____________

46. inflammation of the nose and eustachian tube ____________

D. Diagnostic Procedures

47. What is the diagnostic technique that means listening and tapping?

____

48. What is the laboratory procedure for determining the pathogen present in sputum?

____

49. A Mantoux skin test is done to detect antibodies for what disorder? ______________________

50. What is an endoscopy of the space between the lungs? ______________________

51. An instrument used to listen to sounds within the chest is a/an ______________________.

52. An instrument used to test breathing capacity in a PFT is a/an ______________________.

53. A sweat test is done to diagnose ______________________.

54. A blood test to determine O_2 and CO_2 is ______________________.

55. A lung ventilation scan is done to determine ______________________.

Decode the term.

56. spirometer ______________________

57. bronchoscopy ______________________

58. pulmonary angiography ______________________

Build a term.

59. a visual examination of the voice box ______________________

60. process of measurement of breathing ______________________

61. process of recording with the use of high-frequency sound waves ______________________

E. Therapeutic Interventions

62. What is the purpose of intubation? ______________________

63. Patients with hypoxia who need mechanical assistance may be placed on a ______________ and administered O_2 through a tube to the nose, called a nasal ______________.

64. What is the term for removal of a lobe of a lung? ______________________

65. What is a surgical repair of a bronchial defect? ______________________

66. What is an incision of the windpipe? ______________________

67. What is an excision of the pharyngeal tonsils? ______________________

Decode the term.

68. pleurocentesis ______________________

69. septoplasty ______________________

70. tonsillectomy ______________________

Build a term.

71. surgical repair of the nose ______________________

72. new opening of the windpipe ______________________

73. incision of the sinuses ______________________

F. Pharmacology

74. Someone who has trouble sleeping because of severe coughing due to an upper respiratory infection may be prescribed what type of drug? ______________________
75. An allergic reaction that is causing rhinorrhea, along with itchy eyes, may cause a physician to suggest that the patient take what type of drug? ______________________

76. Antiasthmatic drugs are often routed through a/an ______________________.
77. The generic drug pseudoephedrine is an example of what class of drug?

____

78. Albuterol is an example of what type of drug? ______________________

G. Abbreviations
Write the meanings of the following abbreviations.

79. Mrs. Vaslos is SOB. ______________________

80. Dr. Waskolicz has LLL pneumonia. ______________________

81. On examination, Gregory Sampson's chest is CTA. ______________________

82. The CXR performed for Dr. W is done in an AP view. ______________________

83. Ms. James experienced DOE climbing stairs. ______________________

H. Singulars and Plurals
Change the following terms from singular to plural.

84. sinus ______________________

85. bronchus ______________________

86. alveolus ______________________

87. pleura ______________________

88. larynx ______________________

89. pharynx ______________________

I. Translations

Rewrite the following sentences in your own words.

90. Paroxysmal dyspnea, SOB, and wheezing were signs that Sari had asthma.

91. The patient's dysphonia and laryngitis were associated with a URI.

92. The doctor termed the high-pitched inspiratory sound heard when the baby inhaled as stridor, a sign of croup.

93. The physician noted pyrexia, dyspnea, and thoracodynia before recording a finding of pleural effusion.

94. After 3 days of severe pharyngitis, the patient had a throat culture to determine the pathogen.

J. Cumulative Review

Circle the correct term in the following statements.

95. Patients with a finding of blunting of the apices of the lungs have a flattening of the *(tops, bottoms)* of the lungs.
96. Mr. Walker had a *(complicated, simple)* fracture of one of his ribs that pierced his left lung.
97. The 35-year-old patient was treated for *(psoriasis, cirrhosis)* on her scalp.
98. "I'm having trouble urinating," said the patient who was being seen for difficulty with *(micturition, mastication)*.
99. It was difficult to hear the patient with laryngitis who called, because she was exhibiting *(dysphonia, eupnea)*.

K. Be Careful

What are the differences between the following?

100. bronchi, brachi ______________________

101. ox/i, oxy- ______________________

102. What are the two meanings for salping/o? ______________________

103. Why is the term *stethoscope* a misnomer?

Trinity Hospital
9898 Old Elm Dr.
Portland, OR 97213

ED RECORD

Patient: Casey Sandoval Date: 3/23/02
Physician: Dr. McClintock

Casey Sandoval, an 8-year-old female, presented to the ED in moderately severe respiratory distress. She was accompanied by her mother. Pt appeared pale, anxious, slightly diaphoretic, and had slight nail bed cyanosis. Casey was unable to speak more than two or three word phrases between breaths. She was placed on oxygen per face mask, and connected to cardiac monitor and pulse oximetry. HR was 125, RR was 33, and labored oximetry measured 89% on 6 L/m O_2. Wheezes were auscultated in all lung fields, with prolonged expiratory phase. Pt has frequent nonproductive cough. Physical exam revealed intercostal retractions and use of accessory muscles on inspiration.

Pt was given an immediate nebulization treatment via hand-held nebulizer containing 5 mg Albuterol and 3 cc NS solution driven by 8 L/m O_2. Oximetry increased to 95% by end of nebulization. Peak flows were measured at 100 L/min post-HHN. Respirations had decreased to 25; heart rate was 95. Breath sounds revealed mild, scattered expiratory wheezes and rhonchi bilaterally. Repeat nebulizer treatment was performed 15 min later. Peak flow measurements had increased to 175 L/min, and pt was able to wean off supplemental oxygen and maintained oxygen saturation of 94% on room air.

A third HHN was ordered 30 min later, and repeat peak flows measured 210 L/min. Breath sounds were clear, and pt respiratory rate had decreased to 18 breaths/min, heart rate to 87, and saturation was 97% on room air.

Pt and parent were instructed on use of metered dose inhaler with spacer, and peak flow meter. MDIs containing Albuterol and Flovent 220 were prescribed. Child and parent were instructed to use 4 puffs Albuterol every 4 h, and 2 puffs Flovent bid. Peak flows were to be measured 3 times daily pre- and post-Albuterol and graphed on the diary card.

____
Patricia Fergus, RRT

L. Healthcare Report

104. In your own words, explain the meaning of the symptoms "slightly diaphoretic" and "circumoral cyanosis."

____

105. How is oxygen measured in pulse oximetry?

____

106. Name and define the two abnormal sounds heard on auscultation.

____

107. What was the most likely reason that a spacer was used with the inhaler given to Casey?

____

108. What is the purpose of a peak flow meter?

____

109. What does the abbreviation HHN mean?

____

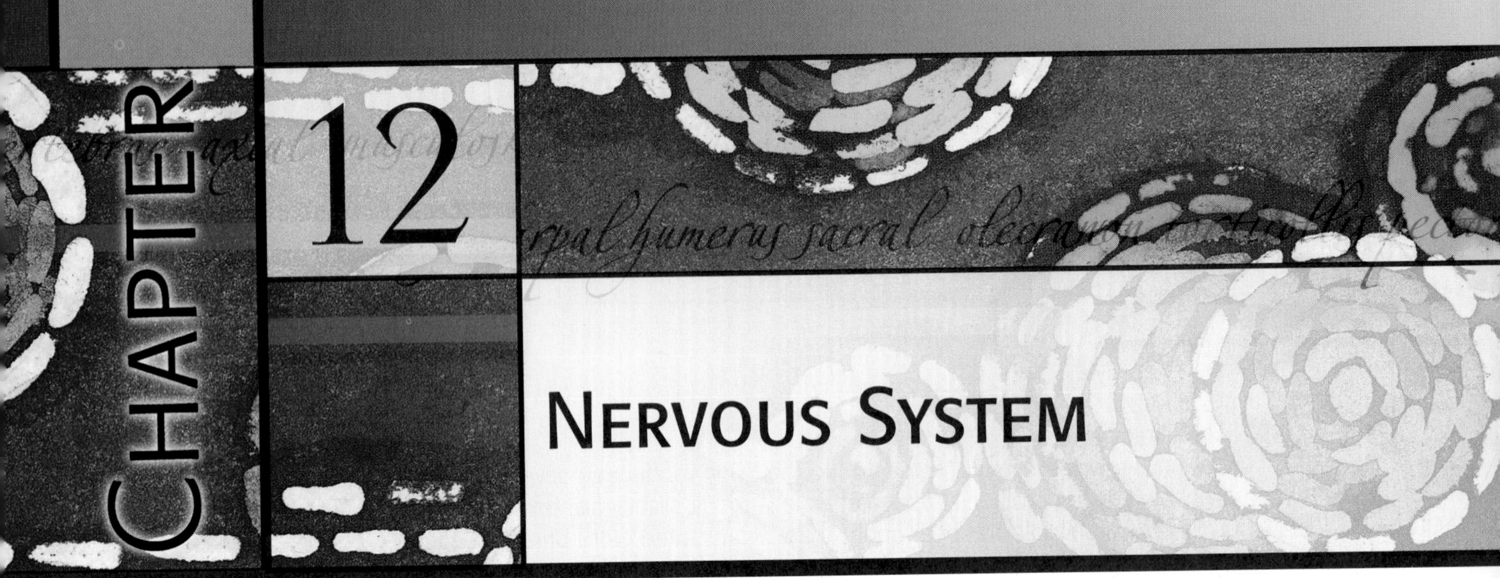

CHAPTER 12 NERVOUS SYSTEM

"Many ambitious people spend the first half of their life ruining their health to earn money and the second half spending that money to regain their health." **—Bashir Quereshi**

Quote

Case Study

Retirement was not going quite the way Max Janovski had planned. The 75-year-old former stockbroker had been visiting his son's family when he became dizzy and fainted. He quickly regained consciousness, only to find that he had difficulty using the right side of his body, and his speech was slurred. The symptoms were of brief duration, and Max insisted that he was fine. However, his son insisted he go to the emergency department (ED). Max was admitted to the hospital and subsequently suffered a stroke while there. The stroke's sequelae required the services of an occupational therapist (OT), Melissa Wood, to help Max take care of himself, and a physical therapist (PT), Eduardo Menendez, to help him regain his physical abilities.

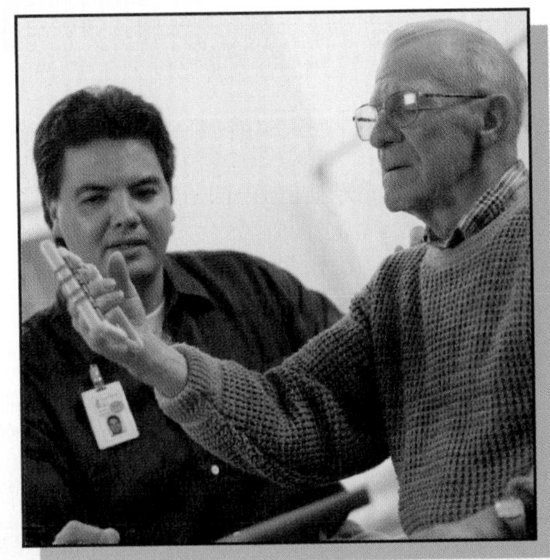

OBJECTIVES

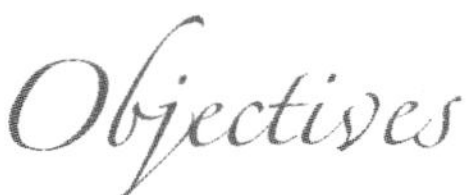

- In your own words, explain the functions of the nervous system.
- Recognize, recall, and apply healthcare terms related to the anatomy and physiology of the nervous system.
- Recognize, recall, and apply healthcare terms related to the pathology of the nervous system.
- Recognize, recall, and apply healthcare terms related to diagnostic procedures of the nervous system.
- Recognize, recall, and apply healthcare terms related to the therapeutic interventions of the nervous system.
- Recognize, recall, and apply the abbreviations introduced in this chapter.
- Recognize, recall, and apply word components used in this chapter to build and decode healthcare terms relevant to the nervous system.
- Demonstrate the ability to change singular terms to plural form.
- Recognize, recall, and apply material learned in previous chapters.

FUNCTIONS OF THE NERVOUS SYSTEM

Possibly the most complex and poorly understood system, the nervous system plays a major role in **homeostasis** (hoh mee oh STAY sis), keeping the other body systems coordinated and regulated to achieve optimum performance. It accomplishes this goal by helping the individual respond to his or her internal and external environments.

The nervous and endocrine systems are responsible for communication and control throughout the body. There are three main **neural** functions, which are as follows:

1. Collecting information about the external and internal environment *(sensing)*.
2. Processing this information and making decisions about action *(interpreting)*.
3. Directing the body to put into play the decisions made *(acting)*.

For example, the sensory function begins with a stimulus (e.g., the uncomfortable pinch of tight shoes). That information travels to the brain, where it is interpreted. The return message is sent to react to the stimulus (e.g., remove the shoes).

Exercise 1: FUNCTIONS OF THE NERVOUS SYSTEM

Circle the correct answer.

1. The action of the nervous system can be divided into three functions: sensing → *(interpreting, controlling)* → acting.
2. The nervous system has the responsibility of communication and control throughout the body, along with the *(gastrointestinal, endocrine)* system.
3. The function of maintaining a steady state is called *(homeostasis, stimulation)*.

ANATOMY AND PHYSIOLOGY

Organization of the Nervous System

In order to carry out its functions, the nervous system is divided into two main subsystems. (See Fig. 12-1 for a schematic of the divisions.) The **central nervous system (CNS)** is composed of the brain and the spinal cord. It is the only site of nerve cells called **interneurons** (in tur NOOR ons), which connect sensory and motor neurons. The **peripheral nervous system (PNS)** is composed of the nerves that extend from the brain and spinal cord to the tissues of the body. These are organized into 12 pairs of cranial nerves and 31 pairs of spinal nerves. The PNS is further divided into voluntary and involuntary neurons, which may be **afferent** (or **sensory**), carrying impulses to the brain and spinal cord, or **efferent** (or **motor**), carrying impulses from the brain and spinal cord to either voluntary or involuntary muscles.

PNS nerves are further categorized into two subsystems:

Somatic (soh MAT ick) **system:** This system is *voluntary* in nature. These nerves collect information from and return instructions to the skin, muscles, and joints.

Autonomic (ah toh NAH mick) **system:** Mostly *involuntary* functions are controlled by this system as sensory information from the internal environment is sent to the CNS, and, in return, motor impulses from the CNS are sent to involuntary muscles: the heart, glands, and organs.

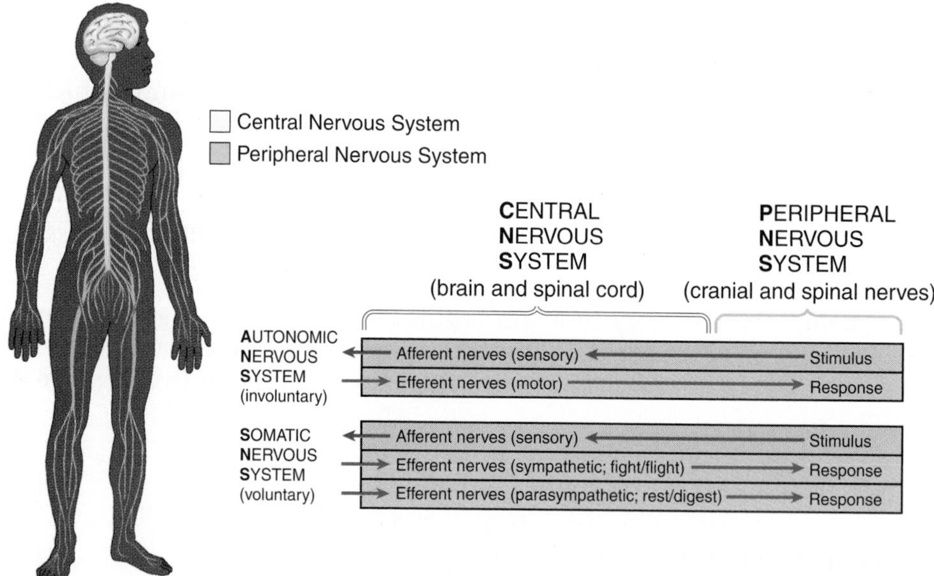

Fig. 12-1 The nervous system. Afferent nerves carry nervous impulses from a stimulus toward the CNS. Efferent nerves carry the impulse away from the CNS to effect a response to the stimulus.

Exercise 2: ORGANIZATION OF THE NERVOUS SYSTEM

Fill in the blanks.

1. The two main divisions of the nervous system are the ______________ and the ______________.

Circle the correct answer.

2. Sensory neurons *(transmit, receive)* information *(to, from)* the CNS.
3. Motor neurons, also called *(efferent, afferent)* neurons, transmit information *(to, from)* the CNS.
4. The *(somatic, autonomic)* nervous system is voluntary in nature, whereas the *(somatic, autonomic)* nervous system is largely involuntary.

Cells of the Nervous System

The nervous system is made up of the following two types of cells:

1. Parenchymal cells, or **neurons**, the cells that carry out the work of the system.
2. Stromal cells, or **glia** (GLEE uh), the cells that provide a supportive function.

Neurons

The basic unit of the nervous system is the nerve cell, or neuron (Fig. 12-2). Not all neurons are the same, but all have the following features in common. **Dendrites** (DEN drytes), projections from the cell body, receive **neural impulses,** also called **action potentials,** from a **stimulus** of some kind. This impulse travels along the dendrite and into the cell body, which is the control center of the cell. This cell body contains the nucleus and surrounding cytoplasm.

From the cell body, the impulse moves out along the **axon** (AX on), a slender, elongated projection that carries the nervous impulse toward the next neuron. The **terminal fibers** are the final branching of the axon and the site of the **axon terminals** that store the chemical **neurotransmitters.** In neurons *outside* the CNS, the axon is covered by a material called **myelin** (MY uh lin), which is a substance produced by **Schwann** (shvahn) **cells** that coat the axons.

From the axon's terminal fibers, the neurotransmitter is released from the cell to travel across the space between these terminal fibers and the dendrites of the next cell. This space is called the **synapse** (SIN aps) (see Fig. 12-2). The impulse continues in this manner until its destination is reached.

Glia

These supportive, or stromal, cells are also called **neuroglia** (noo RAH glee ah). They accomplish their supportive function by physically holding the neurons together and also protecting them. One type of neuroglia, the **astrocytes** (AS troh sites), connect neurons and blood vessels and form a structure called the **blood-brain barrier (BBB)** that prevents or slows the passage of some drugs and disease-causing organisms to the CNS.

DID YOU KNOW?

Small collections of nerve cell bodies outside the brain and spinal cord (i.e., in the PNS) are called **ganglia** (GANG glee uh) (*sing.* ganglion).

DID YOU KNOW?

The myelin sheath that coats the axons gives the neuron a white appearance, which inspired the term *white matter.*

BE CAREFUL!

The abbreviation *BBB* can stand for either *blood-brain barrier* or *bundle branch block,* a cardiac condition.

DID YOU KNOW?

Glia means *glue* because they hold the neurons together. *Dendrite* means *tree* and *astr/o* means *star* because of their appearances.

COMBINING FORMS FOR CELLS OF THE NERVOUS SYSTEM

MEANING	COMBINING FORM
body	somat/o
ganglion	gangli/o
glue	gli/o
nerve	neur/o
star	astr/o
tree	dendr/o

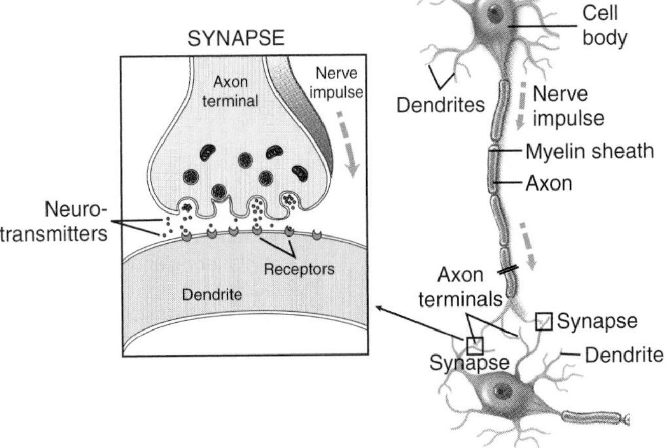

Fig. 12-2 The nerve cell (neuron) with an inset of a synapse.

Exercise 3: Cells of the Nervous System

1. List words connected by arrows to show the path of the action potential from initial stimulus to synapse.

____

Matching.

_____ 2. star
_____ 3. body
_____ 4. nerve
_____ 5. ganglion
_____ 6. glue
_____ 7. tree

A. gangli/o
B. gli/o
C. somat/o
D. dendr/o
E. astr/o
F. neur/o

The Central Nervous System

As stated previously, the CNS is composed of the **brain** and the **spinal cord.**

The Brain

The brain is one of the most complex organs of the body. It is divided into four parts: the **cerebrum** (suh REE brum), the **cerebellum** (sair ih BELL um), the **diencephalon** (dye en SEF fuh lon), and the **brainstem** (Fig. 12-3).

CEREBRUM. The largest portion of the brain, the cerebrum is divided into two halves, or hemispheres (Fig. 12-4). It is responsible for thinking, reasoning, and memory. The surfaces of the hemispheres are covered with **gray matter** and are called the **cerebral cortex.** Arranged into folds, the valleys are referred to as **sulci** (SULL sye) (*sing.* sulcus), and the ridges are **gyri** (JYE rye) (*sing.* gyrus). The cerebrum is further divided into sections called **lobes,** which each have their own functions:

1. The **frontal lobe** contains the functions of speech and the motor area that controls voluntary movement on the contralateral side of the body.
2. The **temporal** (TEM pur rul) **lobe** contains the auditory and olfactory areas.
3. The **parietal** (puh RYE uh tul) **lobe** controls the sensations of touch and taste.
4. The **occipital** (ock SIP ih tul) **lobe** is responsible for vision.

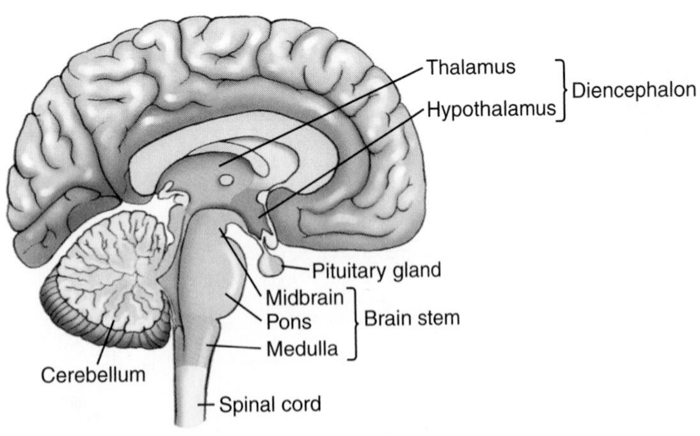

Fig. 12-3 The brain.

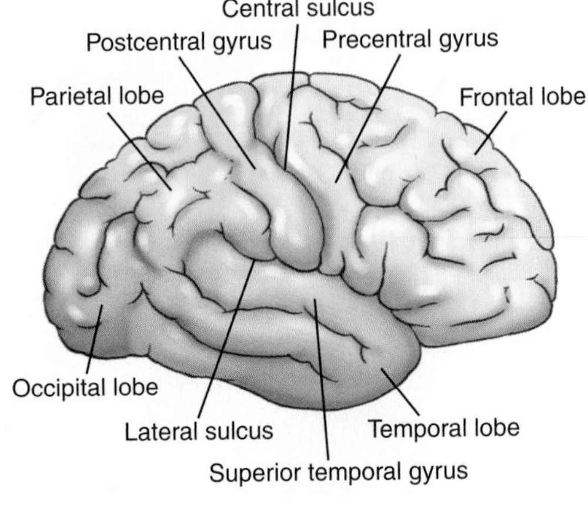

Fig. 12-4 The cerebrum.

Cerebellum. Located inferior to the occipital lobe of the cerebrum, the **cerebellum** coordinates voluntary movement but is involuntary in its function. For example, walking is a voluntary movement. The coordination needed for the muscles and other body parts to walk smoothly is involuntary and controlled by the cerebellum.

Diencephalon. The diencephalon is composed of the **thalamus** (THAL uh mus) and the structure inferior to it, the **hypothalamus** (HYE poh thal uh mus). The thalamus is responsible for relaying sensory information (with the exception of smell) and translating it into sensations of pain, temperature, and touch. The hypothalamus activates, integrates, and controls the peripheral autonomic nervous system, along with many functions such as body temperature, sleep, and appetite.

Brainstem. The brainstem connects the cerebral hemispheres to the spinal cord. It is composed of three main parts: **midbrain, pons** (ponz), and **medulla oblongata** (muh DOO lah ob lon GAH tah). The midbrain connects the pons and cerebellum with the hemispheres of the cerebrum. It is the site of reflex centers for eye and head movements in response to visual and auditory stimuli. The second part of the brainstem, the pons, serves as a bridge between the medulla oblongata and the cerebrum. Finally, the lowest part of the brainstem, the medulla oblongata, regulates heart rate, blood pressure, and breathing.

The Spinal Cord

The spinal cord extends from the medulla oblongata to the first lumbar vertebra (Fig. 12-5). It then extends into a structure called the **cauda equina** (KAH dah eh KWY nah). The spinal cord is protected by the bony vertebrae surrounding it and the coverings unique to the CNS called **meninges** (meh NIN jeez). The spinal cord is composed of **gray matter**, the cell bodies of motor neurons, and **white matter**, the myelin-covered axons or nerve fibers that extend from the nerve cell bodies. The 31 pairs of spinal nerves emerge from the spinal cord at the **nerve roots.**

Be Careful!

Myel/o can mean *bone marrow* or *spinal cord*—memorization and context will be the student's only methods to determine which is which.

Did You Know?

Cauda equina is a Latin term meaning *horse tail.*

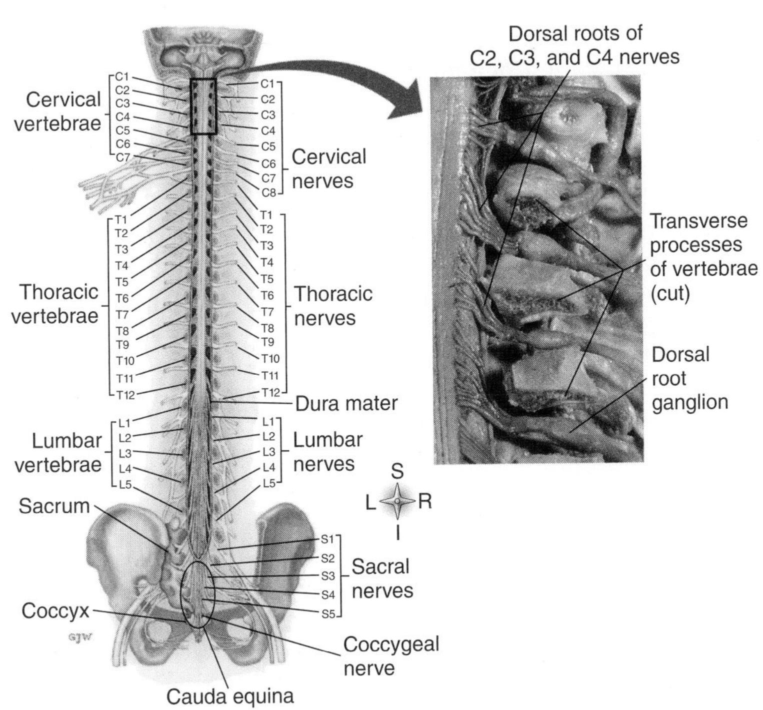

Fig. 12-5 The spinal cord with an inset of a cervical segment showing emerging cervical nerves.

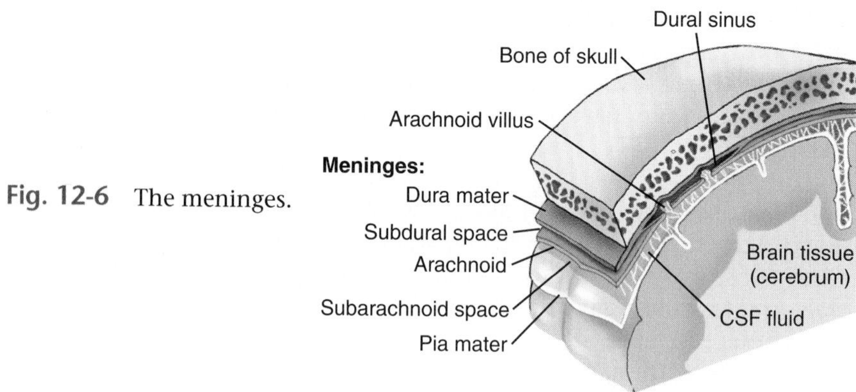

Fig. 12-6 The meninges.

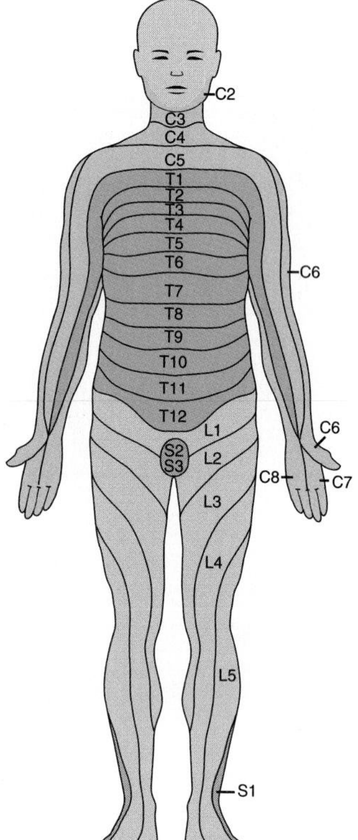

Fig. 12-7 Dermatomes. Each dermatome is named for the spinal nerve that serves it.

MENINGES. Meninges act as protective coverings for the CNS and are composed of three layers separated by spaces (Fig. 12-6). The **dura mater** (DUR ah MAY tur) is the tough, fibrous, outer covering of the meninges; its literal meaning is *hard mother.* The space between the dura mater and arachnoid membrane is called the **subdural space.** Next comes the **arachnoid** (uh RACK noyd) **membrane,** a thin, delicate membrane that takes its name from its spidery appearance. The **subarachnoid space** is the space between the arachnoid membrane and the pia mater, containing **cerebrospinal fluid (CSF).** CSF is also present in cavities in the brain called **ventricles.** Finally, the **pia mater** (PEE uh MAY tur) is the thin, vascular membrane that is the innermost of the three meninges; its literal meaning is *soft mother.*

The Peripheral Nervous System

The **peripheral nervous system** is divided into 12 pairs of **cranial nerves** that conduct impulses between the brain and the head, neck, thoracic, and abdominal areas, and 31 pairs of **spinal nerves** that closely mimic the organization of the vertebrae and provide innervation to the rest of the body. If the nerve fibers from several spinal nerves form a network, it is termed a **plexus** (PLECK sus). Spinal nerves are named by their location (cervical, thoracic, lumbar, sacral, and coccygeal), as well as by number. Cranial nerves are named by their number and also their function or distribution.

Dermatomes (DUR mah tomes) are skin surface areas supplied by a single afferent spinal nerve. These areas are so specific that it is actually possible to map the body by dermatomes (Fig. 12-7). This specificity can be demonstrated in patients with shingles, who show similar patterns as specific peripheral nerves are affected (see Fig. 12-12).

The **autonomic nervous system (ANS)** consists of nerves that regulate involuntary function. Examples include cardiac muscle and smooth muscle. The motor portion of this system is further divided into the sympathetic nervous system and the parasympathetic nervous system, two opposing systems that provide balance in the rest of the body systems:

- The **sympathetic nervous system** is capable of producing a "fight-or-flight" response. This is the one part of the nervous system that helps the individual respond to perceived stress. The heart rate and blood pressure increase, digestive processes slow, and sweat and adrenal glands increase their secretions.
- The **parasympathetic nervous system** tends to do the opposite of the sympathetic nervous system—slowing the heart rate, lowering blood pressure, increasing digestive functions, and decreasing adrenal and sweat gland activity. This is sometimes called the "rest and digest" system.

BE CAREFUL!

The term *dermatome* can be used to describe an instrument that cuts thin slices of skin for grafting, and the term also signifies a mesodermal layer in early development, which becomes the dermal layers of the skin.

An example of a sensory response follows:

"Eight-year-old Joey is hungry. He decides to sneak some cookies before dinner. Afraid his mother will see him, he surreptitiously takes a handful into the hall closet and shuts the door. As he begins to eat, the closet door flies open. Joey's heart begins to race as he whips the cookies out of sight. When he sees it's only his sister, he relaxes and offers her a cookie as a bribe not to tell on him."

Joey's afferent (sensory) somatic neurons carried the message to his brain that he was hungry. This message was interpreted by his brain as a concern, and the response was to sneak cookies from the jar and hide himself as he ate them. When the closet door flew open, his sensory neurons perceived a danger and triggered a sympathetic "fight-or-flight" response, which raised his heart rate and blood pressure and stimulated his sweat glands. When the intruder was perceived to be harmless, his parasympathetic nervous system took over and reduced his heart rate, bringing it back to normal. The same afferent fibers perceived the intruder in two different ways, with two different sets of autonomic motor responses (sympathetic and parasympathetic).

COMBINING FORMS FOR THE NERVOUS SYSTEM

MEANING	COMBINING FORM	MEANING	COMBINING FORM
brain	encephal/o	nerve root	radicul/o, rhiz/o
cerebellum	cerebell/o	skin	dermat/o
cerebrum	cerebr/o	spinal cord	cord/o, myel/o
dura mater	dur/o	spine	spin/o
meninges	mening/o, meningi/o	vertebra	spondyl/o, vertebr/o

Exercise 4: CENTRAL AND PERIPHERAL NERVOUS SYSTEM

Match the following parts of the brain with their functions.

_____ 1. pons

_____ 2. parietal cerebral lobe

_____ 3. hypothalamus

_____ 4. temporal cerebral lobe

_____ 5. midbrain

_____ 6. cerebellum

_____ 7. occipital cerebral lobe

_____ 8. thalamus

_____ 9. frontal cerebral lobe

_____ 10. medulla oblongata

A. auditory and olfactory activity
B. relays sensory information
C. reflex center for eye and head movements
D. sensation of vision
E. regulates heart rate, blood pressure, and breathing
F. regulates temperature, sleep, and appetite
G. speech and motor activity
H. connects medulla oblongata and cerebrum
I. coordinates voluntary movement
J. sensation of touch and taste

Match the CNS part with its combining form.

_____ 11. cerebellum

_____ 12. spinal cord

_____ 13. meninges

_____ 14. nerve root

_____ 15. dura mater

_____ 16. cerebrum

_____ 17. brain

_____ 18. skin

_____ 19. spine

A. meningi/o
B. myel/o
C. dur/o
D. rhiz/o
E. dermat/o
F. cerebr/o
G. spin/o
H. cerebell/o
I. encephal/o

20. Name the five layers of the meninges in order, from innermost to outermost.

____

Circle the correct answer.

21. The peripheral nervous system has *(12, 31)* pairs of cranial nerves and *(12, 31)* pairs of spinal nerves.
22. *(Afferent, Efferent)* nerves carry nerve impulses toward the CNS.
23. The *(sympathetic, parasympathetic)* nervous system is capable of producing a "rest and digest" response.

Case Study Continued

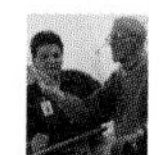

It is likely that one of the arteries in Max's brain was initially temporarily deprived of its blood flow, and hence, its oxygen. This is termed a *transient ischemic attack (TIA)*. The first blood clot either dislodged or disintegrated, only to be replaced by another while Max was in the hospital. This blood clot did not dissolve and subsequently caused his stroke, or cerebrovascular accident (CVA). Depending on the area affected, a neural deficit will develop when a clot lodges in the brain area. In Max's case, the clot on the left side of his brain caused weakness on his right side and slurred speech.

Be Careful!

Don't confuse *dysarthria* (difficulty with speech) and *dysarthrosis* (any disorder of a joint).

PATHOLOGY

The signs and symptoms for this system encompass many systems because of the nature of the neural function: communicating, or failing to communicate, with other parts of the body.

Terms Related to Signs and Symptoms

Term	Word Origin	Definition
Amnesia am NEE zsa		Loss of memory caused by brain damage or severe emotional trauma.
Aphasia ah FAY zsa	*a-* without *phas/o* speech *-ia* condition	Lack or impairment of the ability to form or understand speech. Less severe forms include **dysphasia** (dis FAY zsa) and **dysarthria** (dis AR three ah).
Asthenia as THEE nee ah	*a-* without *-sthenia* condition of strength	Muscle weakness.

Terms Related to Signs and Symptoms—cont'd

TERM	WORD ORIGIN	DEFINITION
Athetosis ath uh TOH sis		Continuous, involuntary, slow, writhing movement of the extremities.
Aura OR uh		Sensation that may precede an epileptic seizure or the onset of some types of headache. May be a sensation of light or warmth.
Dysphagia dis FAY zsa	*dys-* difficult *phag/o* eat *-ia* condition	Condition of difficulty with swallowing.
Fasciculation fah sick yoo LAY shun		Involuntary contraction of small, local muscles.
Gait, abnormal		Disorder in the manner of walking. An example is **ataxia** (uh TACK see uh), a lack of muscular coordination, as in cerebral palsy.
Hypokinesia hye poh kih NEE sza	*hypo-* deficient *kinesi/o* movement *-ia* condition	Decrease in normal movement; may be due to paralysis.
Parasomnia pair uh SOM nee ah	*para-* abnormal *somn/o* sleep *-ia* condition	Disorder of sleep. **Hypersomnia** is excessive depth or length or sleep; **insomnia** is the inability to sleep or stay asleep; and **somnambulism** (som NAM byoo lih zum) is walking in one's sleep.
Paresthesia pair uhs THEE zsa	*para-* abnormal *esthesi/o* feeling *-ia* condition	Feeling of prickling, burning, or numbness.
Seizure SEE zhur		Neuromuscular reaction to abnormal electrical activity within the brain (see Fig. 12-17). Causes include fever or epilepsy, a recurring seizure disorder; also called **convulsions.** Types of seizures include **tonic clonic (grand mal),** accompanied by temporary loss of consciousness and severe muscle spasms; **absence seizures (petit mal)** accompanied by loss of consciousness exhibited by unresponsiveness for short periods without muscle involvement. **Status epilepticus** (STA tis eh pih LEP tih kus) is a condition of intense, unrelenting, life-threatening seizures.
Spasm SPAZ um		Involuntary muscle contraction of sudden onset. Examples are hiccoughs, tics, and stuttering.
Syncope SINK oh pee		Fainting. A **vasovagal** (VAS soh VAY gul) **attack** is a form of syncope that results from abrupt emotional stress involving the vagus nerve's effect on blood vessels.
Tremors TREH murs		Rhythmic, quivering, purposeless skeletal muscle movements seen in some elderly individuals and in patients with various neurodegenerative disorders.
Vertigo	See **Did You Know?** box.	Dizziness.

DID YOU KNOW?

Vertigo is derived from a Latin term meaning *to turn.*

Terms Related to Learning and Perceptual Differences		
TERM	**WORD ORIGIN**	**DEFINITION**
Acalculia ay kal KYOO lee ah	*a-* without *calcul/o* stone *-ia* condition See **Did You Know?** box.	Inability to perform mathematical calculations.
Ageusia ah GOO zsa	*a-* without *geus/o* taste *ia* condition	Absence of the ability to taste. **Parageusia** (pair ah GOO zsa) is an abnormal sense of taste or a bad taste in the mouth.
Agnosia ag NOH zsa	*a-* without *gnos/o* knowledge *-ia* condition	Inability to recognize objects visually, auditorily, or with other senses.
Agraphia ah GRAFF ee ah	*a-* without *graph/o* record *-ia* condition	Inability to write.
Anosmia an NOS mee ah	*an-* without *osm/o* sense of smell *-ia* condition	Lack of sense of smell.
Apraxia ah PRACK see ah	*a-* without *prax/o* purposeful movement *-ia* condition	Inability to perform purposeful movements or to use objects appropriately.
Dyslexia dis LECK see ah	*dys-* bad *lex/o* word *-ia* condition	Inability or difficulty with reading and/or writing.
Romberg's sign		Indication of loss of the sense of position, in which the patient loses balance when standing erect, with feet together and eyes closed.

DID YOU KNOW?

The term *acalculia* comes from the Greek word for *stone.* Shepherds once used stones to keep track of (calculate) the number of sheep in the fields, using one stone for each sheep that went out in the morning and the same number of stones when the sheep returned that evening.

Exercise 5: NEUROLOGIC SIGNS, SYMPTOMS, AND PERCEPTUAL DIFFERENCES

Match the neurologic signs, symptoms, and perceptual differences with their combining forms.

_____ 1. sthen/o

_____ 2. phas/o

_____ 3. somn/o

_____ 4. calcul/o

_____ 5. geus/o

_____ 6. gnos/o

_____ 7. graph/o

_____ 8. lex/o

_____ 9. osm/o

A. taste
B. words
C. knowledge
D. strength
E. stone
F. sense of smell
G. record
H. speech
I. sleep

Match the sign/symptom with its meaning.

_____ 10. syncope	_____ 13. aura	A. dizziness
_____ 11. vertigo	_____ 14. fasciculation	B. involuntary contraction of small muscles
_____ 12. amnesia		C. loss of memory
		D. fainting
		E. premonition

Terms Related to Congenital Disorders

TERM	WORD ORIGIN	DEFINITION
Cerebral palsy (CP) SAIR uh brul PALL zee	*cerebr/o* cerebrum *-al* pertaining to	Motor function disorder as a result of permanent, nonprogressive brain defect or lesion caused perinatally. Neural deficits may include paralysis, ataxia, **athetosis** (a thih TOE sis) (slow, writhing movements of the extremities), seizures, and/or impairment of sensory functions.
Huntington's chorea koh REE ah		Inherited disorder that manifests itself in adulthood as a progressive loss of neural control, uncontrollable jerking movements, and dementia.
Hydrocephalus hye droh SEFF uh lus	*hydr/o* water *-cephalus* head	Condition of abnormal accumulation of fluid in the ventricles of the brain; may or may not result in mental retardation.
Spina bifida SPY nah BIFF uh dah	*bi-* two *-fida* split	Condition in which the spinal column has an abnormal opening that allows the protrusion of the meninges and/or the spinal cord. This is termed a **meningocele** (meh NIN goh seel) or **meningomyelocele** (meh nin go MY eh loh seel) (Fig. 12-8).
Tay-Sachs tay sacks		Inherited disease that occurs mainly in people of Eastern European Jewish origin; characterized by an enzyme deficiency that results in CNS deterioration.

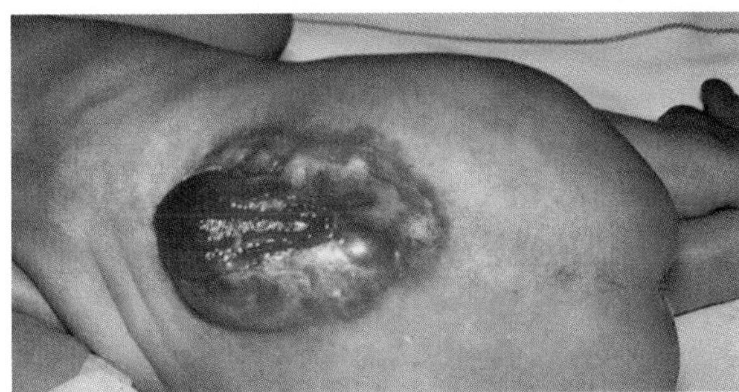

Fig. 12-8 Meningomyelocele.

Terms Related to Traumatic Conditions		
TERM	**WORD ORIGIN**	**DEFINITION**
Coma KOH mah		Deep, prolonged unconsciousness from which the patient cannot be aroused; usually the result of a head injury, neurologic disease, acute hydrocephalus, intoxication, or metabolic abnormalities.
Concussion kun KUH shun		Serious head injury characterized by one or more of the following: loss of consciousness, amnesia, seizures, or a change in mental status.
Contusion, cerebral kun TOO zhun		Head injury of sufficient force to bruise the brain. Bruising of the brain often involves the brain surface and causes extravasation of blood without rupture of the pia-arachnoid; often associated with a concussion.
Hematoma hee muh TOH mah	*hemat/o* blood *-oma* tumor, mass	Localized collection of blood, usually clotted, in an organ, tissue, or space, due to a break in the wall of a blood vessel (Fig. 12-9).

BE CAREFUL!

Although the word origin of the term *hematoma* means a *blood tumor,* this is a misnomer. A hematoma is a mass of blood that has leaked out of a vessel and pooled.

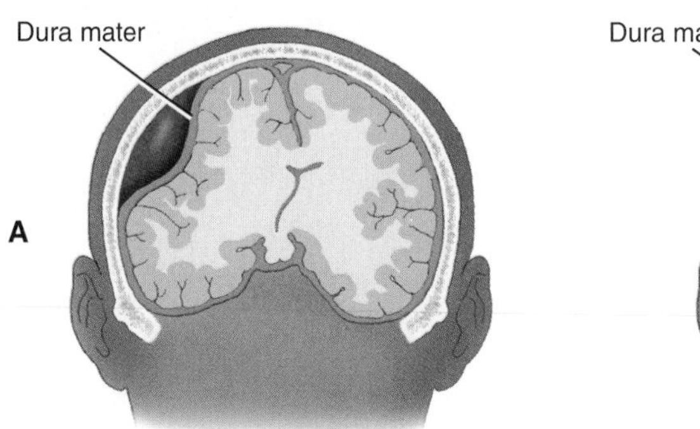

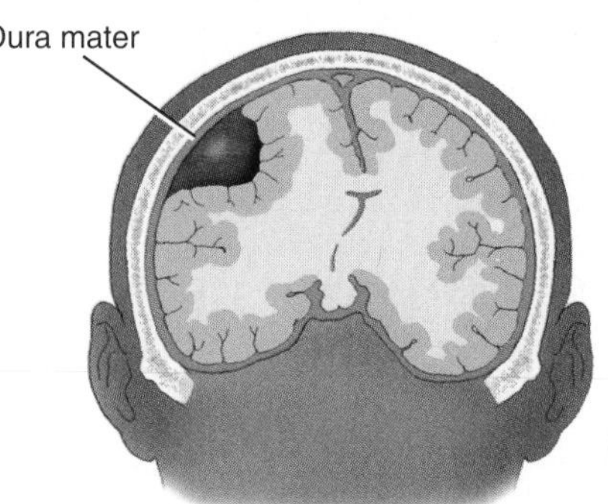

Fig. 12-9 **A,** Epidural hematoma. **B,** Subdural hematoma.

Exercise 6: CONGENITAL AND TRAUMATIC CONDITIONS

Fill in the blanks with the correct congenital disorder term listed below.

Tay-Sachs, hydrocephalus, cerebral palsy, spina bifida, Huntington's chorea

1. A condition characterized by an abnormal opening of the spine, allowing the protrusion of the meninges and possibly the spinal cord. _______________
2. An inherited disorder resulting in dementia and a progressive loss of neural control beginning in adulthood. _______________
3. A condition characterized by an accumulation of fluid in the ventricles of the brain. _______________
4. An inherited disease of people of Eastern European descent that results in a deterioration of the brain and spinal cord as a result of an enzyme deficiency. _______________
5. Permanent motor function disorder as a result of brain damage during the perinatal period. _______________

Fill in the blanks with the correct trauma term listed below.

cerebral contusion, concussion, coma, epidural hematoma, subdural hematoma

6. Prolonged unconsciousness from which the patient cannot be aroused is termed ______________.
7. Head injury accompanied by amnesia, loss of consciousness, seizures, and/or change in mental status is called a/an ______________.
8. Bruising of the brain with hemorrhage and swelling is a/an ______________.
9. Collection of blood, if above the dura mater, is described as a/an ______________, or if below it, a/an ______________.

Terms Related to Degenerative Disorders

TERM	WORD ORIGIN	DEFINITION
Alzheimer's disease (AD) ALLTZ hye murz		Progressive, neurodegenerative disease in which patients exhibit an impairment of cognitive functioning. The cause of the disease is unknown. Alzheimer's is the most common cause of dementia (Fig. 12-10).
Amyotrophic lateral sclerosis (ALS) ay mye oh TROH fick LAT ur ul sklih ROH sis	*a-* no *my/o* muscle *troph/o* development *-ic* pertaining to *later/o* side *-al* pertaining to	Degenerative, fatal disease of the motor neurons, in which patients exhibit progressive asthenia and muscle atrophy; also called **Lou Gehrig's disease.**
Dementia deh MEN sha	*de-* lack of *ment/o* mind *-ia* condition	Chronic, progressive, organic mental disorder characterized by chronic personality disintegration; symptoms include confusion, disorientation, stupor, deterioration of intellectual capacity and function, and impairment of memory, judgment, and impulse control.
Guillain-Barré syndrome GEE on bar AY		Autoimmune disorder of acute polyneuritis producing profound myasthenia that may lead to paralysis.

Continued

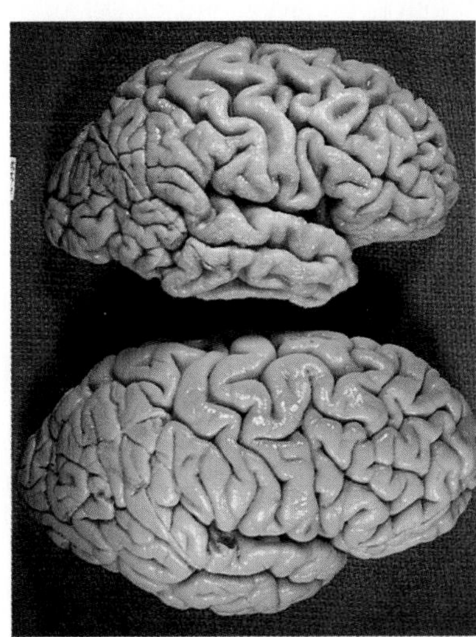

Fig. 12-10 Alzheimer's disease. The affected brain *(top)* is smaller and shows narrow gyri and widened sulci compared with the normal, age-matched brain *(bottom)*.

Terms Related to Degenerative Disorders—cont'd

TERM	WORD ORIGIN	DEFINITION
Multiple sclerosis (MS)	*sclerosis* condition of hardening	Neurodegenerative disease characterized by destruction of the myelin sheaths on the CNS neurons (demyelination) and their abnormal replacement by the gradual accumulation of hardened plaques. The disease may be progressive or characterized by remissions and relapses. Etiology is unknown (Fig. 12-11).
Parkinson's disease (PD)		Progressive neurodegenerative disease characterized by tremors, fasciculations, slow shuffling gait, hypokinesia, dysphasia, and dysphagia.

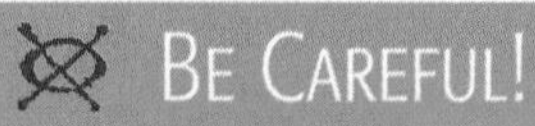

MS stands for both *musculoskeletal system* and *multiple sclerosis.*

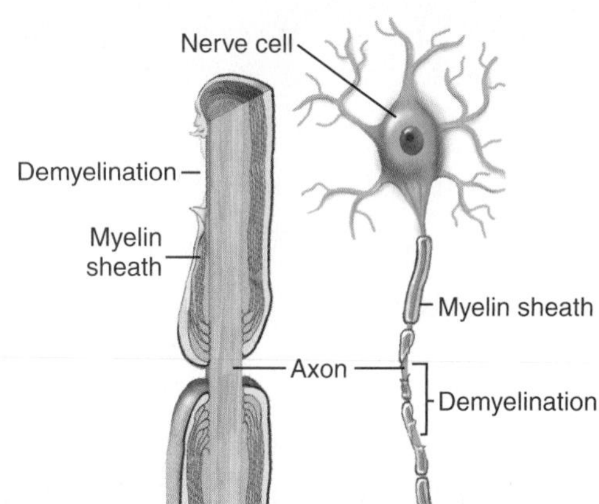

Fig. 12-11 Nerve sheath demyelination seen in multiple sclerosis.

Terms Related to Nondegenerative Disorders

TERM	WORD ORIGIN	DEFINITION
Bell's palsy PALL zee		Paralysis of the facial nerve. Unknown in etiology, the condition usually resolves on its own within 6 months.
Epilepsy EP ih lep see	*epi-* above *-lepsy* seizure	Group of disorders characterized by some or all of the following: recurrent seizures, sensory disturbances, abnormal behavior, and/or loss of consciousness. Causes may be trauma, tumor, intoxication, chemical imbalance, or vascular disturbances.
Narcolepsy NAR koh lep see	*narc/o* sleep *-lepsy* seizure	Disorder characterized by sudden attacks of sleep.
Tourette's syndrome tur ETTS		Abnormal condition characterized by facial grimaces, tics, involuntary arm and shoulder movements, and involuntary vocalizations, including **coprolalia** (kop pro LAYL yah) (the use of vulgar, obscene, or sacrilegious language).

Exercise 7: DEGENERATIVE AND NONDEGENERATIVE DISORDERS

Fill in the blank with the correct disorder listed below.

Alzheimer's disease, Guillain-Barré syndrome, Bell's palsy, amyotrophic lateral sclerosis, Parkinson's disease, Tourette's syndrome

1. A paralysis of a facial nerve. ________________

2. A disease characterized by tics, facial grimaces, and involuntary vocalizations. ________________

3. A progressive disease characterized by a shuffling gait, tremors, and dysphasia. ________________

4. A degenerative fatal disorder of motor neurons. ________________

5. A progressive, degenerative disorder of impairment of cognitive functioning. ________________

6. An autoimmune disorder causing severe muscle weakness, often leading to paralysis. ________________

Matching.

_____ 7. later/o

_____ 8. narc/o

_____ 9. my/o

_____ 10. troph/o

_____ 11. myel/o

A. development
B. muscle
C. sleep
D. spinal cord
E. side

Terms Related to Infectious Diseases

TERM	WORD ORIGIN	DEFINITION
Encephalitis en seff uh LYE tis	*encephal/o* brain *-itis* inflammation	Inflammation of the brain, most frequently caused by a virus transmitted by the bite of an infected mosquito.
Meningitis men in JYE tis	*mening/o* meninges *-itis* inflammation	Any infection or inflammation of the membranes covering the brain and spinal cord, most commonly due to bacterial infection, although more severe strains are viral or fungal in nature.
Neuritis noo RYE tis	*neur/o* nerve *-itis* inflammation	Inflammation of the nerves.
Polyneuritis pall ee noo RYE tis	*poly-* many *neur/o* nerve *-itis* inflammation	Inflammation of many nerves.
Radiculitis rad ick kyoo LYE tis	*radicul/o* nerve root *-itis* inflammation	Inflammation of the root of a spinal nerve.
Sciatica sye AT ick kah		Inflammation of the sciatic nerve. Symptoms include pain and tenderness along the path of the nerve through the thigh and leg (see Fig. 3-14).
Shingles SHIN guls		Acute infection caused by the latent varicella zoster virus (chicken pox), characterized by the development of vesicular skin eruption underlying the route of cranial or spinal nerves; also called **herpes zoster** (HER pees ZAH ster) (Fig. 12-12).

Fig. 12-12 Shingles on dermatome T4.

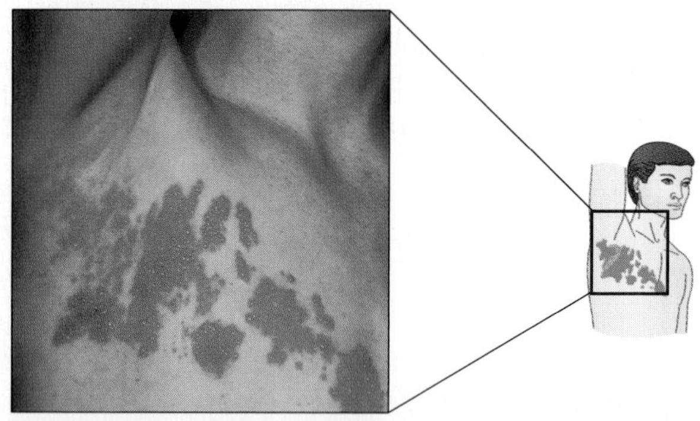

Terms Related to Vascular Disorders

Term	Word Origin	Meaning
Cerebrovascular accident (CVA) seh ree broh VAS kyoo lur	*cerebr/o* cerebrum *vascul/o* vessel *-ar* pertaining to	Ischemia of cerebral tissue due to an occlusion (blockage) from a thrombus (*pl.* thrombi) or embolus (*pl.* emboli), or as a result of a cerebral hemorrhage. Results of a stroke depend on the duration and location of the ischemia. These sequelae may include paralysis, weakness, speech defects, sensory changes that last more than 24 hours, or death. Also called **stroke, brain attack, cerebral infarction,** and **apoplexy** (A poh pleck see) (Fig. 12-13).
Migraine		Headache of vascular origin. May be classified as *migraine with aura* or *migraine without aura.*
Transient ischemic attack (TIA) TRANS ee ent is KEE mick	*ischem/o* hold back *-ia* condition	TIA has the same mechanisms as a CVA, but the sequelae resolve and disappear within 24 hours; also known as a **ministroke.**

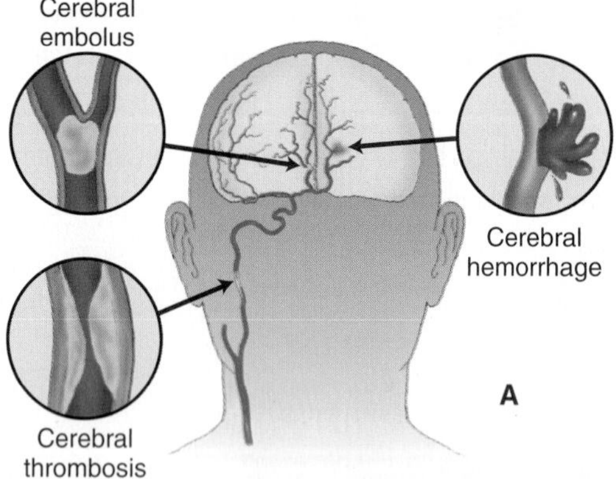

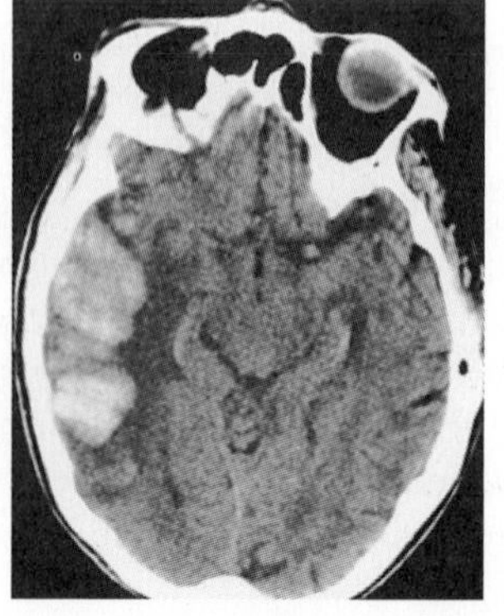

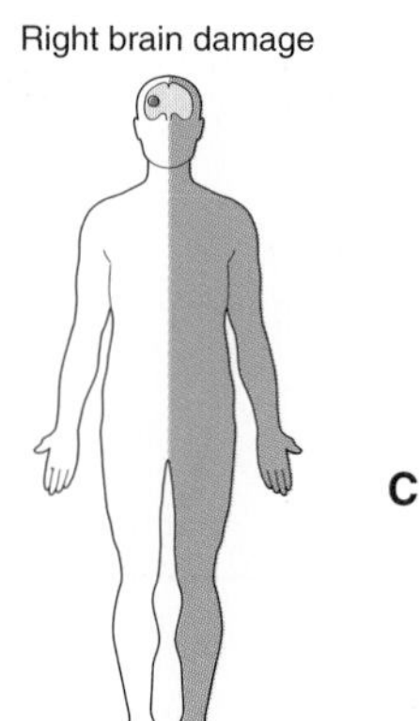

Fig. 12-13 Cerebrovascular accident (CVA). **A,** Events causing stroke. **B,** MRI showing hemorrhagic stroke in right cerebrum. **C,** Areas of the body affected by CVA.

Terms Related to Paralytic Conditions

TERM	WORD ORIGIN	DEFINITIONS
Diplegia dye PLEE jee ah	*di-* two *-plegia* paralysis	Paralysis of the same body part on both sides of the body.
Hemiparesis hem mee puh REE sis	*hemi-* half *-paresis* slight paralysis	Muscular weakness or slight paralysis on the left or right side of the body.
Hemiplegia hem mee PLEE jee ah	*hemi-* half *-plegia* paralysis	Paralysis on the left or right side of the body.
Monoparesis mah noh pah REE sis	*mono-* one *-plegia* paralysis	Weakness or slight paralysis on the left or right side of the body.
Monoplegia mah noh PLEE jee ah	*mono-* one *-plegia* paralysis	Paralysis of one limb on the left or right side of the body.
Paralysis puh RAL ih sis	*para-* abnormal *-lysis* destruction	Loss of muscle function, sensation, or both; may be described according to which side is affected and whether it is the dominant or nondominant side (Fig. 12-14).
Paraparesis pair uh pah REE sis	*para-* abnormal *-paresis* slight paralysis	Slight paralysis of the lower limbs and trunk.
Paraplegia pair uh PLEE jee ah	*para-* abnormal *-plegia* paralysis	Paralysis of the lower limbs and trunk.
Quadriparesis kwah drih pah REE sis	*quadri-* four *-paresis* slight paralysis	Weakness or slight paralysis of the arms, legs, and trunk.
Quadriplegia kwah drih PLEE jee ah	*quadri-* four *-plegia* paralysis	Paralysis of arms, legs, and trunk.

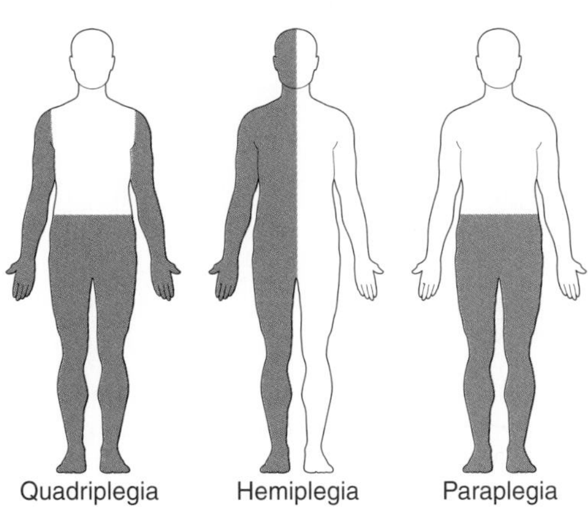

Fig. 12-14 Types of paralysis.

Exercise 8: INFECTIOUS, VASCULAR, AND PARALYTIC DISORDERS

Circle the correct answer.

1. An inflammation of the root of a spinal nerve is called *(polyneuritis, radiculitis)*.
2. An inflammation of the covering of the CNS is called *(meningitis, encephalitis)*.
3. An inflammation of a nerve in the thigh and leg is called *(shingles, sciatica)*.
4. Paralysis on the left or right half of the body is called *(hemiparesis, hemiplegia)*.
5. A ministroke is a *(transient ischemic attack, cerebrovascular accident)*.
6. A slight paralysis from the waist down is called *(para, mono)* paresis.

Match the suffixes and prefixes with their correct meanings.

_____ 7. hemi-
_____ 8. -plegia
_____ 9. mono-
_____ 10. quadri-
_____ 11. para-
_____ 12. -paresis
_____ 13. di-

A. one
B. slight paralysis
C. half
D. abnormal
E. paralysis
F. four
G. two

14. Three causes of occlusion that lead to a CVA are:

____

15. The difference between a CVA and a TIA is that:

____

Case Study Continued

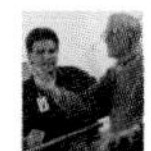

Max was glad that his stroke had occurred in the hospital. He knew that if he hadn't been lucky enough to get help so soon, he could have suffered severe disability or died. As it is, Max has right hemiparesis and is having trouble doing things that he has always taken for granted, such as buttoning his shirt and using a spoon. Melissa, the OT, reassures Max that she will work with him on ways to feed, dress, and toilet himself. Eduardo, the PT, tells Max that he will help him regain his mobility.

DIAGNOSTIC PROCEDURES

Terms Related to Imaging

TERM	WORD ORIGIN	DEFINITION
Brain scan		Nuclear medicine procedure involving intravenous injection of radioisotopes to localize and identify intracranial masses, lesions, tumors, or infarcts. Photography is done by a scintillator or scanner.
Cerebral angiography	*cerebr/o* cerebrum *-al* pertaining to *angi/o* vessel *-graphy* process of recording	X-ray of the cerebral arteries, including the internal carotids, taken after the injection of a contrast medium (Fig. 12-15); also called **cerebral arteriography.**
Computed tomography (CT) scan	*tom/o* slice *-graphy* process of recording	Transverse sections of the CNS are imaged, sometimes after the injection of a contrast medium (unless there is suspected bleeding). Used to diagnose strokes, edema, tumors, and hemorrhage resulting from trauma.
Echoencephalography eh koh en seh fah LAH gruh fee	*echo-* sound *encephal/o* brain *-graphy* process of recording	Ultrasound exam of the brain, usually done only on newborns, because sound waves do not readily penetrate bone.

Terms Related to Imaging—cont'd

TERM	WORD ORIGIN	DEFINITION
Magnetic resonance imaging (MRI)		Medical imaging that uses radiofrequency radiation in a powerful magnetic field. **Magnetic resonance angiography (MRA)** is imaging of the carotid arteries using injected contrast agents.
Myelography mye eh LAH gruh fee	*myel/o* spinal cord *-graphy* process of recording	X-ray of the spinal canal after the introduction of a radiopaque substance.
Positron emission tomography (PET scan)		Use of radionuclides to reconstruct brain sections. Measurements can be taken of blood flow, volume, and oxygen and glucose uptake, enabling radiologists to determine the functional characteristics of specific parts of the brain (Fig. 12-16). PET scans are used to assist in the diagnosis of Alzheimer's disease and stroke.
Radiography		Process of making an x-ray image (with or without contrast media).
Single photon emission computed tomography (SPECT)		An injection of a radioactive sugar substance that is metabolized by the brain, which is then scanned for abnormalities.
Ultrasonography	*ultra-* beyond *son/o* sound *-graphy* process of recording	Noninvasive imaging using high-frequency sound waves.

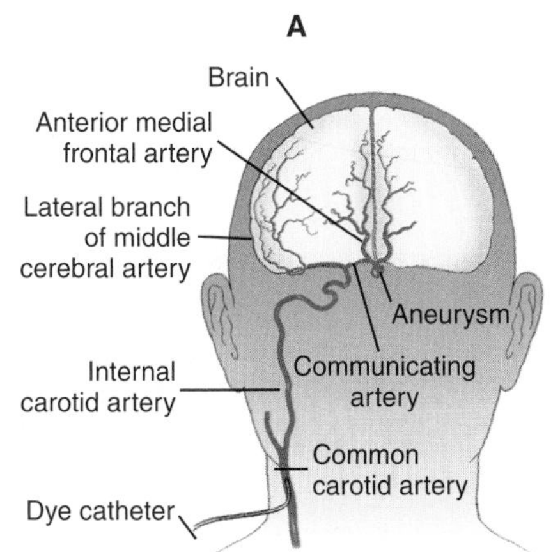

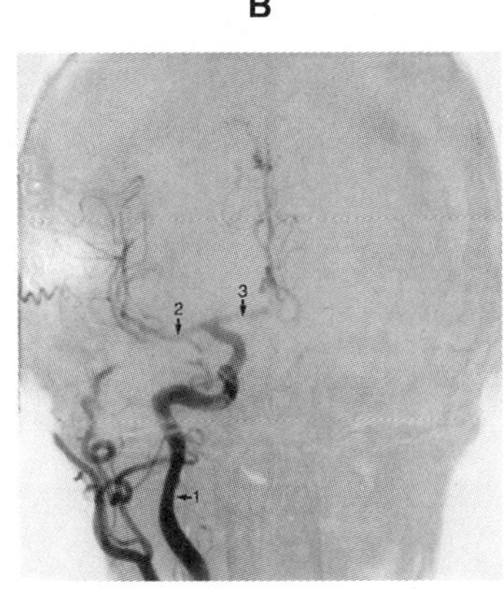

Fig. 12-15 Cerebral angiography. **A,** Insertion of dye through a catheter in the common carotid artery outlines the vessels of the brain. **B,** Angiogram showing vessels. *1,* Internal carotid artery; *2,* middle cerebral artery; *3,* middle meningeal artery.

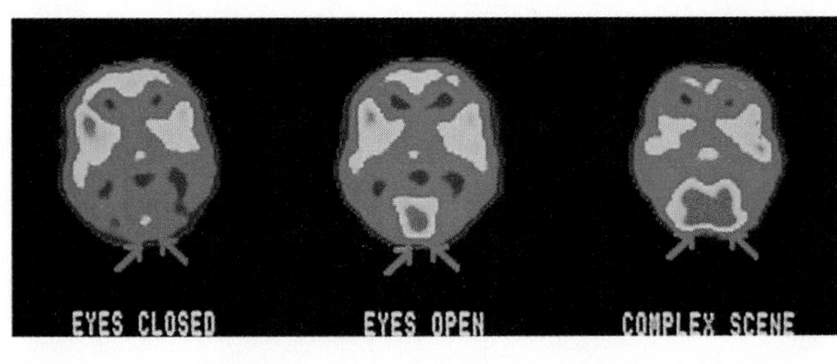

Fig. 12-16 Colorized PET scan.

Terms Related to Electrodiagnostic Procedures

TERM	WORD ORIGIN	DEFINITION
Electroencephalography (EEG) ee leck troh en seff fah LAH gruh fee	***electr/o*** electricity ***encephal/o*** brain ***-graphy*** process of recording	Record of the electrical activity of the brain. May be used in the diagnosis of epilepsy, infection, and coma (Fig. 12-17).
Evoked potential (EP)		Electrical response from the brainstem or cerebral cortex that is produced in response to specific stimuli. This results in a distinctive pattern on an EEG.
Multiple sleep latency test (MSLT)		Test that consists of a series of short, daytime naps in the sleep lab to measure daytime sleepiness and how fast the patient falls asleep; used to diagnose or rule out narcolepsy.
Nerve conduction test		Test of the functioning of peripheral nerves. Conduction time (impulse travel) through a nerve is measured after a stimulus is applied; used to diagnose polyneuropathies.
Polysomnography pah lee som NAH gruh fee	***poly-*** many ***somn/o*** sleep ***-graphy*** process of recording	Measurement and record of a number of functions while the patient is asleep (e.g., cardiac, muscular, brain, ocular, and respiratory functions). Most often used to diagnose sleep apnea.

Fig. 12-17 EEG. **A,** Photograph of person with electrodes attached. **B,** EEG tracing showing activity in four different places in the brain. Compare the normal activity with the explosive activity that occurs during a seizure.

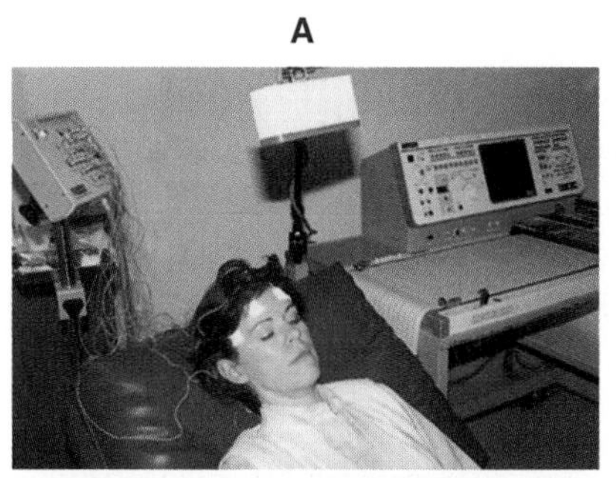

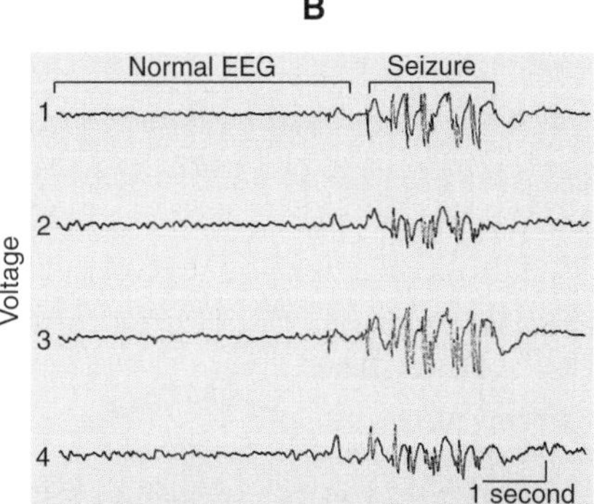

Terms Related to Other Diagnostic Tests

TERM	WORD ORIGIN	DEFINITION
Babinski's reflex bah BIN skeez		In normal conditions, the dorsiflexion of the great toe when the plantar surface of the sole is stimulated. **Babinski's sign** is the loss or diminution of the Achilles tendon reflex seen in sciatica.
Cerebrospinal fluid (CSF) analysis		Examination of fluid from the CNS to detect pathogens and abnormalities. Useful in diagnosing hemorrhages, tumors, and various diseases.
Deep tendon reflexes (DTR)		Assessment of an automatic motor response by striking a tendon. Useful in the diagnosis of stroke.
Gait assessment rating scale (GARS)		Inventory of 16 aspects of gait (how one walks) to determine abnormalities. May be used as one method to evaluate cerebellar function.
Lumbar puncture (LP)		Procedure to aspirate CSF from the lumbar subarachnoid space. A needle is inserted between two lumbar vertebrae to withdraw the fluid for diagnostic purposes. Also called a **spinal tap.**

 Exercise 9: DIAGNOSTIC PROCEDURES

Match the word part with its meaning. Some letters may be used more than once.

_____ 1. electr/o	_____ 10. arteri/o	A. sleep	
		B. sound	
_____ 2. cerebr/o	_____ 11. radi/o	C. artery	
		D. inside	
_____ 3. extra-	_____ 12. tom/o	E. spinal cord	
		F. slice	
_____ 4. somn/o	_____ 13. spin/o	G. outside	
		H. spine	
_____ 5. myel/o	_____ 14. son/o	I. brain	
		J. skull	
_____ 6. crani/o	_____ 15. ultra-	K. record	
		L. cerebrum	
_____ 7. angi/o	_____ 16. poly-	M. electricity	
		N. beyond	
_____ 8. intra-	_____ 17. encephal/o	O. rays	
		P. many	
_____ 9. -gram		Q. vessel	

Circle the correct answer.

18. Walking abnormalities are measured by a *(gait assessment rating scale, deep tendon reflex).*
19. Examination of fluid from CNS is a/an *(evoked potential, cerebrospinal fluid analysis).*
20. Aspiration of CSF for diagnostic purposes is a *(CT scan, spinal tap).*
21. Record of electrical activity of the brain is an *(electroencephalogram, electrocardiogram).*
22. A finding that indicates loss of Achilles tendon reflex is *(Babinski's reflex, Babinski's sign).*
23. *(Multiple sleep latency test, Polysomnography)* is used to diagnose sleep apnea.
24. An x-ray study of cerebral arteries is called *(cerebral angiography, magnetic resonance angiography).*
25. *(Nerve conduction test, echoencephalography)* is an ultrasound study of the brain.
26. *(Myelography, Myography)* is an x-ray of the spinal cord.

THERAPEUTIC INTERVENTIONS

Terms Related to Brain and Skull Interventions

TERM	WORD ORIGIN	DEFINITIONS
Craniectomy kray nee ECK tuh mee	*crani/o* skull, cranium *-ectomy* removal	Removal of part of the skull.
Craniotomy kray nee AH tuh mee	*crani/o* skull, cranium *-tomy* incision	Incision into the skull as a surgical approach or to relieve intracranial pressure; also called **trephination** (treff fin NAY shun).
CSF shunt		Tube implanted in the brain to relieve the pressure of cerebrospinal fluid as a result of hydrocephalus.
Stereotaxic radiosurgery stair ee oh TACK sick	*stere/o* 3-D *tax/o* order, arrangement *-ic* pertaining to	Surgery using radiowaves to localize structures within 3-D space.

Terms Related to Peripheral Nervous System Interventions

Term	Word Origin	Definition
Ganglionectomy gan glee oh NECK tuh mee	*gangli/o* ganglion *-ectomy* removal	Removal of a ganglion (*pl.* ganglions or ganglia).
Vagotomy vay GAH tuh mee	*vag/o* vagus nerve *-tomy* incision	Cutting of the vagus nerve to reduce the secretion of gastric acid.

Terms Related to General Interventions

Term	Word Origin	Definition
Microsurgery	*micro-* small, tiny	Surgery in which magnification is used to repair delicate tissues.
Nerve block		Use of anesthesia to prevent sensory nerve impulses from reaching the CNS.
Neurectomy noo RECK tuh mee	*neur/o* nerve *-ectomy* removal	Excision of part or all of a nerve.
Neurolysis noo RAH lih sis	*neur/o* nerve *-lysis* destruction	Destruction of a nerve.
Neuroplasty noo roh PLAS tee	*neur/o* nerve *-plasty* surgical repair	Surgical repair of a nerve.
Neurorrhaphy noo ROAR ah fee	*neur/o* nerve *-rrhaphy* suture	Suture of a severed nerve.
Neurotomy noo RAH toh mee	*neur/o* nerve *-tomy* incision	Incision of a nerve.

Terms Related to Pain Management

Term	Word Origin	Definition
Carotid endarterectomy kuh RAH tid en dar tur ECK tuh mee	*end-* within *arter/o* artery *-ectomy* removal	Removal of the atheromatous plaque lining the carotid artery to increase blood flow and leave a smooth surface. Done to prevent thrombotic occlusions (Fig. 12-18).
Cordotomy kore DAH tuh mee	*cord/o* spinal cord *-tomy* incision	Incision of the spinal cord to relieve pain.
Rhizotomy rye ZAH tuh mee	*rhiz/o* spinal nerve root *-tomy* incision	Resection of the dorsal root of a spinal nerve to relieve pain.
Sympathectomy sim puh THECK tuh mee	*sympath/o* to feel with *-ectomy* removal	Surgical interruption of part of the sympathetic pathways for the relief of chronic pain or to promote vasodilation.
Transcutaneous electrical nerve stimulations (TENS)	*trans-* through *cutane/o* skin *-ous* pertaining to	Method of pain control effected by the application of electrical impulses to the skin (Fig. 12-19).

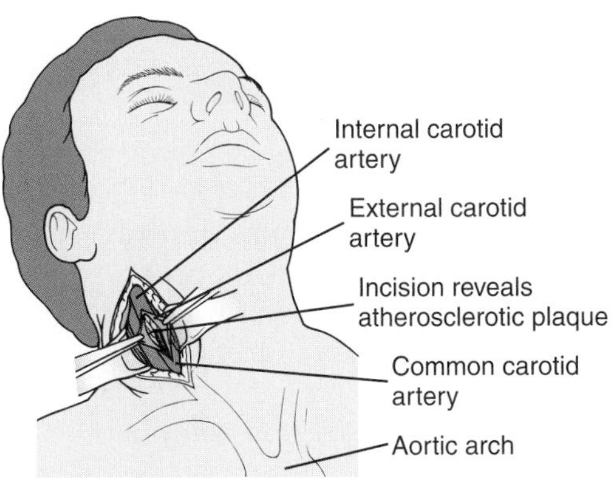

Fig. 12-18 Carotid endarterectomy.

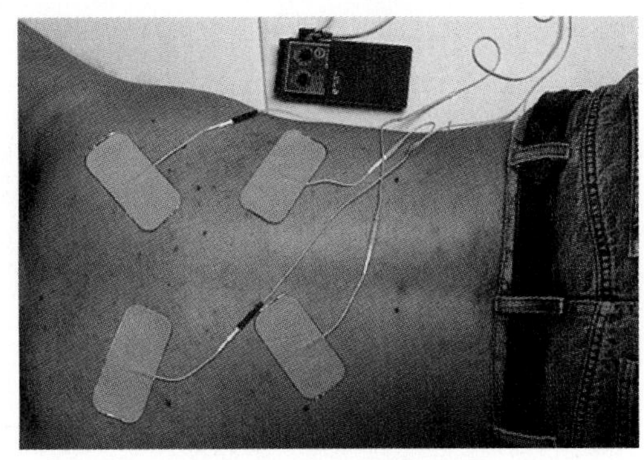

Fig. 12-19 TENS treatment.

Exercise 10: THERAPEUTIC INTERVENTIONS

Match the word part with its meaning.

____ 1. stere/o
____ 2. disk/o
____ 3. tax/o
____ 4. syn-
____ 5. cutane/o
____ 6. sympath/o
____ 7. -desis
____ 8. lamin/o
____ 9. radi/o
____ 10. rhiz/o
____ 11. trans-
____ 12. spondyl/o
____ 13. -tomy
____ 14. lob/o
____ 15. -plasty
____ 16. arter/o
____ 17. gangli/o
____ 18. crani/o
____ 19. -ectomy
____ 20. cord/o
____ 21. -rrhaphy
____ 22. neur/o
____ 23. vag/o
____ 24. end-
____ 25. -lysis

A. stabilization
B. artery
C. suture
D. incision
E. within
F. intervertebral disk
G. nerve root
H. order, arrangement
I. vagus nerve
J. together
K. nerve
L. rays
M. vertebra
N. destruction
O. spinal cord
P. 3-D
Q. to feel with
R. through
S. removal
T. section
U. surgical repair
V. ganglion
W. skull
X. lamina
Y. skin

Circle the correct answer.

26. A method of pain control using electrical impulses is called *(TENS, ADL)*.
27. A method of relieving pressure of CSF from hydrocephalus is through the use of *(stereotaxic radiosurgery, CSF shunt)*.
28. Use of a local anesthetic to prevent sensory nerve impulses from reaching the CNS is called a *(nerve block, rhizotomy)*.
29. A *(cordotomy, vagotomy)* reduces the secretion of gastric acid.

PHARMACOLOGY

Amphetamines: Nervous system stimulants used for narcolepsy. An example is dextroamphetamine (Dexedrine).

Analgesics: Used to relieve pain. Examples include sumatriptan (Imitrex), Fiorinal, aspirin, acetaminophen (Tylenol), and naproxen (Anaprox).

Anticonvulsants: Reduce or prevent the severity of epileptic or other convulsive seizures. Examples include clonazepam (Klonopin) and phenytoin (Dilantin).

Antiinfectives: Reduce CNS infection, such as meningitis. An example is metronidazole (Flagyl).

Antimultiple sclerosis drugs: Used to slow effects of MS. Examples include interferon (Avonex, Betaseron, Rebif), glatiramer acetate (Copaxone), and tizanidine (Zanaflex).

Antiparkinsonian drugs: Effective against Parkinson's disease. Examples include levodopa and carbidopa (Sinemet) and tolcapone (Tasmar).

Antipyretics: Reduce fever. Examples include aspirin, acetaminophen (Tylenol), and naproxen (Anaprox, Aleve).

Hypnotics: Class of drugs often used as sedatives. Cause an insensitivity to pain. Called *soporifics* or *somnifacients* when used to induce sleep. Examples include flurazepam (Dalmane) to treat insomnia.

Neuroprotective drugs: Reduce the effects of ischemia on cells in stroke patients. Examples include nalmefene, lubeluzole, and clomethiazole (Zendra).

Sedatives: Decrease functional activity, diminish irritability, and allay excitement. Examples include flurazepam (Dalmane) and triazolam (Halcion).

Stroke risk-reduction drugs: Thin blood in stroke patients. Examples include aspirin and simvastatin (Zocor).

Thrombolytics: Clot buster drugs (tissue plasminogen activators [TPAs] and streptokinase) used to treat strokes.

Exercise 11: PHARMACOLOGY

Match the drug with its effect.

_____ 1. reduces infection

_____ 2. treats PD

_____ 3. relieves pain

_____ 4. decreases activity irritability and excitement

_____ 5. induces sleep

_____ 6. thins blood

_____ 7. reduces fever

_____ 8. clot buster

_____ 9. reduces severity of seizures

_____ 10. reduces effect of ischemia on cells

_____ 11. slows progression of MS

_____ 12. nervous system stimulant

A. antimultiple sclerosis drug
B. antipyretic
C. soporific
D. thrombolytic
E. anticonvulsant
F. sedative
G. neuroprotective agent
H. amphetamine
I. stroke risk-reduction
J. analgesic
K. antiparkinsonian drug
L. antiinfective

Case Study Continued

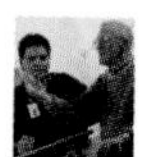

Intravenous thrombolytic (clot buster) therapy was begun soon after Max's stroke to prevent more serious damage. Max is grateful that medicine is available but realizes that his physical and occupational therapy were valuable treatment options too. Melissa has been helping him work toward regaining his activities of daily living (ADLs), and Eduardo has helped him improve his motor skills, strength, and coordination. Their combination of coach, teacher, and cheerleader is helping Max literally and figuratively get back on his feet.

Abbreviations

Abbreviation	Definition
AD	Alzheimer's disease
ADLs	Activities of daily living
ALS	Amyotrophic lateral sclerosis
ANS	Autonomic nervous system
BBB	Blood-brain barrier
C1-C8	Cervical nerves
CNS	Central nervous system
CP	Cerebral palsy
CSF	Cerebrospinal fluid
CT scan	Computerized tomography scan
CVA	Cerebrovascular accident
DTR	Deep tendon reflex
EEG	Electroencephalogram
ICP	Intracranial pressure
L1-L5	Lumbar nerves
LP	Lumbar puncture
MRI	Magnetic resonance imaging
MS	Multiple sclerosis
PD	Parkinson's disease
PET scan	Positron emission tomography scan
PNS	Peripheral nervous system
PSG	Polysomnography
S1-S5	Sacral nerves
SAH	Subarachnoid hemorrhage
SNS	Somatic nervous system
SPECT	Single photon emission computed tomography
T1-T12	Thoracic nerves
TENS	Transcutaneous electrical nerve stimulation
TIA	Transient ischemic attack

Exercise 12: ABBREVIATIONS

Spell out the following abbreviations.

1. Barry had a LP to analyze his CSF for meningitis.

   Lumbar Puncture Cerebro Spinal Fluid

2. Maria became a quadriplegic when she sustained a C2 fracture diving into the shallow end of a swimming pool.

3. Ms. Damjanov had an MRI to aid in the dx of her MS.

4. The patient underwent PSG to detect abnormalities related to hypersomnia.

5. Walter needed help with his ADLs after a CVA that left him with right hemiparesis.

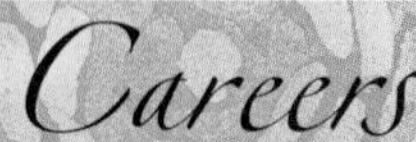

Careers

Occupational Therapists

Occupational therapists (OTs) assist patients who have become mentally, physically, developmentally, or emotionally disabled to live independent, productive, and satisfying lives. OTs help these patients regain and build skills that are important for health and well-being, including activities of daily living (ADLs)—the activities usually performed in the course of a normal day in the person's life, such as eating, toileting, dressing, bathing, or brushing teeth. Aside from hospitals, work sites may include outpatient and community settings, as well as schools. The Bureau of Labor Statistics reports that currently over a third of OTs work part-time.

All 50 states require at least a bachelor's degree; this also holds true in both Puerto Rico and Washington, DC. To become a licensed, registered occupational therapist (OTR), an applicant must graduate from an accredited program and pass a national certification examination.

Employment is expected to increase faster than the average for all occupations through the year 2010. Over the long run, the demand should continue to increase as a result of growth in the number of individuals with disabilities—the baby boom generation's movement into middle age, with the concomitant incidence of heart attack and stroke.

For further information, contact the American Occupational Therapy Association, 4720 Montgomery Lane, PO Box 31220, Bethesda, MD 20824-1220. Internet: http://www.aota.org.

Physical Therapists

Physical therapists (PTs) work with patients who need assistance in restoring or improving their mobility. The treatment may include exercise, electrical stimulation, heat therapy, and/or ultrasound. PTs may be generalists or specialize in cardiopulmonary, sports medicine, neurology, pediatrics, geriatrics, or orthopedic physical therapy areas.

Most PTs work in hospitals or clinics for a 40-hour work week. About one fourth of PTs work part-time.

For further information, contact the American Physical Therapy Association, 111 North Fairfax Street, Alexandria, VA 22314-1488. Internet: http://www.apta.org.

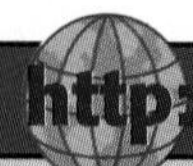

http: INTERNET PROJECT

Using the Websites below to get you started, choose one of the following assignments:

- Make a brochure/flyer on preventive measures and warning signs for strokes. Design it to make friends and/or family aware of the most common signs/ symptoms of CVAs and TIAs, what can be done to avoid them, and current statistics as to who is affected.
- Write a 2-page report on the newest research on treatment options for one of the diseases of the nervous system.
- Write a 2-page report on new techniques in imaging the nervous system.

Be sure to include references (at least three) to the following Websites:

National Stroke Association: http://www.stroke.org
American Stroke Association, a division of the American Heart Association: http://www.strokeassociation.org
National Institute of Neurological Disorders and Stroke: http://www.ninds.nih.gov
Food and Drug Administration: http://www.fda.gov
MEDLINEplus—Brain and Nervous System Topics: http://www.nlm.nih.gov/medlineplus/brainandnervoussystem.html

Chapter Review

A. Functions of the Nervous System

1. In your own words, explain the functions of the nervous system and give an example of how one disorder illustrates a dysfunction of this system.

____

____

____

B. Anatomy and Physiology

2. Explain the two main divisions of the nervous system and how they are organized.

____

____

3. Label the following diagrams of the brain. Include the terms and their respective combining forms where appropriate.

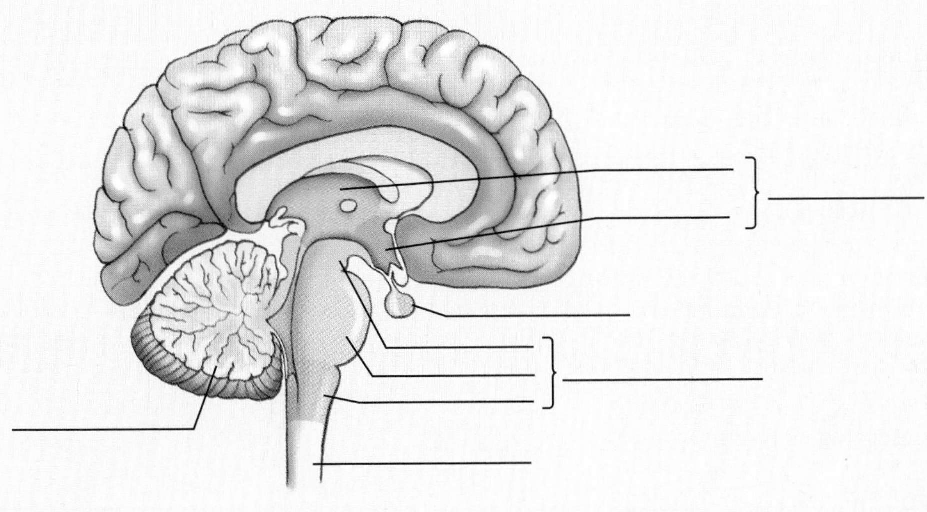

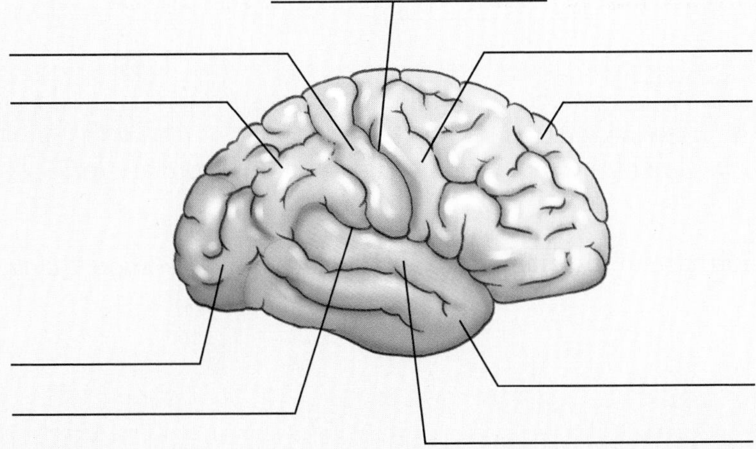

4. What are the names of the nerves that carry impulses toward the brain?

____

5. What is the covering of the CNS? List the layers from outermost to innermost.

____

6. The spinal nerves emerge from the spinal cord at the nerve _______________.

7. A network of spinal nerves is called a/an _______________.

8. What type of chemical moves across the space between two nerve cells? _______________

9. What is the name of the supportive or stromal cells of the nervous system? _______________

10. What part of the brain is responsible for thinking, reasoning, and memory? _______________

11. Which part of the brain is responsible for the coordination of movement? _______________

C. Pathology

12. A patient reports having difficulty remembering; this symptom is termed _______________.

13. Ms. Roberts reports that she has problems falling asleep at night. She has _______________.

14. What form of syncope is associated with abrupt emotional stress? _______________

15. Cara experiences a "warning" before an epileptic seizure. What is this called? _______________

16. Ms. Murphy's speech is slurred after her brain attack. She is exhibiting _______________.

17. A patient who walks very slowly in an incoordinated manner, or shuffles, has an abnormal

_______________.

18. Samantha has lost her sense of taste. She is exhibiting _______________.

19. Zack was born with an abnormal accumulation of CSF in the ventricles of the brain. He has

_______________.

20. A patient who faints is described as having _______________.

21. Patients with infections of the covering of the CNS have _______________.

22. Currently, the most common cause of dementia is _______________.

23. What is the eponym for ALS? _______________

24. A patient with a paralysis of the body from the neck down is _______________.

25. In what disorder is there an abnormal opening of the spine from which the spinal cord and/or meninges protrude? _______________

26. A patient who has a blockage or a hemorrhage in the brain with neural deficits that last more than a day has had a/an _______________.

Build a term.

27. inflammation of many nerves ______________________

28. inflammation of the brain ______________________

29. lack of a sense of smell ______________________

Decode the term.

30. hypersomnia ______________________

31. narcolepsy ______________________

32. radiculitis ______________________

D. Diagnostic Procedures

33. What is the term for an examination of the CSF? ______________________

34. What is SPECT? ______________________
35. What imaging technique is used to diagnose strokes, edema, and tumors?

    ____

36. MSLT stands for ____________ and is used to diagnose ____________.

37. DTR is used to assist in the diagnosis of ____________.

Decode the term.

38. myelography ______________________

39. cerebral arteriography ______________________

40. polysomnography ______________________

E. Therapeutic Interventions

41. Patients are assisted with ADLs to cope with the sequelae of a stroke. What are ADLs?

    ____
42. What type of surgery uses radiowaves to localize structures within 3-D spaces?

    ____
43. A tube implanted in the brain to relieve the pressure of cerebrospinal fluid is called a/an

    ____________.

44. TENS is done for the purpose of ______________________.

Build a term.

45. excision of a nerve ____________________

46. incision of the skull ____________________

47. surgical repair of a nerve ____________________

Decode the term.

48. neurolysis ____________________

49. rhizotomy ____________________

50. spondylosyndesis ____________________

F. Pharmacology

51. Epilepsy is treated by what class of drug? ____________________

52. Blood thinners are what class of drug? ____________________

53. Cells are protected from the effects of ischemia by ____________________.

54. Drugs that relieve pain, such as aspirin, acetaminophen, and Anaprox, are called ____________________.

55. Roslyn took a drug to relieve her fever. That type of drug is called a/an ____________________.

G. Abbreviations

Spell out the abbreviated terms.

56. Susan woke up with a loss of the use of the right side of her body. She was diagnosed with a CVA.

____

57. Rose had an EEG, which was used to diagnose her epilepsy. ____________________

58. A PET scan is especially useful in the diagnosis of AD. ____________________

59. When the LP was done on the patient, the needle was inserted between L3-L4.

____

60. A patient with PD presented with dysphagia, dysphasia, and a shuffling gait.

____

H. Singulars and Plurals

Change the following terms from singular to plural.

61. gyrus ____________________

62. stimulus ____________________

63. sulcus ____________________

64. ganglion ______________________________

65. thrombus ______________________________

I. Translations

Rewrite the following sentences in your own words.

66. Mr. O'Connor had a right-sided brain attack that affected the contralateral side of his body. His symptoms included hemiparesis and dysphasia.

____

____

67. Due to a blow on the head, the patient sustained an epidural hematoma.

____

____

68. The patient reported vertigo and syncope before her arrival at the emergency department.

____

____

69. The baby's spina bifida resulted in a meningomyelocele.

____

____

70. The neonate's hydrocephalus was treated with a CSF shunt.

____

____

J. Cumulative Exercises

71. Oligohydramnios is a condition of ______________________________.
72. What is the term for a backflow of urine from the bladder to the ureters?

____

73. CT scans image what plane? ______________________________

74. What structure is inferior to the thalamus? ______________________________

K. Be Careful

75. What are the different definitions for dermatome?

____

____

76. Myelo- means spinal cord or bone marrow. In the following examples, define each term accurately, using a dictionary if necessary.

A. myelogram ______________________

B. myeloma ______________________

C. osteomyelitis ______________________

D. meningomyelocele ______________________

E. myelitis ______________________

F. myelocyte ______________________

G. myelodysplasia ______________________

77. What is the difference between dysarthria and dysarthrosis?

____

78. What are the two meanings for the following abbreviations?

A. BBB ______________________

B. MS ______________________

South Shore Hospital
2243 Seaspray Dr.
Seacrest Beach, FL 32405

DISCHARGE SUMMARY

Patient Name: Max Janovski
MR#: 349812
Date of Admission: 07/04/02
Date of Discharge: 07/08/02
Admission Diagnosis: Rule out cerebrovascular accident
Discharge Diagnoses: (1) Cerebrovascular accident; (2) emphysema; (3) CAD.

History

This patient is a 75-year-old white male with a history of emphysema, coronary artery disease, and benign prostatic hyperplasia. His BPH was treated with a TURP in 1998. He had a triple CABG in 2000. Patient reports smoking 2 packs per day until 2 years ago. Denies any recent tobacco or alcohol use. He has benefited from oxygen therapy for the last 2 months.

He was admitted for an episode of vertigo and several episodes of syncope that occurred as he was visiting his son's family over the Fourth of July holiday. His son brought him to the ED when he reported a loss of feeling on his left side and his speech became slurred. These symptoms resolved before he arrived at the hospital. He has no history of headaches but has admitted to continued dizziness. Patient was admitted and experienced a right-sided CVA the following morning. Intravenous thrombolytic therapy was administered immediately, but patient remains with a left hemiparesis.

Physical Examination on Admission

Physical examination was largely negative. The patient is quiet, mildly anxious yet cooperative. Pupils are equal and reactive. Neck is negative. There is a normal sinus rhythm with no significant murmurs. Abdomen is negative. There is no peripheral edema. Patient exhibits a minimal amount of ataxia on walking, but there are no other neurologic findings.

The neurologist ordered and reviewed CT scans of head, MRIs, intracranial and extracranial MRAs, and Holter monitor readings. Cerebral hemorrhage was ruled out.

Laboratory findings included mild hypercholesterolemia and a hemoglobin of 12.1. Chest x-ray demonstrated hyperinflation, with vascular markings diminished at the apices. EEG was normal.

Patient appears to be stable at the present time and is discharged to his son's home while continuing his physical and occupational therapy. He has demonstrated a good understanding of his condition and of the need for full cooperation with his therapists to work toward regaining his independence.

An appointment has been scheduled for follow-up in 2 weeks.

_______________ J. M. Smythe, MD

L. Healthcare Report

79. Patient was admitted for vertigo and syncope. Define each.

____

80. What is hypercholesterolemia? _______________

81. What is BPH treated with TURP? _______________

82. Ataxia refers to _______________.

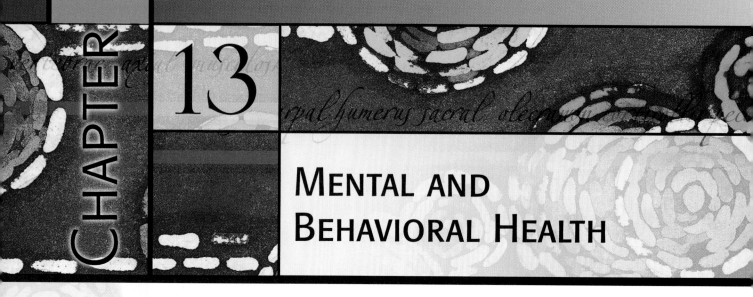

Chapter 13 Mental and Behavioral Health

"Health . . . is not a static condition, but rather is manifested in dynamic responses to the stresses and challenges of life. The more complete the human freedom, the greater the likelihood that new stresses will appear—organic and psychic—because man himself continuously changes his environment through technology, and because endlessly he moves into new conditions during his restless search for adventure."
—René Jules Dubos

Quote

Case Study

Nadine White's husband of 39 years died last spring, and she has been unable to adjust to life without him. According to her daughter, Nadine did not put in a garden this year, stopped volunteering at the local hospital, and has no appetite. Today she is meeting with a psychiatric social worker, Andrew Dawson, to whom she was referred by her family physician, Dr. McGuire. Andrew has read Dr. McGuire's notes on Mrs. White and is prepared to begin his grief counseling with her.

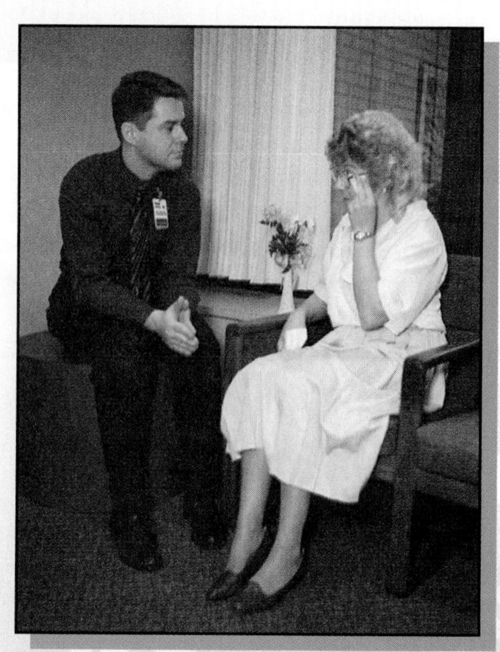

OBJECTIVES

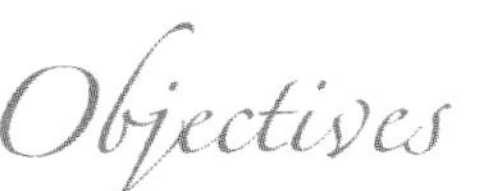

- In your own words, define mental and behavioral health.
- Explain the role of the *Diagnostic and Statistical Manual of Mental Disorders* (DSM) in the definition of mental illness.
- Recognize, recall, and apply healthcare terms related to the pathology of mental and behavioral health.
- Recognize, recall, and apply healthcare terms related to the diagnostic procedures introduced in this chapter.
- Recognize, recall and apply healthcare terms related to the therapeutic interventions introduced in this chapter.
- Recognize, recall, and apply the pharmacology introduced in this chapter.
- Recognize, recall, and apply the abbreviations introduced in this chapter.
- Recognize and recall word components used in this chapter to build and decode healthcare terms relevant to mental and behavioral health.
- Recognize, recall, and apply material learned in previous chapters.

INTRODUCTION TO MENTAL AND BEHAVIORAL HEALTH

Recent national statistics reveal the following:

- One out of every five American adults and children has a mental disorder.
- Over 25% of the 100 top-selling medications are for psychiatric disorders.
- The eighth most common diagnostic category for inpatient admissions is substance-related mental disorders.
- Approximately 19 million Americans are diagnosed with anxiety.
- An estimated 44% of inpatient admissions for mental disorders are for alcohol- and substance-related disorders.
- Approximately 2 to 2.5 million Americans are mentally retarded.*

Given these statistics, behavioral health is a content area that cannot be ignored.

The term *behavioral health* reflects an integration of the outdated concept of the separate nature of the body (physical health/illness) and the mind (mental health/illness). Advances in research continually acknowledge the roles of culture, environment, and spirituality in influencing physical and behavioral health. The use of the term *behavior* refers to observable, measurable activities that may be used to evaluate the progress of treatment.

Similar to previous chapters, this chapter examines disorders that result when an individual has a maladaptive response to his or her environment (internal or external). (See Chapter 12 for an explanation of the anatomy and physiology of the brain and nervous system.) However, even though some mental illnesses have organic causes in which neurotransmitters and other known brain functions play a role, there is no mental "anatomy" per se. Instead, behavioral health is a complex interaction among an individual's emotional, physical, mental, and behavioral processes in an environment that includes cultural and spiritual influences.

Mental health may be defined as a relative state of mind in which a person who is healthy is able to cope with and adjust to the recurrent stresses of everyday living in a culturally acceptable way. Thus mental illness may be generally

*It should be noted that mental retardation is not an illness; it is a condition characterized by developmental delays and difficulty with learning and social situations.

defined as a functional impairment that substantially interferes with or limits one or more major life activities for a significant duration.

The American Psychiatric Association (APA) publishes the official listing of diagnosable mental disorders: the *Diagnostic and Statistical Manual of Mental Disorders* (DSM). The codes that are used within the DSM are coordinated with the International Classification of Diseases (ICD), which provides acceptable billing codes in the United States. Major revisions to the DSM occur at approximately 10-year intervals, with minor updates about every 5 years. The current edition as this book goes to press is DSM IV-TR (text revision), published in the year 2000.

COMBINING FORMS FOR MENTAL AND BEHAVIORAL HEALTH

MEANING	COMBINING FORM
mind	psych/o, thym/o
study	log/o
treatment	iatr/o

Exercise 1: INTRODUCTION TO MENTAL AND BEHAVIORAL HEALTH

Circle the correct answer.

1. Who publishes the official listing of mental disorders for the United States? *(American Medical Association, American Psychiatric Association)*
2. What is the abbreviation of the name for this listing? *(DSM, ICD)*
3. Major revisions for the official listing of mental disorders for the United States are accomplished approximately every *(5, 10)* years.
4. Current thinking acknowledges the influence of *(spirituality, climate)* on behavioral health.
5. The term *(behavioral, mental)* refers to observable, measurable activities that may be used to evaluate treatment.

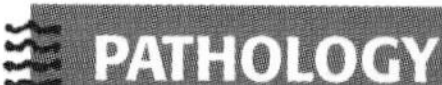

PATHOLOGY

Terms Related to General Symptoms

TERM	WORD ORIGIN	DEFINITION
Akathisia ack uh THEE zsa	*a-* lack of *kathis/o* sitting *-ia* condition	Inability to remain calm, still, and free of anxiety.
Amnesia am NEE zsa		Inability to remember either isolated parts of the past or one's entire past; may be caused by brain damage or severe emotional trauma.
Anhedonia an hee DOH nee ah	*an-* without *hedon/o* pleasure *-ia* condition	Absence of the ability to experience either pleasure or joy, even in the face of causative events.

Terms Related to General Symptoms—cont'd

TERM	WORD ORIGIN	DEFINITION
Catatonia kat tah TOH nee ah	*cata-* down *ton/o* tension *-ia* condition	Paralysis or immobility from psychological or emotional rather than physical causes.
Confabulation kon fab byoo LAY shun		Effort to conceal a gap in memory by fabricating detailed, often believable stories.
Defense mechanism		Unconscious mechanism for psychological coping, adjustment, or self-preservation in the face of stress or a threat. Examples include **denial** of an unpleasant situation or condition and **projection** of intolerable aspects onto another individual.
Delirium dih LEER ree um		Condition of confused, unfocused, irrational agitation. In mental disorders, agitation and confusion may also be accompanied by a more intense disorientation, incoherence, or fear, as well as illusions, hallucinations, and delusions.
Delusion dih LOO zhun		Persistent belief in a demonstrable untruth or a provably inaccurate perception despite clear evidence to the contrary.
Dementia dih MEN shah		Mental disorder in which the individual experiences a progressive loss of memory, personality alterations, confusion, loss of touch with reality, and **stupor** (seeming unawareness of, and disconnection with, one's surroundings).
Echolalia eh koh LAYL yuh	*echo* reverberation *-lalia* condition of babbling	Repetition of words or phrases spoken by others.
Hallucination hah loo sih NAY shun		Any unreal sensory perception that occurs with no external cause.
Illusion ill LOO zhun		Inaccurate sensory perception based on a real stimulus; examples include mirages or interpreting music or wind as voices.
Libido lih BEE doh		Normal psychological impulse drive associated with sensuality, expressions of desire, or creativity. Abnormality occurs only when such drives are excessively heightened or depressed.
Psychosis sye KOH sis	*psych/o* mind *-osis* abnormal condition	Disassociation with or impaired perception of reality; may be accompanied by hallucinations, delusions, incoherence, akathisia, and/or disorganized behavior.
Somnambulism som NAM byoo liz um	*somn/o* sleep *ambul/o* walking *-ism* condition	Sleepwalking.

Case Study Continued

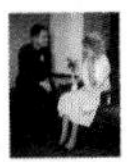

Andrew gently questions Mrs. White about how her life is different now after her husband's death. In a voice barely above a whisper and devoid of emotion, she states that she is unable to be happy anymore. "I used to be so pleased to work in my garden, or read, or volunteer at the hospital. I didn't need to have my husband with me every minute; it wasn't like that. It's just—" she hesitates—"it's just that I knew I could always come home to him. We were best friends."

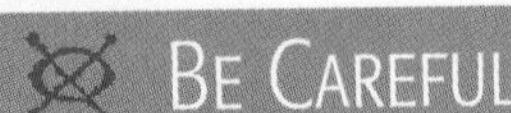

Be Careful!

The suffix *-thymia* means *a condition of the mind,* but *thym/o* refers to the *thymus gland* and the *mind.*

Affects

Affects are observable demonstrations of emotion that can be described in terms of quality, range, and appropriateness. The following list defines the most significant affects encountered in behavioral health:

Blunted: Moderately reduced range of affect.
Flat: The diminishment or loss of emotional expression sometimes observed in schizophrenia, mental retardation, and some depressive disorders.
Labile: Multiple, abrupt changes in affect seen in certain types of schizophrenia and bipolar disorder.
Full/wide range of affect: Generally appropriate emotional response.

Terms Related to Moods

Term	Word Origin	Definition
Anger		As a symptom, anger is pathologic in nature if it is inappropriate for the situation.
Anxiety		Anticipation of impending danger and dread accompanied by restlessness, tension, tachycardia, and breathing difficulty not associated with an apparent stimulus.
Dysphoria dis FOR ree ah	*dys-* abnormal *phor/o* to carry, to bear *-ia* condition	Generalized negative mood characterized by depression.
Euphoria you FOR ee ah	*eu-* good, well *phor/o* to carry, to bear *-ia* condition	Exaggerated sense of physical and emotional well-being not based on reality, disproportionate to the cause, or inappropriate to the situation.
Euthymia yoo THIGH mee ah	*eu-* good, well *thym/o* mind *-ia* condition	Normal range of moods and emotions.

Exercise 2: Symptoms, Affects, and Moods of Mental Illness

Did You Know?

Euphoria comes from *eu-*, meaning *good* or *well,* and *-phoria,* a condition of *carrying* or *bearing.* Originally from the Greek meaning *well-bearing,* it now has the connotation of an inappropriate sense of elation, or an exaggerated sense of well-being.

Matching.

_____ 1. anhedonia
_____ 2. delusion
_____ 3. hallucination
_____ 4. dementia
_____ 5. dysphoria
_____ 6. euthymia
_____ 7. amnesia
_____ 8. akathisia

A. sleepwalking
B. paralysis from psychological causes
C. normal range of moods and emotions
D. lack of memory
E. restlessness, inability to sit still
F. normal drive of sensuality, creativity, desire
G. mental condition characterized by confusion and agitation
H. inaccurate sensory perception based on a real stimulus
I. belief in a falsehood
J. lack of ability to experience pleasure
K. negative mood characterized by depression
L. condition characterized by dissociation with reality

_____ 9. confabulation

_____ 10. delirium

_____ 11. catatonia

_____ 12. illusion

_____ 13. psychosis

_____ 14. somnambulism

_____ 15. libido

M. making up stories to conceal lack of memory
N. unreal sensory perception
O. condition characterized by loss of memory, personality changes, confusion, and loss of touch with reality

Circle the correct answer.

16. Anger, anxiety, and dysphoria are examples of a patient's *(affect, mood).*
17. Individuals whose emotions change rapidly are said to have a *(labile, blunted)* affect.
18. Patients who subconsciously blame another person for their own problems are using a defense mechanism called *(denial, projection).*

Terms Related to Disorders Usually First Diagnosed in Childhood

TERM	WORD ORIGIN	DEFINITION
Asperger's disorder		Disorder characterized by impairment of social interaction and repetitive patterns of inappropriate behavior.
Attention deficit/hyperactivity disorder (ADHD)		Series of syndromes that includes impulsiveness, inability to concentrate, and short attention span.
Autism AH tiz um		Condition of abnormal development of social interaction, impaired communication, and repetitive behaviors.
Conduct disorder		Any of a number of disorders characterized by patterns of persistent aggressive and defiant behaviors. **Oppositional defiant disorder (ODD),** an example of a conduct disorder, is characterized by hostile, disobedient behavior.
Mental retardation		Condition of subaverage intellectual ability, with impairments in social and educational functioning. The "intelligence quotient" (IQ) is a measure of an individual's intellectual functioning compared to the general population. **Mild mental retardation:** IQ range of 50-69; learning difficulties result. **Moderate mental retardation:** IQ range of 35-49; support needed to function in society. **Severe mental retardation:** IQ of 20-34; continuous need of support to live in society. **Profound mental retardation:** IQ <20; severe self-care limitations.
Rett's disorder		Condition characterized by initial normal functioning followed by loss of social and intellectual functioning.
Tourette's syndrome too RETTS		Group of involuntary behaviors that includes the vocalization of words or sounds (sometimes obscene) and repetitive movements; vocal and multiple tic disorder.

 Exercise 3: DISORDERS USUALLY FIRST DIAGNOSED IN CHILDHOOD

Choose the correct answer from the following list.

attention deficit/hyperactivity disorder, mild mental retardation, severe mental retardation, autism, Rett's disorder, Asperger's disorder, conduct disorder, oppositional defiant disorder, moderate mental retardation, Tourette's syndrome

1. Type of mental retardation in which the IQ range is 20 to 34. ________________
2. Disorder characterized by impairment of social interaction due to repetitive patterns of behavior. ________________
3. Group of involuntary behaviors that include tics, vocalizations, and repetitive movements. ________________
4. Group of disorders characterized by persistent aggressive and defiant behaviors. ________________
5. IQ range of 50 to 69. Most prevalent form of mental retardation, which manifests itself in learning difficulties. ________________
6. IQ range of 35 to 49. Adults will need support in living in society. ________________
7. A series of syndromes that include impulsiveness, inability to concentrate, and a short attention span. ________________
8. Condition of pathologic social withdrawal, impairment of communication, and repetitive behaviors. ________________
9. Persistent negative behavior characterized by hostile, disobedient behavior. ________________
10. Condition characterized by initial normal functioning followed by loss of social and intellectual functioning. ________________

Terms Related to Cognitive Impairment

Disorders in this category manifest significant cognitive (thinking) changes from previous functioning.

TERM	WORD ORIGIN	DEFINITION
Amnesia am NEE zsa		Memory impairment without other significant cognitive impairments.
Delirium deh LEER ee um		Characterized by short-term impairment of consciousness and change in cognition; may be associated with drug abuse or a medical condition.
Dementia deh MEN sha		Characterized by memory deficits, along with other cognitive deficits of long-term duration. May be associated with Alzheimer's disease or vascular or other medical conditions.

Substance-Related Disorders

The most rapidly increasing group of disorders are substance-related disorders. These include abuse of a number of substances, including alcohol, opioids, cannabinoids, sedatives or hypnotics, cocaine, stimulants (including caffeine), hallucinogens, tobacco, and volatile solvents (inhalants). Classifications for substance abuse include psychotic, amnesiac, and late-onset disorders. It is important to be aware that addiction is not a character flaw. Rather, addiction has a neurologic basis; the effects of specific drugs are localized to equally specific areas of the brain.

An individual is considered an "abuser" if he or she uses substances in ways that threaten health or impair social or economic functioning. Levels of abuse vary.

DID YOU KNOW?

The term *delirium* is taken from the Latin *de-*, meaning *away from,* and *lira,* meaning a *furrow;* thus someone who is mentally confused cannot "plow a straight furrow."

Terms Related to Substance Abuse

TERM	WORD ORIGIN	DEFINITION
Acute intoxication		Episode of behavioral disturbance following ingestion of alcohol or psychotropic drugs.
Delirium tremens (DTs) deh LEER ee um TREM uns	See **Did You Know?** box.	Acute and sometimes fatal delirium induced by the cessation of ingesting excessive amounts of alcohol over a long period of time.
Dependence syndrome		Difficulty in controlling use of a drug.
Harmful use		Pattern of drug use that causes damage to health.
Tolerance		State in which the body becomes accustomed to the substances ingested; hence the user requires greater amounts to create the desired effect.
Withdrawal state		Group of symptoms that occurs during the cessation of the use of a regularly taken drug.

Schizophrenia, Schizotypal, and Delusional Disorders

These disorders are not always easy to classify but carry with them some common characteristics. Roughly, these disorders can be grouped as follows:

Acute and transient psychotic disorders: Heterogeneous group of disorders characterized by the acute onset of psychotic symptoms such as delusions, hallucinations, and perceptual disturbances, and by the severe disruption of ordinary behavior. *Acute onset* is defined as a crescendo from a normal perceptual state to a clearly abnormal clinical picture in about 2 weeks or less. For these disorders, there is no evidence of organic causation. Perplexity and puzzlement are often present, but disorientation for time, place, and person is not persistent or severe enough to justify a diagnosis of organically caused delirium. The disorder may or may not be associated with acute stress (usually defined as stressful events preceding the onset by 1 or 2 weeks).

Persistent delusional disorders: Variety of disorders in which long-standing delusions constitute the only, or the most conspicuous, clinical characteristic and cannot be classified as organic, schizophrenic, or affective.

Schizophrenic disorders: Disorders characterized by fundamental distortions of thinking and perception, coupled with affects that are inappropriate or blunted. The patient exhibits characteristic inability to recognize an appropriate perception of reality (Fig. 13-1). The patient's intellectual capacity is usually intact. Symptoms may include hallucinations, delusions, and thought disorder.

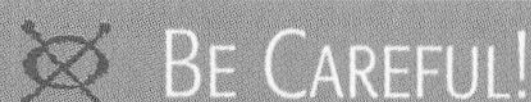

BE CAREFUL!

The combining form *phren/o* can mean *mind* or *diaphragm.*

- **Catatonic schizophrenia** (kat tah TAH nick skit zoh FREH nee uh) is dominated by prominent psychomotor disturbances that may alternate between extremes such as hyperkinesis and stupor, and may be accompanied by a dreamlike (oneiric) state and hallucinations.
- **Disorganized schizophrenia** is characterized by prominent affective changes, fleeting and fragmentary delusions and hallucinations, and irresponsible and unpredictable behavior. Shallow, inappropriate mood, flighty thoughts, social isolation, and incoherent speech are also present.
- **Paranoid schizophrenia** is dominated by relatively stable, persistent delusions, usually accompanied by auditory hallucinations and perceptual disturbances in affect, volition (will), and speech.
- **Schizotypal** (skiz zoh TIE pull) **disorder,** although sometimes described as borderline schizophrenia, has none of the characteristic schizophrenic anomalies. Patients may exhibit anhedonia, eccentric behavior, cold affect, and social isolation.

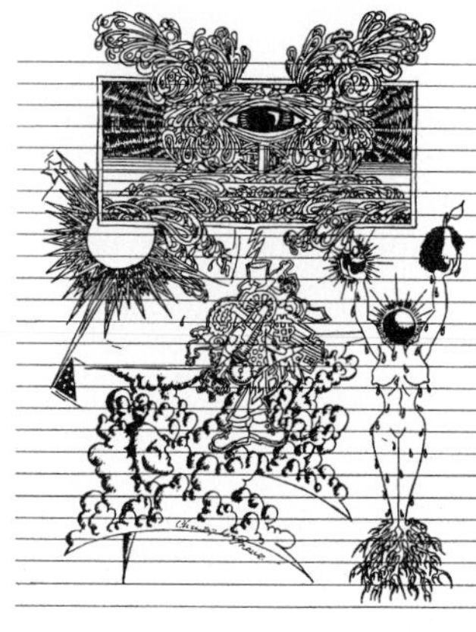

A

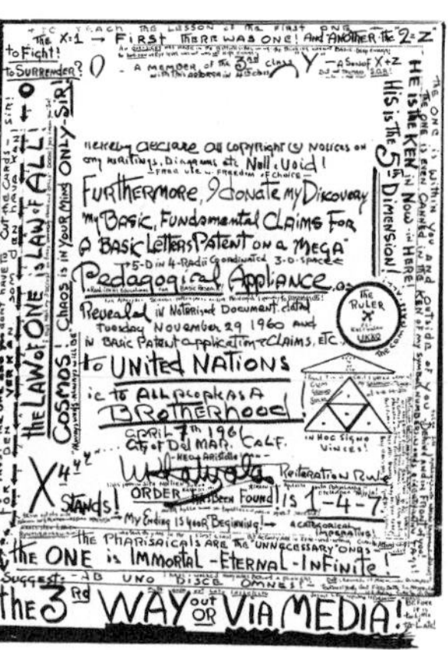

B

Fig. 13-1 **A,** This drawing by a patient with schizophrenia demonstrates thought disorder. **B,** Drawing by a delusional patient with schizophrenia.

Exercise 4: COGNITIVE DISORDERS, SUBSTANCE ABUSE, AND SCHIZOPHRENIC DISORDERS

Fill in the blanks with the following terms.

schizophrenia, hallucinations, persistent delusional, disorganized, dementia, delusions, alcohol, inhalants, dream, controlling substance use

1. Alzheimer's patients exhibit which type of disorder? ________________
2. A patient with the DTs is showing withdrawal symptoms from ________________.
3. Volatile solvents are included under ________________.
4. Dependence syndrome is a condition in which the patient has difficulty ________________.
5. Auditory hallucinations, delusions, and thought disturbances are characteristic of ________________.
6. A patient with oneiric symptoms acts as if he or she is in a ________________-like state.
7. The difference between schizophrenic and schizotypal disorders is that the schizotypal patient does not have sustained ________________ or ________________.

8. The only, or most conspicuous, clinical characteristic of patients with ________________ disorders is the presence of long-standing aberrant beliefs or perceptions.
9. Shallow, inappropriate mood, flighty thought, social isolation, and incoherent speech are all symptoms of which type of schizophrenia? ________________

Case Study Continued

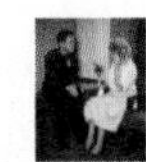

Andrew notes that Nadine's generally flattened affect is punctuated by bouts of tearfulness and anxiety. She says, "I know I'm unhappy—how else should I be? I'm tired, but I can't sit still. I go to sleep and then I wake up in the middle of the night. I try to read to take my mind off of feeling bad, and I just can't concentrate. I know he's not coming back. It just worries me that I'm never going to feel any better than I do now. And I don't know what to do."

Mood Disorders

Patients with mood disorders, also called *affective disorders,* show a disturbance of affect ranging from depression (with or without associated anxiety) to elation. The mood change is usually accompanied by a change in the overall level of activity; most of the other symptoms are either secondary to, or easily understood in the context of, the change in mood and activity. Most of these disorders tend to be recurrent, and the onset of individual episodes can often be related to stressful events or situations.

Terms Related to Mood Disorders

Term	Word Origin	Definition
Bipolar disorder (BP) bye POH lur	*bi-* two *pol/o* pole *-ar* pertaining to	Disorder characterized by swings between an elevation of mood, increased energy and activity (hypomania and mania), and a lowering of mood and decreased energy and activity (depression).
Cyclothymia sye kloh THIGH mee ah	*cycl/o* cycling *thym/o* mind *-ia* condition of	Disorder characterized by recurring episodes of mild elation and depression that are not severe enough to warrant a diagnosis of bipolar disorder.
Depressive disorder		Depression typically characterized by its degree (minimal, moderate, severe) or number of occurrences (single or recurrent, persistent). Patient exhibits dysphoria, reduction of energy, and decrease in activity. Symptoms include anhedonia, lack of ability to concentrate, and fatigue. Patient may experience **parasomnias** (abnormal sleep patterns), diminished appetite, and loss of self-esteem.
Dysthymia dis THIGH mee ah	*dys-* difficult *thym/o* mind *-ia* condition	Mild, chronic depression of mood that lasts for years but is not severe enough to justify a diagnosis of depression.
Hypomania hye poh MAY nee ah	*hypo-* decreased *man/o* madness *-ia* condition	Disorder characterized by an inappropriate elevation of mood that may include positive as well as negative aspects. Patient may report increased feelings of well-being, energy, and activity, but may also report irritability and conceit.

Continued

Terms Related to Mood Disorders—cont'd

TERM	WORD ORIGIN	DEFINITION
Persistent mood disorders		Group of long-term, cyclic mood disorders in which the majority of the individual episodes are not sufficiently severe to warrant being described as hypomanic or mild depressive episodes.
Seasonal affective disorder (SAD)		Weather-induced depression resulting from decreased exposure to sunlight in autumn and winter.

Terms Related to Anxiety Disorders

TERM	WORD ORIGIN	DEFINITION
Acrophobia ack roh FOH bee ah	*acr/o* heights, extremes *-phobia* fear	Fear of heights.
Agoraphobia ah gore uh FOH bee ah	*agor/a* marketplace *-phobia* fear	Fear of leaving home and entering crowded places.
Anthropophobia an throh poh FOH bee ah	*anthrop/o* man *-phobia* fear	Fear of scrutiny by other people; also called **social phobia.**
Claustrophobia klos troh FOH bee ah	*claustr/o* a closing *-phobia* fear	Fear of enclosed spaces.
Generalized anxiety disorder (GAD)		One of the most common diagnoses assigned, but not specific to any particular situation or circumstance. Symptoms may include persistent nervousness, trembling, muscular tensions, sweating, lightheadedness, palpitations, dizziness, and epigastric discomfort.
Obsessive-compulsive disorder (OCD)		Characterized by recurrent, distressing, and unavoidable preoccupations or irresistible drives to perform specific rituals (e.g., constantly checking locks or excessive handwashing) that the patient feels will prevent some harmful event.
Panic disorder (PD)		Recurrent, unpredictable attacks of severe anxiety (panic) that are not restricted to any particular situation. Symptoms may include vertigo, chest pain, and heart palpitations.
Posttraumatic stress disorder (PTSD)		Extended emotional response to a traumatic event. Symptoms may include flashbacks, recurring nightmares, anhedonia, insomnia, hypervigilance, anxiety, depression, suicidal thoughts, and emotional blunting.

Terms Related to Adjustment Disorder, Dissociative Identity Disorder, and Somatoform Disorder

TERM	WORD ORIGIN	DEFINITION
Adjustment disorder		Disorder that tends to manifest during periods of stressful life changes (e.g., divorce, death, relocation, job loss). Symptoms include anxiety, impaired coping mechanisms, social dysfunction, and a reduced ability to perform normal daily activities.
Dissociative identity disorder		Maladaptive coping with severe stress by developing one or more separate personalities. A less severe form, **dissociative disorder** or **dissociative reaction,** results in identity confusion accompanied by amnesia, a dreamlike state, and somnambulism.
Somatoform disorder soh MAT toh form	*somat/o* body	Any disorder that presents as unfounded physical complaints by the patient, despite medical assurance that no physiologic problem exists. One type of somatoform disorder is **hypochondriacal disorder,** which is the preoccupation with the possibility of having one or more serious and progressive physical disorders.

Terms Related to Eating Disorders

TERM	WORD ORIGIN	DEFINITION
Anorexia nervosa an oh RECKS see ah nur VOH sah	*an-* without *orex/o* appetite *-ia* condition	Prolonged refusal to eat adequate amounts of foods and an altered perception of what constitutes a normal minimal body weight, caused by an intense fear of becoming obese. Primarily affects adolescent females; emaciation and amenorrhea result (Fig. 13-2).
Bulimia nervosa boo LIM ee ah nur VOH sah		Eating disorder in which the individual eats large quantities of food and then purges the body through self-induced vomiting or inappropriate use of laxatives.

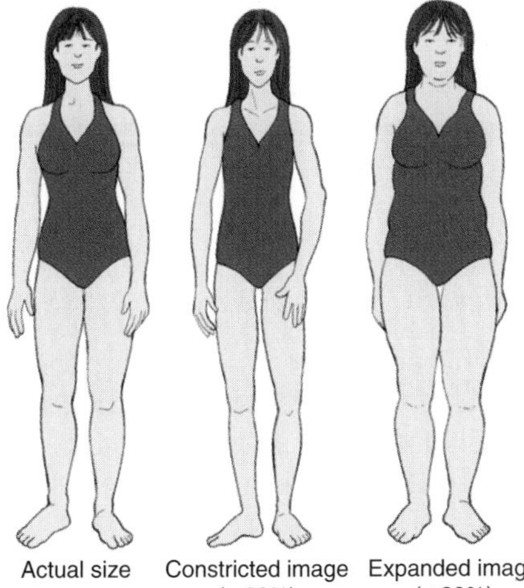

Fig. 13-2 The perception of body shape and size can be evaluated with the use of special computer drawing programs that allow a subject to distort (increase or decrease) the width of an actual picture of a person's body by as much as 20%. Subjects with anorexia consistently adjusted their own body picture to a size 20% larger than its true form, which suggests that they have a major problem with the perception of self-image.

DID YOU KNOW?

Anorexia has the highest mortality rate of any psychiatric disorder (7% to 24%).

Sleep Disorders

Sleep disorders are called **dyssomnias** (dih SOM nee ahs), or difficulties with the sleep-wake cycle, and **parasomnias** (pair ah SOM nee ahs), or abnormal activation of physiologic functions during the sleep cycle. **Nightmare disorder** and **sleep terrors** are examples of parasomnias, and insomnia and hypersomnia are examples of dyssomnias. They may take a variety of forms.

Terms Related to Sleep Disorders

Term	Word Origin	Definition
Dyssomnia	*dys-* bad *somn/o* sleep *-ia* condition	Difficulty with the sleep-wake cycle. Examples include **insomnia,** the chronic struggle either to fall asleep or stay asleep, and **hypersomnia,** abnormally deep or lengthy periods of sleep.
Parasomnia	*para-* abnormal *somn/o* sleep *-ia* condition	Abnormal activation of physiologic functions during the sleep cycle. Examples include **sleep terrors,** in which repeated episodes of sudden awakening are accompanied by intense anxiety, agitation, and amnesia.

Terms Related to Sexual Dysfunction

Term	Word Origin	Definition
Frigidity frij ID ih tee		Indifference or unresponsiveness to sexual stimuli; inability to achieve orgasm during intercourse. Also called **hypoactive sexual desire disorder.**
Nymphomania nim foh MAY nee ah	*nymph/o-* woman *-mania* madness	Relentless drive to achieve sexual orgasm in the female. In the male the condition is called **satyriasis** (sat tih RYE ah sis).
Premature ejaculation		Involuntary, anxiety-induced ejaculation of semen during sexual activity.
Sexual anhedonia an hee DOH nee ah	*an-* without *hedon/o* pleasure *-ia* condition	Inability to enjoy sexual pleasure.

Personality Disorders

Personality disorders have several common characteristics, including long-standing, inflexible, dysfunctional behavior patterns and personality traits that result in an inability to function successfully in society. These characteristics are not due to stress, and affected patients have very little to no insight into their disorder.

Terms Related to Personality Disorders

TERM	WORD ORIGIN	DEFINITION
Borderline personality disorder		Disorder characterized by impulsive, unpredictable mood and self-image, resulting in unstable interpersonal relationships and a tendency to see and respond to others as unwaveringly good or evil.
Dissocial personality disorder		Disorder in which the patient shows a complete lack of interest in social obligations, to the extreme of showing antipathy for other individuals. Patients frustrate easily, are quick to display aggression, show a tendency to blame others, and do not change their behavior even after punishment.
Paranoid personality disorder		State in which the individual exhibits inappropriately suspicious thinking, self-importance, a lack of ability to forgive perceived insults, and an extreme sense of personal rights.
Schizoid personality disorder		Condition in which the patient withdraws into a fantasy world, with little need for social interaction. Most patients have a limited capacity to experience pleasure or to express their feelings.

Terms Related to Habit and Impulse Disorders

TERM	WORD ORIGIN	DEFINITION
Kleptomania klep toh MAY nee ah	*klept/o* steal *-mania* madness	Uncontrollable impulse to steal.
Pyromania pye roh MAY nee ah	*pyr/o* fire *-mania* madness	Uncontrollable impulse to set fires.
Trichotillomania trick oh till oh MAY nee ah		Uncontrollable impulse to pull one's hair out by the roots.

Terms Related to Paraphilias (Sexual Perversion) or Disorders of Sexual Preference

TERM	WORD ORIGIN	DEFINITION
Exhibitionism eck sih BISH uh niz um		Condition in which the patient derives sexual arousal from the exposure of his or her genitals to strangers.
Fetishism FET ish iz um		Reliance on an object as a stimulus for sexual arousal and pleasure.
Pedophilia ped oh FILL ee ah	*ped/o* child *phil/o* attraction *-ia* condition	Sexual preference, either in fantasy or actuality, for children as a means of achieving sexual excitement and gratification.
Sadomasochism say doh MASS oh kiz um		Preference for sexual activity that involves inflicting or receiving pain and/or humiliation.
Voyeurism VOY yur iz um		Condition in which an individual derives sexual pleasure and gratification from surreptitiously looking at individuals engaged in intimate behavior.

Exercise 5: MISCELLANEOUS BEHAVIORAL DISORDERS

Fill in the blanks with the following terms.

kleptomania, posttraumatic stress disorder, anorexia nervosa, hypomania, satyriasis, somnambulism, sadomasochism, dysthymia, bipolar disorder, obsessive-compulsive disorder, social phobia, cyclothymia, hypersomnia, paranoid personality disorder, premature ejaculation, pyromania, depressive disorder, hypochondriacal disorder, dissociative identity disorder, generalized anxiety disorder, claustrophobia

1. An alternative name for anthropophobia is _______________.
2. Fear of enclosed spaces is called _______________.
3. Patients who experience symptoms of persistent nervousness, trembling, muscular tension, sweating, lightheadedness, palpitations, dizziness, and epigastric discomfort may be diagnosed with _______________.
4. Patients who are compelled to have repetitive thoughts or repeat specific rituals may have a diagnosis of _______________.
5. Extreme trauma that may result in flashbacks, nightmares, hypervigilance, or reliving the trauma is called _______________.
6. Patients who develop separate personalities as a result of a severely stressful situation are diagnosed with what disorder? _______________
7. Patients who continually express physical complaints that have no real basis have a type of _______________.
8. Episodes of mood changes from depression to mania are called _______________.
9. Patients who have a loss of energy, of pleasure, and of interest in life may be experiencing _______________.
10. An inappropriate, persistent elevation of mood that may include irritability is called _______________.
11. Patients with chronic, extremely mild depression that varies to mild elation may suffer from _______________.
12. A chronic depression that lasts for years but does not warrant a diagnosis of depression, may be termed _______________.
13. What is the healthcare term for walking in one's sleep? _______________
14. What is the term for an insatiable sexual desire in men? _______________
15. Male patients who experience uncontrollable ejaculation due to anxiety may be diagnosed with _______________.
16. What is the healthcare term for sleep that is excessive in depth or duration? _______________
17. What is the disorder in which patients refuse to maintain a body weight that is a minimum weight for height? _______________

18. What is the healthcare term for the pathologic impulse to set fires? ________________
19. What is the healthcare term for a severe, enduring personality disorder with paranoid tendencies?

    ____

20. A preference for sexual activity that involves pain and humiliation is called ________________.

21. Uncontrollable stealing is called ________________.

Case Study Continued

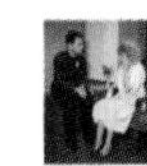

Andrew recognizes that Mrs. White is exhibiting classic signs of depression: fatigue, anhedonia, insomnia, and inability to concentrate. He empathizes with her about how hard it is to accept the death of a loved one, especially a life partner. "I want you to know, Mrs. White, that your symptoms are not unusual or untreatable. I think I can help you get back on track and enjoy life again. The bad news is, although you say you don't want to 'talk about it,' talking may be the best way to get through this. Let's try that first."

DIAGNOSTIC PROCEDURES

Behavioral diagnoses must take into account underlying healthcare abnormalities that may cause or influence a patient's mental health. Some of the common laboratory and imaging procedures are mentioned here, along with procedures that are traditionally considered to be psychological.

Diagnostic Criteria

DSM-IV-TR multiaxial assessment diagnosis: Diagnostic tool measuring mental health of the individual across five axes. The first three (if present) are stated as diagnostic codes, whereas Axis IV is a statement of factors influencing the patient's mental health (e.g., lack of social supports, unemployment), and Axis V is a numerical score that summarizes a patient's overall functioning.

1. Axis I: Clinical Disorders
2. Axis II: Personality Disorders and/or Mental Retardation
3. Axis III: General Medical Conditions
4. Axis IV: Psychosocial and Environmental Problems
5. Axis V: Global Assessment of Functioning Scale (GAF)

Mental status examination: A diagnostic procedure to determine a patient's current mental state. It includes assessment of the patient's appearance, affect, thought processes, cognitive function, insight, and judgment.

Laboratory Tests

Patients may have blood counts (complete blood cell count [CBC] with differential), blood chemistry, thyroid function panels, screening tests for syphilis (rapid plasma reagin [RPR] or microhemagglutination-*Treponema pallidum* [MHA-TP]), urinalyses with drug screen, urine pregnancy checks for females with childbearing potential, blood alcohol levels, serum levels of medications, and human immunodeficiency virus (HIV) tests in high-risk patients.

Imaging

Imaging is most helpful in ruling out neurologic disorders and in research; it is less helpful in diagnosing or treating psychiatric problems. Computed tomography (CT) scans and magnetic resonance imaging (MRI) can be used to screen for brain lesions. Positron emission tomography (PET) scans can be used to examine and map the metabolic activity of the brain.

Psychological Testing

Bender Gestalt Test: A test of visuomotor and spatial abilities; useful for children and adults.

Draw-a-Person (DAP) Test: Analysis of patient's drawings of male and female individuals. Used to assess personality.

Minnesota Multiphasic Personality Inventory (MMPI): Assessment of personality characteristics through a battery of forced-choice questions.

Rorschach: A projective test using inkblots to determine the patient's ability to integrate intellectual and emotional factors in his or her perception of the environment.

Thematic apperception test (TAT): Test in which patients are asked to make up stories about the pictures they are shown. This test may provide information about a patient's interpersonal relationships, fantasies, needs, conflicts, and defenses.

Wechsler Adult Intelligence Scale (WAIS): Measure of verbal IQ, performance IQ, and full-scale IQ.

Exercise 6: Diagnostic Procedures

Matching.

_____ 1. WAIS

_____ 2. TAT

_____ 3. PET scan

_____ 4. MMPI

_____ 5. Rorschach

_____ 6. GAF

_____ 7. Bender Gestalt

A. numerical measure of overall mental health
B. provides information about needs, fantasies, interpersonal relationships
C. measures personality characteristics
D. IQ test
E. test of visuomotor and spatial skills
F. imaging of metabolic activity (in brain)
G. examines integration of emotional and intellectual factors

THERAPEUTIC INTERVENTIONS

Terms Related to Psychotherapy

TERM	WORD ORIGIN	DEFINITION
Behavioral therapy		Therapeutic attempt to alter an undesired behavior by substituting a new response or set of responses to a given stimulus.
Cognitive therapy		Wide variety of treatment techniques that attempt to help the individual alter inaccurate or unhealthy perceptions and patterns of thinking.
Psychoanalysis sye koh uh NAL ih sis		Behavioral treatment developed initially by Sigmund Freud to analyze and treat any dysfunctional effects of unconscious factors on a patient's mental state.

Terms Related to Other Therapeutic Methods

TERM	WORD ORIGIN	DEFINITION
Detoxification		Removal of a chemical substance (drug or alcohol) as an initial step in treatment of a chemically dependent individual.
Electroconvulsive therapy (ECT)		Method of inducing convulsions to treat affective disorders in patients who have been resistant or unresponsive to drug therapy.
Light therapy		Exposure of the body to light waves to treat patients with depression due to seasonal fluctuations (Fig. 13-3).

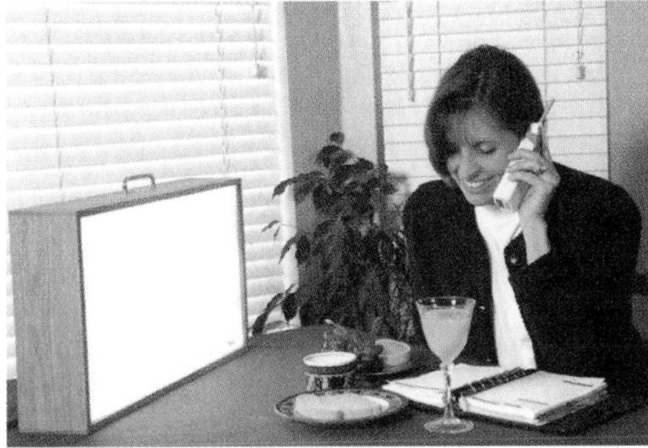

Fig. 13-3 Broad-spectrum, fluorescent lamps like this one are used in daily therapy sessions from autumn into spring for people with SAD. Patients report feeling less depressed within 3 to 7 days. (Courtesy Apollo Light Systems.)

DID YOU KNOW?

Frontal lobotomy (incision and/or removal of the frontal lobes of the brain) was a popular treatment in the 1940s for patients with depression or schizophrenia. Although most of the negative symptomatology was diminished, patients appeared to have flattened affects. When Thorazine, a tranquilizer without sedative properties, was developed in the 1950s, the number of lobotomies declined tremendously. Today the surgery is seldom performed; it is done only to relieve intractable pain or depression.

Exercise 7: THERAPEUTIC INTERVENTIONS

Fill in the blanks with the following terms.

cognitive therapy, ECT, behavioral, light therapy, psychoanalysis

1. Patients are treated with ________________ therapy when an attempt is made to replace maladjusted patterns with a new response to a given stimulus.
2. What type of therapy uses exposure of the body to light waves to treat patients with depression due to seasonal fluctuations? ________________
3. What is a method of inducing convulsions to treat affective disorders in patients who have been resistant or unresponsive to drug therapy? ________________
4. What therapy is used to analyze and treat any dysfunctional effects of unconscious factors or a patient's mental state? ________________
5. What are any of the various methods of treating mental and emotional disorders that help a person change attitudes, perceptions, and patterns of thinking? ________________

PHARMACOLOGY

A major part of treatment for behavioral disorders is the use of drug therapy. For example, patients may be prescribed a type of selective serotonin reuptake inhibitor (SSRI) for major depression or depression in bipolar disorder. Serotonin is one type of neurotransmitter in many synapses in the brain. In depressed patients, there is not enough serotonin available at the postsynaptic neuron. SSRIs prevent the presynaptic neuron from taking the serotonin back up, thereby increasing the amount of serotonin available in the synapse. (For a review of synapses and neurotransmitter action, see Chapter 12.) The psychiatric medications described appear in the top 100 prescribed medications in the United States. Medications are continually being developed and reevaluated and are closely regulated by the Food and Drug Administration. Examples include the following:

Antialcoholics: Drugs intended to discourage use of alcohol. An example is naltrexone hydrochloride (ReVia), used for alcohol and narcotic withdrawal. Disulfiram (Antabuse) is used to deter alcohol consumption.

Anticonvulsants: Drugs to control or prevent seizures. Examples include clonazepam (Klonopin), phenytoin (Dilantin), and phenobarbital (Tedral preparations).

Antidepressants: Medications intended to relieve symptoms of depressed mood. Many classes are available, including SSRIs, tricyclics, and tetracyclics. Examples include fluoxetine (Prozac), sertraline (Zoloft), bupropion (Wellbutrin), and imipramine (Tofranil).

Antimanics: Drugs intended to control mental disorders characterized by euphoria. One example is lithium (Lithobid).

Antipsychotics (also referred to as **neuroleptics** and **major tranquilizers**): Medications intended to control psychotic symptoms such as hallucinations and delusions. Examples include chlorpromazine (Thorazine), olanzapine (Zyprexa), and clozapine (Clozaril).

DID YOU KNOW?

The Office of Alternative Medicine at the National Institutes of Health (NIH) discusses several therapies not included in this chapter. Notable are culturally based therapies (e.g., acupuncture, yoga, Native American traditional practices, and *cuentos,* or Puerto Rican folk tales), relaxation and stress reduction techniques, pastoral counseling, self-help groups, expressive therapies, and diet and nutrition.

Anxiolytics: Drugs whose effect is to relieve symptoms of anxiety. Examples are lorazepam (Ativan), buspirone (BuSpar), and diazepam (Valium).

Hypnotics: These drugs promote sleep. Sedatives, sedative-hypnotics, and anxiolytics, which are similar in effect and are often used interchangeably, overlap with this category. Examples include zolpidem (Ambien) and flurazepam (Dalmane).

Nosotropics: These drugs combat the cognitive deterioration seen in disorders characterized by dementia, such as Alzheimer's disease. Examples are tacrine (Cognex) and donepezil (Aricept).

Sedatives: This term may be used to describe a class of central nervous system depressant drugs or the calming effect or action a drug may exert. An example is promethazine hydrochloride (Phenergan).

Sedative-hypnotics: A combination of two drug classes, these drugs are central nervous system depressants intended to calm patients. An example is meprobamate (Equanil, Miltown).

Stimulants: Generally intended to increase synaptic activity of targeted neurons, these drugs are amphetamine-like in nature and are used to treat narcolepsy, as well as ADHD. An example is methylphenidate (Ritalin, Concerta).

Exercise 8: PHARMACOLOGY

Match the drug class with the drug name.

_____ 1. antimanic

_____ 2. antidepressant

_____ 3. nosotropic

_____ 4. sedative

_____ 5. anticonvulsant

_____ 6. anxiolytic

_____ 7. stimulant

_____ 8. sedative-hypnotic

_____ 9. hypnotic

A. Miltown
B. Ritalin
C. fluoxetine, bupropion
D. clonazepam, Dilantin, phenobarbital
E. tacrine, donepezil
F. Ambien, Dalmane
G. lithium
H. BuSpar, diazepam
I. Phenergan

Case Study Continued

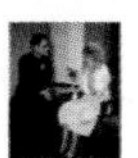

At the end of the scheduled session, Adam suggests that Mrs. White participate in a bereavement group for women and men who have lost their partners. "I think you'd find it useful to hear how other people are coping with their losses. That group meets here one evening a week. I'd also like you to come back and see me once a week, so that we can continue to get to know each other and work on a new start for you. How do you feel about that?" Mrs. White offers a glimmer of a smile as she clutches her well-used tissue and says, "I must admit that I was angry with my daughter when she brought me to Dr. McGuire, but now that we've talked, I think I'd like to give it a try. When do we meet again?"

Abbreviations

Abbreviation	Definition	Abbreviation	Definition
ADHD	Attention deficit/hyperactivity disorder	O × 3	Oriented to time, place, and person
BD	Bipolar disorder	O × 4	Oriented to time, place, person, and objects
DT	Delirium tremens	OCD	Obsessive-compulsive disorder
GAD	Generalized anxiety disorder	ODD	Oppositional defiant disorder
ECT	Electroconvulsive therapy	PTSD	Posttraumatic stress disorder
GAF	Global Assessment of Functioning	SAD	Seasonal affective disorder
IQ	Intelligence quotient	SSRI	Selective serotonin reuptake inhibitor
MR	Mental retardation	Sx	Symptoms
O × 1	Oriented to time	WAIS	Weschler Adult Intelligence Scale
O × 2	Oriented to time and place		

Exercise 9: ABBREVIATIONS

Write out the abbreviations in the following sentences.

1. Michele was being treated with light therapy for her SAD. ____________________
2. John was diagnosed with GAD after exhibiting sx of difficulty concentrating, excessive worry, and disturbed sleep over the last year. ____________________
3. The patient had a diagnosis of mild MR, with an IQ of 55, as determined by the WAIS.
   ____
4. Roger was referred to the school psychologist by his teacher to be evaluated for the possibility of an ADHD diagnosis after many behavioral problems at school and at home.
   ____
5. The patient was diagnosed with PTSD after she was assulted. ____________________

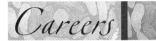

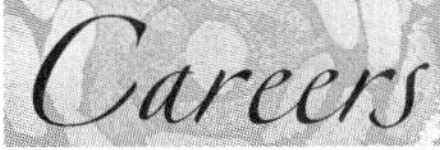

Social Workers

Although many professions are involved in working with psychiatric and substance abuse patients, the career predicted to grow faster than average in the next few years in this area is that of social worker. Although a bachelor's degree is a minimum requirement, most positions require a master's degree—that is, a master's of social work (MSW). Individuals who choose social work as a profession tend to have a strong desire to help their clients overcome difficulties and solve personal or family problems. Because this is an extremely broad profession, most social workers specialize. Those who work with patients with mental or emotional problems may provide such services as crisis intervention, individual or group therapy, social rehabilitation, or training in everyday living skills. Substance abuse social workers assist drug and alcohol abusers in recovery from their dependencies. A common adjunct to this treatment includes employment counseling. For more information about the field of social work, please contact the National Association of Social Workers at http://www.naswdc.org.

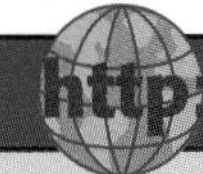

INTERNET PROJECT

Depression

Almost 10% of American adults experience a form of depression each year. Choose from the following disorders:

- Major depressive disorder
- Dysthymic disorder
- Bipolar disorder
- Postpartum depression

Write a 4-page, double-spaced paper on one of these forms of depression that includes the following:

- Causes
- Risk factors
- Symptoms
- Treatment options
- Statistics of occurrence
- Alternative and complementary treatments

To start your research, you may use the following resources:

Mayo Foundation for Medical Information and Research: Depression
http://www.mayoclinic.com/invoke.cfm?id=DS00175
National Center for Complementary and Alternative Medicine
http://nccam.nih.gov/health/stjohnswort/index.htm
National Institute of Mental Health: Statistics
http://www.nimh.nih.gov/publicat/numbers.cfm
National Mental Health Association: Symptoms of Depression
http://www.nmha.org/ccd/support/symptoms.cfm
National Institute of Mental Health: Medications. Check out their Website for medications for the disorder chosen.
http://www.nimh.nih.gov/publicat/medicate.cfm
MEDLINEplus: Depression
http://www.nlm.nih.gov/medlineplus/depression.html

Chapter Review

A. Introduction

1. Who publishes the official listing of diagnosable mental disorders for the United States, and what is this listing called?

____

2. Describe behavioral health.

____

____

B. Pathology

3. The therapist records the symptoms of a patient who reports seeing lizards in her bathroom that are trying to attack her. She is having visual ______________.
4. Since the death of her brother, Kate has been crying constantly and experiencing a great deal of difficulty eating, sleeping, and working. Her diagnosis is ______________.
5. The counselor interviewed a client who expressed the belief that she is the current queen of England. Her symptom is considered a/an ______________.
6. John reported that the sound of the wind coming down his chimney was actually a voice. He was experiencing a/an ______________.
7. What is the term for a progressive, organic mental disorder characterized by disorientation, stupor, and loss of cognitive abilities? ______________
8. What is the term for an appropriate range of emotion? ______________
9. What is the healthcare term that describes restlessness and an inability to sit still? ______________
10. Someone with a blunt affect has a ______________ range of emotions.
11. What is a "labile affect"? ______________________________
12. What is the term for a person's normal psychological impulse drive? ______________
13. A state of psychologically induced immobility is called ______________.
14. Denial and projection are examples of ______________.
15. An unreal sensory perception that does not result from an external stimulus and occurs in the waking state is a/an ______________.
16. What is a condition of confused, unfocused, and irrational agitation? ______________
17. A dysphoric mood is characterized by ______________.

18. What is the difference between euphoria and euthymia?

____

____

19. A false interpretation of an external sensory stimulus is a/an _______________.

20. What is the term for difficulty in controlling use of a drug? _______________

21. In what disorder does a patient have fundamental distortions of thinking and perception but with intact intellectual capacity? _______________

22. Another term for borderline schizophrenia is _______________.

23. When a patient experiences an acute onset of symptoms such as delusions, hallucinations, perceptual disturbances, and a severe disruption of ordinary behavior, he or she has an acute, transient _______________ disorder.

24. Mood disorders are also referred to as _______________ disorders.

25. Bipolar affective disorder is characterized by two extremes of behavior: _______________ and _______________.

26. Give an example of a dyssomnia: _______________

27. Give an example of a parasomnia: _______________

28. Dysthymia is _______________.

29. Give an example of a healthcare term for a "fear" disorder and explain what it is.

____

30. Patients who have recurrent, involuntary patterns of thought and meaningless activity may be diagnosed with _______________.

31. Patients who have an extended emotional response to a traumatic event may experience _______________.

32. Patients who develop multiple personalities as a result of severe stress are diagnosed with _______________.

33. An eating disorder characterized by an insatiable craving for food, followed by purging through vomiting or use of laxatives, is called _______________.

34. A group of disorders that have characteristics of long-standing, inflexible, dysfunctional behavior patterns and personality traits is what type of disorder? _______________

35. An IQ range of 50 to 69 is considered what type of retardation? _______________

36. Patterns of persistent aggressive and defiant behaviors may result in a diagnosis of _______________.

37. A group of involuntary behaviors that include vocalizations and repetitive movements is called _______________.

Decode the term.

38. acrophobia ______________________________

39. pedophilia ______________________________

40. euthymia ______________________________

41. anhedonia ______________________________

42. echolalia ______________________________

43. akathisia ______________________________

44. pyromania ______________________________

Build a term.

45. excessive sleep ______________________________

46. excessive movement ______________________________

47. condition of normal range of mood ______________________________

48. pertaining to dreams ______________________________

49. fear of enclosed spaces ______________________________

C. Diagnostic Procedures

50. What form of imaging uses a computerized nuclear medicine technique to examine the metabolic activity of the brain? ______________________________
51. What are the five axes of the DSM-IV-TR multiaxial evaluation?

    ____

52. Personality characteristics are assessed through which test? ______________________________
53. Which test has the patient tell a story to go with a picture that is presented?

    ____

54. The WAIS measures ______________________________.

D. Therapeutic Interventions

55. ECT is ______________________________ and is used to treat ______________________________.
56. A type of treatment that is used to help people change attitudes, perceptions, and patterns of thinking is ______________ therapy.
57. An attempt at substituting a new response to a given stimulus occurs in what type of therapy?

    ____

58. Detoxification is an initial step in treating ______________.

59. Light therapy is used to treat which disorder? ______________________________

E. Pharmacology

Fill in the blank next to the generic term with the type of medication.

anticonvulsant, stimulant, anxiolytic, antidepressant, nosotropic, sedative-hypnotic, antipsychotic

60. diazepam ______________

61. sertraline ______________

62. clonazepam ______________

63. chlorpromazine ______________

64. tacrine ______________

65. methylphenidate ______________

66. meprobamate ______________

67. What agency controls the medications that are distributed in this country?

____

F. Abbreviations

68. If the patient is described as being O × 3, you know that ____________________________.

69. If the abbreviation MR appears on a healthcare report, you know that it stands for

____________________________, but you do not know to what degree.

70. Patients who exhibit OCD have which disorder? ____________________________

71. DTs are used to abbreviate a finding that occurs in patients undergoing withdrawal from which type of substance abuse? Identify the abbreviation and the substance. ____________________________

72. Patients who exhibit GAD have which disorder? ____________________________

G. Translations

Write the following in your own words.

73. The patient presented with blunted affect, dysthymic mood, and complained of insomnia.

____

74. The 15-year-old patient was admitted with a diagnosis of anorexia nervosa.

____

75. Ariel explained that it would be difficult to go to school because she was agoraphobic.

____

76. The patient was referred to a sleep therapist for somnambulism.

____

77. The patient was diagnosed with pyromania after detectives had arrested him in connection with three intentionally set fires in his community.

____

H. Be Careful

Provide meanings for each of the following word parts.

78. phren/o ______________ or ______________

79. thym/o ______________

80. -thymia ______________

I. Cumulative Review

81. Patients with ADHD may exhibit hyperkinesis. What is hyperkinesis?

____

82. Patients with an inability to speak due to a physical impairment exhibit motor ______________.

83. Patients with GAD may exhibit a rapid heart rate, which is called ______________.

84. A patient who has bulimia and has been vomiting for a prolonged time may develop varicose veins of the esophagus, which are called ______________.

85. Patients who have "seizures of sleep" have a disorder termed ______________.

86. Discontinuation of chronic cocaine use may be associated with EEG changes. What is an EEG?

____

The problem-oriented medical record (POMR) was proposed by Lawrence Weed, MD, in the *New England Journal of Medicine* in the late 1960s. The record is composed of a problem list of health concerns organized by SOAP notes:

S subjective (the patient's complaints)
O objective (the physician's findings)
A assessment (interpretation by the physician)
P plan (action plan for what can be done for that particular problem)

This method is still being used, and applications have been extended to all disciplines, including veterinary medicine.

Castlewood Clinic
14037 Marion St.
Reno, NV 89512

Patient: Nadine White
DOB: 3/24/34
MR#: 23-45-69
Date: 8/12/02

S: This 68-year-old white female was brought here today by her daughter. She has a history of hypertension, GERD, and constipation. Her daughter states, "Nadine has been sleeping a lot, eating very poorly, and seems uninterested in life" since the death of her husband. The patient says that she has come only because her daughter insisted and admits that she has not been eating or sleeping well. She has been using Correctol for her constipation but says that it causes runny stools.

O: General: The patient is an older white female who appears to be fatigued and somewhat sad and tearful. HEENT: Tympanic membranes were clear bilaterally. Nose had some pale mucosa, otherwise clear. Throat was clear. Neck was supple. Lungs: Clear to auscultation. Cardiovascular: Regular rate and rhythm without murmur. Abdomen: Soft and diffusely tender to a mild degree. Bowel sounds were active.

A: (1) Depression. (2) Hypertension. (3) GERD. (4) Constipation.

P: (1) She will be referred to a psychiatric social worker for cognitive therapy. If she does not seem improved within the month, a prescription for Zoloft or Prozac will be considered. (2) Her hypertension has been controlled through diet and is within normal limits today. (3) Her GERD is being treated with Tagamet. (4) For her constipation, I recommended Citrucel or some similar type of fiber, increasing her fluid intake, and closely monitoring her diet for additional roughage.

____
Patrick McGuire, MD

J. Healthcare Report

87. If the multiaxial format had been used, which diagnosis would have been included in Axis I?

____

88. Would the patient have had a diagnosis appropriate for Axis II (with the information you have been given)? ________________________

89. What is the meaning of GERD? ________________________

90. Zoloft and Prozac are what types of medications? ________________________

91. What type of therapy has been suggested for Mrs. White? ________________________

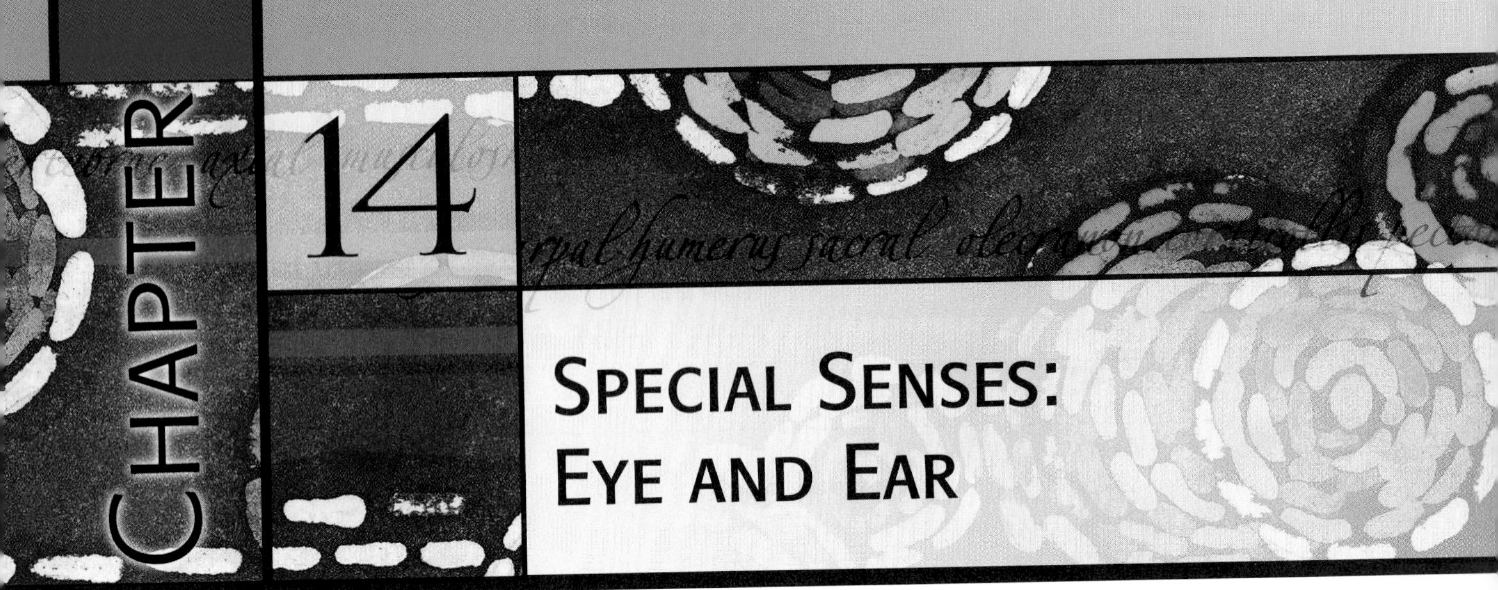

CHAPTER 14

SPECIAL SENSES: EYE AND EAR

"A beautiful eye makes silence eloquent, a kind eye makes contradiction an assent, an enraged eye makes beauty deformed. This little member gives life to every part about us." **—Joseph Addison**

Quote

Case Study

Mary Ellen Wright has had moderate vision problems for much of her life. She has worn glasses since she was 10 years old. She tried contacts a couple of times but could not get used to them. Today she is visiting her optometrist, Dr. Roland O'Connor, for her annual checkup. She is planning to ask him if he thinks she is a candidate for LASIK surgery.

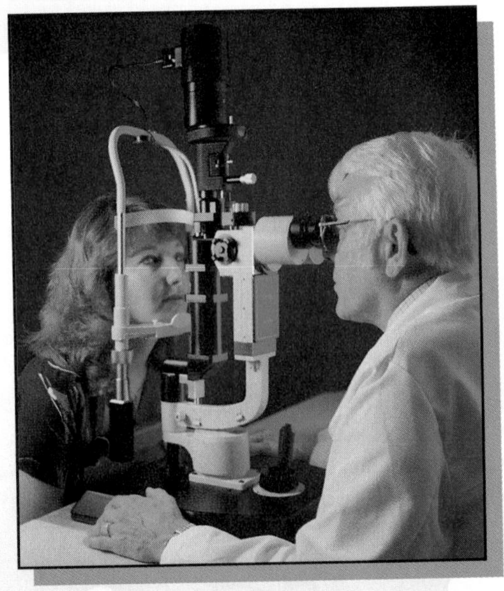

OBJECTIVES

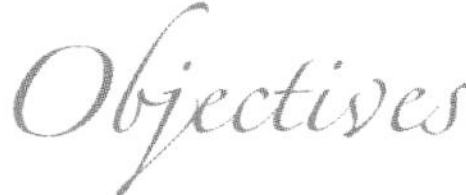

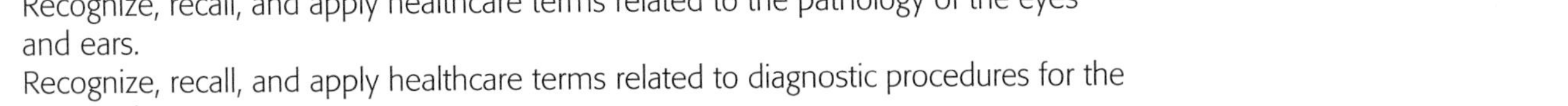

- In your own words, explain the functions of the special senses.
- Recognize, recall, and apply healthcare terms related to the anatomy and physiology of the eyes and ears.
- Recognize, recall, and apply healthcare terms related to the pathology of the eyes and ears.
- Recognize, recall, and apply healthcare terms related to diagnostic procedures for the eyes and ears.
- Recognize, recall, and apply healthcare terms related to the therapeutic interventions of the eyes and ears.
- Recognize, recall, and apply the abbreviations introduced in this chapter.
- Recognize, recall, and apply word components used in this chapter to build and decode healthcare terms relevant to eyes and ears.
- Demonstrate ability to change terms from singular to plural and vice versa.
- Recognize, recall, and apply material learned in previous chapters.

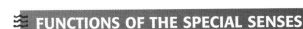

FUNCTIONS OF THE SPECIAL SENSES

When we want to relate our understanding of how someone is feeling, we say, "I hear you" or even "I see what you're saying!" Our experience in the world is filtered through our senses and our interpretations of them.

The senses include vision, hearing, taste, smell, and touch. They allow us to experience our environment through specific nervous tissue that transmits, processes, and then acts on our perceptions. This chapter covers the eyes and ears.

THE EYE

ANATOMY AND PHYSIOLOGY

The eye can be divided into the ocular adnexa—the structures that surround and support the function of the eyeball—and the structures of the globe of the eye itself.

Ocular Adnexa

Each of our paired eyes is encased in a protective, bony socket called the **orbit.** Our **binocular** vision sends two slightly different images to the brain that produce depth of vision. The right eye is called the *oculus dextra (OD),* the left eye is called the *oculus sinistra (OS),* and each eye is called the *oculus uterque (OU).* Within the orbit, the eyeball is protected by a cushion of fatty tissue. The **eyebrows** mark the supraorbital area and provide a modest amount of protection from perspiration and sun glare. Further protection is provided by the upper and lower eyelids and the eyelashes that line their edges (Fig. 14-1).

The corners of the eyes are referred to as the **canthi** (KAN thy) (*sing.* canthus); the inner canthus is termed *medial* (toward the middle of the body), and the outer canthus is *lateral.* The area where the upper and lower eyelids meet is referred to as the **palpebral fissure** (PAL puh brul FISH ur). This term comes from the function of blinking, called **palpebration** (pal puh BRAY shun). The eyelids are lined with a protective, thin mucous membrane called the **conjunctiva**

> **BE CAREFUL!**
>
> OD can mean many things. Check with your hospital/healthcare facility for a list of approved definitions—each abbreviation should be used for only one definition.

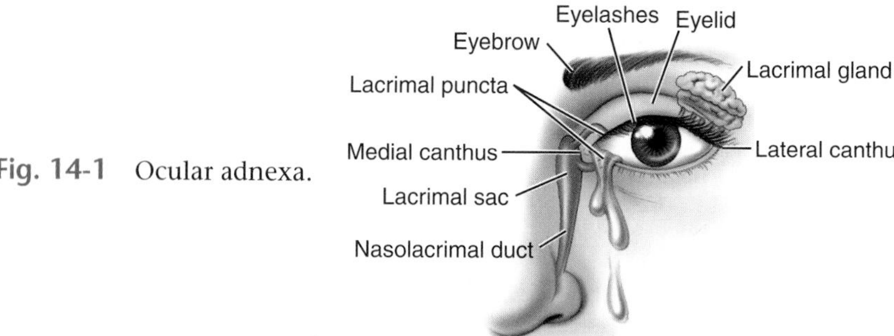

Fig. 14-1 Ocular adnexa.

(kun jungk TYE vuh) (*pl.* conjunctivae) that spreads to coat the anterior surface of the eyeball as well.

Also surrounding the eye are two types of glands. Sebaceous glands in the eyelid secrete oil to lubricate the eyelashes, and lacrimal glands above the eyes produce tears. The sebaceous glands for the eyelashes are called **meibomian** (mye BOH mee un) **glands.** These glands can be a common source of complaint when they become blocked or infected. The other type of gland, the **lacrimal** (LACK rih mul) **gland,** or tear gland, provides a constant source of cleansing and lubrication for the eye. The process of producing tears is termed **lacrimation** (lack rih MAY shun). The lacrimal glands are located in the upper outer corners of the orbit. The constant blinking of the eyelids spreads the tears across the eyeball. They then drain into two small holes (the lacrimal puncta) in the medial canthus, into the lacrimal sacs, and then into the **nasolacrimal ducts,** which carry the tears to the nasal cavity.

The **extraocular** (eck strah OCK yoo lur) **muscles** attach the eyeball to the orbit and, on impulse from the cranial nerves, move the eyes. These six voluntary (skeletal) muscles are made up of four rectus (straight) and two oblique (diagonal) muscles.

BE CAREFUL!

The term *palpebrate* means *to blink or wink.* Do not confuse this with the terms *palpate* or *palpitate.*

COMBINING FORMS FOR ACCESSORY EYE STRUCTURES

MEANING	COMBINING FORM
conjunctiva	conjunctiv/o
eye	ophthalm/o, ocul/o
eyelids	palpebr/o, blephar/o
tear	lacrim/o, dacry/o
vision	opt/o, optic/o

PREFIXES FOR ACCESSORY EYE STRUCTURES

PREFIX	MEANING
bi-, bin-	two
extra-	outside
supra-	above

Exercise 1: ACCESSORY EYE STRUCTURES

Match the term with its correct combining form or prefix. More than one answer may be correct.

_____ 1. membrane that lines eyelids and covers the surface of the eyes

_____ 2. eyelid

_____ 3. tear

_____ 4. vision

_____ 5. two

_____ 6. eye

_____ 7. outside

_____ 8. above

A. lacrim/o
B. conjunctiv/o
C. optic/o, opt/o
D. ophthalm/o
E. palpebr/o
F. ocul/o
G. blephar/o
H. bin-
I. dacry/o
J. supra-
K. extra-

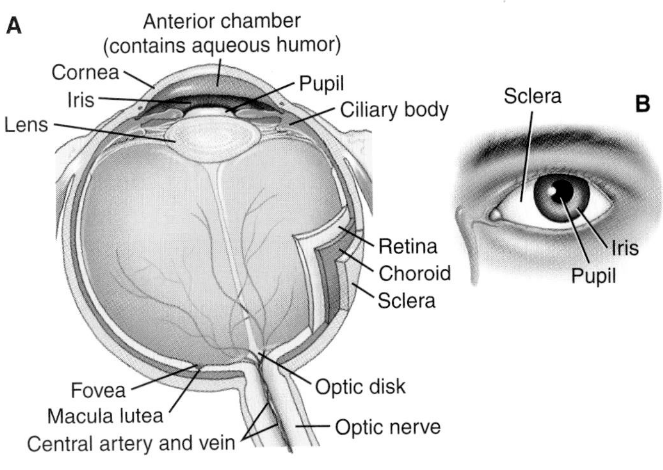

Fig. 14-2 **A,** The eyeball viewed from above. **B,** The anterior view of the eyeball.

Circle the correct answer.

9. The eyeball is located in a bony structure termed the *(adnexa, orbit).*
10. The corners of the eyes are referred to as the medial and lateral *(canthi, fissures).*
11. The process of blinking is called *(palpitation, palpebration).*
12. The sebaceous glands for the eyelashes are called *(meibomian, Bartholin)* glands.
13. The process of producing tears is called *(lacrimation, lactation).*
14. The eyes move as the result of six voluntary *(intra-, extra-)* ocular muscles.

The Eyeball

The anatomy of the eyeball itself is traditionally explained in three layers or **tunics** (TOO nicks) (Fig. 14-2). The outer layer, or **fibrous tunic**, consists of the **sclera** (SKLIR uh) and **cornea** (KOR nee uh). The middle layer, or **vascular tunic**, consists of the **uvea** (YOO vee uh), which is made up of the **choroid** (KOR oyd), **ciliary** (SILL ih air ee) **body**, and **iris** (EYE ris). The inner layer, or **nervous tunic**, consists of the **retina** (RET in uh). These three layers are essential to the process of seeing. All parts work together with impressive harmony. The eye muscles coordinate their movements with one another; the cornea and pupil control the amount of light that enters the eye; the lens focuses the image on the retina; and the optic nerve transmits the image to the brain.

Two important mechanisms also contribute to the ability to see. As light hits the eye, it passes first through the cornea, which bends the rays of light **(refraction)** so that they are projected properly onto receptor cells in the eye. Then, muscles in the ciliary body adjust the shape of the lens to aid in this refraction. The lens flattens to adjust to something seen at a distance, or thickens for close vision—a process called **accommodation.** Errors of refraction are the most common reason for lens prescriptions.

The Sclera

The outermost lateral and posterior portion of the eye, the white of the eye, is called the **sclera,** which means *hard.* The portion of the sclera that covers the anterior section of the eye is transparent and is called the **cornea.** The border of the cornea, between it and the sclera, is called the **limbus** (LIM bus). The cornea is where refraction (the bending of light) begins.

The Uvea

The **uvea** is the middle, highly vascular layer of the eye. It includes the **iris**, the **ciliary body,** and the **choroid.** The iris (*pl.* irides), pupil, lens (*pl.* lenses), and ciliary body are located directly behind the cornea. The iris is a smooth muscle that contracts and relaxes to moderate the amount of light that enters the eye. In most individuals, this is the colored part of the eye (brown, gray, hazel, blue) because of its pigmentation. Individuals with albinism, however, have reddish-pink irides (*sing.* iris), because a lack of pigment makes visible the blood cells traveling through the vessels supplying the iris.

The **pupil** is the dark area in the center of the iris, where the light continues its progress through the lens. The **lens** is an avascular structure made of protein and covered by an elastic capsule. It is held in place by the thin strands of muscle that make up the ciliary body. The fluid produced by the capillaries of the ciliary body is called the **aqueous** (AY kwee us) **humor.** It nourishes the cornea, gives shape to the anterior eye, and maintains an optimal intraocular pressure. It normally drains through tiny veins called the canals of Schlemm. The aqueous humor circulates in both the anterior chamber, between the cornea and the iris, and the posterior chamber, behind the iris and in front of the lens. Between the lens and the retina is a jellylike substance, the **vitreous** (VIT ree us) **humor,** which holds the choroid membrane against the retina to ensure an adequate blood supply.

BE CAREFUL!

Core/o, meaning *pupil of the eye,* and *corne/o,* meaning *cornea,* are easy to confuse.

DID YOU KNOW?

The combining form *kerat/o* means *hard* or *horny* and refers to both the skin and the cornea. This is because the cornea is formed from the same tissue as the epidermis.

The Retina

The inner layer of the eye, called the **retina,** contains the sensory receptors for the images carried by the light rays. These sensory receptors are either **rods,** which appear throughout the retina and are responsible for vision in dim light, or **cones,** which are concentrated in the central area of the retina and are responsible for color vision.

During daylight, the area of the retina on which the light rays focus is called the **macula lutea** (MACK yoo lah LOO tee uh). The **fovea** (FOH vee uh), is an area within the macula that contains only cones and provides the sharpest image. The area that allows a natural blind spot in our vision is the **optic disk,** where the optic nerve leaves the retina to travel to the brain. There are no light receptors there.

COMBINING FORMS FOR THE EYEBALL

MEANING	COMBINING FORM	MEANING	COMBINING FORM
choroid	choroid/o	optic disk	papill/o
ciliary body	cycl/o	pupil	pupill/o, cor/o, core/o
cornea	kerat/o, corne/o	retina	retin/o
iris	ir/o, irid/o	sclera	scler/o
lens	phac/o, phak/o, lent/i	uvea	uve/o
macula lutea	macul/o	vitreous body	vitre/o

Exercise 2: THE EYEBALLS

Match the parts of the eye with the correct combining forms. More than one answer may be correct.

_____ 1. ir/o, irid/o

_____ 2. papill/o

_____ 3. retin/o

_____ 4. cor/o, core/o

_____ 5. pupill/o

_____ 6. macul/o

_____ 7. phac/o, phak/o

_____ 8. choroid/o

A. hard, outer covering of the eye
B. dark center of iris
C. substance between retina and lens
D. middle, highly vascular layer of the eye
E. choroid
F. ciliary body
G. transparent, anterior portion of sclera

____ 9. cycl/o	____ 13. scler/o	H. lens
		I. made up of rods and cones
____ 10. lent/i	____ 14. corne/o	J. pigmented muscle that allows light in eye
		K. light focuses on this retinal structure
____ 11. uve/o	____ 15. vitre/o	L. optic disk
		M. inner layer of eye
____ 12. kerat/o		

Circle the correct answer.

16. The order of the layers of the eyes from outside to inside are fibrous → vascular → *(nervous, muscular).*
17. The vascular tunic consists of the *(uvea, retina).*
18. The tough, outer covering is composed of the iris, ciliary body, and *(choroid membrane, sclera).*
19. Optimal intraocular pressure is maintained by the *(aqueous, vitreous)* humor.
20. The sensory receptors of the retina responsible for color vision are the *(rods, cones).*
21. The area within the macula lutea that provides the sharpest image is the *(optic disk, fovea).*

PATHOLOGY

Terms Related to Eyelid Disorders

TERM	WORD ORIGIN	DEFINITION
Blepharedema bleff ah ruh DEE mah	*blephar/o* eyelid *-edema* swelling	Swelling of the eyelid.
Blepharitis bleff ah RYE tis	*blephar/o* eyelid *-itis* inflammation	Inflammation of the eyelid.
Blepharochalasis bleff ah roh KAL luh sis	*blephar/o* eyelid *-chalasis* relaxation, slackening	Hypertrophy of the skin of the eyelid.
Blepharoptosis bleff ah rop TOH sis	*blephar/o* eyelid *-ptosis* drooping	Drooping of the upper eyelid.
Ectropion eck TROH pee on	*ec-* out *trop/o* turning *-ion* process of	Turning outward (eversion) of the eyelid, exposing the conjunctiva.
Entropion en TROH pee on	*en-* in *trop/o* turning *-ion* process of	Turning inward of the eyelid toward the eye.

Terms Related to Eyelash Disorders

TERM	WORD ORIGIN	DEFINITION
Chalazion kuh LAY zee on		Hardened swelling of a meibomian gland resulting from a blockage. Also called **meibomian cyst** (Fig. 14-3).
Hordeolum hor DEE uh lum		Stye; infection of one of the sebaceous glands of an eyelash.

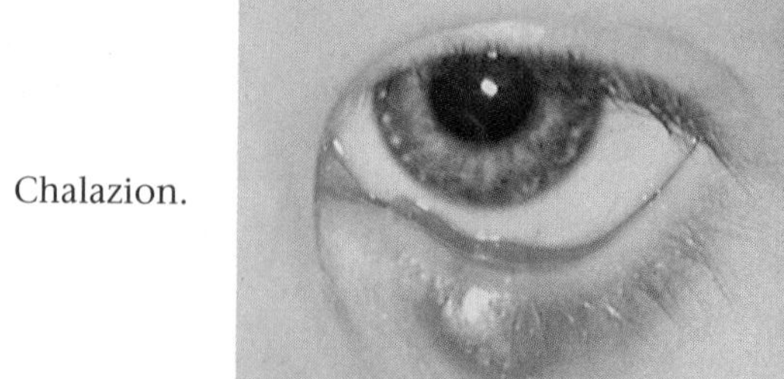

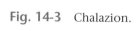

Fig. 14-3 Chalazion.

Terms Related to Tear Gland Disorders

TERM	WORD ORIGIN	DEFINITION
Dacryoadenitis dack ree oh add eh NYE tis	*dacry/o* tear *aden/o* gland *-itis* inflammation	Inflammation of a lacrimal gland.
Dacryocystitis dack ree oh sis TYE tis	*dacry/o* tear *cyst/o* sac *-itis* inflammation	Inflammation of a lacrimal sac.
Epiphora eh PIFF or ah		Overflow of tears; excessive lacrimation.
Keratoconjunctivitis sicca kair ah toh kun junk tih VYE tis SICK ah	*kerat/o* cornea *conjunctiv/o* conjunctiva *-itis* inflammation *sicca* dry	Dryness and/or inflammation of the cornea and conjunctiva due to inadequate tear production. Usually the result of an immune disorder.
Xerophthalmia zeer off THAL mee ah	*xer/o* dry *ophthalm/o* eye *-ia* condition	Dry eye; lack of adequate tear production to lubricate the eye. Usually the result of vitamin A deficiency.

Terms Related to Conjunctiva Disorders

TERM	WORD ORIGIN	DEFINITION
Conjunctivitis kun junk tih VYE tis	*conjunctiv/o* conjunctiva *-itis* inflammation	Inflammation of the conjunctiva, commonly known as *pinkeye,* a highly contagious disorder.
Ophthalmic neonatorum off THAL mick nee oh nay TORE um	*ophthalm/o* eye *-ic* pertaining to *neo-* new *nat/o* born	Severe, purulent conjunctivitis in the newborn, usually due to gonorrheal or chlamydial infection. Routine introduction of an antibiotic ophthalmic ointment (erythromycin) prevents most cases.

Terms Related to Eye Muscle and Orbital Disorders

TERM	WORD ORIGIN	DEFINITION
Amblyopia am blee OH pee ah	*ambly/o* dull, dim *-opia* vision	Dull or dim vision due to disuse.
Diplopia dih PLOH pee ah	*dipl/o* double *-opia* vision	Double vision. **Emmetropia** means normal vision.
Esotropia eh soh TROH pee ah	*eso-* inward *trop/o* turning *-ia* condition	Turning inward of one or both eyes.
Exophthalmia eck soff THAL mee ah	*ex-* out *ophthalm/o* eye *-ia* condition	Protrusion of the eyeball from its orbit; may be congenital or the result of an endocrine disorder (Fig. 14-4).
Exotropia eck so TROH pee ah	*exo-* outward *trop/o* turning *-ia* condition	Turning outward of one or both eyes.
Strabismus strah BISS mus		General term for a lack of coordination between the eyes, usually due to a muscle weakness or paralysis. Sometimes called a "squint," which refers to the patient's effort to correct the disorder.

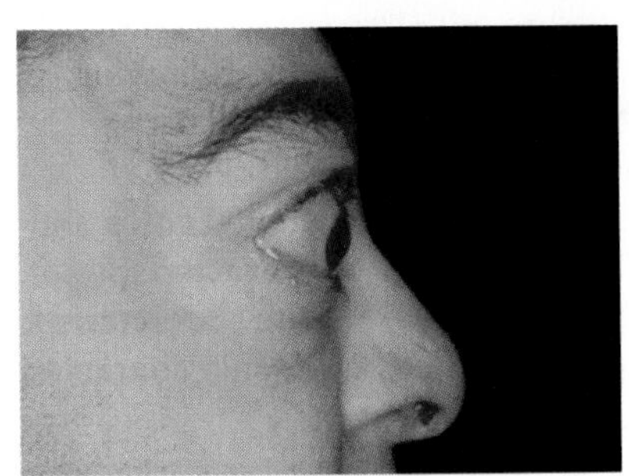

Fig. 14-4 Exophthalmia.

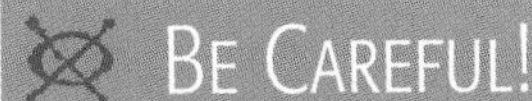

BE CAREFUL!

Do not confuse these similar terms: *esotropia, exotropia, entropion,* and *ectropion.*

Exercise 3: DISORDERS OF THE OCULAR ADNEXA

Matching.

_____ 1. epiphora
_____ 2. xerophthalmia
_____ 3. hordeolum
_____ 4. ectropion
_____ 5. diplopia
_____ 6. blepharoptosis
_____ 7. chalazion
_____ 8. exotropia
_____ 9. conjunctivitis
_____ 10. exophthalmia

A. double vision
B. eversion of the eyelid
C. pinkeye
D. excessive lacrimation
E. drooping of an upper eyelid
F. stye
G. meibomian cyst
H. outward protrusion of the eyeball
I. dry eye
J. outward turning of the eye

Circle the correct answer.

11. Normal vision is called *(amblyopia, emmetropia).*
12. A turning inward of one or both eyes is called *(esotropia, entropion).*
13. A swelling of an eyelid is called *(blepharitis, blepharedema).*

14. An inflamed lacrimal sac is called *(dacryoadenitis, dacryocystitis).*
15. Dryness and inflammation of the cornea and conjunctiva due to inadequate tear production is called *(ophthalmic neonatorium, keratoconjunctivitis sicca).*

Terms Related to Refraction and Accommodation Disorders

Term	Word Origin	Definition
Asthenopia as thuh NOH pee ah	*a-* lack of *sthen/o* strength *-opia* visual condition	Visual impairment due to weakness of ocular or ciliary muscles.
Astigmatism ah STIG mah tiz um		Malcurvature of the cornea leading to blurred vision. If uncorrected, asthenopia may result (Fig. 14-5, *A*).
Hyperopia hye pur OH pee ah	*hyper-* excessive *-opia* vision	Farsightedness; refractive error that does not allow the eye to focus on nearby objects (Fig. 14-5, *B*).
Myopia mye OH pee ah	*my/o* muscle *-opia* vision	Nearsightedness; refractive error that may be treated with corrective lenses or surgery (Fig. 14-5, *C*).
Presbyopia press bee OH pee ah	*presby/o* old age *-opia* vision	Progressive loss of elasticity of the lens (usually accompanies aging), resulting in hyperopia.

Terms Related to Sclera Disorders

Term	Word Origin	Definition
Corneal ulcer	*corne/o* cornea *-al* pertaining to	Trauma to the outer covering of the eye, resulting in an abrasion.
Keratitis kair uh TYE tis	*kerat/o* cornea *-itis* inflammation	Inflammation of the cornea.
Keratoconus kair uh toh KOH nus	*kerat/o* cornea *con/o* cone	Malformation of the cornea that appears as a protrusion of the center of the cornea. More prevalent in females than males, this condition may cause astigmatism.

Terms Related to Uvea Disorders

Term	Word Origin	Definition
Anisocoria an nye soh KORE ee ah	*an-* not *iso-* equal *cor/o* pupil *-ia* condition	Condition of unequally sized pupils, sometimes due to pressure on the optic nerve as a result of trauma or lesion.
Hyphema hye FEE mah	*hypo-* under *hem/o* blood	Blood in the anterior chamber of the eye as a result of hemorrhaging due to trauma.
Iritis eye RYE tis	*ir/o* iris *-itis* inflammation	Inflammation of the iris.
Uveitis yoo vee EYE tis	*uve/o* uvea *-itis* inflammation	Inflammation of the uvea (iris, ciliary body, and choroids).

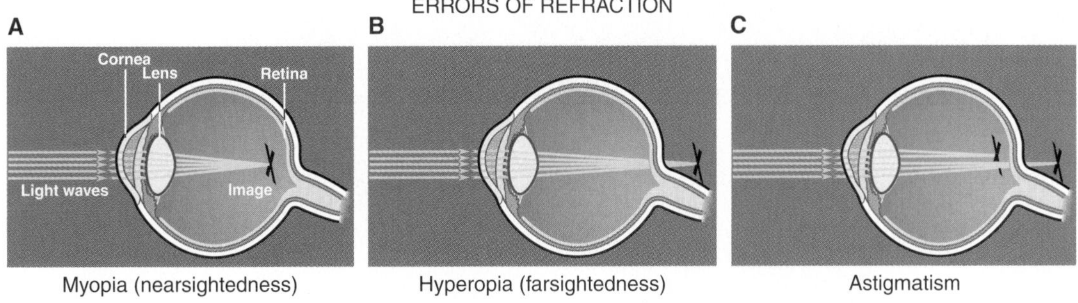

Fig. 14-5 Refraction errors. **A,** Myopia. **B,** Hyperopia. **C,** Astigmatism.

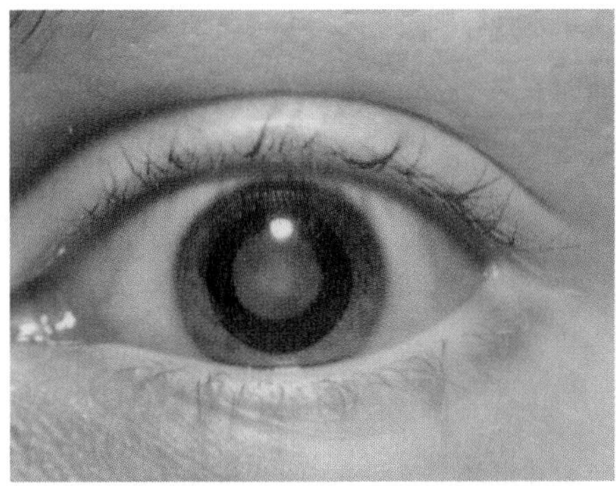

Fig. 14-6 The cloudy appearance of a lens affected by a cataract.

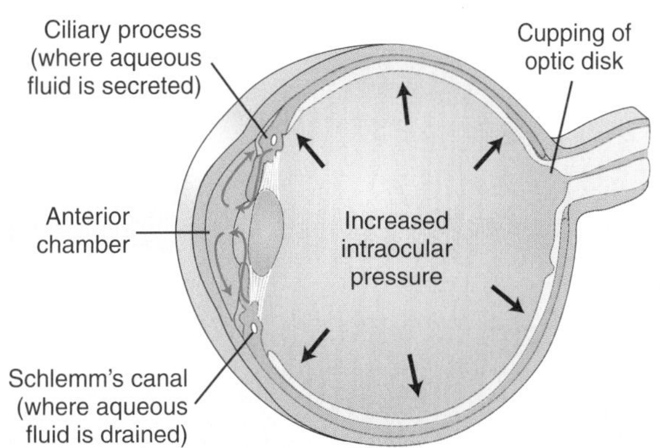

Fig. 14-7 Open-angle glaucoma.

Terms Related to Lens Disorders

TERM	WORD ORIGIN	DEFINITION
Aphakia ah FAY kee ah	*a-* without *phak/o* lens *-ia* condition	Condition of no lens, either congenital or acquired.
Cataract KAT ur ackt		Progressive loss of transparency of the lens of the eye (Fig. 14-6).
Glaucoma glah KOH mah	*glauc/o* gray, bluish green *-oma* mass, swelling	Abnormal intraocular pressure due to the obstruction of the outflow of the aqueous humor. **Chronic** or **primary open-angle glaucoma** (Fig. 14-7) is characterized by an open anterior chamber angle. **Angle-closure** or **narrow-angle glaucoma** is characterized by an abnormally narrowed anterior chamber angle.
Synechia sin ECK kee ah		Adhesion of the iris to the lens and the cornea.

Terms Related to Retina Disorders

TERM	WORD ORIGIN	DEFINITION
Achromatopsia ah kroh mah TOPE see ah	*a-* without *chromat/o* color *-opsia* vision	Impairment of color vision. Inability to distinguish between certain colors because of abnormalities of the photopigments produced in the retina. Also called **color blindness.**
Age-related macular degeneration (ARMD or AMD)		Progressive destruction of the macula, resulting in a loss of central vision. This is the most common visual disorder after the age of 75 (Fig. 14-8).
Diabetic retinopathy dye ah BET ick ret in OP ah thee	*retin/o* retina *-pathy* disease	Damage of the retina due to diabetes; the leading cause of blindness (Fig. 14-9).
Hemianopsia hem ee an NOP see ah	*hemi-* half *an-* without *-opsia* vision	Loss of half the visual field, often the result of a cerebral vascular accident.
Nyctalopia nick tuh LOH pee ah	*nyct/o* night *-opia* vision	Inability to see well in dim light. May be due to a vitamin A deficiency, retinitis pigmentosa, or choroidoretinitis.
Retinal tear, retinal detachment		Separation of the retina from the choroid layer. May be due to trauma, inflammation of the interior of the eye, or aging. A hole in the retina allows fluid from the vitreous humor to leak between the two layers.
Retinitis pigmentosa ret in EYE tis pig men TOH sah	*retin/o* retina *-itis* inflammation	Hereditary, degenerative disease marked by nyctalopia and a progressive loss of the visual field.
Scotoma skoh TOH mah	*scot/o* darkness *-oma* mass, tumor	Area of decreased vision in the visual field. Commonly called a **blind spot.**

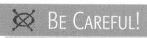

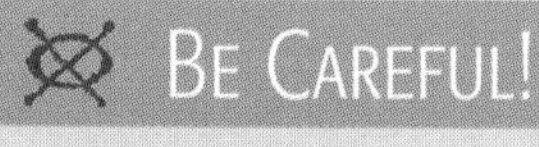

Nyctalopia is night blindness, not night vision.

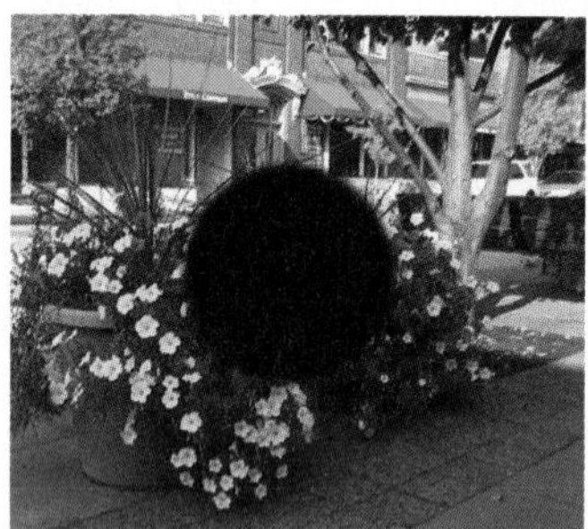

Fig. 14-8 Macular degeneration.

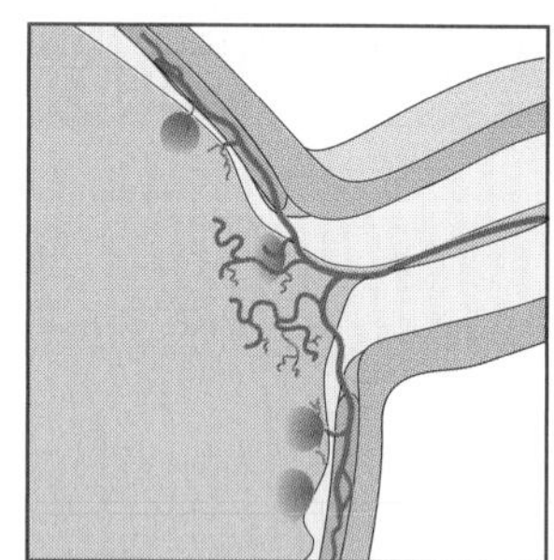

Fig. 14-9 Diabetic retinopathy.

Terms Related to Optic Nerve Disorders

TERM	WORD ORIGIN	DEFINITION
Nystagmus nye STAG mus		Involuntary, back-and-forth eye movements due to a disorder of the labyrinth of the ear and/or parts of the nervous system associated with rhythmic eye movements.
Optic neuritis OP tick nyoo RYE tis	*opt/o* vision *-ic* pertaining to *neur/o* nerve *-itis* inflammation	Inflammation of the optic nerve resulting in blindness; often mentioned as a predecessor to the development of multiple sclerosis.

Exercise 4: DISORDERS OF THE EYEBALL

Matching.

_____	1. cataract	_____	6. myopia	A. abrasion of the outer eye
_____	2. ARMD	_____	7. hyperopia	B. farsightedness
_____	3. glaucoma	_____	8. corneal ulcer	C. lack of a lens
_____	4. anisocoria	_____	9. astigmatism	D. hemorrhage within the eye
_____	5. aphakia	_____	10. hyphema	E. malcurvature of the cornea
				F. increased intraocular pressure
				G. unequally sized pupils
				H. nearsightedness
				I. loss of central vision
				J. loss of transparency of the lens

Circle the correct answer.

11. Patients with an inflammation of the cornea have *(keratitis, uveitis).*
12. An impairment of color vision is called *(scotoma, achromatopsia).*
13. The inability to see well in dim light is called *(amblyopia, nyctalopia).*
14. Adhesion of the iris to the lens and cornea is called *(synechia, macular degeneration).*
15. Loss of half of the visual field is called *(optic neuritis, hemianopsia).*

DIAGNOSTIC PROCEDURES

Terms Related to Diagnostic Procedures

TERM	WORD ORIGIN	DEFINITION
Amsler grid		Test to assess central vision and to assist in the diagnosis of age-related macular degeneration.
Diopters DYE op turs		Level of measurement that quantifies **refraction errors,** including the amount of nearsightedness (negative numbers), farsightedness (positive numbers), and astigmatism.
Fluorescein angiography FLOO res seen an jee AH gruh fee	***angi/o*** vessel ***-graphy*** process of recording	Procedure to confirm suspected retinal disease by injection of a fluorescein dye into the eye, and use of a camera to record the vessels of the retina.
Fluorescein staining		Use of a dye dropped into the eyes that allows differential staining of abnormalities of the cornea.
Gonioscopy goh nee AH skuh pee	***goni/o*** angle ***-scopy*** visual exam	Visualization of the angle of the anterior chamber of the eye; used to diagnose glaucoma and inspect ocular movement.
Ophthalmic ultrasonography	***ophthalm/o*** eye ***-ic*** pertaining to ***ultra-*** beyond ***son/o*** sound ***-graphy*** process of recording	Use of high-frequency sound waves to image the interior of the eye when opacities prevent other imaging techniques. May be used for diagnosing retinal detachments, inflammatory conditions, vascular malformations, and suspicious masses.
Ophthalmoscopy off thal MAH skuh pee	***ophthalm/o*** eye ***-scopy*** visual exam	Any visual examination of the interior of the eye with an ophthalmoscope.

Continued

Terms Related to Diagnostic Procedures—cont'd

TERM	WORD ORIGIN	DEFINITION
Schirmer tear test		Test to determine the amount of tear production; useful in diagnosing dry eye (xerophthalmia).
Slit lamp examination		Part of a routine eye examination; used to examine the various layers of the eye. Medications may be used to dilate the pupils (mydriatics), numb the eye (anesthetics), or to dye the eye (fluorescein staining).
Tonometry toh NAH meh tree	*ton/o* tone, tension *-metry* process of measurement	Measurement of intraocular pressure; used in the diagnosis of glaucoma. In **Goldmann applanation tonometry,** the eye is numbed and measurements are taken directly on the eye. In **air-puff tonometry,** a puff of air is blown onto the cornea.
Visual acuity (VA) assessment		Test of the clearness or sharpness of vision; also called the **Snellen test.** Normal vision is described as being 20/20. The top figure is the number of feet the examinee is standing from the Snellen chart (Fig. 14-10); the bottom figure is the number of feet a normal person would be from the chart and still be able to read the smallest letters. Thus if the result is 20/40, the highest line that the individual can read is what a person with normal vision can read at 40 feet.
Visual field (VF) test		Test to determine the area of physical space visible to an individual. A normal visual field (VF) is 65 degrees upward, 75 degrees downward, 60 degrees inward, and 90 degrees outward (Fig. 14-11).

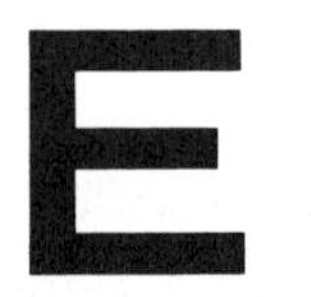

Fig. 14-10 Snellen chart.

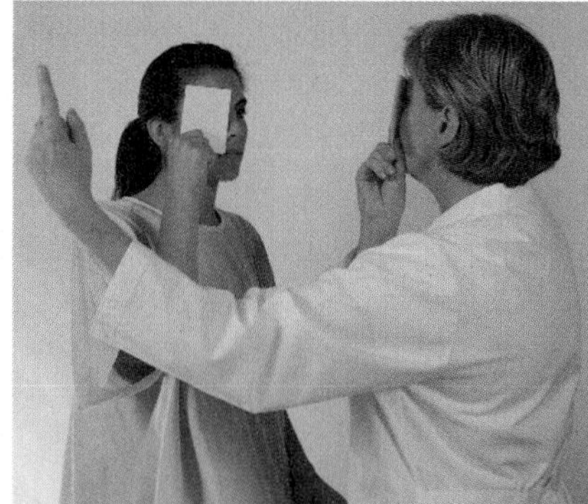

Fig. 14-11 Assessment of visual fields.

Exercise 5: DIAGNOSTIC PROCEDURES

Matching.

_____ 1. measure of the area of physical space visible to an individual

_____ 2. exam of intraocular pressure

_____ 3. visual exam of interior of eye

_____ 4. test of sharpness of vision

_____ 5. visualization of angle of anterior chamber

_____ 6. test to measure central vision

_____ 7. test to determine amount of tear production

_____ 8. exam of abnormalities of cornea

_____ 9. part of routine eye exam of layers of the eye

_____ 10. use of injected dye to record suspected retinal disease

_____ 11. instrument used to measure refraction errors

A. slit lamp exam
B. VA test
C. Schirmer test
D. fluorescein staining
E. VF test
F. ophthalmoscopy
G. Amsler grid
H. tonometry
I. gonioscopy
J. fluorescein angiography
K. diopters

Case Study Continued

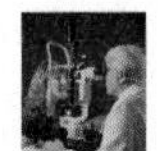

Mary Ellen has astigmatism. Because it has always been diligently treated with eyeglasses, she has no asthenopia, or muscle weakening, but her blurred vision is beginning to get worse. Dr. O'Connor performs routine ophthalmoscopy and slit lamp exam on Mary Ellen. Then the doctor uses a fluorescein staining to visualize the abnormalities on Mary Ellen's cornea.

THERAPEUTIC PROCEDURES

Terms Related to Interventions of the Eyeball and Adnexa

Term	Word Origin	Definition
Blepharoplasty BLEFF ar oh plas tee	*blephar/o* eyelid *-plasty* surgical repair	Surgical repair of the eyelids. May be done to correct blepharoptosis or blepharochalasis.
Blepharorrhaphy BLEFF ar oh rah fee	*blephar/o* eyelid *-rrhaphy* suture	Suture of the eyelids.
Enucleation of the eye eh noo klee AY shun		Removal of the entire eyeball.
Evisceration of the eye eh vis uh RAY shun		Removal of the contents of the eyeball, leaving the outer coat (the sclera) intact.
Exenteration of the eye eck sen tur RAY shun		Removal of the entire contents of the orbit.

Terms Related to Refractive Surgery

TERM	WORD ORIGIN	DEFINITION
Astigmatic keratotomy (AK) as tig MAT ick kair uh TAH tuh mee	*kerat/o* cornea *-tomy* incision	Corneal incision process that treats astigmatism by effecting a more rounded cornea.
Corneal incision procedure		Any keratotomy procedure in which the cornea is cut to change shape, correcting a refractive error (AK, RK, PRK).
Flap procedure		Any procedure in which a segment of the cornea is cut as a means of access to the structures below (LASIK, LASEK).
Laser-assisted in situ keratomileusis (LASIK) kair uh toh mih LOO sis	*kerat/o* cornea	Flap procedure in which an excimer laser is used to remove material under the corneal flap. Corrects astigmatism, myopia, and hyperopia (Fig. 14-12).
Laser epithelial keratomileusis (LASEK)	*kerat/o* cornea	Flap procedure that differs from the LASIK procedure only in the amount of tissue cut. LASEK incises the epithelium and only part of the stroma, with an advantage of the opportunity for more easily treated possible infections.
Photoablation foh toh ah BLAY shun	*photo-* light *ablation* removal	Use of ultraviolet radiation to destroy and remove tissue from the cornea.
Photorefractive keratectomy (PRK) foh toh ree FRACK tiv kair uh TECK tuh mee	*kerat/o* cornea *-ectomy* removal	Treatment for astigmatism, hyperopia, and myopia that uses an excimer laser to reshape the cornea.
Radial keratotomy (RK) RAY dee ul kair uh TAH tuh mee	*radi/o* rays *-al* pertaining to *kerat/o* cornea *-tomy* incision	Corneal incision process that treats myopia by incising the cornea in a spokelike pattern.

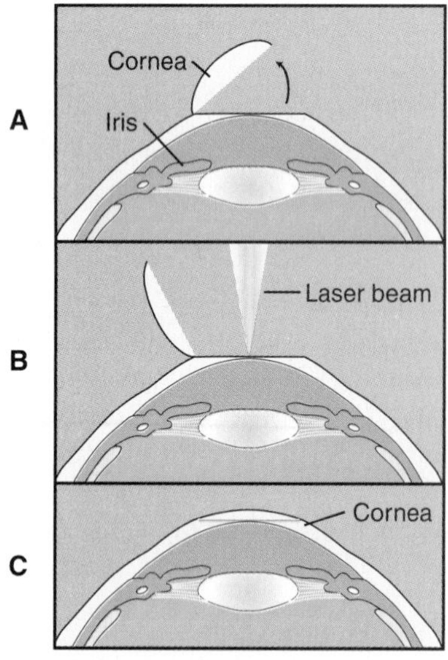

Fig. 14-12 LASIK surgery. **A,** A microkeratome is used to create a hinged cap of tissue, which is lifted off the cornea. **B,** An excimer laser is used to vaporize and reshape underlying tissue. **C,** Tissue cap is replaced.

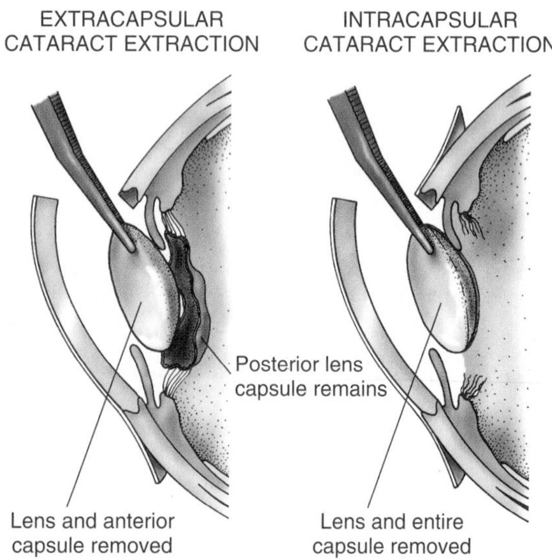

Fig. 14-13 Lens removal.

Terms Related to Limbal, Scleral, and Corneal Procedures

Term	Word Origin	Definition
Anterior ciliary sclerotomy (ACS) sklair AH tuh mee	*scler/o* sclera *-tomy* incision	Incision in the sclera to treat presbyopia.
Corneal transplant		Transplantation of corneal tissue from a donor or the patient's own (autograft) cornea. May be either full- or partial-thickness grafts; also called **keratoplasty** (kair uh toh PLAS tee).
Epikeratophakia eh pee kair uh toh FAY kee ah	*epi-* above *kerat/o* cornea *phak/o* lens *-ia* condition	Replacement of lens function with the use of a donor corneal graft. May be used for myopia, hyperopia, astigmatism, and, occasionally, keratoconus.
Implantation of corneal ring segments		Procedure to correct myopia with the addition of pieces of the cornea.
Laser thermal keratoplasty (LTK)	*therm/o* heat *-al* pertaining to *kerat/o* cornea *-plasty* surgical repair	Use of heat and a holmium laser to treat hyperopia in patients over 40.
Limbal relaxing incision (LRI)		Incision of the limbus to treat astigmatism.

Terms Related to Lens Interventions

Term	Word Origin	Definition
Extraction of the lens		Removal of the lens to treat cataracts. May be **intracapsular,** in which the entire lens and capsule are removed, or **extracapsular,** in which the lens capsule is left in place (Fig. 14-13).
Implantable contact lenses (ICL)		Use of an artificial lens implanted behind the iris and in front of the natural abnormal lens to treat myopia and farsightedness.
Phacoemulsification and aspiration of cataract fay koh ee MULL sih fih KAY shun	*phac/o* lens	Vision correction accomplished through the destruction and removal of the contents of the capsule by breaking it into small pieces and removing them by suction.

Terms Related to Iris Interventions

Term	Word Origin	Definition
Coreoplasty kore ee oh PLAS tee	*core/o* pupil *-plasty* surgical repair	Surgical repair to form an artificial pupil.
Goniotomy goh nee AH tuh mee	*goni/o* angle *-tomy* incision	Incision of Schlemm's canal to correct glaucoma by providing an exit for the aqueous humor.
Iridotomy eye rih DOT tuh mee	*irid/o* iris *-tomy* incision	Incision of the iris to treat postoperative glaucoma or to gain access for cataract surgery.
Trabeculotomy truh beck kyoo LAH tuh mee		External excision of the eye to promote intraocular circulation.

Terms Related to Retina Interventions

TERM	WORD ORIGIN	DEFINITION
Retinal photocoagulation RET in ul foh toh koh agg yoo LAY shun	*retin/o* retina *-al* pertaining to *phot/o* light *coagulation* to clot	Destruction of retinal lesions using light rays to solidify tissue.
Scleral buckling SKLAIR ul BUCK ling	*scler/o* sclera *-al* pertaining to	Reattachment of the retina with a cryoprobe and the use of a silicone sponge to push the sclera in toward the retinal scar; includes the removal of fluid from the subretinal space (Fig. 14-14).
Vitrectomy vih TRECK tuh mee	*vitr/o* vitreous humor, glassy *-ectomy* removal	Removal of part or all of the vitreous humor.

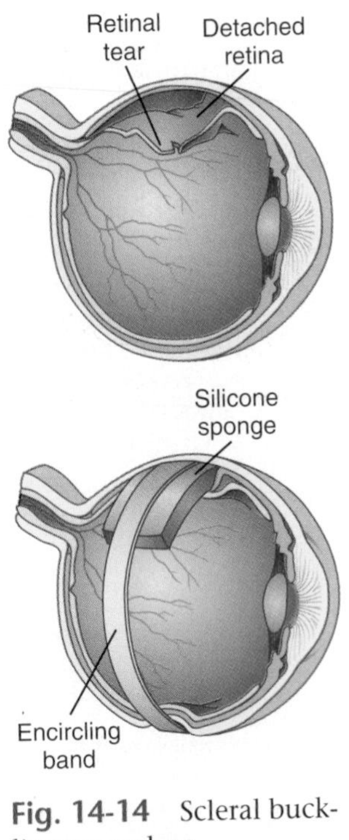

Fig. 14-14 Scleral buckling procedure.

Exercise 6: THERAPEUTIC INTERVENTIONS

Matching.

_____ 1. suture of the eyelids

_____ 2. removal of vitreous humor

_____ 3. surgical repair of a pupil defect

_____ 4. destruction of retinal lesions with light

_____ 5. incision of Schlemm's canal to correct glaucoma

_____ 6. incision of the iris to treat glaucoma

_____ 7. removal of contents of eyeball, except for outer coat

_____ 8. any keratotomy procedure to correct a refractive error

_____ 9. procedure to cut cornea to access deeper structures

_____ 10. use of UV radiation to destroy tissue

_____ 11. corneal transplant

_____ 12. removal of entire orbital contents

_____ 13. reattachment of retina

_____ 14. removal of entire eyeball

_____ 15. surgical repair of eyelids

A. retinal photocoagulation
B. blepharoplasty
C. scleral buckling
D. enucleation of eye
E. corneal incision procedure
F. exenteration of the eye
G. flap procedure
H. vitrectomy
I. blepharorrhaphy
J. iridotomy
K. goniotomy
L. photoablation
M. evisceration of eye
N. coreoplasty
O. keratoplasty

Case Study Continued

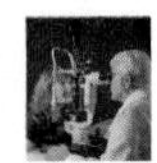

After a thorough examination, Dr. O'Connor talks to Mary Ellen about LASIK. He thinks she is an excellent candidate for such a procedure. He gives her a list of recommended doctors that perform LASIK and other procedures. Mary Ellen has the procedure done and very soon is seeing 20/20 again. She gratefully donates her glasses to charity.

PHARMACOLOGY

Antibiotics: Medications used to treat bacterial infections. Examples include erythromycin, gentamicin, and ciprofloxacin.

Antihistamines: Medications used to treat allergy-induced inflammation characterized by pain, redness, or photophobia. May be steroids or nonsteroidal. Examples include prednisolone, dexamethasone, and ketorolac.

Cycloplegics: Pharmaceutical agents that induce paralysis of the ciliary body to allow examination of the eye.

Lubricants: Medications that keep the eyes moist, mimicking natural tears.

Medications to treat glaucoma: Medications used to decrease the intraocular pressure by decreasing the amount of fluid in the eye or increasing the drainage include carbonic anhydrase inhibitors (dorzolamide), osmotics, anticholinergics (pilocarpine), beta blockers (levobunolol), and alpha agonists (lopidine).

Miotics: Drugs that cause the pupils to constrict; often used to treat glaucoma.

Mydriatics: Drugs that cause the pupils to dilate; used in diagnostic and refractive examination of the eye.

Topical anesthetics: Medications used to temporarily anesthetize the eye for the purpose of examination.

DID YOU KNOW?

Photophobia may mean *sensitivity to light* when used to describe the eyes, or *fear of light* when used to describe a psychiatric condition.

DID YOU KNOW?

The term *mydriatic* comes from a Greek word meaning *hot mass.* The Greeks thought that grasping something hot would cause one's pupils to widen.

Exercise 7: PHARMACOLOGY

Matching.

_____ 1. used for exposure to allergens

_____ 2. used to constrict pupils

_____ 3. used to allow examination of eye by paralyzing ciliary body

_____ 4. used to dilate pupils

_____ 5. used to keep eyes moist

A. mydriatics
B. cycloplegics
C. antihistamines
D. lubricants
E. miotics

Abbreviations

Abbreviation	Meaning	Abbreviation	Meaning
Acc	Accommodation	NVA	Near visual acuity
ARMD, AMD	Age-related macular degeneration	OD	Oculus dextra (right eye)
Astigm, As, Ast	Astigmatism	Ophth	Ophthalmology
c̄ gl	Correction with glasses	OS	Oculus sinistra (left eye)
ECCE	Extracapsular cataract extraction	OU	Oculus uterque, each eye
EM, Em	Emmetropia	PERRLA	Pupils equal, round, reactive to light and accommodation
EOM	Extraocular movements	PRK	Photorefractive keratectomy
ICCE	Intracapsular cataract extraction	RE	Right eye
IOL	Intraocular lens	RK	Radial keratotomy
IOP	Intraocular pressure	s̄ gl	Correction without glasses
L & A	Light and accommodation	VA	Visual acuity
LASIK	Laser in situ keratomileusis	VF	Visual field
LE	Left eye	WNL	Within normal limits
MY	Myopia		

Exercise 8: ABBREVIATIONS

Write out the following abbreviations.

1. Jonathan Sobel was diagnosed with MY in his OS and was prescribed c̄ gl.

____

2. Marlena decided to consider the merits of LASIK and PRK before she had her prescription filled.

____

3. Katsuko's vision was described as 20/300 on his VA test.

____

4. The patient presented with AMD. ______________________________
5. Arielle was prescribed eye drops to be used OU. ______________________________
6. The patient's IOP is described as being WNL. ______________________________
7. An Amsler grid is used to test the patient's VF. ______________________________

THE EAR

ANATOMY AND PHYSIOLOGY

The ear is regionally divided into the outer, middle, and inner ear (Fig. 14-15). Sound is conducted through air, bone, and fluid through these divisions. The majority of the ear is contained within the **petrous** (PEH trus) portion of the temporal bone.

Outer (External) Ear

Sound waves are initially gathered by the flesh covered cartilage of the outer ear called the **pinna** (PIN nuh), or **auricle** (ORE ick kul). The gathered sound is then funneled into the **external auditory canal.** Ear wax, or **cerumen** (sih ROO mun), is secreted by modified sweat glands within the external auditory canal and protects the ear with its antiseptic property and its stickiness, trapping foreign debris and moving it out of the ear. The opening of the outer ear is the **external auditory meatus** (AH dih tor ee mee AY tus). The **tympanic** (tim PAN ick) **membrane,** or eardrum, marks the end of the external ear and the beginning of the middle ear.

Middle Ear

The eardrum conducts sound to three tiny bones in the middle ear called the **ossicles** (AH sick kuls), or the **ossicular chain.** These ossicles are named for their shapes: the **malleus** (MAL ee us), or hammer; the **incus** (ING kus), or anvil; and the **stapes** (STAY peez) (*pl.* stapedes), or stirrup. The ossicles transmit the sound to the **oval window** through the stapes. Within the middle ear is the opening for the **eustachian** (yoo STAY shun) **tube,** also called the auditory tube, a mucous membrane-lined connection between the ears and the throat that equalizes pressure within the middle ear.

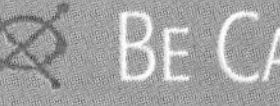

BE CAREFUL!

The combining form *salping/o* means both *fallopian tube* and *eustachian tube.*

Inner Ear

Once sound is conducted to the oval window, it is transmitted to a structure called the **labyrinth** (LAB uh rinth), or the inner ear. A membranous labyrinth is enclosed within a bony labyrinth. Between the two, and surrounding the inner labyrinth, is a fluid called **perilymph** (PAIR ee limf). Within the membranous labyrinth is a fluid called **endolymph** (EN doh limf). Hair cells within the inner ear fluids act as nerve endings that function as sensory receptors for hearing and

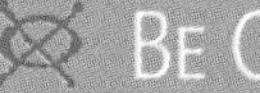

BE CAREFUL!

Malleus means *an ossicle. Malleolus* means *a process on the tibia and fibula.*

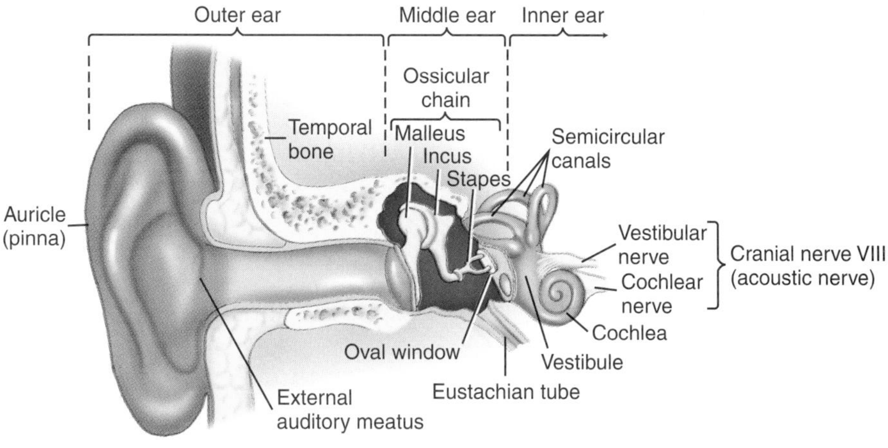

Fig. 14-15 The ear.

equilibrium. The outer, bony labyrinth is composed of three parts: the vestibule, the semicircular canals, and the cochlea. The **vestibule** (VES tih byool) and **semicircular canals** function to provide information about the body's sense of equilibrium, whereas the **cochlea** (KAH klee ah) is an organ of hearing.

Within the vestibule, two structures called the **utricle** (YOO trick ul) and the **saccule** (SACK yool) function to determine the body's static equilibrium. A specialized patch of epithelium called the **macula** (MACK yoo lah), found in both the utricle and the saccule, provides information about the position of the head and a sense of acceleration and deceleration. The semicircular canals detect dynamic equilibrium, or a sense of sudden rotation, through the function of a structure called the **crista ampullaris** (KRIS tah am pyoo LAIR is).

The cochlea receives the vibrations from the perilymph and transmits them to the cochlear duct, which is filled with endolymph. The transmission of sound continues through the endolymph to the **organ of Corti**, where the hearing receptor cells (hairs) stimulate a branch of the eighth cranial nerve, the vestibulocochlear nerve, to transmit the information to the temporal lobe of the brain.

BE CAREFUL!

Do not confuse *oral*, meaning *by mouth*, with *aural*, meaning *by ear.*

COMBINING FORMS FOR ANATOMY OF THE EAR

MEANING	COMBINING FORM	MEANING	COMBINING FORM
ear	ot/o, aur/o, auricul/o	inner ear	labyrinth/o
eardrum	tympan/o, myring/o	nose	rhin/o
earwax	cerumin/o	ossicles	ossicul/o
eustachian tube	salping/o	stapes	staped/o
hearing	audi/o, acous/o	temporal bone	tempor/o

Exercise 9: ANATOMY OF THE EAR

Match the combining forms with the correct parts of the ear. More than one letter may be correct.

_____ 1. eardrum

_____ 2. bones of the ear

_____ 3. earwax

_____ 4. inner ear

_____ 5. hearing

_____ 6. eustachian tube

_____ 7. ear

_____ 8. stirrup-shaped ear bone

_____ 9. temporal bone

A. tempor/o
B. labyrinth/o
C. ossicul/o
D. cerumin/o
E. staped/o
F. myring/o
G. salping/o
H. ot/o
I. audi/o
J. tympan/o
K. aur/o

Fill in the blanks.

10. Fill in the missing structures. Pinna → _______________ → tympanic membrane → _______________ → oval window → _______________ → eighth cranial nerve.

11. Name the three bones in the ossicular chain. _______________

12. Which structure of the labyrinth is responsible for hearing? ______________________________

13. Which structures of the labyrinth are responsible for equilibrium? ______________________________

Case Study

Sarah, a 3-year-old girl, is usually energetic and talkative. Over the last 18 months, however, she has had a series of earaches and ear infections that have slowed her down. Her preschool teacher notices that Sarah interacts less with the other children. Both the teacher and Sarah's parents have noticed that she does not seem to hear as well as she once did.

This morning, Sarah has awakened with yet another earache, and her parents are pretty sure it is going to be yet another diagnosis of middle ear inflammation. They get her in to the pediatrician right away. Along with a prescription for an antibiotic, Sarah is given a referral to an audiologist.

PATHOLOGY

Terms Related to Symptomatic Disorders

Term	Word Origin	Definition
Otalgia oh TAL juh	*ot/o* ear *-algia* pain	Earache, pain in the ear; also called **otodynia** (oh toh DIN nee ah).
Otorrhea oh tuh REE ah	*ot/o* ear *-rrhea* discharge	Discharge from the auditory canal; may be serous, bloody, or purulent.
Tinnitus tin EYE tis		Abnormal sound heard in one or both ears caused by trauma or disease; may be a ringing, buzzing, or jingling.
Vertigo VUR tih goh		Abnormal sensation of movement when there is none, either of one's self moving, or of objects moving around oneself. May be caused by middle ear infections or the toxic effects of alcohol, sunstroke, and certain medications.

Terms Related to Outer Ear Disorders

Term	Word Origin	Definition
Impacted cerumen		Blockage of the external auditory canal with cerumen.
Macrotia mah KROH sha	*macro-* large *ot/o* ear *-ia* condition	Condition of abnormally large auricles.
Microtia mye KROH sha	*micro-* small *ot/o* ear *-ia* condition	Condition of abnormally small auricles.
Otitis externa oh TYE tis eck STER nah	*ot/o* ear *-itis* inflammation *externa* outer	Inflammation of the outer ear.

Terms Related to Middle Ear Disorders

TERM	WORD ORIGIN	DEFINITION
Cholesteatoma koh less tee ah TOH mah	*chol/e* bile *steat/o* fat *-oma* tumor	Cystic mass composed of epithelial cells and cholesterol. Mass may occlude middle ear and destroy adjacent bones.
Infectious myringitis meer in JYE tis	*myring/o* eardrum *-itis* inflammation	Inflammation of the eardrum and vesicles are due to a bacterial or viral infection.
Otitis media (OM) oh TYE tis MEE dee ah	*ot/o* ear *-itis* inflammation *media* middle	Inflammation of the middle ear. Common in young children, it is usually secondary to an upper respiratory infection. Treatment usually includes administration of antibiotics (Fig. 14-16).
Otosclerosis oh toh sklair ROH sis	*ot/o* ear *-sclerosis* condition of hardening	Development of bone around the oval window with resulting ankylosis of the stapes to the oval window; usually results in progressive deafness.

Terms Related to Inner Ear Disorders

TERM	WORD ORIGIN	DEFINITION
Acoustic neuroma ah KOO stick noo ROH mah	*acous/o* hearing *-tic* pertaining to *neur/o* nerve *-oma* tumor	Benign tumor that grows in the auditory canal; may result in hearing loss, dizziness, and unsteady gait.
Labyrinthitis lab uh brinth EYE tis	*labyrinth/o* labyrinth *-itis* inflammation	Inflammation of the inner ear that may be due to infection or trauma; symptoms may include vertigo, nausea, and nystagmus.
Ménière's disease may nee URZ		Chronic condition of the inner ear characterized by vertigo, hearing loss, and tinnitus. The etiology (cause) is unknown.
Ruptured tympanic membrane		Tear (perforation) of the eardrum due to trauma or disease process (Fig. 14-17).

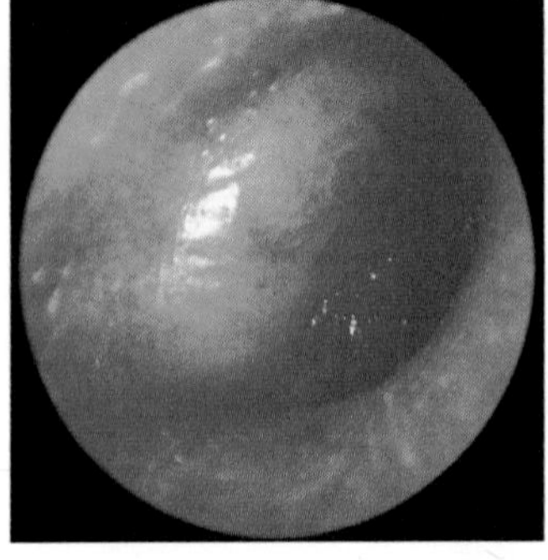

Fig. 14-16 Otitis media. Tympanic membrane is erythematous, opaque, and bulging.

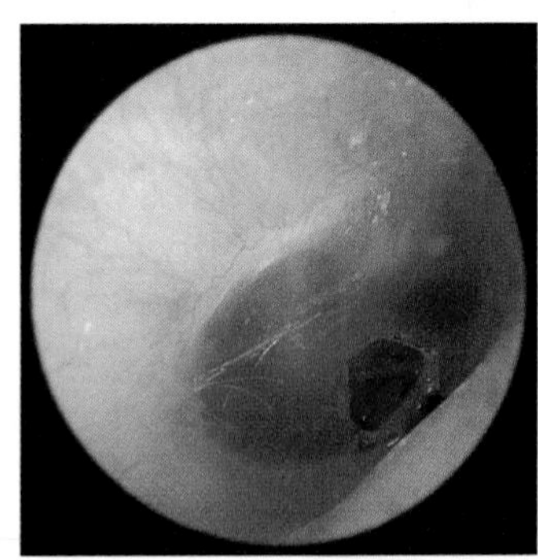

Fig. 14-17 Tympanic membrane perforation.

Terms Related to Hearing Loss Disorders

TERM	WORD ORIGIN	DEFINITION
Anacusis an uh KYOO sis	*an-* without *-cusis* hearing	General term for hearing loss or deafness.
Conductive hearing loss		Hearing loss resulting from damage to or malformation of the middle or outer ear.
Paracusis pair uh KYOO sis	*para-* abnormal *-cusis* hearing	Abnormality of hearing.
Presbycusis prez bee KYOO sis	*presby/o* old age *-cusis* hearing	Loss of hearing common in old age.
Sensorineural hearing loss Sen suh ree NOOR ul		Hearing loss resulting from damage to the inner ear (cochlea) or the auditory nerve.

Exercise 10: PATHOLOGY

Matching.

_____ 1. cholesteatoma

_____ 2. vertigo

_____ 3. otorrhea

_____ 4. macrotia

_____ 5. labyrinthitis

_____ 6. otitis media

_____ 7. tinnitus

_____ 8. presbycusis

_____ 9. otalgia

_____ 10. anacusis

_____ 11. otitis externa

_____ 12. acoustic neuroma

A. cystic mass in the middle ear composed of cholesterol
B. ringing in the ears
C. earache
D. loss of hearing typical of aging
E. hearing loss
F. inflammation of inner ear
G. abnormally large auricles
H. abnormal sense of movement
I. middle ear infection
J. inflammation of outer ear
K. discharge from the ear
L. benign tumor that grows in the auditory canal

Circle the correct answer.

13. Hearing loss due to damage of the inner ear or auditory nerve is *(conductive hearing loss, sensorineural hearing loss).*
14. Blockage of the external auditory canal with earwax is called *(impacted cerumen, otosclerosis).*
15. A patient who exhibits a chronic condition of the inner ear characterized by ringing in the ear, hearing loss, and vertigo may have *(infectious myringitis, Ménière's disease).*

DIAGNOSTIC PROCEDURES

Terms Related to Hearing Tests		
TERM	**WORD ORIGIN**	**DEFINITION**
Audiometric testing	*audi/o* hearing *-metric* pertaining to measurement	Measurement of hearing, usually with an instrument called an **audiometer** (ah dee AH met tur). The graphic representation of the results is called an **audiogram** (Fig. 14-18).
Otoscopy oh TAH skuh pee	*ot/o* ear *-scopy* process of visual examination	Visual examination of the external auditory canal and the tympanic membrane using an **otoscope.**
Pure tone audiometry	*audi/o* hearing *-metry* process of measurement	Measurement of perception of pure tones with extraneous sound screened out.
Rinne tuning fork test RIH nuh		Method of distinguishing conductive from sensorineural hearing loss.
Speech audiometry	*audi/o* hearing *-metry* process of measurement	Measurement of ability to hear and understand speech.

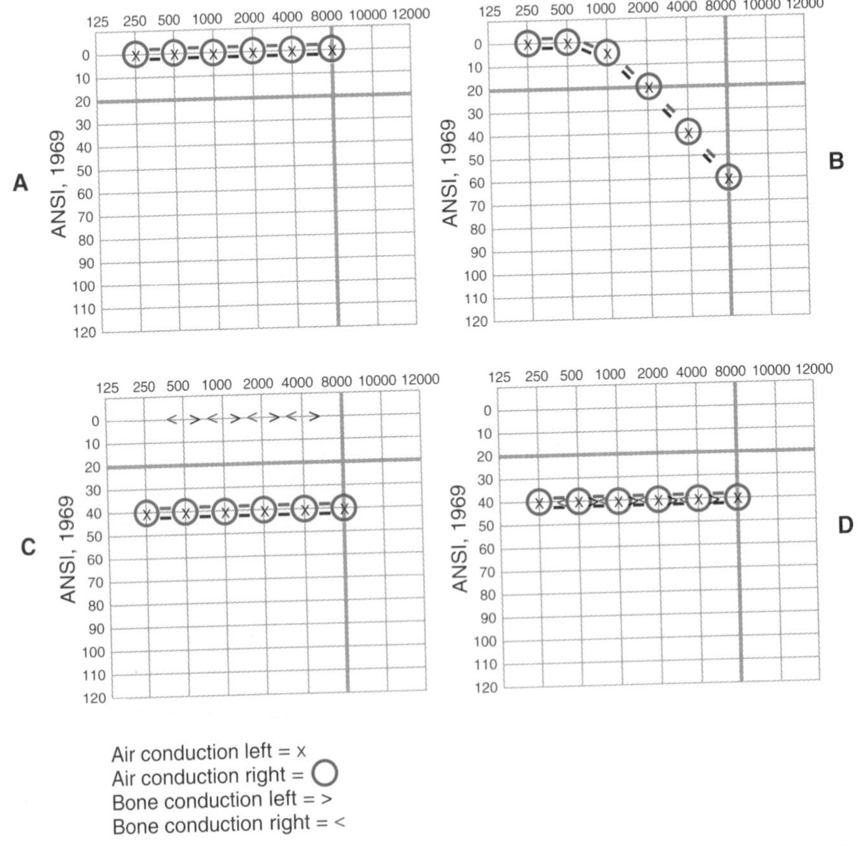

Fig. 14-18 Audiograms. **A,** Normal hearing. **B,** Conductive hearing loss. **C,** High-frequency hearing loss. **D,** Sensorineural hearing loss.

Terms Related to Hearing Tests—cont'd		
TERM	**WORD ORIGIN**	**DEFINITION**
Tympanometry tim pan NAH muh tree	*tympan/o* eardrum *-metry* process of measurement	Measurement of the condition and mobility function of the eardrum. The resultant graph is called a **tympanogram.**
Universal Newborn Hearing Screening (UNHS)		Test that uses **otoacoustic emissions (OAEs)** measured by the insertion of a probe into the baby's ear canal, and **auditory brainstem response (ABR),** which involves the placement of four electrodes on the baby's head to measure the change in the electrical activity of the brain in response to sound while the baby is sleeping.
Weber tuning fork test WEB ur		Method of testing auditory acuity.

Exercise 11: Diagnostic Procedures

Matching.

_____ 1. instrument to measure hearing

_____ 2. test of auditory acuity

_____ 3. record of function of eardrum

_____ 4. instrument to visually examine the ears

_____ 5. test to distinguish between conductive and sensorineural hearing loss

_____ 6. measurement of ability to hear and understand speech

A. otoscope
B. Rinne tuning fork test
C. speech audiometry
D. Weber tuning fork test
E. audiometer
F. tympanogram

THERAPEUTIC PROCEDURES

Terms Related to Therapeutic Interventions		
TERM	**WORD ORIGIN**	**DEFINITION**
Cochlear implant KAH klee ur	*cochle/o* cochlea *-ar* pertaining to	Implanted device that assists those with hearing loss by electrically stimulating the cochlea (Fig. 14-19).
Hearing aid		Electronic device that amplifies sound.
Otoplasty OH toh plas tee	*ot/o* ear *-plasty* surgical repair	Surgical or plastic repair and/or reconstruction of the external ear.
Stapedectomy stay puh DECK tuh mee	*staped/o* stapes *-ectomy* removal	Removal of the third ossicle, the stapes, from the middle ear.
Tympanoplasty tim PAN oh plas tee	*tympan/o* eardrum *-plasty* surgical repair	Surgical repair of the eardrum, with or without ossicular chain reconstruction. Some patients may require a prosthesis (an artificial replacement) for one or more of the ossicles.

Continued

Terms Related to Therapeutic Interventions—cont'd

TERM	WORD ORIGIN	DEFINITION
Tympanostomy tim pan AH stuh mee	*tympan/o* eardrum *-stomy* new opening	Surgical creation of an opening through the eardrum to promote drainage and/or allow the introduction of artificial tubes to maintain the opening (Fig. 14-20); also called a **myringostomy** (mir ring AH stoh mee).
Tympanotomy tim pan AH tuh mee	*tympan/o* eardrum *-tomy* incision	Incision of an eardrum; also called a **myringotomy** (mir ring AH toh mee).

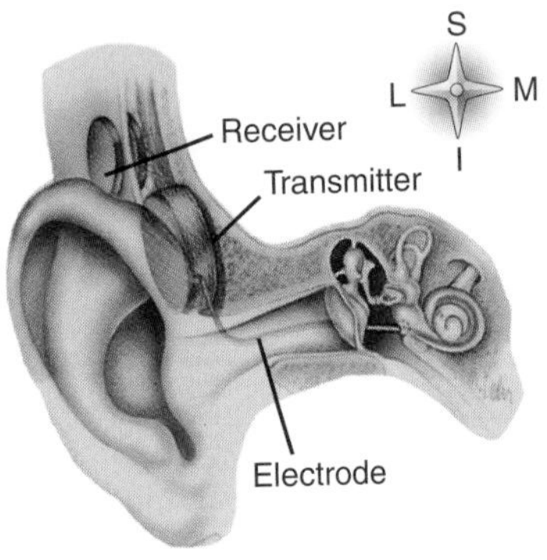

Fig. 14-19 Cochlear implant.

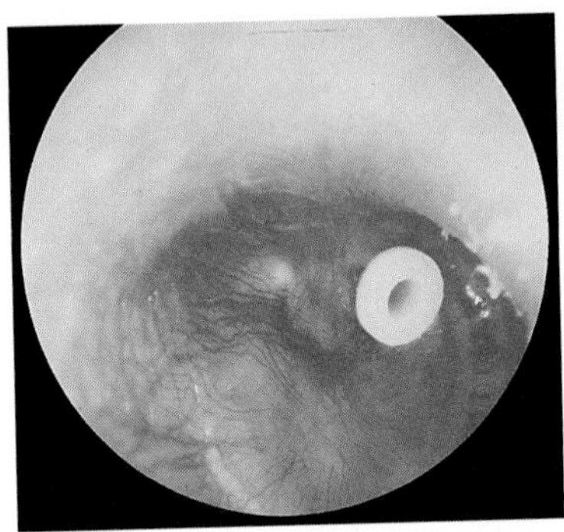

Fig. 14-20 Tympanostomy tube in place.

Exercise 12: THERAPEUTIC INTERVENTIONS

Matching.

_____ 1. incision of eardrum

_____ 2. surgical reconstruction of the external ear

_____ 3. surgical creation of a new opening through the ear drum

_____ 4. device implanted in inner ear to stimulate hearing

_____ 5. excision of ossicle that strikes the oval window

A. cochlear implant
B. otoplasty
C. tympanostomy
D. stapedectomy
E. myringotomy

Case Study Continued

Sarah is diagnosed with otitis media, presenting with otodynia. Her otoscopy shows moderate cerumen buildup and inflammation; her audiogram demonstrates some degree of paracusis; and finally, her tympanogram shows significant reduction in mobility of the eardrum. The ear, nose, and throat (ENT) doctor recommends a tympanostomy. Two weeks after the procedure, Sarah is her usual energetic self; she is free of inflammation, and her hearing has improved.

PHARMACOLOGY

Antibacterials: Drugs used to treat bacterial infections.
Antihistamines/decongestants: Drugs used to treat allergic conditions by reducing swelling or congestion.
Ceruminolytics: Medications used to soften and break down earwax.
Otics: Drugs used to treat the external ear canal or to remove earwax.

Exercise 13: PHARMACOLOGY

Matching.

_____ 1. otics
_____ 2. ceruminolytics
_____ 3. antibacterials
_____ 4. antihistamines

A. drugs used to treat infections
B. drugs used to treat allergic conditions
C. drugs used to treat external ear canal or remove earwax
D. medications to soften and break down earwax

Abbreviations

Abbreviation	Meaning	Abbreviation	Meaning
ABR	Auditory brain response	BC	Bone conduction
AC	Air conduction	ENT	Ear, nose, throat
AD	Auris dextra, right ear	OAE	Otoacoustic emission
AS	Auris sinistra, left ear	OM	Otitis media
ASL	American sign language	Oto	Otology
AU	Auris uterque, each ear	PHL	Permanent hearing loss

Exercise 14: ABBREVIATIONS

Matching.

_____ 1. OM
_____ 2. AS
_____ 3. BC
_____ 4. ENT
_____ 5. OAE

A. bone conduction
B. otoacoustic emissions
C. left ear
D. ear, nose, throat
E. otitis media

Careers

Optometrists

Optometrists monitor the visual health of their patients by diagnosing vision disorders. When the disorder is a refractive one, they may prescribe corrective lenses (either glasses or contacts) or discuss possible surgical interventions. Increasingly, optometrists are given the responsibility of prescribing medications for nonrefractive types of visual disorders.

To be an optometrist, a student must complete at least 3 years of college, taking courses in biology, chemistry, physics, mathematics, and English. Application to one of the accredited schools in optometry requires the completion of the Optometry Admissions Test. On graduation from optometric school (4 years), the graduate becomes a Doctor of Optometry. Before beginning to practice, the optometrist must take a written and clinical state board examination in order to be licensed to work in any of the States or the District of Columbia.

The job outlook for optometrists is good; opportunities are expected to increase as fast as the average for healthcare. The competing factors influencing the outlook are an aging population with more visual impairments versus improved technology allowing the quicker treatment of a greater number of patients. Optometrists are currently able to do preoperative and postoperative care for patients who have the different types of laser surgery, and although the number of glasses prescriptions may decrease, it is expected that surgical intervention will increase.

For more information, contact the following:

Association of Schools and College of Optometry at http://www.opted.org

American Optometric Association at http://www.aoanet.org

Audiologists

Audiologists work with patients who have hearing and balance problems. They are responsible for measuring an individual's hearing loss and devising a treatment plan to deal with the diagnosis.

The number of audiologists needed is expected to grow much faster than average for all occupations through the year 2010 because of the increasing proportion of middle-aged and older adults. Most of those interested in this profession will need to pursue a graduate-level degree and licensure. Courses may include anatomy and physiology, genetics, math, physics, communication development, auditory balance and neural systems assessment and treatment, audiologic rehabilitation, and ethics.

If interested, contact the American Academy of Audiology, 8201 Greensboro Dr., Suite 300, McLean, VA 22102. General information on audiology is available from the American Speech-Language-Hearing Association at http://professional.asha.org.

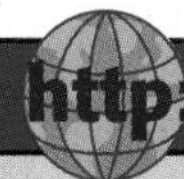

http: INTERNET PROJECT

Eyes and Ears

Technology is providing healthcare with a multitude of new possibilities for therapeutic interventions and diagnostic techniques in the area of vision and hearing. For this project, choose one of the following (or a topic assigned by your instructor) and write a 3-page, double-spaced report:

- Glaucoma
- Hearing loss
- Cataracts
- Refractive errors
- AMD

Be sure to list at least three of the following sources for your information:

The government's MEDLINEplus Website (http://www.nlm.nih.gov/medlineplus/) is a good overview of links to the general topics of vision or hearing.

At the Food and Drug Administration Website (http://www.fda.gov/), check the "Hot Topics" section, as well as news on a variety of healthcare topics, including laser surgery, contact lenses, hearing aids, and new drugs.

Healthfinder.gov is a Website for general information on healthcare conditions that you can use to start you on a search for a topic of interest. Visit it at http://www.healthfinder.gov.

At the National Eye Institute Website (http://www.nei.nih.gov/health/clinicaltrials_facts/index.htm), look into the clinical trials for visual disorders. Explain what a clinical trial is, what participation entails, and which ones are currently in effect for visual disorders.

At the Glaucoma Research Foundation Website (http://www.glaucoma.org/), check out the news on glaucoma research.

Check the National Institutes of Health Website (http://clinicaltrials.gov) for clinical trials focused on hearing and deafness.

The National Institute on Deafness and other Communication Disorders Website (http://www.nidcd.nih.gov/health/pubs_hb/coch.htm) is especially useful for information on cochlear implants.

Chapter Review

A. Functions, Anatomy, and Physiology of Eyes and Ears

1. What is the term for the process of blinking? ______________
2. What is the term for the production of tears? ______________
3. Kerat/o is the combining form for which structure of the eye? ______________
4. The muscles that hold the eye in place are the ______________ muscles.
5. What type of error is due to an inability of the lens to focus accurately? ______________
6. The eardrum is called the ______________.
7. The ossicular chain is made up of the ______________.
8. The part of the inner ear that is responsible for hearing is the ______________.
9. Which part of the middle ear strikes the oval window? ______________
10. The combining form for the temporal bone is ______________.

B. Pathology

11. The term for nearsightedness is ______________.
12. Label the following illustrations, including combining forms.

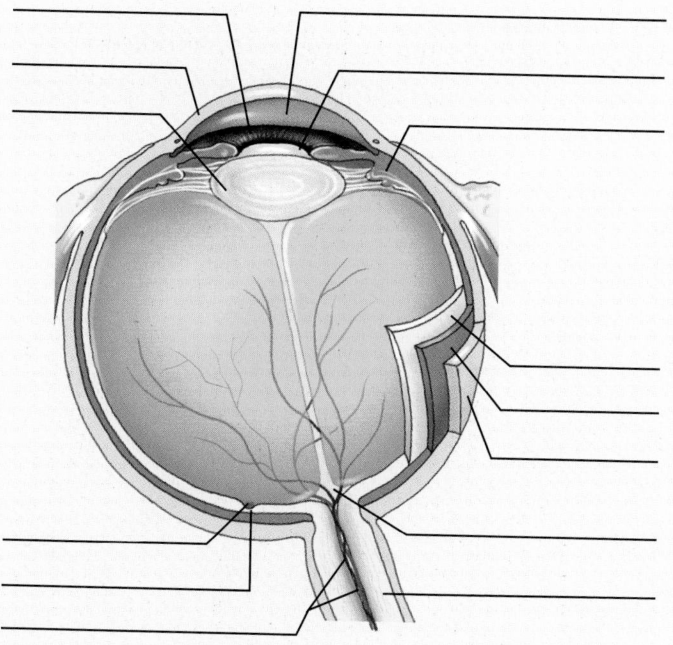

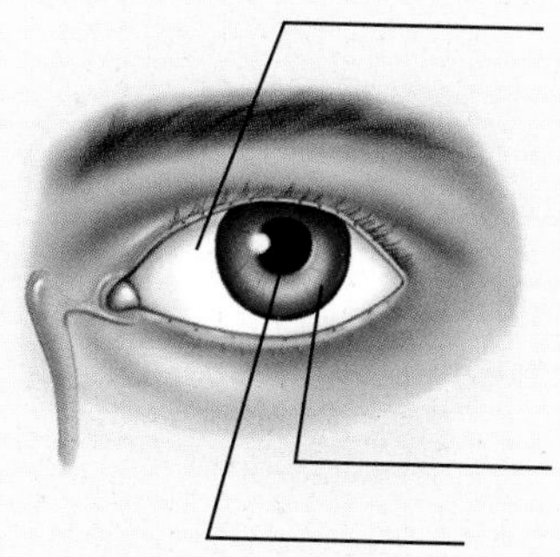

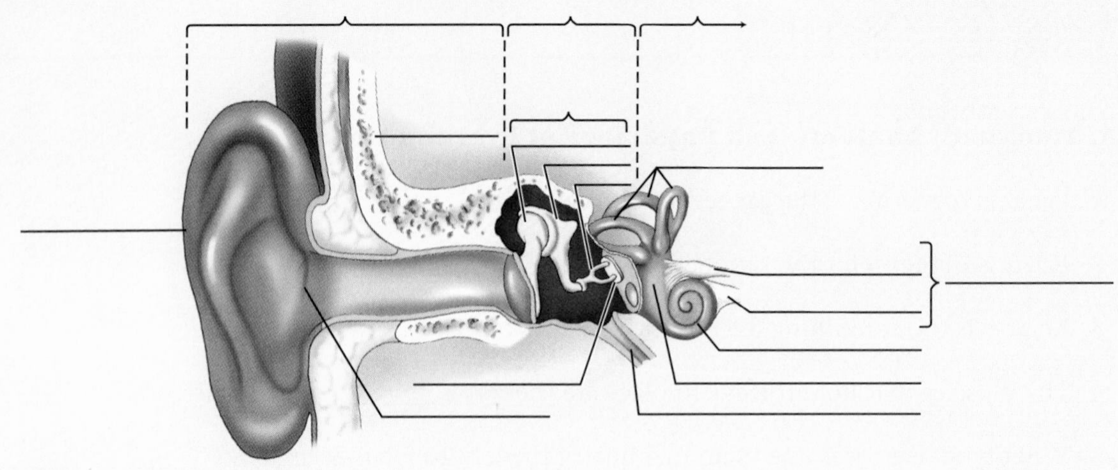

13. The other term for a stye is ________________.

14. An overflow of tears is called ________________.

15. Disease of the retina due to diabetes is termed ________________.

16. Ringing in the ears is called ________________.

17. The term for a blockage of the external auditory canal with earwax. ________________

18. Inflammation of the outer ear is called ________________.
19. Development of bone around the oval window resulting in an ankylosis of the stapes is called

________________.

20. Loss of hearing common in old age is called ________________.
21. A chronic condition of the inner ear characterized by hearing loss, tinnitus, and vertigo is called

________________.

Build a term.

22. condition of abnormally large auricles ________________________________

23. pain in the ear ________________________________

24. discharge of the ear ________________________________

25. condition of dry eyes ________________________________

26. double vision ________________________________

Decode the term.

27. anisocoria ______________________________

28. otitis media ______________________________

29. paracusis ______________________________

30. aphakia ______________________________

31. achromatopsia ______________________________

C. Diagnostic Procedures

32. Term for the use of high-frequency sound waves to image the interior of the eye. ______________

33. What is a test of the clearness of vision? ______________

34. What is a visualization of the angle of the anterior chamber of the eye? ______________

35. What test is used to screen for ARMD? ______________

36. Term for the visual examination of the interior of the eye with an ophthalmoscope. ______________

37. What is the measurement of intraocular pressure called? ______________

38. What is a method of testing auditory acuity? ______________

39. What is a measurement of the condition and mobility function of the eardrum? ______________

40. What is a test of an individual's ability to hear and understand speech? ______________

41. What is the placement of electrodes on babies to measure their response to sound? ______________

D. Therapeutic Interventions

42. What is a suture of the eyelids? ______________
43. What is the abbreviation for the use of an excimer laser to remove material under a corneal flap?

    ____

44. What is the removal of the entire contents of the orbit called? ______________

45. What is the replacement of lens function by the use of a donor corneal graft? ______________

46. Term for removal of the entire lens and its capsule. ______________

47. Term for an incision of the eardrum. ______________

48. Term for surgical repair of the external ear. ______________

49. What is an opening of the eardrum to insert tubes called? ______________

50. What is an implanted device that assists those with hearing loss? ______________

Build a term.

51. relaxation of the eyelids ____________________

52. incision of the iris ____________________

53. loss of half of the visual field ____________________

Decode the term.

54. keratotomy ____________________

55. blepharoplasty ____________________

56. stapedectomy ____________________

E. Pharmacology

57. What class of medications keep the eyes moist? ____________

58. What class of medications are used to dilate the pupils? ____________

59. What class of medications temporarily numb the eyes? ____________

60. What class of medications paralyze the ciliary muscle? ____________

61. What disorder is treated with carbonic anhydrase inhibitors, osmotics, anticholinergics, beta blockers, and alpha agonists? ____________

62. What type of medication is used to dissolve earwax? ____________

63. What type of drugs are used to treat external ear conditions and/or remove earwax? ____________

64. What type of medications are used to treat allergic conditions by reducing swelling and/or congestion? ____________ and ____________

65. What type of medication is used to reduce infection? ____________

66. What type of medication is used to constrict the pupils? ____________

F. Abbreviations

67. What is the abbreviation for correct vision? ____________

68. What is the abbreviation for the left eye? ____________

69. A patient with a diagnosis of As has ____________________.

70. Eulalia had a notation in her chart that said PERRLA. What does this mean? ____________________

71. The ophthalmologist measures a patient's IOP. What exactly is he or she measuring? ____________________

72. What is the abbreviation for the right ear? ____________

73. What is the diagnosis for a patient with OM? ________________

74. What is the abbreviation for the study of the ear? ________________

75. A patient has her hyperopia treated c̄ gl. What does this mean? ________________

76. What does the Snellen test measure? ________________

G. Singulars and Plurals

Change the following singular terms to plural.

77. pinna ________________________________

78. stapes ________________________________

79. malleus ________________________________

80. iris ________________________________

81. canthus ________________________________

82. conjunctiva ________________________________

83. sclera ________________________________

84. cornea ________________________________

H. Translations

Rewrite the following sentences in your own words.

85. Maria appeared at the ED complaining of photophobia, epiphora, and conjunctivitis.

____

86. The baby appeared inconsolable when her mother brought her to the pediatrician for what was diagnosed as otitis media.

____

87. An auto accident victim presented at the ED with anisocoria, hyphema, and a closed ear injury after being thrown from his vehicle.

____

88. When the child had his first full eye examination, it was discovered that he had slight red/green achromatopsia and emmetropia.

____

89. The 80-year-old patient evaluated by an audiologist was found to have presbycusis.

____

90. The patient with glaucoma was tested with tonometry to measure her intraocular pressure.

____

I. Cumulative Review

Circle the correct answer.

91. The *(medial, lateral)* canthus is near the nose.
92. The cornea is part of the *(anterior, posterior)* part of the eye.

93. One possible sign of an overactive thyroid gland is a protrusion of the eyes from their orbits, which is called *(exophthalmos, ectopic ophthalmia).*
94. The 45-year-old patient had her annual gynecologic visit, which included a *(Pap test, HPV)* test for vaginal or cervical cancer and a *(hysterosalpingography, mammography)* x-ray to detect breast cancer.
95. The middle-aged patient presented to his physician with a complaint of *(borborygmus, dyspepsia)*, or chronic indigestion.
96. An abnormal increase in the number of white blood cells is termed *(leukocytosis, leukopenia).*

J. Be Careful

97. What is the difference between oral and aural?

____

98. What is the difference between exotropia and esotropia?

____

99. Photophobia, as a symptom of a corneal abrasion, means ____________________.
100. Give two meanings for the combining form salping/o.

____

101. Explain the difference between palpebrate, palpate, and palpitate.

____

102. What is the difference between malleus and malleous?

____

O'Connor Eye Associates
456 Humphrey St.
St. Augustine, FL 32084

Morgan Optometric Associates
789 Henry Ave.
Philadelphia, PA 19118

August 12, 2002

Re: Mary Ellen Wright, DOB: 4/1/1970

Dear Dr. Morgan:

I have had the pleasure of treating Mary Ellen Wright for the past 11 years. She has asked me to summarize her treatment for you. She tells me that she is moving across the country next month and has expressed an interest in surgical correction of her refractive disorders.

Ms. Wright had received comprehensive optometric care from her previous optometrist from 1985 to 1991. Her previous records reflected good binocular oculomotor function and good ocular health, including the absence of posterior vitreous detachment, retinal breaks, or peripheral retinal degeneration OU. She specifically denies any incidence of trauma, diplopia, asthenopia, or cephalgia. She also denies any personal or family history of glaucoma, strabismus, retinal disease, diabetes, hypertension, heart disease, or breathing problems. She is on no medications. Entrance tests, such as EOMs, pupils, color vision, confrontation fields, and cover test appeared unchanged from previously reported exams. Refractive correction for compound myopic astigmatism contained the following parameters:

Spectacle Correction: OD −7.50−1.00 × 165 20/20
OS −7.50−1.00 × 180 20/20
Contact Lenses: OD 20/15; OS 20/15

The contact lens fit showed a stable paralimbal soft lens fit with good centration, 360 degree corneal coverage, and 0.50 mm movement OU. Each lens surface contained a trace amount of scattered protein deposits.

She presented for her last comprehensive examination without any visual or ocular complaints. She desired a new supply of disposable contact lenses. She reported clear and comfortable vision at distance, intermediate, and near with both her glasses and contact lenses.

Eye Health Assessment: Slit lamp examination revealed clean lids with good tonicity and apposition to the globe. The lashes and lid margins were clear of debris. There was no discharge OU. The corneas were clear with no fluorescein staining OU. Pupils were equal, round, and reactive to light and accommodation without afferent defect. Intraocular pressures measured 10 mmHg OD,OS at 1:30 PM with Goldmann applanation tonometry.

If any further information is needed, please feel free to contact me regarding this patient.

Sincerely,

Roland O'Connor, OD

K. Healthcare Report

103. Mary Ellen denies diplopia, asthenopia, and cephalgia. Explain these terms.

____

____

104. Explain the abbreviations EOM, OU, OS, and OD.

____

105. Mary Ellen has been diagnosed with myopic astigmatism. In your own words, explain this visual disorder.

____

106. What is the name of the test for glaucoma? ____________________

107. Explain the term *paralimbal.* ____________________

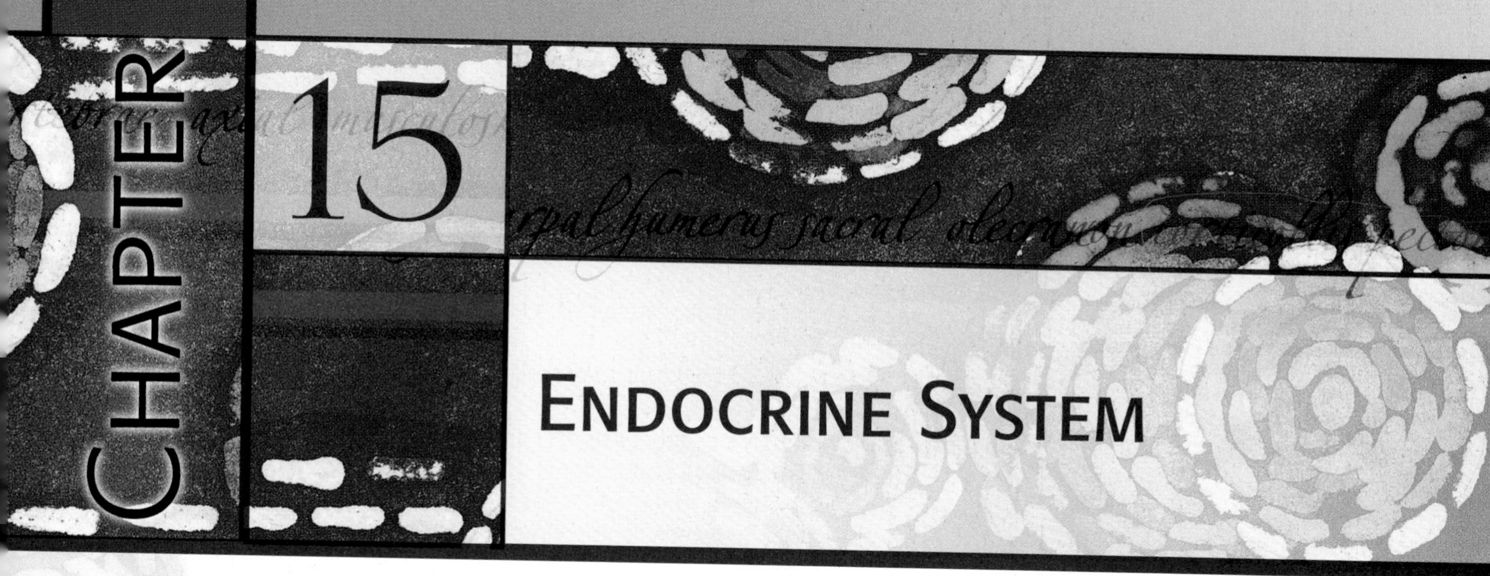

Chapter 15

Endocrine System

"If I'd known I was gonna live this long, I'd have taken better care of myself." ***—Eubie Blake at age 100***

Quote

Case Study

Darren Williams has just been diagnosed with type II diabetes mellitus. Besides prescribing oral insulin, his physician has referred him to Hillary Gorman, a dietitian, to discuss necessary diet and lifestyle changes. Darren fears that Hillary will tell him that he will not be able to eat any of the foods that he likes—ever again.

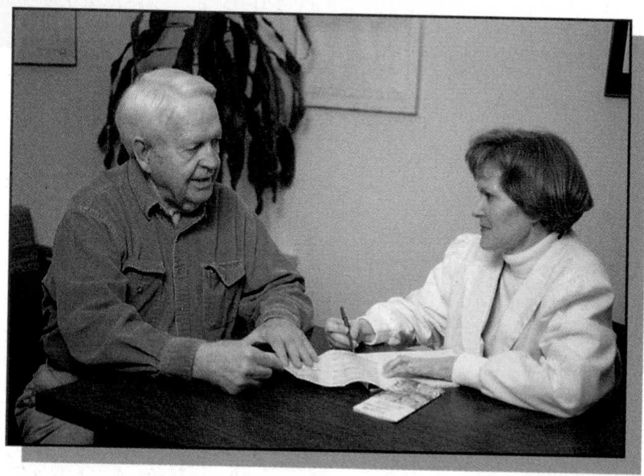

OBJECTIVES

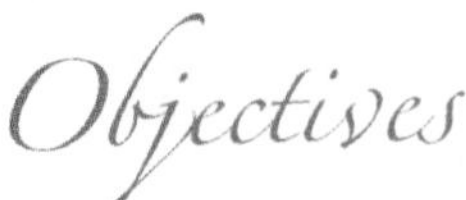

- In your own words, explain the functions of the endocrine system.
- Recognize, recall, and apply healthcare terms related to the anatomy and physiology of the endocrine system.
- Recognize, recall, and apply healthcare terms related to the pathology of the endocrine system.
- Recognize, recall, and apply healthcare terms related to diagnostic procedures of the endocrine system.
- Recognize, recall, and apply healthcare terms related to the therapeutic interventions of the endocrine system.
- Recognize, recall, and apply the abbreviations introduced in this chapter.
- Recognize, recall, and apply word components used in this chapter to build and decode healthcare terms relevant to the endocrine system.
- Recognize, recall, and apply material learned in previous chapters.

FUNCTIONS OF THE ENDOCRINE SYSTEM

The **endocrine** (EN doh krin) system assists in the function of achieving the delicate physiologic balance necessary for survival. The endocrine system uses the circulatory system and chemical messengers called **hormones** to regulate a number of body functions, including metabolism, growth, reproduction, and water and electrolyte balances.

 Exercise 1: FUNCTIONS OF THE ENDOCRINE SYSTEM

Circle the correct answer.

1. The endocrine system uses the *(nervous, circulatory)* system to send chemical messengers called *(neurotransmitters, hormones)* to regulate body functions.

ANATOMY AND PHYSIOLOGY

The endocrine system is composed of several single and paired ductless glands that secrete hormones into the bloodstream. The hormones regulate specific body functions by acting on target cells with receptor sites for those particular hormones only. See Fig. 15-1 for an illustration of the body with the locations of the endocrine glands.

Pituitary Gland

The **pituitary** (pih TOO ih tare ree) **gland**, also known as the **hypophysis** (hye POFF ih sis), is a tiny gland located behind the optic nerve in the cranial cavity. Sometimes called the *master gland* because of its role in controlling the functions of other endocrine glands, it is composed of anterior and posterior lobes, each with their own functions.

The **anterior lobe**, or **adenohypophysis** (add uh noh hye POFF ih sis), is composed of glandular tissue and secretes myriad hormones in response to stimulation by the hypothalamus. The hypothalamus sends hormones through blood vessels, which cause the adenohypophysis either to release or to inhibit the re-

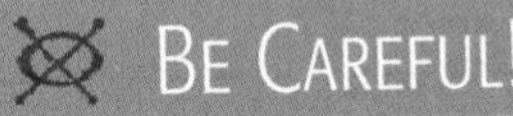

Do not confuse *aden/o,* which means *gland,* with *adren/o,* which means *the adrenal gland.*

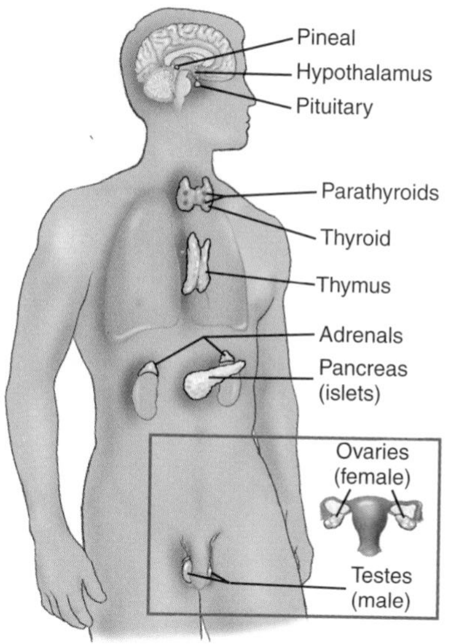

Fig. 15-1 Location of the endocrine glands.

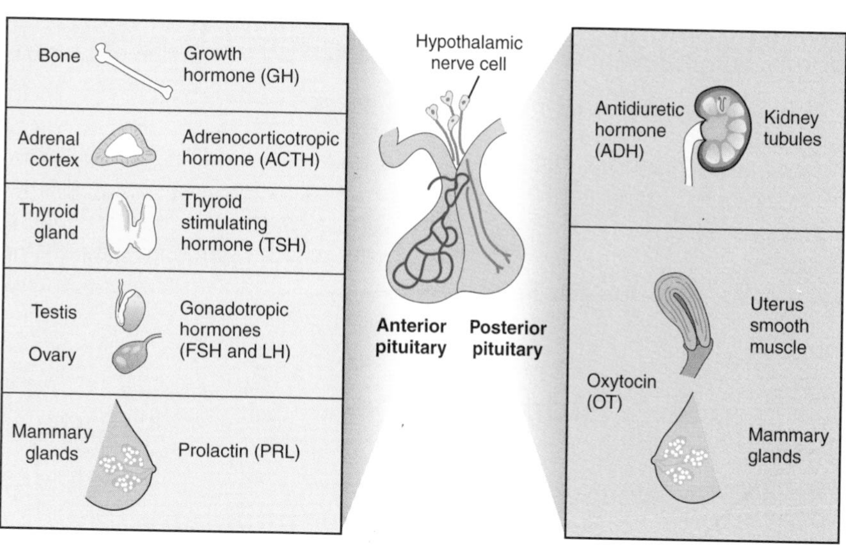

Fig. 15-2 Pituitary hormones. Principal anterior and posterior pituitary hormones and their target organs.

Adenohypophysis Hormones and Their Effects

ADENOHYPOPHYSIS HORMONES	EFFECT
Growth hormone (GH) (also called **human growth hormone [hGH]** or **somatotropin hormone [STH]**)	Stimulates growth of long bones and skeletal muscle; converts proteins to glucose.
Prolactin (PRL) (also called **lactogenic hormone**)	Stimulates milk production in the breast.
Thyrotropin (also called **thyroid stimulating hormone [TSH]**)	Stimulates thyroid to release two other thyroid hormones.
Adrenocorticotropic hormone (ACTH)	Stimulates the adrenal cortex to release steroids.
Gonadotropic hormones (include **follicle-stimulating hormone [FSH], luteinizing hormone [LH],** and **interstitial cell-stimulating hormone [ICSH]**)	FSH stimulates the development of gametes in the respective sexes. LH stimulates ovulation in the female and the secretion of sex hormones in both the male and female. ICSH stimulates production of reproductive cells in the male.

lease of specific hormones. The adenohypophysis has a wide range of effects on the body, as Fig. 15-2 and the table above illustrate.

The **posterior lobe (neurohypophysis)** of the pituitary gland is composed of nervous tissue. The hormones that it secretes are produced in the hypothalamus, transported to the neurohypophysis directly through the tissue connecting the organs, and released from storage in the posterior lobe by neural stimulation from the hypothalamus. The two hormones released by this lobe are **antidiuretic hormone (ADH)** and **oxytocin.** See the following table and Fig. 15-2 for the hormones secreted by the neurohypophysis and their effects.

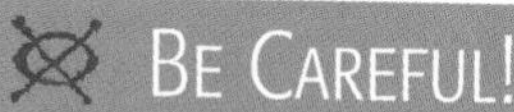

The combining form *trop/o* means *turning,* whereas *troph/o* means *development* or *nourishment.*

Neurohypophysis Hormones and Their Effects

NEUROHYPOPHYSIS HORMONES	EFFECT
Antidiuretic hormone (ADH) (also called **vasopressin**)	Stimulates the kidneys to reabsorb water and return it to circulation; is also a vasoconstrictor, resulting in higher blood pressure.
Oxytocin (OT)	Stimulates the muscles of the uterus during the delivery of an infant and the muscles surrounding the mammary ducts to contract, releasing milk.

Exercise 2: PITUITARY FUNCTIONS

Circle the correct answer.

1. The pituitary gland, the *(pineal, hypophysis)*, is called the master gland because of its control over other endocrine glands.
2. The pituitary gland is controlled by what other gland? *(thalamus, hypothalamus)*
3. The anterior lobe of the pituitary gland is also known as the *(adenohypophysis, neurohypophysis)*.
4. The hormone that stimulates bone growth is called *(somatotropin, thyrotropin)*.
5. PRL is a hormone responsible for stimulating *(ovulation, milk production)*.
6. The hormone that stimulates the kidneys to reabsorb water and return it to circulation is *(ADH, FSH)*, secreted by the *(neurohypophysis, adenohypophysis)*.
7. ACTH is responsible for stimulating the *(adrenal cortex, thyroid gland)* to release steroids.

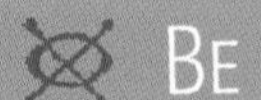

BE CAREFUL!

Oxytocin should not be confused with *oxytocia*, which means *a rapid birth*.

Thyroid Gland

The **thyroid gland** is a single organ located on the anterior of the neck. It regulates the metabolism of the body and normal growth and development, and controls the amount of calcium deposited into bone. The following table describes the hormones secreted by the thyroid and their effects.

Thyroid Gland Hormones and Their Effects

THYROID GLAND HORMONE	EFFECT
Triiodothyronine (T_3)	Increases cell metabolism.
Tetraiodothyronine (also called **thyroxine [T_4]**)	Increases cell metabolism.
Calcitonin	Regulates the amount of calcium in the bloodstream.

Parathyroid Glands

The **parathyroids** (pair uh THIGH royds) are four small glands located on the posterior surface of the thyroid gland in the neck. They secrete **parathyroid hormone (PTH)** in response to a low level of calcium in the blood. When low calcium is detected, the PTH increases calcium by causing it to be released from the bone, which results in calcium reabsorption by the kidneys and the digestive system. PTH is inhibited by high levels of calcium.

 Exercise 3: THYROID AND PARATHYROID GLANDS

Circle the correct answer.

1. The thyroid gland is responsible for the regulation of the body's *(metabolism, circulation)* and controls the amount of *(phosphorus, calcium)* deposited into bone.
2. What is an alternate name for tetraiodothyronine (T_4)? *(calcitonin, thyroxine)*
3. *(Calcitonin, Triiodothyronine)* regulates the amount of calcium in the bloodstream.
4. The parathyroid glands produce a hormone called *(parathyroid hormone, thyroxine)* that increases the levels of *(phosphorus, calcium)* in the blood when low levels are detected.

Adrenal Glands (Suprarenals)

The **adrenal** (uh DREE nuls) **glands,** also called the **suprarenals,** are paired, one on top of each kidney. Different hormones are secreted by the two different parts of these glands: the external portion called the **adrenal cortex** (uh DREE nul KORE tecks) and an internal portion called the **adrenal medulla** (uh DREE nul muh DOO lah).

The adrenal cortex secretes three hormones that are called steroids.

The **adrenal medulla** is the inner portion of the adrenal gland. It produces sympathomimetic hormones that stimulate the fight-or-flight response to stress, similar to the action of sympathetic nervous system.

Adrenal Cortex Hormones and Their Effects

ADRENAL CORTEX HORMONES	EFFECT
Mineralocorticoids (e.g., aldosterone)	Regulate blood volume, blood pressure, and electrolytes.
Glucocorticoids (e.g., cortisol [hydrocortisone])	Respond to stress; have antiinflammatory properties.
Sex hormones (e.g., estrogen, androgen)	Responsible for secondary sex characteristics.

Adrenal Medulla Hormones and Their Effects

ADRENAL MEDULLA HORMONES (CATECHOLAMINES)	EFFECT
Epinephrine (also called **adrenaline**)	Dilates bronchi, increases heart rate, raises blood pressure, dilates pupils, and elevates blood sugar levels.
Norepinephrine (also called **noradrenaline**)	Increases heart rate and blood pressure and elevates blood sugar levels for energy use.
Dopamine	Dilates arteries and increases production of urine, blood pressure, and cardiac rate. Acts as a neurotransmitter in the nervous system.

Exercise 4: THE ADRENAL GLANDS

Circle the correct answer.

1. Adrenal glands are named for their location either near or above the *(liver, kidneys).*
2. The inner part of the adrenal gland is the adrenal *(cortex, medulla),* whereas the outer part of the adrenal gland is the adrenal *(cortex, medulla).*
3. The types of hormones secreted by the adrenal cortex are called *(catecholamines, steroids).*
4. The action of the hormones of the adrenal medulla is similar to the function of the sympathetic nervous system. They are referred to as *(sympathomimetic, efferent)* hormones.
5. Aldosterone regulates blood volume, blood pressure, and *(vitamins, electrolytes).*
6. Androgens secreted by the adrenal cortex are responsible for the development of *(secondary sex, stress response)* characteristics.
7. What hormone has an antiinflammatory effect? *(cortisol, adrenalin)*
8. Which hormone acts as a neurotransmitter in the nervous system? *(norepinephrine, dopamine)*

Pancreas

The pancreas, located inferior and posterior to the stomach, has both exocrine and endocrine functions. The exocrine function is to release digestive enzymes through a duct into the small intestines. The endocrine function, accomplished through a variety of types of cells called **islets of Langerhans** (EYE lets) of (LANG gur hahnz), is to regulate the level of glucose in the blood. The two main types of islets of Langerhans cells are alpha and beta cells. Alpha cells produce the hormone glucagon that increases the level of glucose in the blood when levels are low. Beta cells secrete **insulin** (IN suh lin) that decreases the level of glucose in the blood when levels are high. These hormones regulate glucose levels through the metabolism of fats, carbohydrates, and proteins.

Thymus Gland

The **thymus** (THIGH mus) gland is located in the mediastinum above the heart. It releases a hormone called **thymosin** that is responsible for stimulating key cells in the immune response. For more detail, see Chapter 9 on the blood, lymphatic, and immune systems.

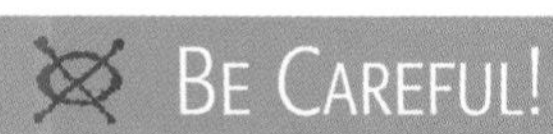

Do not confuse *thyr/o,* which means *thyroid,* and *thym/o,* which means *thymus.*

Ovaries and Testes

The **ovaries** and **testes**, the female and male gonads, also act as endocrine glands, which influence reproductive functions.

Pineal Gland

The **pineal** (PIH nee ul) gland is located in the center of the brain, functioning to secrete the hormone **melatonin**, thought to be responsible for inducing sleep.

COMBINING FORMS FOR ANATOMY AND PHYSIOLOGY

MEANING	COMBINING FORM	MEANING	COMBINING FORM
adrenal gland	adren/o	pressure	press/o
body	somat/o	sugar	gluc/o, glyc/o
delivery, labor	toc/o	thalamus	thalam/o
gland	aden/o	thyroid gland	thyr/o, thyroid/o
gonad	gonad/o	to grow	phys/o
lobe, section	lob/o	to secrete	crin/o
milk	lact/o	to turn	trop/o
nerve	neur/o	urinary system, urine	ur/o
origin	gen/o	vessel	vas/o
pituitary gland	hypophys/o		

PREFIXES AND SUFFIXES FOR ANATOMY AND PHYSIOLOGY

PREFIX/SUFFIX	MEANING	PREFIX/SUFFIX	MEANING
anti-	against	oxy-	rapid
endo-	within	pro-	in front of
exo-	outside	-crine	to secrete
hypo-	under		

Exercise 5: PANCREAS, THYMUS, OVARIES, TESTES, PINEAL GLANDS

Circle the correct response.

1. The endocrine gland that functions to effect an immune response is the *(pineal, thymus)*.
2. The islets of Langerhans in the *(pancreas, kidneys)* function to regulate the amount of *(calcium, glucose)* in the bloodstream.
3. Sleep is thought to be induced by the hormone *(thymosin, melatonin)*.
4. The metabolism of carbohydrates, fats, and proteins is regulated by *(insulin and glucagon, epinephrine and norepinephrine)*.

Match the word parts with their correct terms.

_____ 5. crin/o	_____ 11. gen/o	A.	to turn
		B.	section
_____ 6. phys/o	_____ 12. thyr/o	C.	body
		D.	thymus
_____ 7. aden/o	_____ 13. adren/o	E.	reproductive gland
		F.	thyroid gland
_____ 8. somat/o	_____ 14. gonad/o	G.	growth
		H.	outside
_____ 9. trop/o	_____ 15. neur/o	I.	nerve
		J.	thalamus
_____ 10. lact/o	_____ 16. thalam/o	K.	vessel

_____ 17. lob/o
_____ 18. ur/o
_____ 19. vas/o
_____ 20. press/o
_____ 21. toc/o
_____ 22. thym/o
_____ 23. gluc/o
_____ 24. pancreat/o
_____ 25. pro-
_____ 26. exo-
_____ 27. endo-
_____ 28. hypo-
_____ 29. oxy-

L. gland
M. sugar
N. pressure
O. urinary system
P. delivery
Q. rapid
R. origin
S. to secrete
T. before, in front of
U. below
V. pancreas
W. milk
X. adrenal gland
Y. within

PATHOLOGY

Most of the pathology of the endocrine system is the result of either hyper- (too much) or hypo- (too little) hormonal secretion. Developmental issues also play a role as to when the malfunction occurs and the results.

Terms Related to Signs and Symptoms of Endocrine Disorders

Term	Word Origin	Definition
Anorexia an oh RECK see ah	*an-* without *orex/o* appetite *-ia* condition	Lack of appetite.
Exophthalmia eck soff THAL mee ah	*ex-* out *ophthalm/o* eye *-ia* condition	Protrusion of eyeballs from their orbits (see Fig. 14-4).
Goiter GOY tur		Enlargement of the thyroid gland, not due to a tumor (Fig. 15-3).
Hirsutism HUR soo tiz um		Abnormal hairiness, especially in women (Fig. 15-4).

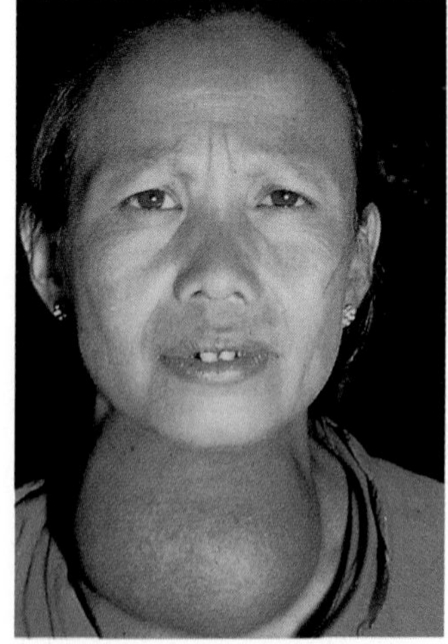

Fig. 15-3 Goiter.

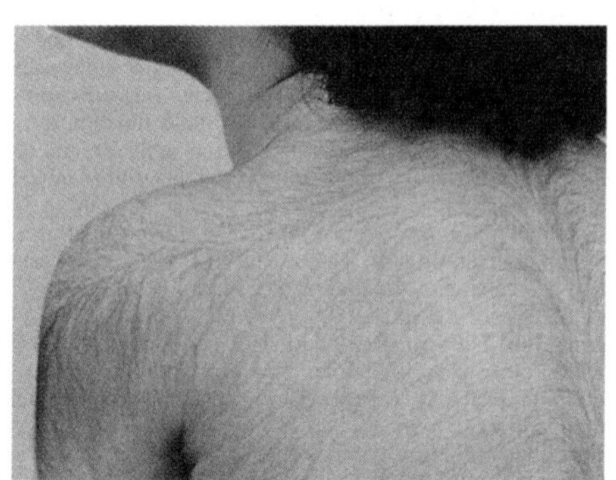

Fig. 15-4 Hirsutism.

Terms Related to Signs and Symptoms of Endocrine Disorders—cont'd

TERM	WORD ORIGIN	DEFINITION
Hypocalcemia hye poh kal SEE mee ah	*hypo-* deficient *calc/o* calcium *-emia* blood condition	Condition of deficient calcium in the blood. The opposite would be **hypercalcemia**—excessive calcium in the blood.
Hypoglycemia hye poh gly SEE mee ah	*hypo-* deficient *glyc/o* sugar *-emia* blood condition	Condition of deficient sugar in the blood. The opposite would be **hyperglycemia**—excessive sugar in the blood.
Hypokalemia hye poh kuh LEE mee ah	*hypo-* deficient *kal/i* potassium *-emia* blood condition	Condition of deficient potassium in the blood. The opposite would be **hyperkalemia**—excessive potassium in the blood.
Hyponatremia hye poh nuh TREE mee ah	*hypo-* deficient *natr/o* sodium *-emia* blood condition	Condition of deficient sodium in the blood. The opposite would be **hypernatremia**—excessive sodium in the blood.
Paresthesia pair uh STHEE zsa	*par-* abnormal *esthesi/o* feeling *-ia* condition	Abnormal sensation, such as prickling.
Polydipsia pah lee DIP see ah	*poly-* excessive *dips/o* thirst *-ia* condition	Condition of excessive thirst.
Polyphagia pah lee FAY jee ah	*poly-* excessive *phag/o* to eat, swallow *-ia* condition	Condition of excessive appetite.
Polyuria pah lee YOO ree ah	*poly-* excessive *ur/o* urine *-ia* condition	Condition of excessive urination.
Tetany TET uh nee		Continuous muscle spasms.

Terms Related to Pituitary Gland Disorders

TERM	WORD ORIGIN	DEFINITION
Acromegaly ack ruh MEG uh lee	*acr/o* extremities *-megaly* enlargement	Hypersecretion of somatotropin from adenohypophysis during adulthood; leads to an enlargement of the extremities (hands and feet) jaw, nose, and forehead (Fig. 15-5).

Continued

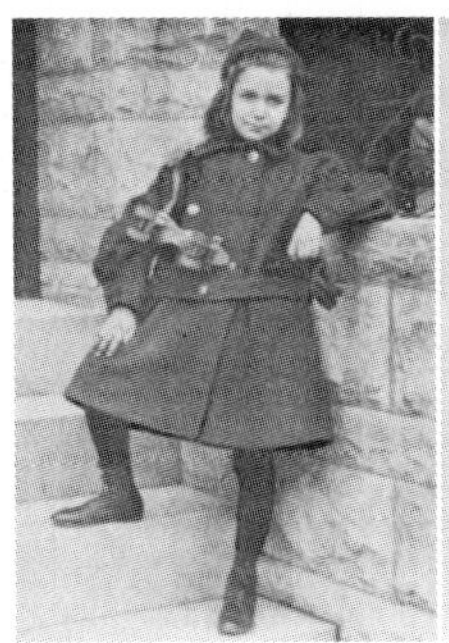
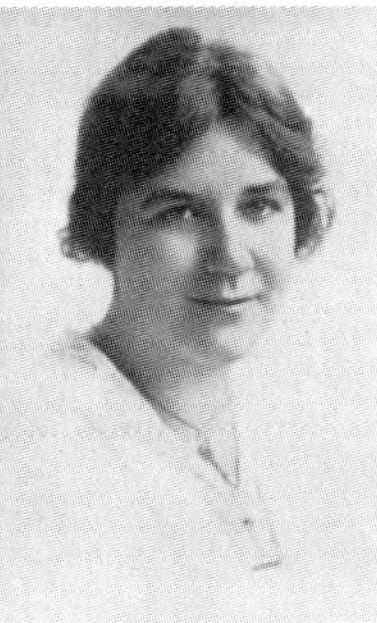
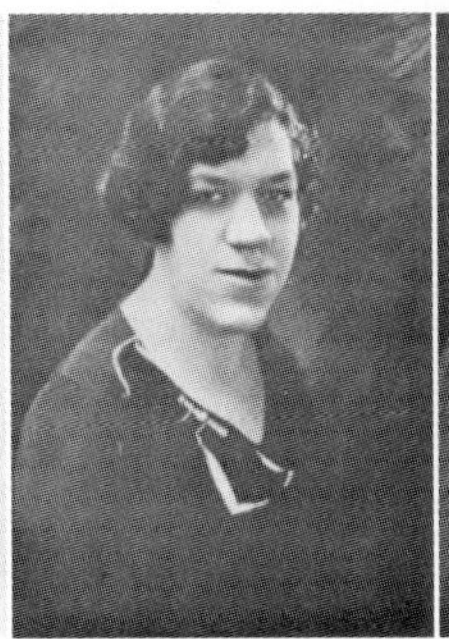
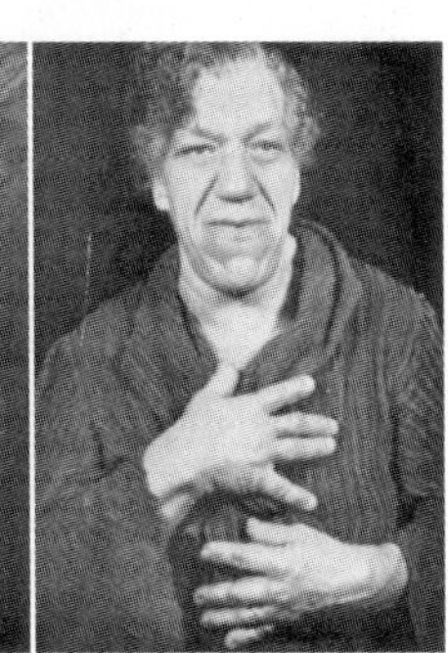

Fig. 15-5 The progression of acromegaly.

Terms Related to Pituitary Gland Disorders—cont'd

TERM	WORD ORIGIN	DEFINITION
Diabetes insipidus dye ah BEE teez in SIP ih dus		Undersecretion of ADH from the neurohypophysis resulting in polydipsia and polyuria.
Gigantism jye GAN tiz um		Hypersecretion of somatotropin from adenohypophysis during childhood, leading to excessive growth.
Growth hormone deficiency (GHD)		Somatotropin deficiency due to adenohypophysis during childhood results in dwarfism (Fig. 15-6). If during adulthood, patients may develop obesity, and experience weakness and cardiac difficulties.
Panhypopituitarism pan hye poh pih TOO ih tur iz um	*pan-* all *hypo-* deficient *pituitar/o* pituitary *-ism* condition	Deficiency or lack of all pituitary hormones causing hypotension, weight loss, weakness, and loss of libido; also called **Simmond's disease.**
Syndrome of inappropriate antidiuretic hormone (SIADH)		Oversecretion of ADH from the neurohypophysis leading to the inability to excrete concentrated urine.

Terms Related to Thyroid Disorders

TERM	WORD ORIGIN	DEFINITION
Hyperthyroidism hye pur THIGH roy diz um	*hyper-* excessive *thyroid/o* thyroid gland *-ism* condition	Excessive thyroid hormone production; also called **thyrotoxicosis,** the most common form of which is **Graves' disease,** which may be accompanied by exophthalmia.
Hypothyroidism hye poh THIGH roy diz um	*hypo-* deficient *thyroid/o* thyroid gland *-ism* condition	Deficient thyroid hormone production. If it occurs during childhood, it causes a condition called **cretinism,** which results in stunted mental and physical growth. The extreme adult form is called **myxedema** (mick suh DEE mah), which is characterized by facial and orbital edema.

Terms Related to Parathyroid Disorders

TERM	WORD ORIGIN	DEFINITION
Hyperparathyroidism hye pur pair uh THIGH roy diz um	*hyper-* excessive *parathyroid/o* parathyroid gland *-ism* condition	Overproduction of parathyroid hormone; symptoms include polyuria, hypercalcemia, hypertension, and kidney stones.
Hypoparathyroidism hye poh pair uh THIGH roy diz um	*hypo-* deficient *parathyroid/o* parathyroid gland *-ism* condition	Deficient parathyroid hormone production results in tetany, hypocalcemia, irritability, and muscle cramps.

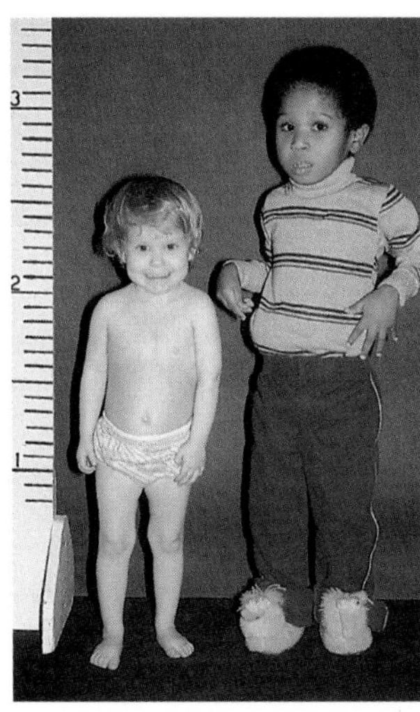

Fig. 15-6 The normal 3½-year-old boy is in the 50th percentile for height. The short, 3-year-old girl exhibits the characteristic "Kewpie" doll appearance, suggesting diagnosis of GH deficiency.

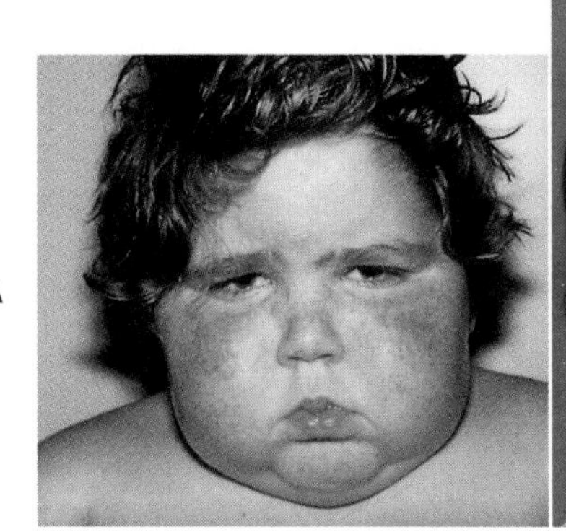

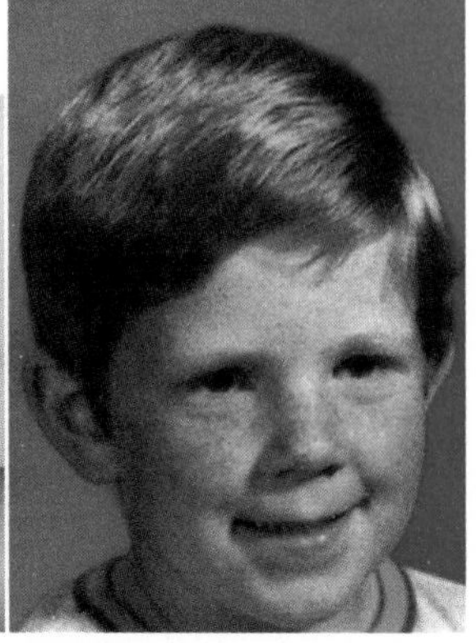

Fig. 15-7 Cushing's disease. **A,** First diagnosed with Cushing's syndrome. **B,** Four months later after treatment.

Terms Related to Adrenal Gland Disorders

TERM	WORD ORIGIN	DEFINITION
Addison's disease		Insufficient secretion of adrenal cortisol from the adrenal cortex is manifested by gastric complaints, hypotension, and dehydration.
Cushing's disease		Excessive secretion of cortisol by the adrenal cortex causes symptoms of obesity, leukocytosis, hirsutism, hypokalemia, hyperglycemia, and muscle wasting (Fig. 15-7).
Pheochromocytoma fee oh kroh moh sye TOH mah	*pheo-* dark *chrom/o* color *cyt/o* cell *-oma* tumor, mass	Tumor of the adrenal medulla that causes oversecretion of epinephrine and norepinephrine.

Terms Related to Pancreas (Islets of Langerhans) Disorders

TERM	WORD ORIGIN	DEFINITION
Type I diabetes		Total lack of insulin production resulting in glycosuria, polydipsia, polyphagia, polyuria, blurred vision, fatigue, and frequent infections. Thought to be an autoimmune disorder. Also called **insulin-dependent diabetes mellitus (IDDM).**
Type II diabetes		Deficient insulin production, with symptoms similar to Type I diabetes. Etiology unknown but associated with obesity and family history; also called **non–insulin-dependent diabetes mellitus (NIDDM).**
Hyperinsulinism hye pur IN suh lin iz um	*hyper-* excessive *insulin/o* insulin *-ism* condition	Oversecretion of insulin; seen in some newborns of diabetic mothers. Causes severe hypoglycemia.

Case Study Continued

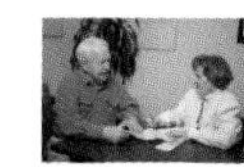

After talking over his diagnosis, Hillary discusses Darren's need to change his diet. "I know you're disappointed that your diet needs to be modified, Mr. Williams. But diabetes is not a disease that you want to ignore. The good news is that it can be managed; the bad news is that if it isn't, complications can occur, ranging from loss of sight, to kidney failure, to loss of limbs. So let's make a plan to get you eating and exercising to manage this disease."

Hillary explains the nutritional recommendations for persons with diabetes as she talks to Darren about his new diet.

Nutritional Recommendations for Persons with Diabetes

RECOMMENDATION	DESCRIPTION
Calories	Sufficient to achieve and maintain reasonable weight.
Carbohydrates	May be up to 45%-55% of total calories. Emphasis is on unrefined carbohydrates with fiber; modest amounts of sucrose and other refined sugars may be acceptable contingent on diabetes control and body weight.
Protein	Usual intake is double the amount needed; exact ideal percentage of total calories is unknown; usually, intake is 10%-20%.
Fat	Ideally, less than 30% of total calories; must be individualized, because 30% may be too low for some individuals. • Polyunsaturated fats: 6%-8% • Saturated fats: <10% • Monounsaturated fats: remaining percentage.
Fiber	Up to 40 g/day; 25 g/1000 cal for low-calorie diet.
Alternative sweeteners	Use of various nutritive and nonnutritive sweeteners is acceptable.
Sodium	1000 mg/1000 cal, not to exceed 3000 mg/day; modified for those with special medical conditions.
Vitamins/minerals	No evidence that diabetes influences vitamin/mineral needs.

Exercise 6: PATHOLOGY

Circle the correct answer.

1. Most endocrine disorders are the result of an abnormal secretion of *(hormones, neurotransmitters).*
2. Pheochromocytoma is a tumor of the adrenal *(cortex, medulla).*
3. Graves' disease is a disorder of the *(thyroid, parathyroid)* gland(s).
4. Addison's and Cushing's diseases are endocrine disorders of the adrenal *(cortex, medulla).*
5. Diabetes insipidus is a disorder of the *(pancreas, pituitary).*
6. *(Hypoparathyroidism, Hyperparathyroidism)* is characterized by tetany.
7. Cretinism and myxedema are disorders that result from a hypofunction of the *(parathyroid, thyroid)* gland(s).
8. Glycosuria, polydipsia, polyuria, and polyphagia are symptoms of a hypofunction of the *(adenohypophysis, islets of Langerhans).*

Match the word part with the correct term.

_____ 9. trop/o	_____ 18. tachy-	A.	thirst
		B.	all
_____ 10. somat/o	_____ 19. acro-	C.	calcium
		D.	fast
_____ 11. natr/o	_____ 20. dips/o	E.	eye
		F.	abnormal
_____ 12. glyc/o	_____ 21. phag/o	G.	appetite
		H.	turning
_____ 13. calc/o	_____ 22. poly-	I.	sugar
		J.	potassium
_____ 14. ophthalm/o	_____ 23. orex/o	K.	sodium
		L.	body
_____ 15. brady-	_____ 24. kal/i	M.	many
		N.	eat, swallow
_____ 16. esthesi/o	_____ 25. pan-	O.	extremities
		P.	slow
_____ 17. para-		Q.	feeling

DIAGNOSTIC PROCEDURES

Terms Related to Imaging

TERM	WORD ORIGIN	DEFINITION
Computed tomography (CT) scan	*tom/o* slice *-graphy* process of recording	May be used to test for bone density in hypoparathyroidism and the size of the adrenal glands in Addison's disease.
Magnetic resonance imaging (MRI)		May be used to examine changes in the size of soft tissues, for example, the pituitary, pancreas, or hypothalamus.
Radioactive iodine (RAI) uptake scan		May be used to test thyroid function by measuring the gland's ability to concentrate and retain iodine. Useful to test for hyperthyroidism.
Radiography	*radi/o* ray *-graphy* process of recording	X-rays are done to examine suspected endocrine changes that affect the density or thickness of bone; also may reveal underlying causes of an endocrine disorder.
Ultrasonography (US)	*ultra* beyond *son/o* sound *-graphy* process of recording	Aside from visualizing the pancreas (Fig. 15-8), US may also be used to guide biopsies of the thyroid gland to discern the differences between solid or fluid-filled cysts.

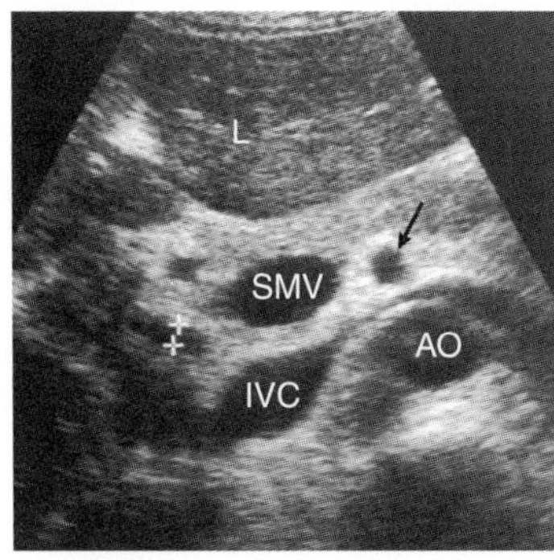

Fig. 15-8 Transverse scan over the epigastric region of the abdomen, demonstrating a normal pancreas *(calipers)*. *L,* Left lobe of the liver; *AO,* aorta; *IVC,* inferior vena cava; *SMV,* superior mesenteric vein; *arrow,* superior mesenteric artery.

Terms Related to Laboratory Tests		
TERM	**WORD ORIGIN**	**DEFINITION**
A1c		Measure of average blood glucose during a 3-month time span. Used to monitor response to diabetes treatment. Formerly called HbA1c.
Fasting blood sugar (FBS)		After a period of fasting, blood is drawn. The amount of glucose present is used to measure the body's ability to break down and utilize glucose.
Glucose tolerance test (GTT)		Blood test to measure the body's response to a concentrated glucose solution. May be used to diagnose diabetes mellitus.
Hormone tests		Measures the amount of antidiuretic hormone (ADH), cortisol, growth hormone, or parathyroid hormone in the blood.
Radioimmunoassay studies (RIA)		Nuclear medicine test used to tag and detect hormones in the blood through the use of radionuclide.
Thyroid function tests (TFTs)		Blood tests done to assess T_3, T_4, and calcitonin. May be used to evaluate abnormalities of thyroid function.
Total calcium		Measures the amount of calcium in the blood. Results may be used to examine parathyroid function, calcium metabolism, or cancerous conditions.
Urine glucose		Used as a screen for or to monitor diabetes mellitus; a urine specimen is tested for the presence of glucose.
Urine ketones KEE tones		Presence of ketones in a urine specimen may indicate diabetes mellitus or hyperthyroidism.

Exercise 7: DIAGNOSTIC PROCEDURES

Circle the correct answer.

1. High-frequency sound waves may be used to image the pancreas, adrenals, or thyroid in a procedure called a/an *(CT scan, ultrasonography).*
2. Detailed images of soft tissues, such as the pituitary, pancreas, or hypothalamus, may be acquired from a technique called *(magnetic resonance imaging, RAI).*
3. A test used to monitor a patient's response to diabetes is *(urine ketone test, A1c).*
4. Parathyroid dysfunction may be detected through a blood test for parathyroid hormone or a test for *(urine glucose, total calcium).*
5. Which type of test can be used to screen for diabetes mellitus? *(urine glucose, total calcium)*

Case Study Continued

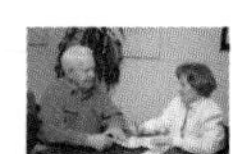

Hillary has Darren look at his lab results with her. She explains the normal range for blood sugar and points to his result. Hillary explains that he will be responsible for keeping track of his blood sugar levels at home and making adjustments to his diet and insulin intake, depending on the results.

THERAPEUTIC INTERVENTIONS

The majority of the therapeutic interventions for endocrine system disorders are excisions. Unlike the case in other body systems, incisions, repairs, or new openings are not as helpful as the removal of part, or all, of the malfunctioning gland.

Terms Related to Excisions

TERM	WORD ORIGIN	DEFINITION
Adrenalectomy uh dree nuh LECK tuh mee	*adren/o* adrenal gland *-ectomy* excision	Bilateral removal of the adrenal glands to reduce excess hormone secretion.
Hypophysectomy hye poff uh SECK tuh mee	*hypophys/o* pituitary gland *-ectomy* excision	Excision of the pituitary gland; usually done to remove a pituitary tumor (Fig. 15-9).
Pancreatectomy pan kree uh TECK tuh mee	*pancreat/o* pancreas *-ectomy* excision	Excision of all or part of the pancreas to remove a tumor or to treat an intractable inflammation of the pancreas.
Parathyroidectomy pair uh THIGH roy DECK tuh mee	*parathyroid/o* parathyroid gland *-ectomy* excision	Removal of the parathyroid glands.
Thyroidectomy thy roy DECK tuh mee	*thyroid/o* thyroid gland *-ectomy* excision	Removal of part or all of the thyroid gland to treat goiter, tumors, or hyperthyroidism that does not respond to medication. Removal of the majority, but not all, of this gland will result in a regrowth of the gland with normal function. If cancer is detected, a total thyroidectomy is performed.

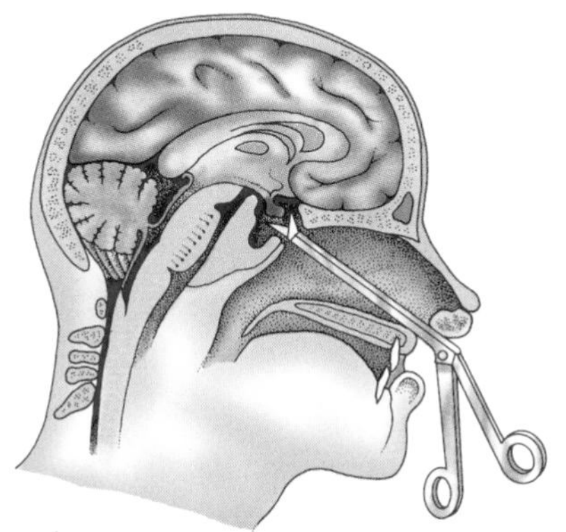

Fig. 15-9 Hypophysectomy.

Exercise 8: THERAPEUTIC INTERVENTIONS

Circle the correct answer.

1. Removal of the gland that is directly above the kidneys. *(adrenalectomy, pancreatectomy)*
2. Removal of the four glands located on the back of the thyroid gland. *(thymectomy, parathyroidectomy)*
3. Removal of the gland that includes the islets of Langerhans. *(adrenalectomy, pancreatectomy)*
4. The procedure to remove part of a gland will result in a regrowth of normal tissue. *(hypophysectomy, thyroidectomy)*

DID YOU KNOW?

Some pharmacologic therapy can cure one disease while causing another. For example, long-term cortisone use, such as that for patients with Crohn's disease or ulcerative colitis, can result in Addison's disease.

PHARMACOLOGY

Most of the pharmacologic interventions for endocrine disorders are to correct imbalances, either inhibiting or replacing abnormal hormone levels.

Corticosteroids: Underfunctioning adrenal cortices (Addison's disease) may be treated with prednisone (Deltasone).

Insulin replacement therapy: Used to compensate for impaired pancreatic functioning. May be used for either type I or II diabetes and is available in either oral, injectable, an oral spray, or pump form (Figs. 15-10 and 15-11). Examples include insulin, tolazamide (Tolinase), metformin (Glucophage), rosiglitazone (Avandia), and glyburide (Micronase).

Thyroid hormone replacement: Used to treat hypothyroidism. Examples include natural thyroid hormones (Armour Thyroid) and levothyroxine (Levoxyl, Synthroid). Methimazole (Tapazole) is used to treat hyperthyroidism.

Vasopressin, desmopressin acetate: Used to treat diabetes insipidus; available in a nasal spray form.

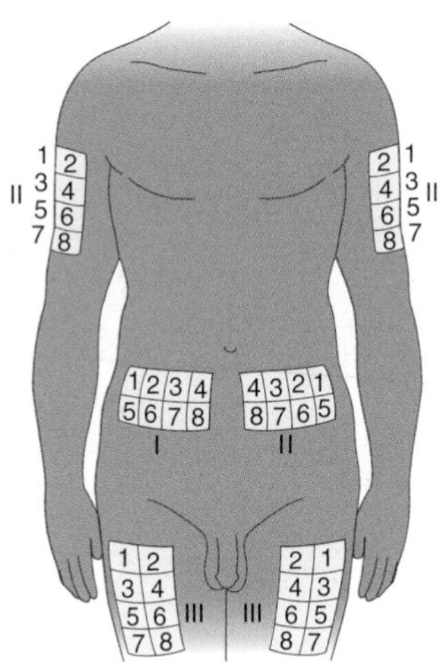

Fig. 15-10 Sites for insulin injection.

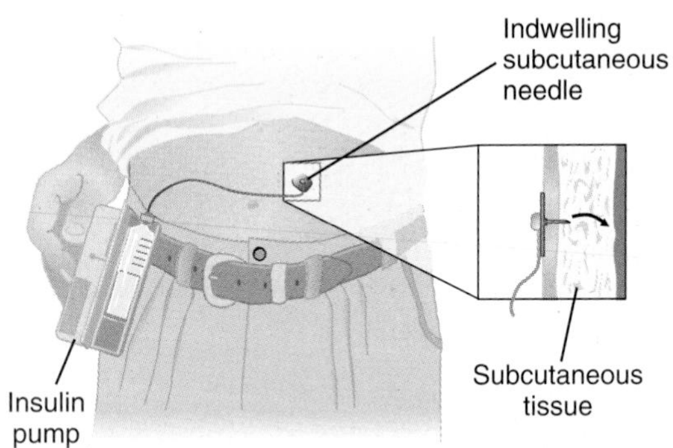

Fig. 15-11 Insulin pump. The device is worn externally and connected to an indwelling subcutaneous needle, usually inserted in the abdomen.

Exercise 9: PHARMACOLOGY

Match the pharmacologic agent with the correct disease or disorder.

_____ 1. insulin

_____ 2. prednisone

_____ 3. vasopressin

_____ 4. synthroid

A. Addison's disease
B. hypothyroidism
C. diabetes mellitus
D. diabetes insipidus

Abbreviations

Abbreviation	Meaning	Abbreviation	Meaning
ACTH	Adrenocorticotropic hormone	NIDDM	Non–insulin-dependent diabetes mellitus
ADH	Antidiuretic hormone	OT	oxytocin
Ca	Calcium	PGH	Pituitary growth hormone
DI	Diabetes insipidus	PTH	Parathyroid hormone
FBS	Fasting blood sugar	RAIU	Radioactive iodine uptake
FSH	Follicle-stimulating hormone	RIA	Radioimmunoassay
GTT	Glucose tolerance test	T_3	Triiodothyronine
HGH	Human growth hormone	T_4	Thyroxine
IDDM	Insulin-dependent diabetes mellitus	T_7	Thyroid-stimulating hormone
K	Potassium	TFT	Thyroid function test
LH	Luteinizing hormone	TSH	Thyroid-stimulating hormone
Na	Sodium	VP	Vasopressin (also known as ADH)

Exercise 10: ABBREVIATIONS

Matching.

_____ 1. Ca

_____ 2. K

_____ 3. Na

_____ 4. OT

_____ 5. VP

_____ 6. NIDDM

_____ 7. IDDM

A. type II diabetes
B. oxytocin
C. potassium
D. type I diabetes
E. calcium
F. sodium
G. ADH

Careers

Dietitians and Dietetic Technicians

Healthcare professionals who work with patients to prevent, treat, and manage disorders through diet planning are dietitians, dietetic technicians, and nutritionists. Dietitians and nutritionists must complete at least a bachelor's level American Dietetic Association (ADA)-approved program, whereas dietetic technicians are required to complete an ADA-approved associate's level program. Both professions have licensing, certification, and registration requirements that vary from state to state.

Dietitians may work with individual patients, evaluating and suggesting dietary changes to prevent or treat disorders. They may also work at an institutional level, running a hospital food service program, for example. Some dietitians may choose to become involved in community outreach programs centered around education. Others may choose to work in schools, managing the food service program and being involved in education. Health clubs; women, infants, and children (WIC) programs; day care centers; restaurants; and correctional facilities are all alternative sources of employment.

Through the year 2010, these jobs are expected to grow as fast as the average healthcare career, with opportunities decreasing in traditional hospital settings as they increase with contractual providers of similar services.

For more information on these careers and schools providing ADA-approved programs, contact the American Dietetic Association at http://www.eatright.org.

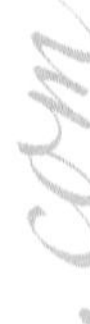

INTERNET PROJECT

Diabetes Mellitus

The incidence of diabetes mellitus is increasing at a rapid pace in the United States. Research one of the following topics regarding this disorder:

- Current statistics, noting sex, age, race, and ethnicity within your state.
- Complications of diabetes mellitus and reasons why these develop.
- New medications/treatments, along with clinical trials.
- Create a brochure intended to inform a particular target population (your choice) on general information, including warning signs and complications. Provide contact information with phone numbers or Websites for individuals to obtain more information.

Limit your presentation to 3 pages, citing your references. Obtain information at the following Websites:

World Health Organization: Diabetes Mellitus
http://www.who.int/inffs/en/fact138.html
The Endocrine Society
http://www.endo-society.org/pubrelations/patientInfo/diabetes2.htm
MEDLINEplus
http://www.nlm.nih.gov/medlineplus/ency/article/000313.htm

Case Study Continued

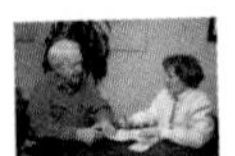

Hillary explains to Darren that the dose of oral insulin he has been prescribed is dependent on his blood sugar results, which will depend on several factors, including the kind and amount of food he eats. She tells him that his new diet will take a while to get used to, but that his health will depend on adhering as closely as possible to it.

"And, to help motivate you further," Hillary says with a smile, "it is possible that by following this diet you will lose enough weight that you will no longer need medication."

Darren releases his pent-up breath. "That's enough for me," he says. "I'll do it."

Chapter Review

A. Functions of the Endocrine System

1. In your own words, explain the functions of the endocrine system.

____

____

____

B. Anatomy and Physiology

2. Label the diagram provided with the endocrine glands and their combining forms.

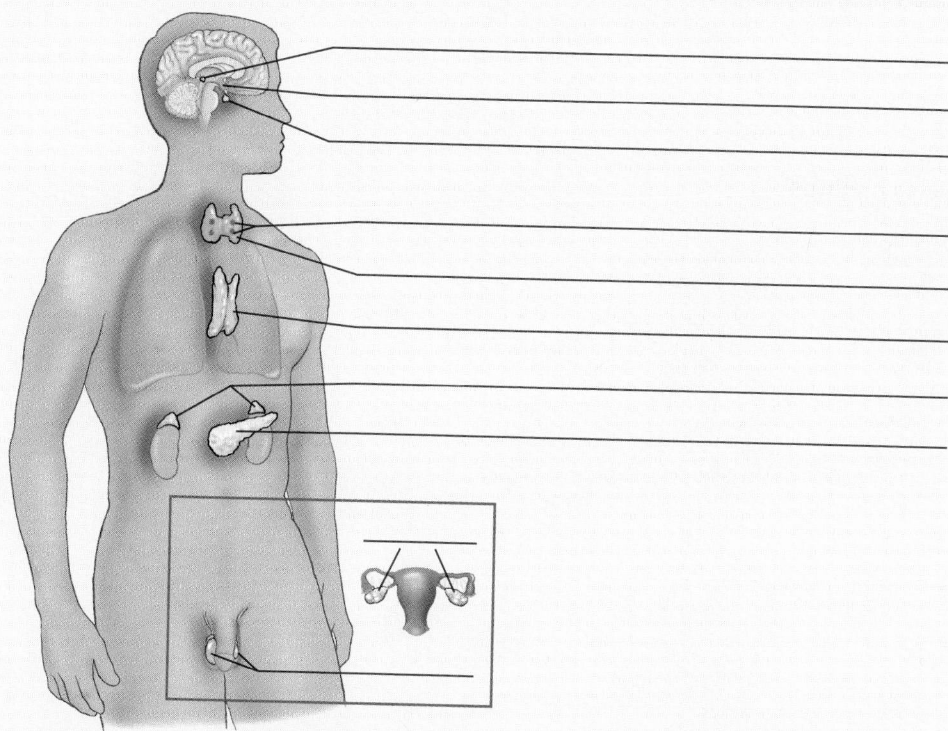

3. Describe the anatomy of the pituitary, listing all of its names, and explain why it is referred to as the *master gland.*

____

____

4. What feature of target cells allows hormonal action? ______________________________

5. What are the functions of the following glands?

A. thyroid ______

B. parathyroids ______

C. adrenal cortex ______

D. adrenal medulla ______

E. islets of Langerhans ______

F. thymus ______

G. ovaries/testes ______

H. pineal ______

C. Pathology

Name the gland (and part of the gland, if appropriate) involved in each of the following disorders.

6. Addison's disease ______
7. pheochromocytoma ______
8. insulin-dependent diabetes mellitus ______
9. Cushing's disease ______
10. thyrotoxicosis ______
11. diabetes insipidus ______
12. gigantism ______

Decode the term.

13. acromegaly ______
14. hypokalemia ______
15. paresthesia ______
16. anorexia ______
17. hypernatremia ______

Build a term.

18. excessive blood sugar ______
19. deficient calcium in the blood ______
20. condition of sugar in urine ______

ties of ________________.

he ________________.

ɪgnose ________________.
hickness or density of which bones in acromegaly?

ɪg.

32. pancreas ________________________________

F. Pharmacology
Name a medication used to treat the following disorders.

33. diabetes insipidus ________________

34. hypothyroidism ________________

35. Addison's disease ________________

36. Type I or II diabetes ________________

G. Abbreviations

37. A patient was given an FBS followed by a GTT. What are these tests, and what disorder is most likely suspected?

____

38. Ms. Wolfe was sent to a lab to have TFTs done for suspected hypothyroidism. What are TFTs?

____

39. A 45-year-old man was diagnosed with DI after a deficiency of ADH was detected. What is ADH?

____

40. The 38-year-old patient was diagnosed with acromegaly when an excessive amount of ________________ was detected (give abbreviation).

H. Singulars and Plurals

Change the following from singular to plural.

41. cortex ______________________________

42. thyrotoxicosis ______________________________

I. Translations

Rewrite the following in your own words.

43. After experiencing polyuria, polyphagia, and polydipsia, Tilda was diagnosed with diabetes mellitus.

____

____

44. Victor was treated for hyperthyroidism with symptoms of exophthalmos, tachycardia, anxiety, and anorexia.

____

____

45. Soo Lin presented with hirsutism, easy bruising, hyperglycemia, and hypokalemia. She was subsequently diagnosed with Cushing's disease.

____

____

46. A 45-year-old patient was seen with complaints of hypertension, hypercalcemia, renal calculi, and polyuria.

____

____

47. A female patient is being treated with Synthroid for hypothyroidism. Symptoms were fatigue, xeroderma, bradycardia, and weight gain.

____

____

J. Cumulative Exercises

48. Michael's father was admitted for difficulty breathing due to a form of pneumoconiosis he had acquired from his career as a coal miner. Decode the term *pneumoconiosis*.

____

49. One of Maureen's midwifery patients needed a C-section due to placenta previa. Explain the terms *C-section* and *placenta previa*.

____

50. The pituitary and hypothalamus are located in which body cavity? ______________

51. The term *tetralogy of Fallot* includes an eponym and a decodable term. Decode tetralogy. To what does the entire term refer?

___

52. A patient with a UTI had a UA that showed pyuria. What do the abbreviations UTI and UA mean? Decode pyuria.

___

K. Be Careful

Define each of the following.

53. aden/o ___

54. adren/o ___

55. trop/o ___

56. troph/o ___

57. thyr/o ___

58. thym/o ___

59. oxytocin ___

60. oxytocia ___

Mercy Memorial Doctors' Building
3037 Amity Way
San Jose, CA 95112

OFFICE VISIT SUMMARY

Mr. Williams returned today to review results of a previous visit. At that time, he presented with complaints of polyuria over the last few months, a significant increase in thirst, and unusual fatigue. He has a family history of diabetes mellitus (father and paternal grandmother). Weight at that time was 198 lb, an increase of 12 lb over last office visit on 3/20/03. Patient admitted to increased appetite and an "abandonment" of his exercise program due to the addition of a second job.

Patient underwent FBS, GTT, and UA and was diagnosed with NIDDM. Micronase 3.0 mg daily was prescribed. Patient was referred to our dietitian, Ms. Gorman, who will help him develop a management plan. Patient has been advised to call if difficulties develop or symptoms do not lessen.

____
Christopher Burns, MD

L. Healthcare Report

61. Mr. Williams initially complained of a symptom called polyuria. What is that?

    ____

62. What is the healthcare term for his other symptom of "increased thirst"? ________________

63. Explain the abbreviations used for testing in this note:

    A. FBS ________________

    B. GTT ________________

    C. UA ________________

64. Micronase is being prescribed to replace which missing (or ineffective) hormone? ________________

65. NIDDM is what type of diabetes? ________________

CHAPTER 16

ONCOLOGY

"While there are several chronic diseases more destructive to life than cancer, none is more feared." **—Charles Horace Mayo**

Quote

Case Study

Edwinna Smith, the cancer registrar at City Medical Center, is interviewing 45-year-old Clifford Walker, newly diagnosed with colon cancer, as part of a research project regarding familial patterns of cancer occurrence. Although Edwinna's job seldom brings her in contact with patients, the research project has included the cancer registrar as a primary information gatherer. During the course of the interview, Clifford tells Edwinna that his father and brother both died of colon cancer before their fiftieth birthdays. He hopes that the information he is providing can be used to help future colon cancer patients.

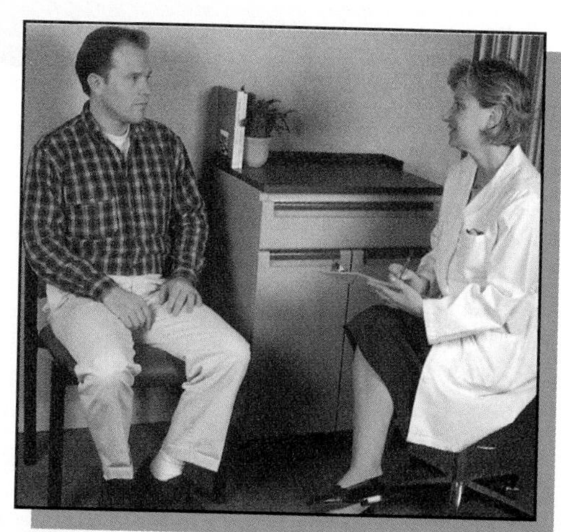

OBJECTIVES

Objectives

- Explain how the process of carcinogenesis is different from the normal process of cell replication.
- Identify and list some of the factors that are currently thought to trigger the process of carcinogenesis.
- Explain the different characteristics of malignant and benign tumors.
- Explain one method of categorizing malignant cancers.
- Explain the difference between grading and staging, and discuss their importance in the cancer treatment process.
- Recognize, recall, and apply healthcare terms related to diagnostic techniques.
- Recognize, recall, and apply healthcare terms related to neoplasia of the different body systems.
- Recognize, recall, and apply healthcare terms related to therapeutic techniques used to treat cancer.
- Recognize, recall, and apply healthcare terms related to pharmacologic techniques used to treat cancer.
- Recognize, recall, and apply the abbreviations used in oncology.
- Integrate the material in this chapter with material covered in previous chapters.

Where there is life, there is cancer. Although the types of cancer and their incidence (the number of new types diagnosed each year) may vary by geography, sex, race, age, and ethnicity, cancer exists in every population and has since ancient times. Archeologists have found evidence of cancer in dinosaur bones and human mummies. Written descriptions of cancer treatment have been discovered dating back to 1600 BC. The name itself comes from the Greek word for *crab,* used by Hippocrates to describe the appearance of the most common type of cancer, carcinoma.

CARCINOGENESIS

Cancer is not *one* disease but a group of hundreds of diseases with similar characteristics. The shared characteristics are uncontrolled cell growth and a spread of altered cells. Different types of cancers have different occurrence rates and different causes.

Current research suggests that there is no single cause of cancer. Radiation, bacteria, viruses, genetics, diet, smoking (or exposure to tobacco smoke), alcohol, and other factors all contribute to the development of cancer. Each of these factors is instrumental in disrupting the normal balance of cell growth and destruction within the body by causing a mutation in the DNA of cells (Fig. 16-1). Once this mutation takes place, a process of uncontrolled cell growth may begin. It is important to note that the cancer cells that replace normal cells no longer function to keep the body working. The only mission of cancer cells is to reproduce. Fig. 16-2 illustrates the process of **apoptosis** (ah pop TOH sis), the body's normal restraining function to keep cell growth in check. Fig. 16-3 shows the progression from normally functioning skin tissue to hyperplasia, to dysplasia, and finally to carcinoma in situ (CIS). Cancer is a continuum—from tissue made up of normally functioning cells fulfilling their role to keep the body healthy, to tissue replaced by cancerous cells that no longer perform the work of the tissue and now perform only the function of reproducing themselves. Cancers are capable of destroying not only the tissue in which they originate (the primary site), but also other tissues, through the process of **metastasis.** This spread of the cancer can occur by direct extension to contiguous organs and tissues, or to distant sites through blood (Fig. 16-4) or lymphatic involvement.

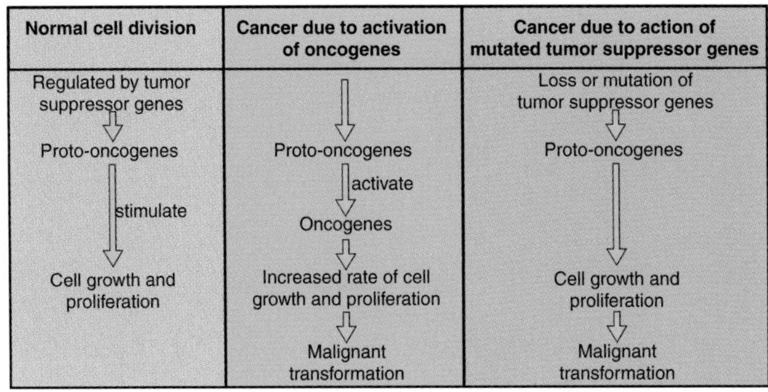

Fig. 16-1 Normal cell growth vs. oncogenesis.

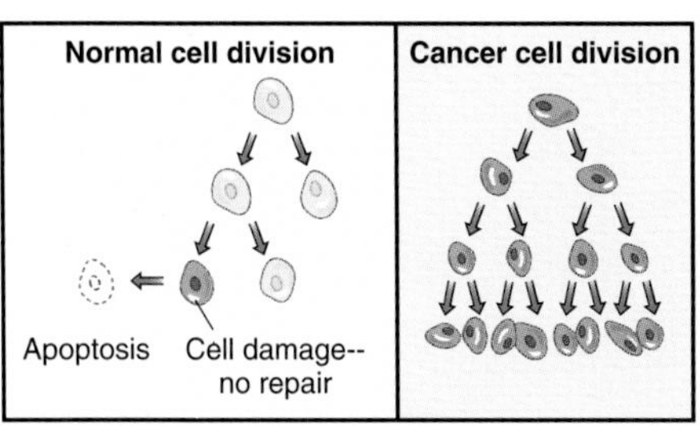

Fig. 16-2 Apoptosis.

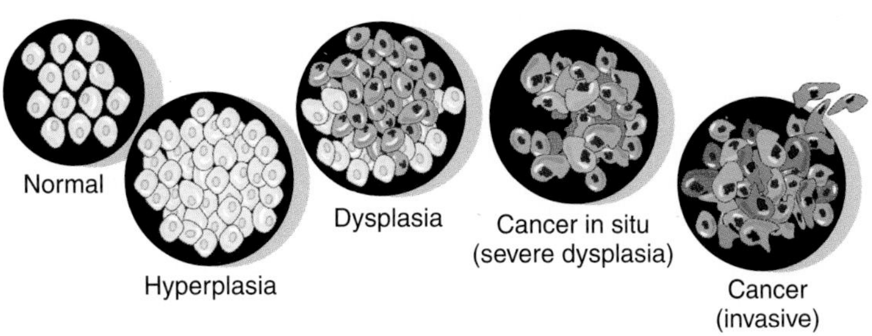

Fig. 16-3 Progression of skin cancer from hyperplasia to cancer.

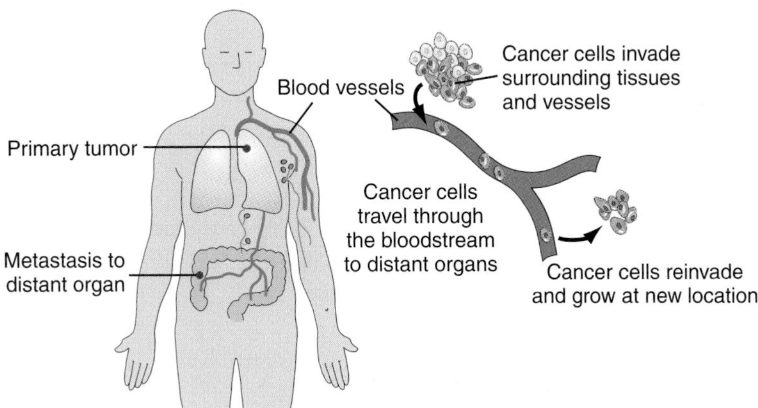

Fig. 16-4 Metastasis.

NAMING MALIGNANT TUMORS

Oncology is the study of tumors, or neoplasms. All cancers are neoplasms (new growths), but not all neoplasms are cancerous. Cancerous tumors are termed *malignant,* whereas noncancerous tumors are termed *benign.*

Although the hundreds of known types of malignant tumors commonly share the characteristics listed previously, the names that they are given reflect their differences. All tissues (and hence organs) are derived from the progression of three embryonic germ layers that differentiate into specific tissues and organs. Tumors are generally divided into two broad categories and a varying number of other categories, based on their embryonic origin. Fig. 16-5 illustrates the different types of cancers and where they occur.

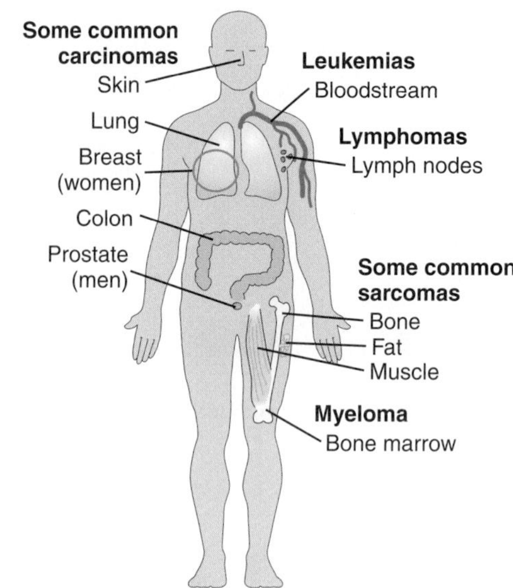

Fig. 16-5 Common cancers and where they occur.

- **Carcinomas:** Approximately 80% to 90% of malignant tumors are derived from the outer (ectodermal) and inner (endodermal) layers of the embryo that develop into epithelial tissue that either covers or lines the surfaces of the body. This category of cancer is divided into two main types. If derived from an organ or gland, it is an adenocarcinoma; if derived from squamous epithelium, it is a squamous cell carcinoma. Examples include gastric adenocarcinoma and squamous cell carcinoma of the lung.
- **Sarcomas** are derived from the middle (mesodermal) layer that becomes connective tissue (bones, muscle, cartilage, blood vessels, and fat). Most end in the suffix *-sarcoma*. Examples include osteosarcoma, chondrosarcoma, hemangiosarcoma, mesothelioma, and glioma.
- **Lymphomas** develop in lymphatic tissue (vessels, nodes, and organs, including the spleen, tonsils, and thymus gland). Lymphomas are solid cancers and may also appear outside of the sites of lymphatic organs in the stomach, breast, or brain; these are called *extranodal lymphomas.* All lymphomas may be divided into two categories: Hodgkin's lymphoma and non-Hodgkin's lymphoma.
- **Leukemia** is cancer of the bone marrow. An example is acute myelocytic leukemia.
- **Myelomas** arise from the plasma cells in the bone marrow. An example is multiple myeloma.
- **Mixed-cell tumors** are a combination of cells from within one category or between two cancer categories. An example is teratocarcinoma.

DID YOU KNOW?

The term *leukemia* means a *condition of the white blood cells,* but leukemia may also involve red blood cells, such as in polycythemia vera.

DID YOU KNOW?

Cancer is the second most frequent cause of death in the United States.

STAGING AND GRADING

To treat cancer, the treating physician must determine the severity of the cancer, the grade, and its stage, or size and spread. Cancers at different grades and stages react differently to various treatments.

Grading is a means of affixing a value to a clinical opinion of the degree of **dedifferentiation (anaplasia)** of the cancer cells, or how much the cells appear different from their original form. Healthy cells are well differentiated; cancer cells are poorly differentiated. The pathologist determines this difference and assigns a grade ranging from I to IV. The higher the grade, the more cancerous, or dedifferentiated, the tissue sample. Grading is a measure of the cancer's *severity.*

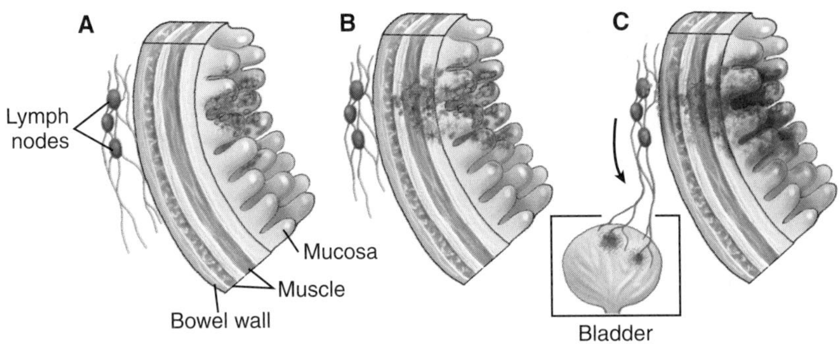

Fig. 16-6 Staging of colon cancer. **A,** stage I; **B,** stage II; **C,** stage III.

The other factor is determining the *size and spread* of the cancer from its original site, which is called **staging.** A number of systems are used to describe this. Some are specific to the type of cancer; others are general systems. If staging is determined by various diagnostic techniques, it is referred to as *clinical staging.* If it is determined by the pathologist's report, it is called *pathologic staging.* An example is TNM staging. In this system, **T** usually stands for the **size** of the tumor, **N** stands for the number of lymph **nodes** positive for cancer, and **M** stands for the presence of distant **metastases** (meh TAS tuh seez). Summary staging puts together the TNM to give one number as a stage. Again, this helps determine the type of treatment that is most effective. Fig. 16-6 illustrates a staging system. If the cancer cells appear only at the original site and have not invaded the organ of origin, it is called **carcinoma in situ (CIS).**

COMBINING FORMS FOR NEOPLASMS

MEANING	COMBINING FORM
cancer of connective tissue origin, flesh	sarc/o
cancer of epithelial origin	carcin/o
formation	plas/o
tumor	onc/o

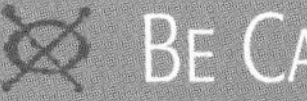

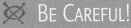

BE CAREFUL!

Don't confuse *sacr/o,* meaning *flesh,* and *sarc/o,* meaning *sacrum.*

PREFIXES FOR NEOPLASMS

PREFIX	MEANING	PREFIX	MEANING
ana-	up, apart	hyper-	excessive
apo-	separate, away	meso-	middle
dys-	abnormal	meta-	beyond, change
ecto-	outer	neo-	new
endo-	inner		

SUFFIXES FOR NEOPLASMS	
SUFFIX	**MEANING**
-oma	tumor, mass
-ptosis	falling
-stasis	stopping, controlling

Exercise 1: General Oncology Terms

Match the word part with its correct meaning.

____ 1. -stasis

____ 2. -oma

____ 3. plas/o

____ 4. meta-

____ 5. dys-

____ 6. carcin/o

____ 7. ana-

____ 8. hyper-

____ 9. neo-

____ 10. sarc/o

A. up, apart
B. abnormal
C. cancer of connective tissue origin
D. new
E. cancer of epithelial tissue origin
F. stopping, controlling
G. beyond, change
H. tumor
I. excessive
J. formation

Circle the correct answer.

11. Tumors that have characteristics of rapid growth, recurrence, and invasiveness are *(benign, malignant).*
12. The most common type of malignant cancer is *(carcinoma, sarcoma, leukemia, lymphoma, myeloma, mixed-cell cancer).*
13. Cancer composed of connective tissue is classified as *(carcinoma, sarcoma, leukemia, lymphoma, myeloma, mixed-cell cancer).*
14. Cancer cells that derive from plasma cells in the bone marrow are classified as *(carcinoma, sarcoma, leukemia, lymphoma, myeloma, mixed-cell tumors).*
15. Healthy cells are *(well, poorly)* differentiated.
16. A determination of the degree of dedifferentiation of cancer cells is called *(grading, staging).*
17. A system of determining how far a cancer has spread from its original site is called *(grading, staging).*
18. The site where the cancer originates is referred to as the *(primary, metastatic)* site.

PATHOLOGY

Signs and Symptoms

The signs and symptoms of cancer are manifestations of how cancer cells replace the functions of healthy tissue. Some examples include anorexia, bruising, leukocytosis, fatigue, cachexia (wasting), and thrombocytopenia.

Neoplasia by Body System

The following tables summarize characteristics of benign and malignant tumors, and cancers by body system. Note that a particular system does not always have all one type of cancer, because organs are composed of a variety of tissues with different embryonic origins. The integumentary system has both carcinomas and sarcomas.

Comparison of Benign and Malignant Tumors

CHARACTERISTICS	BENIGN	MALIGNANT
Mode of growth	Relatively slow growth by expansion; encapsulated; cells adhere to each other	Rapid growth; invades surrounding tissue by infiltration
Cells under microscopic examination	Resemble tissue of origin; well differentiated; appear normal	Do not resemble tissue of origin; vary in size and shape; abnormal appearance and function
Spread	Remains isolated	Metastasis; cancer cells carried by blood and lymphatics to one or more other locations; secondary tumors occur
Other properties	No tissue destruction; not prone to hemorrhage; may be smooth and freely movable	Ulceration and/or necrosis; prone to hemorrhage; irregular and less movable
Recurrence	Rare after excision	A common characteristic
Pathogenesis	Symptoms related to location with obstruction and/or compression of surrounding tissue or organs; usually not life threatening unless inaccessible	Cachexia; pain; fatal if not controlled

From Frazier MS, Drzymkowski JW: *Essentials of human diseases and conditions,* ed 2, Philadelphia, 2000, WB Saunders.

Tumors by Body System

BODY SYSTEM	ORGAN	BENIGN TUMORS	MALIGNANT TUMORS
Musculoskeletal	Bone	Osteoma	Ewing's sarcoma, osteosarcoma
	Cartilage	Chondroma	Chondrosarcoma (Fig. 16-7)
	Muscle	Rhabdomyoma, leiomyoma	Rhabdomyosarcoma, leiomyosarcoma
Integumentary	Skin	Dermatofibroma	Basal cell carcinoma, squamous cell carcinoma, malignant melanoma (Fig. 16-8), Kaposi's sarcoma
Gastrointestinal	Esophagus Stomach Pancreas Colon/rectum	Leiomyoma Polyp Gastric adenoma	Adenocarcinoma of the esophagus (Fig. 16-9), stomach, pancreas, colon, and/or rectum

Continued

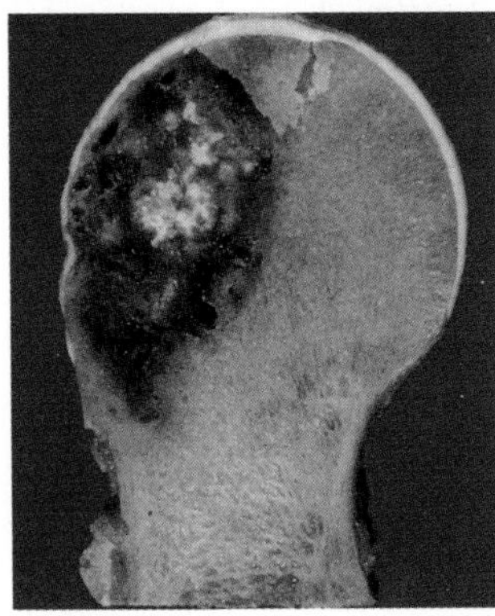

Fig. 16-7 Chondrosarcoma of femur.

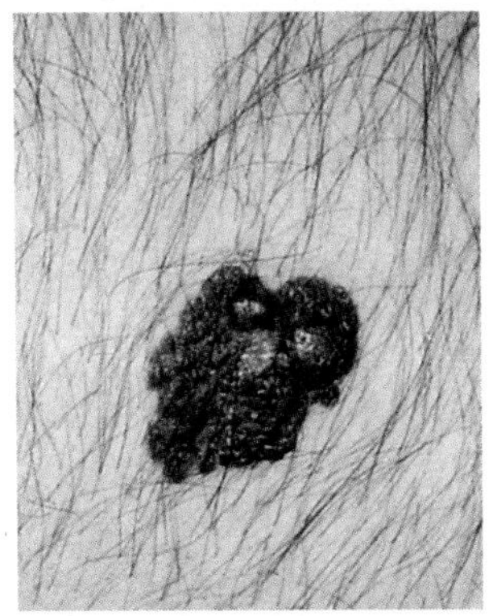

Fig. 16-8 Malignant melanoma on arm.

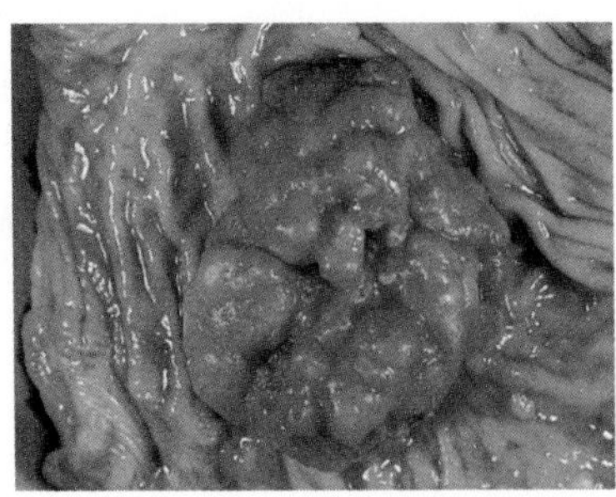

Fig. 16-9 Adenocarcinoma of the esophagus.

Tumors by Body System—cont'd

Body System	Organ	Benign Tumors	Malignant Tumors
Urinary	Kidney	Nephroma	Hypernephroma/renal cell carcinoma, Wilm's tumor/nephrosarcoma
	Bladder		Transitional cell carcinoma (bladder cancer) (Fig. 16-10)
Male Reproductive	Testis		Seminoma (Fig. 16-11), teratoma
	Prostate	Benign prostatic hyperplasia	Prostatic cancer
Female Reproductive	Breast	Fibrocystic disease	Infiltrating ductal adenocarcinoma of the breast
	Uterus	Fibroids (Fig. 16-12)	Stromal endometrial carcinoma
	Ovaries	Ovarian cyst	Epithelial ovarian carcinoma
	Cervix	Cervical dysplasia	Squamous cell carcinoma of the cervix
Blood/Lymphatic/ Immune	Blood		Leukemia (Fig. 16-13)
	Lymph vessels		Non-Hodgkin's lymphoma, Hodgkin's lymphoma
	Thymus gland	Thymoma	Malignant thymoma
Cardiovascular	Blood vessels	Hemangioma	Hemangiosarcoma
	Heart	Myxoma	Myxosarcoma (Fig. 16-14)
Respiratory	Epithelial tissue of respiratory tract, lung, bronchus	Papilloma	Adenocarcinoma of the lung, small cell carcinoma, mesothelioma (Fig. 16-15), bronchogenic carcinoma
Nervous	CNS (brain, spinal cord, meninges)	Neuroma, neurofibroma	Glioblastoma, meningioma (Fig. 16-16), astrocytoma
	PNS		
Endocrine	Pituitary	Benign pituitary tumor (Fig. 16-17)	
	Thyroid		Thyroid carcinoma
	Adrenal medulla		Pheochromocytoma
Eyes and Ears	Retina		Retinoblastoma (Fig. 16-18)
	Acoustic nerve	Acoustic neuroma	
	Middle ear	Cholesteatoma	

Combining Forms Related to Oncology

Meaning	Combining Form	Meaning	Combining Form
base	bas/o	kidney	nephr/o
bone	oste/o	lymph	lymph/o
carcinoma, epithelial tissue cancer	carcin/o	sarcoma, connective tissue cancer	sarc/o
cartilage	chondr/o	scale	squam/o
change	mut/a	semen	semin/i
embryonic	blast/o	skeletal muscle	rhabdomy/o
fiber	fibr/o	skin	dermat/o
gland	aden/o	smooth muscle	leiomy/o
glue	gli/o	star	astr/o

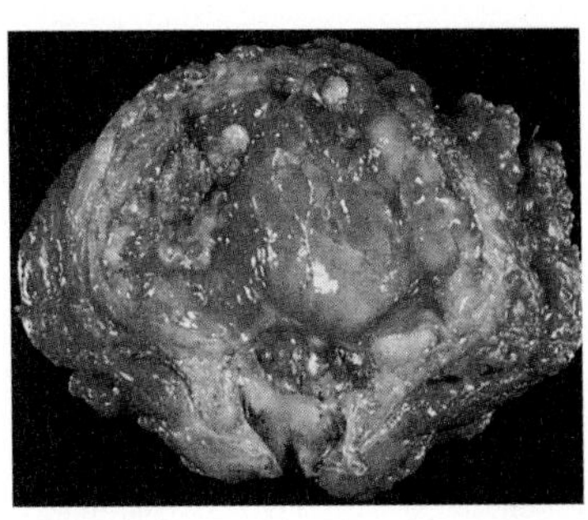

Fig. 16-10 Carcinoma of the bladder.

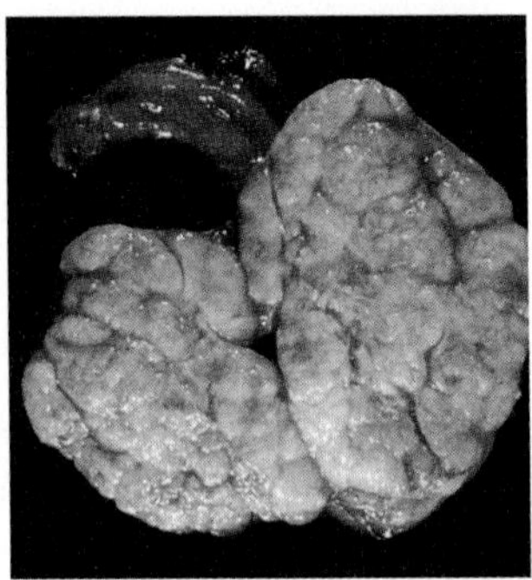

Fig. 16-11 Seminoma of the testicle.

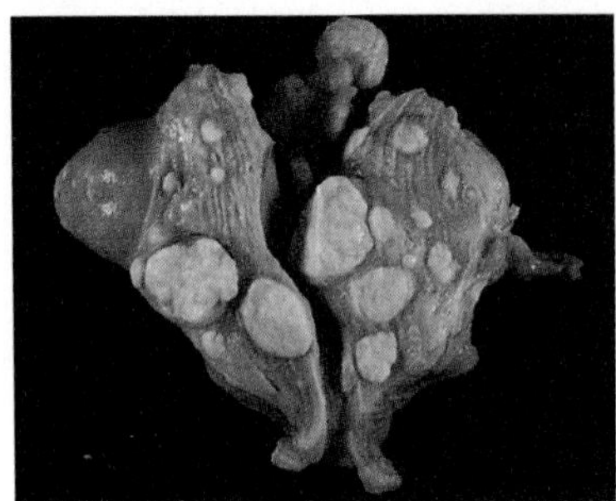

Fig. 16-12 Leiomyomas of the uterus.

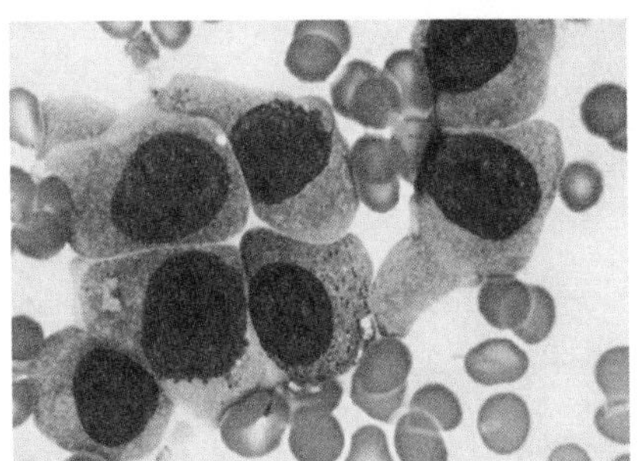

Fig. 16-13 Micrograph of leukemia.

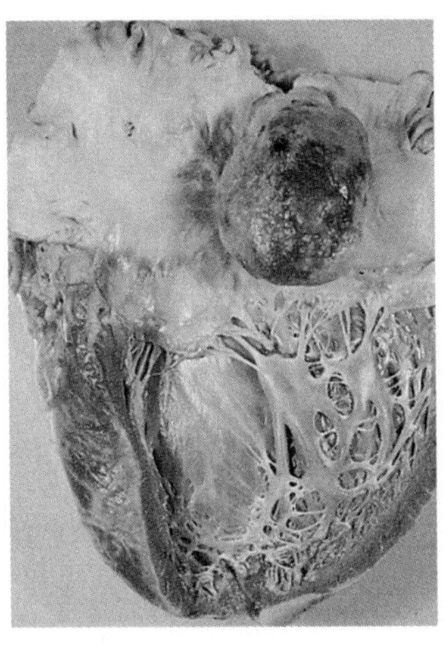

Fig. 16-14 Myxosarcoma of the heart.

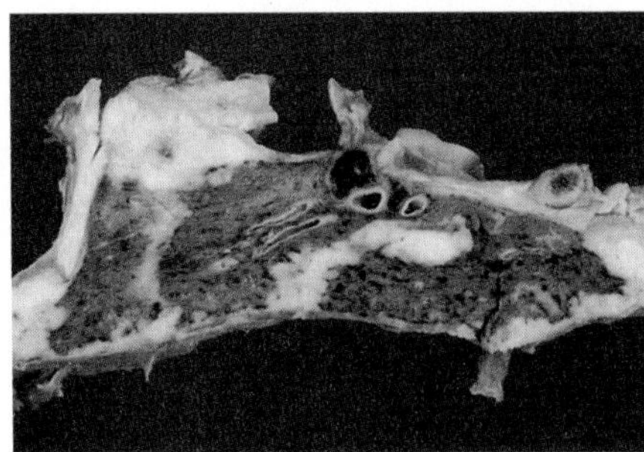

Fig. 16-15 Mesothelioma of the lung.

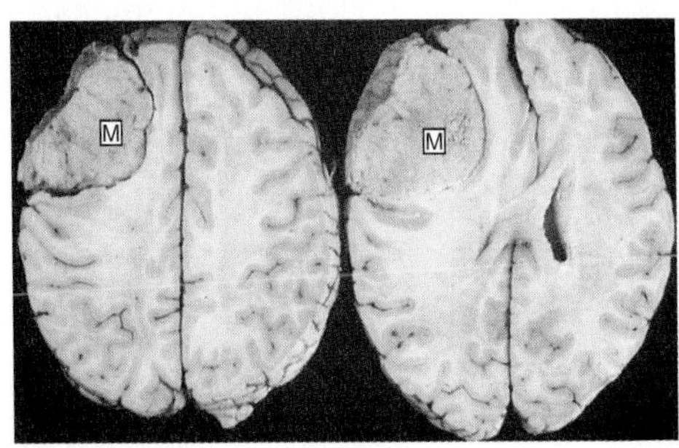

Fig. 16-16 Meningioma of the meninges of the brain.

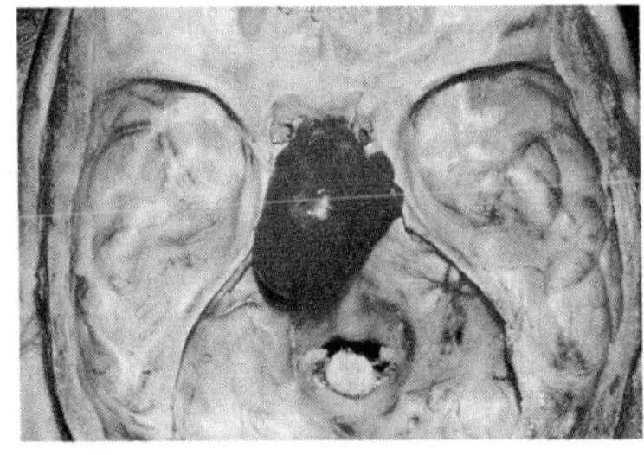

Fig. 16-17 Pituitary tumor.

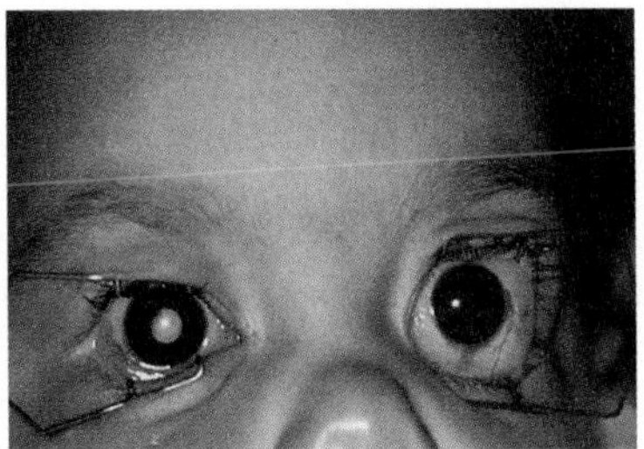

Fig. 16-18 Retinoblastoma. White pupil is a classic sign.

Exercise 2: PATHOLOGY

Match the combining form with its correct meaning.

____ 1. nephr/o
____ 2. astr/o
____ 3. gli/o
____ 4. fibr/o
____ 5. aden/o
____ 6. squam/o
____ 7. carcin/o
____ 8. sarc/o
____ 9. rhabdomy/o
____ 10. chondr/o
____ 11. blast/o
____ 12. semin/i
____ 13. oste/o
____ 14. leiomy/o
____ 15. bas/o

A. bone
B. semen
C. smooth muscle
D. embryonic
E. cartilage
F. skeletal muscle
G. kidney
H. base
I. scale
J. star
K. epithelial tissue cancer
L. glue
M. fiber
N. connective tissue cancer
O. gland

Circle the correct answer.

16. An example of a benign muscle tumor is a *(rhabdomyoma, leiomyosarcoma).*
17. Which of the following is a malignant tumor of the skin? *(dermatofibroma, basal cell carcinoma)*
18. A patient with fibroids has a *(benign, malignant)* growth.
19. Which of the following is NOT a malignancy? *(nephroma, lymphoma, seminoma, thymoma)*
20. An astrocytoma is a *(benign, malignant)* tumor of the nervous system.

Case Study Continued

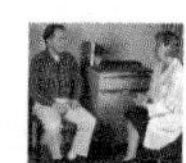

Clifford Walker's cancer was diagnosed by colonoscopy and pathologic testing. The following pathology report states that he has colonic tissue with adenocarcinoma, moderately to poorly differentiated.

Type:	Sigmoid colon
Tumor type:	Infiltrating adenocarcinoma
Tumor grade:	Grade II
Tumor size:	4.5 × 3.8 × 1.2 cm
Depth of invasion:	Through thickness of bowel wall into serosal fat
Lymphatic/vascular invasion:	No
All 12 lymph nodes:	Negative for carcinoma
Margins of resection:	Free of tumor

DIAGNOSTIC PROCEDURES

Patient History

Along with the various clinical techniques described, the patient's history is especially important, including information regarding family history (for genetic information) and social history, such as tobacco and alcohol use, diet, and sexual history. A patient's smoking history is described in terms of "pack years." Pack years equals the average number of packs smoked per day multiplied by the number of years of smoking. For example: 25 pack years represents 1 pack/day × 25 years of smoking. A patient's current or former occupation may also shed light on the type of cancer. For example, exposure to asbestos, through an occupation of ship building or working with brake repair, may lead to a rare type of lung cancer, mesothelioma.

Tumor Markers

Tumor marker tests measure the levels of a variety of biochemical substances detected in the blood, urine, or body tissues that often appear in higher than normal amounts in individuals with certain neoplasms. Because other factors may influence the amount of the tumor marker present, they are not intended to be used as a sole means of diagnosis. Examples include the following:

AFP: Increased levels may indicate liver or germ cell cancer.
CA125: Used for ovarian cancer detection and management.
CA15-3: Levels are measured to determine the stage of breast cancer.
CA19-9: Levels are elevated in stomach, colorectal, and pancreatic cancers.
CA27-29: Used to monitor breast cancer; especially useful to test for recurrences.
CEA: Monitors colorectal cancer when the disease has spread or after treatment to measure the patient's response.
HCG: Used as a screen for choriocarcinoma.
LDH: Levels may be used to monitor Ewing's sarcoma, non-Hodgkin's lymphoma, testicular cancer, and some forms of leukemia.
NSE: Used to measure the stage and/or patient's response to treatment of small cell cancer and neuroblastoma.
PAP: May be higher in patients with prostate cancer.
PSA: Increased levels may be due to BPH or prostate cancer.

Biopsy (bx)

See Chapter 4 for information on biopsies.

Imaging

Radiography: Because tumors are usually more dense than the tissue surrounding them, they may appear as a lighter shade of gray (blocking more radiation). Abdominal x-rays may reveal tumors of the stomach, liver, kidneys, and so on, whereas chest x-rays are useful in detecting lung cancer. If a contrast medium is used, as in an upper or lower gastrointestinal (GI) series or intravenous urogram (IVU), tumors of the esophagus, rectum, colon, or kidneys may be detected. Another special type of x-ray is a **mammogram**, useful in the early detection of breast cancer. **Stereotactic (3-D) mammography** may be used for an image-guided biopsy.

Computed tomography (CT) scans: CT scans provide information about a tumor's shape, size, and location, along with the source of its blood supply. They are useful in detecting, evaluating, and monitoring cancer, especially liver, pancreatic, bone, lung, and adrenal gland cancers. CT scans are also useful in staging cancer and guiding needles for aspiration biopsy (Fig. 16-19).

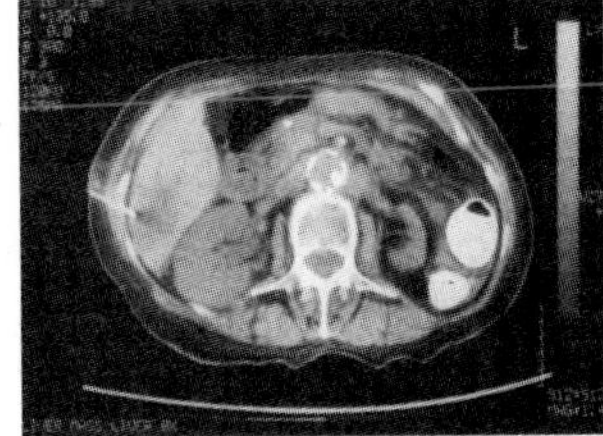

Fig. 16-19 CT scan of needle biopsy of the liver clearly shows the needle in the liver on the left. (Courtesy Riverside Methodist Hospitals, Columbus, Ohio.)

Magnetic resonance imaging (MRI): Areas of the body that are often difficult to image are possible to see with MRI because of its three-dimensional capabilities. MRI is useful in detecting cancer in the central nervous system

(CNS) and musculoskeletal (MS) system. It is also used to stage breast and endometrial cancer before surgery and to detect metastatic spread of cancer to the liver.

Nuclear scans: Nuclear scans are useful in locating and staging cancer of the thyroid and the bone. A *positron emission tomography (PET) scan* provides information about the metabolism of an internal structure, along with its size and shape. It is used for images of the brain, colon, rectum, ovary, and lung. It may also help to identify more aggressive tumors. *Single photon emission computed tomography (SPECT)* uses a rotating camera to create three-dimensional images with the use of radioactive substances. It is useful to determine metastases to the bone. *Monoclonal antibodies* are used to evaluate cancer of the prostate, colon, breast, and ovaries, as well as melanoma.

Self-Detection

Self-detection remains the most important method of discovering cancer. The American Cancer Society (ACS) has developed a series of reminders and rules to help individuals become aware of cancer signs and symptoms. For general detection of cancer, they have developed the following CAUTION criteria:

CAUTION Criteria

Change in bowel or bladder habits
A sore that does not heal
Unusual bleeding or discharge
Thickening or lump in the breast, testicles or elsewhere
Indigestion or difficulty swallowing
Obvious change in the size, shape, color, or thickness of a wart, mole, or mouth sore
Nagging cough or hoarseness

For discovering skin cancer, the ACS has come up with the following ABCDE rule:

ABCDE Rule

A for **asymmetry:** A mole that, when divided in half, does not look the same on both sides.
B for **border:** A mole with edges that are blurry or jagged.
C for **color:** Changes in the color of a mole, including darkening, spread of color, loss of color, or the appearance of multiple colors such as blue, red, white, pink, purple, or gray.
D for **diameter:** A mole larger than ¼ inch in diameter.
E for **elevation:** A mole that is raised above the skin and has an uneven surface.

The ACS also has criteria for breast and testicular self-examination.

Exercise 3: DIAGNOSTIC PROCEDURES

Circle the correct answer.

1. A patient's history of smoking may be described as pack years, which is the number of *(cigarettes, packs)* smoked per day × the number of years smoking.
2. Information regarding previous diet, alcohol use, and family members with cancer may be found in the *(history, pathology)* section of a patient's medical record.
3. Levels of biochemical substances present in the blood that may indicate neoplastic activity are referred to as *(monoclonal antibodies, tumor markers)*.
4. Removal of a sample of tissue to be examined for signs of cancer is a *(tomography, biopsy)*.
5. Mammography may be done to test for cancer of the *(breast, colon)*.

Case Study *Continued*

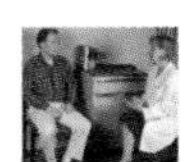

Part of Edwinna's job is to stage cancers. She stages Clifford's cancer by looking at the pathology report. From the size and level of invasion of the tumor recorded on the pathology report, she chooses T4. Because there were no lymph nodes positive for cancer, she chooses N0; because there were no metastases, she chooses M0. Using the rubric provided, she finds that a T4 N0 M0 is the equivalent of a stage II colon cancer. She notes that the pathologist has determined that the cancer is a grade II, moderately to poorly differentiated.

THERAPEUTIC INTERVENTIONS

Surgery

The primary treatment for cancer has always been and remains the removal of the tumor. When the tumor is relatively small and present only in the organ that is removed, surgery is most effective.

The amount of tissue removed varies with the stage and grade of the cancer. In breast cancer surgery, for example, the types of surgery are as follows:

Lumpectomy: removal of the tumor only.

Simple mastectomy: removal of the breast containing the cancer.

En bloc resection: removal of the cancerous tumor and the lymph nodes.

Radical mastectomy: removal of the breast containing the cancer, along with the lymph nodes and the muscle under the breast. When the surgical report discusses **margins**, it refers to the borders of normal tissue surrounding the cancer. A **wide margin resection** means that the cancer is removed with a significant amount of tissue around the tumor to ensure that all the cancer cells are removed. If the margins are reported as negative, no cancer cells are seen. If positive, cancer cells have been detected by the pathologist.

Lymph node dissection: the removal of clinically involved lymph nodes. **Lymph node mapping** determines a pattern of spread from the primary tumor site through the lymph nodes. The **sentinel node** is the first node in which lymphatic drainage occurs in a particular area. If this node is negative for cancer upon dissection, then the lymph system is free of cancer.

Radiotherapy

Approximately half of all cancer patients receive radiation. The goal of radiation is to destroy the nucleus of the cancer cells, thereby destroying their ability to reproduce and spread.

Although radiation is usually started after removal of the tumor, sometimes it is done before, in order to shrink the tumor. Some cancers may be treated solely with radiation.

Brachytherapy (brah kee THAYR uh pee): the use of radiation placed directly on or within the cancer through the use of needles or beads containing radioactive gold or cobalt, or radium.

Systemic Therapy

Chemotherapy: Chemotherapy is the circulation of cancer-destroying medicine throughout the body. Chemotherapy may also be used as an adjuvant (aid) to other forms of treatment to relieve symptoms or slow down the spread of cancer. See the Pharmacology section for more details on chemotherapy drugs.

Immunotherapy: Immunotherapy is the use of the body's own defense system to attack cancer cells. See the description of interleukins in the Pharmacology section.

Bone marrow transplant (BMT): Patients who are incapable of producing healthy blood cells are given bone marrow from a matching donor to stimulate normal blood cell growth. Patients with specific types of leukemia may receive bone marrow transplants after chemotherapy has effectively destroyed the functioning of their own bone marrow.

Complementary and alternative medicine (CAM) techniques: Prayer, massage, diet, exercise, and mind-body techniques encompass the majority of CAM methods used in cancer treatment. The U.S. government has established the National Center for Complementary and Alternative Medicine, which reports on results of research studies on the use of CAM techniques for various disorders (http://www.nccam.nih.gov).

Exercise 4: THERAPEUTIC INTERVENTIONS

Circle the correct response.

1. Treatment with radioactive beads near or inside the cancer is called *(chemotherapy, brachytherapy).*
2. A determination of the spread of the primary tumor through the lymph nodes is referred to as lymph node *(dissection, mapping).*
3. The first node in which lymphatic drainage occurs is the *(sentinel, primary)* node.
4. Removal of the tumor and lymph nodes is *(lumpectomy, en bloc resection).*
5. The borders of normal tissue surrounding the cancer are called *(stages, margins).*
6. Use of the body's own defense system to attack cancer cells is called *(immunotherapy, BMT).*
7. Prayer, massage, exercise, and mind-body techniques are examples of *(CAM, adjuvant therapy).*

PHARMACOLOGY

Chemotherapy works by disrupting the cycle of cell replication. All cells go through a cycle of reproducing themselves, but, unlike cancer cells, they have a built-in mechanism that limits their growth. The side effects of cancer therapy, such as hair loss or nausea, are due to the inability of chemotherapeutic agents to differentiate between normal and cancerous cells. Thus cells that reproduce rapidly, such as hair cells or those that line the stomach, are also affected. It should also be noted that two or more chemotherapeutic agents are usually used together to effectively attack the cancer at various stages. This is referred to as a drug *protocol* or plan.

The majority of the pharmaceuticals prescribed to treat cancer are referred to as *antineoplastic agents*. They accomplish the goal of slowing or stopping the progression of cancer in different ways:

Alkylating agents: Prevent cells from multiplying and dividing. Examples include nitrosoureas and nitrogen mustards.
Antimetabolites: Prevent cancer cells from obtaining necessary nutrients. An example is methotrexate fluorouracil (5-FU).
Antineoplastic antibiotics: Prevent or delay cell replication. Examples include doxorubicin and megestrol.
Antineoplastic hormones: Interfere with receptors for growth stimulating proteins. Examples include leuprolide and tamoxifen.
Interleukins: Stimulate cells of the immune system to recognize and attack cancer cells. An example is aldesleukin (interleukin-2).
Mitotic inhibitors: Prevent cell division. An example is etoposide injection.
Plant alkaloids: Prevent formation of chromosome spindles necessary for cell duplication. Examples include vincristine and vinblastine.

Exercise 5: PHARMACOLOGY

Circle the correct answer.

1. Patients who are prescribed chemotherapy receive a drug *(protocol, adjuvant).*
2. Side effects of chemotherapy frequently occur because the drugs used to kill cancer cells often *(stimulate, kill)* normal cells.
3. Most chemotherapeutic agents work by disrupting a phase of the cell *(cycle, movement).*
4. Drugs that interfere with receptors for growth-stimulating proteins are *(antineoplastic hormones, antimetabolites).*
5. Drugs that prevent cells from multiplying and dividing are called *(antineoplastic antibiotics, alkylating agents).*
6. Drugs that prevent cancer cells from obtaining necessary nutrients to live are *(interleukins, antimetabolites).*
7. Cell division is prevented by *(plant alkaloids, mitotic inhibitors).*

Case Study Continued

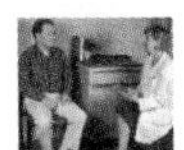

The information Edwinna has collected on the familial pattern study will be used to devise better screening for cancers with suspected genetic components. The registry information she collects is continually merged with national data to determine the most efficient treatment protocols. Like so many other health professionals at the end of a work day, Edwinna can honestly feel that she is making a difference in someone's life.

Abbreviations

Abbreviation	Meaning	Abbreviation	Meaning
AFP	Alpha-fetoprotein test	hCG	Human chorionic gonadotropin
BSE	Breast self-examination	LDH	Lactate dehydrogenase (may be used to detect presence of cancer or to monitor certain cancers)
bx	Biopsy	mets	Metastases
CA	Cancer	NSE	Neuron-specific enolase (used to detect neuroblastoma, small cell cancer)
CA125	Tumor marker primarily for ovarian cancer	PAP	Prostatic acid phosphatase
CA15-3	Tumor marker to monitor breast cancer	PAP	Papanicolaou test for cervical/vaginal cancer
CA19-9	Tumor marker for pancreatic, stomach, and bile duct cancer	PSA	Prostatic-specific antigen
CA27-29	Tumor marker to check for recurrence of breast cancer	SPECT	Single photon emission computed tomography
CEA	Carcinoembryonic antigen (used to monitor colorectal cancer)	TNM	Tumor, nodes, metastases
CTR	Certified tumor registrar	TSE	Testicular self-examination
FOBT	Fecal occult blood test		
G	Grade		

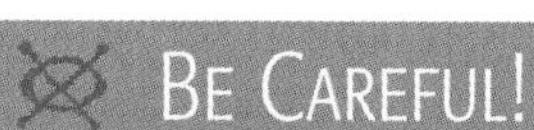

PAP is an abbreviation for two diagnostic tests.

Exercise 6: ABBREVIATIONS

Write the meaning of the following abbreviations.

1. The patient appeared for a bx of a suspicious mole.

   ____

2. The prognosis was poor for the lung cancer patient with a G IV finding on his path report. ______________________________
3. The 50-year-old woman made an appointment for a colonoscopy to check for CA after she had a positive finding on a home FOBT.

   ____

4. The CTR at Montgomery Memorial recorded the TNM stage for the patient's abstract.

   ____

5. SPECT was used to detect bone mets in the patient with advanced breast cancer.

   ____

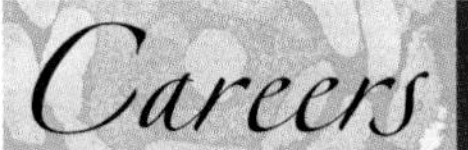

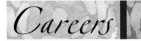

Careers

Cancer Registrars

Cancer registrars (also called tumor registrars) are specialists in cancer data management. Their primary responsibility is to report and track patients with cancer who are diagnosed and/or treated at the registrar's healthcare facility. Registrars identify cancer patients, abstract demographic and medical information, and perform lifetime follow-up on these patients. Most registrars work in hospitals, but some work in regional or state registries. Patient contact is the exception, not the rule.

Cancer registrars are trained on the job, through workshops or formal education programs. Students take courses in healthcare terminology, anatomy and physiology, cancer management, statistics, and cancer registry procedures. Individuals with the appropriate amount of education and/or experience may sit for a certification examination offered by the National Board for Certification of Registrars. A passing score earns a certified tumor registrar (CTR) credential.

Students interested in finding out more about the profession may check out the Website of the National Cancer Registrars Association at http://www.ncra~usa.org.

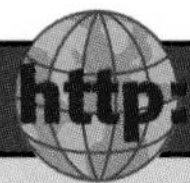

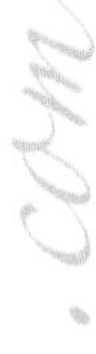

http: INTERNET PROJECT

Using the following Websites to get started, choose a cancer from one of the body systems and report on the most recent findings in one of the following areas:

- Incidence with regard to sex, race, age, ethnicity, and geographic location
- Diagnostic techniques
- Causes of cancer
- Treatment
- Clinical trials

Citing at least three sources, write a 3-page paper using the following Websites:

National Cancer Institute: http://www.cancer.gov/cancerinformation/
American Cancer Society: http://www.cancer.org
CDC Cancer Prevention and Control: http://www.cdc.gov/cancer/
College of American Pathologists: http://www.cap.org/html/public/pathrep.html
Texas Cancer Online: http://www.jasper-web.com/texascanceronline/
American Academy of Family Physicians: http://www.familydoctor.org
WebMD: http://webmd.lycos.com/content/article/1680.54508

Chapter Review

A. Carcinogenesis

1. In your own words, explain the process of carcinogenesis.

   ____

2. Compare the differences between benign and malignant cancers.

   ____

3. Explain how the terms *anaplasia* and *dedifferentiation* are key to the concept of grading.

   ____

4. What is staging, and why it is important in the initial diagnosis of a cancer?

   ____

5. What are the differences among carcinoma, sarcoma, and lymphoma/leukemia?

   ____

6. What do you know about terms that end with *-carcinoma* or *-sarcoma?*

   ____

7. What is usually true about terms ending with the suffix *-oma?*

   ____

8. What are some cancerous tumors that do not end with *-sarcoma?*

   ____

B. Pathology

Build a term.

9. a connective tissue cancer of bone ______________________

10. a benign tumor of skeletal muscle ______________________

11. a glandular cancer of epithelial tissue ______________________

Decode the term.

12. chondroma ______________________________

13. neoplasm ______________________________

14. hyperplasia ______________________________

C. Diagnostic Procedures

15. A patient smokes two packs a day for 10 years. How many pack years is that?

    ____

16. Which tumor markers are used to detect prostate cancer? ______________________

17. Which tumor marker is used to detect ovarian cancer? ____________________
18. Which tumor marker is used to monitor colon cancer patients posttreatment?

____

19. Which tumor marker is used as a screen for choriocarcinoma? ____________________
20. Which tumor marker is used to detect neuroblastoma or small cell carcinoma?

____

21. Samples of friable lesions may be obtained by scraping with sharp instruments in which type of biopsy?

____________________ (see Chapter 4)

22. Which type of biopsy removes fluid from lesions for culture and examination?

____________________ (see Chapter 4)

23. What is a 3-D image-guided breast biopsy called? ____________________
24. Which type of imaging uses low-level radionuclides to locate and stage tumors?

____

D. Therapeutic Interventions

25. A patient who has a lumpectomy has what type of tissue removed?

____

26. A patient with an en bloc resection has had which types of tissue removed?

____

27. To what does the term *lymph node dissection* refer? ____________________

28. What is a sentinel node? ____________________
29. If the margins of the tissue surrounding a cancer are negative, what does that mean?

____

30. Brachytherapy is what type of therapeutic technique? ____________________

31. ____________ is the circulation of cancer-destroying medicine systemically.

32. Immunotherapy uses the body's own ____________ to attack cancer cells.

33. A bone marrow transplant may be done to replace normal production of ____________.

34. Massage, spiritual counseling, and diet are used in what category of treatment? ____________

E. Pharmacology

35. A plan of treatment for a patient's chemotherapy regimen is called a/an ____________.

36. Interleukins are chemotherapeutic agents used to ____________________.

37. Antimetabolites work by ____________________.

38. Alkylating agents prevent cells from ______________________.
39. Cell replication is delayed or prevented by which type of antineoplastic agent?

____

40. Vincristine and vinblastine are plant alkaloids that prevent the formation of chromosome spindles for cell ______________________.

F. Abbreviations
Define the following abbreviations.

41. John was dx with CA of the nose after a punch bx.

____

42. After a monthly BSE, Sara discovered a lump in her breast.

____

43. The lung tumor was staged T1 N0 M0, summary stage I.

____

44. The CTR at the local hospital reviewed a patient in the cancer registry who had recently been diagnosed with brain mets.

____

45. As a result of a FOBT, the patient's colon cancer was diagnosed in an early stage.

____

G. Translations
Rewrite the following in your own words.

46. The cancer registry student had four cases to abstract: one seminoma, one multiple myeloma, and two adenocarcinomas of the lung.

____

47. The pathologist described the cancer as grade I, well-differentiated.

____

48. The patient was diagnosed with metastatic breast cancer.

____

49. The PAP smear revealed severe dysplasia of the cervical cells.

____

50. The breast cancer patient was treated with a lumpectomy, radiotherapy, and chemotherapy.

____

H. Cumulative Exercises

Define the underlined terms.

51. The patient who reported chronic pain in the distal aspect of his femur was found to have an osteosarcoma.

 ____

52. The patient called to report a lump located in the upper outer quadrant of her left breast, which she discovered during her monthly BSE. ______________________________

53. A former patient seen for suspected melanoma had several dysplastic nevi removed.

 ____

54. A patient in his 20s called the office to report a unilateral swelling on his testicle.

 ____

55. A patient had an abnormal finding of a mass in the apex of his left lung.

 ____

I. Be Careful

56. Describe the difference between sarc/o and sacr/o

 ____

57. What are the two meanings of PAP?

 ____

Hamstead Memorial Hospital
532 13th St.
Hamstead, TX 75201

DISCHARGE SUMMARY

Patient Name: Clifford Walker
Physician: Albert Schwartz, MD

MR#: 163544
Adm: 12/01/02
Disch: 12/04/02

Diagnosis: Sigmoid colon cancer by colonoscopy
Procedure: Sigmoid colectomy and appendectomy
History: This 45-year-old male with a significant family history of colon cancer presented to my office after a colonoscopy demonstrated a carcinoma at 18 cm. He presents now after having an outpatient bowel preparation.
Hospital Course: The patient was admitted, and a sigmoid colectomy was performed. At that time, an appendectomy was also done. His postoperative course was unremarkable. His diet was slowly advanced, and by day 4, he was able to be discharged to home.

His pathology report demonstrated a carcinoma through the wall with a microperforation. He had 12 nodes examined, all negative for carcinoma. His appendix was also positive for subacute appendicitis. He was scheduled for follow-up in my office in 10 days.
Discharge Medications: Percocet, Tylenol

Albert Swartz, MD

J. Healthcare Report

58. What was the patient's diagnosis?

59. How was his cancer diagnosed?

60. What procedures were done?

61. How do we know that there was no cancer in the lymph nodes?

Illustration Credits

Ballinger PW, Frank ED: *Merrill's atlas of radiographic positions and radiologic procedures,* ed 9, St Louis, 1999, Mosby (Figs. 1-3, 2-2, 2-3, 3-18, 5-17, 5-18, 9-13, 10-17, *C,* 10-18, 10-19, 15-8).

Barkauskas VH: *Health and physical assessment,* ed 3, St Louis, 2002, Mosby (Case Study Fig. Ch. 4, *A*).

Beare PG, Myers JL: *Adult health nursing,* ed 3, St Louis, 1998, Mosby (Figs. 5-19, *A,* 11-16, *D*).

Black JM, Hawks JH, Keene A: *Medical-surgical nursing: clinical management for positive outcomes,* ed 6, Philadelphia, 2001, WB Saunders (Figs. 5-9, 6-15, 6-16, 8-11, 9-11, 11-13, *A,* 11-15, 12-13, *B,* 12-15, *B,* 14-6, 14-11, 14-18, 15-11).

Bonewit-West K: *Clinical procedures for medical assistants,* ed 3, Philadelphia, 2000, WB Saunders (Figs. 6-8, 6-9, 9-15).

Bontrager KL: *Textbook of radiographic positioning and related anatomy,* ed 5, St Louis, 2001, Mosby (Fig. 6-11).

Bork K, Brauninger W: *Skin diseases in clinical practice,* ed 2, Philadelphia, 1999, WB Saunders (Fig. 4-11).

Brody HJ: *Chemical peeling,* ed 2, St Louis, 1997, Mosby (Fig. 4-23).

Callen JP, Greer KE, Saller AS, et al: *Color atlas of dermatology,* ed 2, Philadelphia, 2000, WB Saunders (Figs. 4-5, 4-10, 4-14, 4-15).

Canobbio MM: *Cardiovascular disorders,* St Louis, 1991, Mosby (Fig. 10-17, *A-B*).

Damjanov I, Linder J: *Anderson's pathology,* ed 10, St Louis, 1996, Mosby (Figs. 5-12, 10-14, 10-15, *B-C,* 11-6, 11-10, 12-10, 16-7 to 16-14, 16-17, 16-18).

Damjanov I, Linder J: *Pathology: a color atlas,* St Louis, 2000, Mosby (Figs. 5-10, 5-12, 5-13, 5-14, 10-14, 10-15, *B-C,* 11-6, 11-10, 12-10).

Early PJ, Sodee DB: *Nuclear medicine: principles and practice,* ed 2, St Louis, 1994, Mosby (Fig. 11-14).

Eisen D, Lynch DP: *The mouth: diagnosis and treatment,* St Louis, 1998, Mosby (Figs. 5-7, 5-8).

Eisenberg RL, Dennis CA: *Comprehensive radiographic pathology,* ed 2, St Louis, 1995, Mosby (Fig. 11-13, *B*).

Elkin MK, Perry AG, Potter PA: *Nursing intervention and clinical skills,* ed 2, St Louis, 2000, Mosby (Fig. 6-13).

Epstein E: *Common skin disorders,* ed 5, Philadelphia, 2001, WB Saunders (Fig. 4-7).

Frazier MS, Drzymkowski JW: *Essentials of human diseases and conditions,* ed 2, Philadelphia, 2000, WB Saunders (Figs. 4-9, 5-15, 6-6, *B*).

Habif TP: *Clinical dermatology,* ed 3, St Louis, 1996, Mosby (Figs. 4-18, 4-22, 9-14).

Hagen-Ansert SL: *Textbook of diagnostic ultrasonography,* ed 5, St Louis, 2001, Mosby (Figs. 8-8, 8-10).

Herlihy B, Maebius NK: *The human body in health and illness,* Philadelphia, 2002, WB Saunders (Figs. 9-6, 9-9, 10-6, 14-1, 14-5).

Hill MJ: *Skin disorders,* St Louis, 1994, Mosby (Figs. 4-8, 4-12).

Ignatavicius DD, Workman ML: *Medical-surgical nursing: critical thinking for collaborative care,* ed 4, Philadelphia, 2002, WB Saunders (Figs. 4-21, 6-7, 11-18, 14-10, 14-13, 14-14, 15-5, 15-9).

LaFleur Brooks M: *Exploring medical terminology: a student-directed approach,* ed 5, St Louis, 2000, Mosby (Figs. 5-20, 6-14).

Lewis SM: *Medical-surgical nursing: assessment and management of clinical problems,* ed 5, St Louis, 2000, Mosby (Figs. 3-12, 3-17, 3-22, 3-23, 4-13, 6-5, 6-10, 10-8, *B-C,* 10-16, 12-18, 12-19, Case Study Fig. Ch. 4, *B*).

Lowdermilk DL, Perry SE, Bobak IM: *Maternity and women's health care,* ed 7, St Louis, 2000, Mosby (Figs. 1-7, 8-4, 8-15, 8-17, Case Study Fig. Ch. 8).

Mace JD, Kowalczyk N: *Radiographic pathology for technologists,* ed 3, St Louis, 1998, Mosby (Fig. 16-19).

McCance KL, Huether SE: *Pathophysiology: the biologic basis for disease in adults and children,* ed 4, St Louis, 2002, Mosby (Fig. 4-20).

Mosby's medical nursing and allied health dictionary, ed 5, St Louis, 1998, Mosby (Figs. 7-7, 15-4).

O'Neill WC: *Atlas of renal ultrasonography,* Philadelphia, 2001, WB Saunders (Fig. 6-6, *A*).

Potter PA, Perry AG: *Fundamentals of nursing,* ed 5, St Louis, 2001, Mosby (Figs. 4-24, 5-19, *B,* 11-16, *A-C,* Case Study Fig. Ch. 13).

Seidel HM, Ball JW, Dains JI, et al: *Mosby's guide to physical examination,* ed 5, St Louis, 2003, Mosby (Figs. 1-4, 3-11, 4-19, 7-4, 7-5, 13-2, *A,* 14-4).

Stevens A, Lowe J: *Pathology: illustrated review in color,* ed 2, St Louis, 2000, Mosby (Fig. 9-10, 16-15, 16-16).

Stuart GW, Laraia MT: *Principles and practice of psychiatric nursing,* St Louis, 2001, Mosby (Figs. 13-2, *B,* 13-3).

Thibodeau GA, Patton KT: *Anatomy and physiology,* ed 5, St Louis, 2002, Mosby (Figs. 8-12, 9-4, 9-7, 10-8, *A,* 14-19).

Thibodeau GA, Patton KT: *The human body in health and disease,* ed 3, St Louis, 2002, Mosby (Figs. 12-5, 12-12, 12-16, 12-17, 15-3, 15-7).

Wilson SF, Giddens JF: *Health assessment for nursing practice,* ed 2, St Louis, 2001, Mosby (Figs. 3-13, 4-6, Case Study Fig. Ch. 15).

Zitelli BJ, Davis HW: *Atlas of pediatric physical diagnosis,* ed 4, St Louis, 2002, Mosby (Figs. 3-7, 3-8, 3-9, 5-6, 5-11, 5-16, 7-2, 11-4, 11-5, 12-8, 14-3, 14-16, 14-17, 14-20, 15-6).

References

Chapter 1

Beers MH, Berkow R, Burs M, editors: *Merck manual diagnosis and therapy,* Whitehouse Station, NJ, 1999, Merck & Co.

Haubrich WS, editor: *Medical meanings: a glossary of word origins,* Philadelphia, 1997, American College of Physicians.

Plato: *The republic,* New York, 1955, Viking Press (Translated by D Lee).

Chapter 2

Shakespeare W: Hamlet. In Montgomery W, Jowet J, Wells S, et al, editors: *Oxford Shakespeare: the complete works of William Shakespeare,* New York, 1999, Oxford University Press.

Chapter 3

Anderson GP: *Healing wisdom: wit, insight, and inspiration for anyone facing illness,* New York, 1994, EP Dutton.

Bureau of Labor Statistics: *Occupational outlook handbook,* Washington, DC, 2002-2003, U.S. Department of Labor.

Davis NM: *Medical abbreviations: 14,000 conveniences at the expense of communication and safety,* ed 9, Huntingdon Valley, Penn, 1999, Neil M. Davis Associates.

Haubrich WS, editor: *Medical meanings: a glossary of word origins,* Philadelphia, 1997, American College of Physicians.

Chapter 4

Edison TA: Life. In Bartlett J, Kaplan J, editors: *Bartlett's familiar quotations: a collection of passages, phrases, and proverbs traced to their sources in ancient and modern literature,* ed 16, New York, 1992, Little, Brown.

Micozzi MS: *Fundamentals of complementary and alternative medicine,* ed 2, New York, 2001, Churchill Livingstone.

Novey DW: *Clinician's complete reference to complementary and alternative medicine,* St Louis, 2000, Mosby.

Chapter 5

Cousins N: *Head first: the biology of hope and the healing power of the human spirit,* New York, 1989, EP Dutton. Available online: ACP-ASIM Medicine in Quotations, http://www.acponline.org/cgi-bin/medquotes.pl.

Franklin B: Letter to Jean-Baptiste Leroy (November 13, 1789). In Bartlett J, Kaplan J, editors: *Bartlett's familiar quotations: a collection of passages, phrases, and proverbs traced to their sources in ancient and modern literature,* ed 16, New York, 1992, Little, Brown.

Rybacki J, Pharm D, Long J: *The essential guide to prescription drugs 2001: everything you need to know for safe drug use,* New York, 2000, Harper Collins.

Chapter 6

Beers MH, Berkow R, Burs M, editors: *Merck manual diagnosis and therapy,* 1999, Merck & Co.

Dinesen I (Karen Blixen): The dreamers. In *Seven gothic tales,* New York, 1934, Random House.

Smith H: *Lectures on the kidney,* Lawrence, 1943, University of Kansas. Available online: ACP-ASIM Medicine in Quotations, http://www.acponline.org/cgi-bin/medquotes.pl.

Chapter 7

Bureau of Labor Statistics: *Occupational outlook handbook,* Washington, DC, 2002-2003, U.S. Department of Labor.

Freeman L, Lawlin GF: *Mosby's complementary and alternative medicine: a research-based approach,* St Louis, 2001, Mosby.

Richardson B: Congressional record, 43905-43906, May 24, 1994.

Chapter 8

Dylan B: Lyrics from "It's alright, ma (I'm only bleeding)" from the album *Bringing it all back home,* 1965, Columbia Records.

Fischbach F: *A manual of laboratory and diagnostic tests,* ed 6, Philadelphia, 2000, Lippincott Williams & Wilkins.

Chapter 9

Quote from http://www.quoteablequotes.net.

Prescott L: Novel anti-IgE monoclonal antibody promising against allergic diseases, *Inpharma* 1232:7-8, 2000.

Chapter 10

Quote from http://www.quoteablequotes.net.

Chapter 11

American College of Physicians—American Society of Internal Medicine: A pulmonologist's valentine, *N Engl J Med* 304:739, 1981. Available online: ACP-ASIM Medicine in Quotations, http://www.acponline.org/cgi-bin/medquotes.pl.

Chapter 12

Quereshi B: Review of Jones L, Sidell M: The challenge of promoting health: exploration and action, *J R Soc Med* 90:705, 1997. Available online: ACP-ASIM Medicine in Quotations, http://www.acponline.org/cgi-bin/medquotes.pl.

Chapter 13

Dubos RJ: The three faces of medicine, *Bull Am Coll Phys* 2:162-166, 1961.

Chapter 14

Quote from http://www.quoteablequotes.net.

Chapter 16

Mayo CH, Hendricks WA: Carcinomas of the right segment of the colon, *Ann Surg* 83:357-363, 1926.

Resources on the World Wide Web

Chapter 1

National Center for Health Statistics
http://www.cdc.gov/nchs/fastats

National Center for Infectious Diseases
http://www.cdc.gov/ncidod/diseases

National Library of Medicine—Drug Information
http://www.nlm.nih.gov/medlineplus/druginformation.html

United States Pharmacopeia
http://www.usp.org

World Health Organization
http://www.who.int/health-topics

Chapter 3

Centers for Disease Control
http://www.cdc.gov/mmwr/

National Institute of Arthritis and Musculoskeletal and Skin Diseases
http://www.nih.gov/niams/healthinfo/artrheu.htm

Chapter 4

American Health Information Management Association
http://www.ahima.org
For CCS and CCS-P eligibility requirements, visit http://www.ahima.org/certification/

Consumer Product Safety Commission
http://www.cpsc.gov/

Shriners
http://www.shrinershg.org/prevention
Information on burn prevention is available.

Chapter 5

American Dietetic Association
http://www.eatright.org

American Heart Association
http://www.americanheart.org
Site includes information on cholesterol-reducing drugs.

Food and Drug Administration
http://www.fda.gov/medwatch/
Lists drugs removed from the market by the government.

Chapter 6

American Academy of Family Physicians
http://www.aafp.org
Available articles include "Urinary Tract Infections in Adults."

Medical Transcription Networking Center
http://www.mtdaily.com
Site includes the values and the explanations for a wide variety of laboratory tests in a format for allied health professionals.

The National Institute of Diabetes and Digestive and Kidney Diseases
http://www.niddk.nih.gov
Site includes statistics on diabetes and digestive and kidney diseases and information on related health topics. Spanish language versions of the resources are available.

Chapter 7

Association of Surgical Technologists
http://www.ast.org

Men's Health Network
http://www.menshealthnetwork.org
Educational and informational resources, including links and activities.

Chapter 8

American Academy of Pediatrics
http://www.aap.org/

American College of Nurse-Midwives
http://www.midwife.org

Doulas of North America
http://www.dona.com

HCUP Healthcare Cost and Utilization Project
http://www.ahrq.gov/data/hcup/hcupnet.htm
Tool for identifying, tracking, analyzing, and comparing statistics on hospitals at the national, regional, and state levels.

March of Dimes
http://www.marchofdimes.com/HealthLibrary/fact_sheets.htm

National Center for Health Statistics
http://www.cdc.gov/nchs/fastats/default.htm

Chapter 9

AIDS Treatment News
http://www.aids.org
Fact sheets and news regarding HIV/AIDS.

Allernet
http://www.allernet.com/FAQ
Allergy FAQ provides an overview of what allergies are and how to treat symptoms.

American Association of Blood Banks
http://www.aabb.org/All About Blood/
This address presents facts about blood and blood banking, including "Highlights of Transfusion Medicine History."

American Red Cross
http://www.redcross.org/
This address provides information about blood donations, testing, and usage.

Food and Drug Administration
http://www.fda.gov/oashi/aids/hiv.html
This address provides information on HIV/AIDS and AIDS-related conditions.

National Center for Health Statistics
http://www.cdc.gov.nchs/fastats/anemia.htm
This address gives information on anemia in the United States.

National Center for HIV, STD and TB Prevention: A division of the Centers for Disease Control
http://www.cdc.npin.org

National Heart, Lung, and Blood Institute Information Center
http://www.nhlbi.nih.gov/health/infoctr/index.htm
Provides information on the prevention and treatment of heart, lung, and blood diseases.

The Sickle Cell Information Center
http://www.emory.edu/PEDS/SICKLE/

WebMDHealth
http://www.my.webmd.com/
General medical site that has an interesting section on allergies, including a quiz.

Chapter 10

American Heart Association
http://www.americanheart.org/statistics/cvd.html
This address provides statistical CAD comparisons of age, sex, race, and ethnicity.

Food and Drug Administration Center for Drug Evaluation and Research
http://www.fda.gov/cder/
Information on new and generic drug approvals and drug warnings. National Drug Code Directory.

HCUP Healthcare Cost and Utilization Project
hcup.ahrq.gov/HCUPnet.asp
This address lets you choose from a selection of databases with the option of starting your own queries. For example, you can find statistics on the cardiovascular system by diagnoses or procedures.

National Heart, Lung and Blood Institute
http://www.nhlbi.nih.gov

Chapter 11

American Academy of Allergy, Asthma, and Immunology Online
http://www.aaaai.org

American Lung Association
http://www.lungusa.org
National organization with many sources of information, including statistics on lung disease by race and ethnicity.

National Heart, Lung, and Blood Institute
http://www.nhlbi.nih.gov/health/public/lung/other/bpd/glossary.htm
A glossary of respiratory terms resides at this address.

National Library of Medicine—Respiratory Diseases
http://www.nlm.nih.gov/medlineplus/respiratorydiseases-general.html

National Women's Health Information Center
http://www.4woman.gov/faq/lung_disease.htm

University of Virginia Health Sciences Center—Children's Medical Center
http://www.hsc.virginia.edu/medicine/clinical/pediatrics/chmedctr/pedpharm/v7n4.html
Click on "Tutorials for Families" to find asthma tutorial.

Chapter 12

Alzheimer's Association
http://www.alz.org

Epilepsy Foundation of America
http://www.efa.org

National Institute of Neurological Disorders and Stroke
http://www.ninds.nih.gov

National Library of Medicine—Brain and Nervous System
http://www.nlm.nih.gov/medlineplus/brainandnervous-system.html

National Library of Medicine—Parkinson's Disease
http://www.nlm.nih.gov/medlineplus/parkinsonsdisease.html
http://www.nmss.org

National Stroke Association
http://www.stroke.org
This site is in English, French, and Spanish.

Parkinson's Disease Foundation, Inc.
http://www.pdf.org

Chapter 13

Department of Health and Human Services National Clearinghouse for Alcohol and Drug Information
http://www.health.org

National Association of Social Workers
http://www.naswdc.org

National Institute on Alcohol Abuse and Alcoholism
http://www.niaaa.nih.gov

National Institute on Drug Abuse
http://www.nida.nih.gov
To gain access to the listserv on research on how drugs affect the brain, visit this address: Announce-NIDA@lists.nida.nih.gov.
This address provides a Spanish language version of the NIDA research report on Methamphetamine Abuse and Addiction: 165.112.78.61/ResearchReports/metanfetamina/metanfeta.html.

Office on National Drug Control Policy
http://www.whitehousedrugpolicy.gov

Chapter 14

American Academy of Otolaryngology—Head and Neck Surgery
http://www.entnet.org
Click on "Public and Patients" to find an online 5-minute hearing test under "Hearing Resources."

American Foundation for the Blind
http://www.afb.org

National Eye Institute
http://www.nei.nih.gov/photo/sims/sims.htm
This site provides images of various scenes as they would be experienced by people with normal vision and how they would be seen by people glaucoma, cataract, diabetic retinopathy, macular degeneration, myopia, and retinitis pigmentosa. Spanish version available on same page.

National Institute on Deafness and Other Communication Disorders
http://www.nidcd.nih.gov/health/hb.htm
Site includes online publications on topics such as American Sign Language, early hearing screening, hearing aids, and Ménière's disease.

National Library of Medicine—Vision Disorders/Blindness
http://www.nlm.nih.gov/medlineplus/visiondisorders-blindness.html

Appendix A

Combining Forms Alphabetized by Meaning

Meaning	Combining Form
abdomen	abdomin/o, celi/o, lapar/o
addition	prosthes/o
adenoid	adenoid/o
adrenal gland	adren/o, adrenal/o
aging	ger/o, presby/o
air	pneum/o
alveolus	alveol/o
amnion	amni/o
angle	goni/o
antrum	antr/o
anus	an/o
anus and rectum	proct/o
aorta	aort/o
apex	apic/o
appendix	append/o, appendic/o
armpit	axill/o
arrangement	tax/o
arrow	sagitt/o
arteriole	arteriol/o
artery	arteri/o
atrium	atri/o
attraction	phil/o
back of body	dors/o, poster/o
bacteria	bacteri/o
Bartholin's glands	bartholin/o
base	bas/o
behind	poster/o
bend	flex/o
bile	bil/i, chol/e
bile vessel	cholangi/o
birth; born	nat/o
black	melan/o
bladder (urinary)	vesic/o
blood serum	ser/o
blood	hem/o, hemat/o
blue	cyan/o
bluish green	glauc/o
body	som/o, corpor/o, somat/o
bone	oss/i, osse/o, oste/o
bone marrow	myel/o
brain	encephal/o
breast	mamm/o, mast/o
breath	halit/o
breathing	spir/o
bronchiole	bronchiol/o
bronchus	bronch/o, bronchi/o
bunion	bunion/o
burn	cauter/o
bursa	burs/o
calcium	calc/o
calyx	cali/o, calic/o
cancer (connective tissue); flesh	sarc/o
cancer (epithelial origin)	carcin/o
capillary	capillar/o
carbon dioxide	capn/o
carpal (wrist bone)	carp/o
carry; bear	phor/o
cartilage	cartilag/o, chondr/o
cast	bol/o
cecum	cec/o
cell	cellul/o, cyt/o
cerebellum	cerebell/o
cerebrum	cerebr/o
cervix	cervic/o
change	mut/a
cheek	bucc/o
chest	pector/o, thorac/o, steth/o
child	ped/o
chloride	chlor/o
chorion	chori/o, chorion/o
choroid	choroid/o
ciliary body	cycl/o

Continued

Combining Forms Alphabetized by Meaning—cont'd

Meaning	Combining Form	Meaning	Combining Form
clavicle	cleid/o	earwax	cerumin/o
closing	claustr/o	eat	phag/o
clot	thromb/o	egg	ov/o, ovi/o
clumping	agglutin/o	elbow	olecran/o
coccyx (tailbone)	coccyg/o	electricity	electr/o
cochlea	cochle/o	embryonic	blast/o
colon	col/o, colon/o	endocardium	endocardi/o
color	chrom/o, chromat/o	endometrium	endometri/o
common bile duct	choledoch/o	epicondyle	epicondyl/o
complete	tel/o	epididymis	epididym/o
condyle	condyl/o	epiglottis	epiglott/o
cone	con/o	epithelium	epitheli/o
conjunctiva	conjunctiv/o	equal	is/o
connective tissue	sarc/o	esophagus	esophag/o
cord	cord/o	ethmoid	ethmoid/o
cornea	corne/o	extreme	pol/o
cortex	cortic/o	extreme cold	cry/o
crooked	ankyl/o	extremes	acr/o
cul-de-sac	culd/o	eye	ocul/o, ophthalm/o, opt/o
curvature	scoli/o	eyelid	blephar/o, palpebr/o
cutting	tom/o	fallopian tube	salping/o
cycling	cycl/o	false	pseud/o
cyst	cyst/o	far	dist/o
dark	melan/o, phe/o	fascia	fasci/o
darkness	scot/o	fat	adip/o, ather/o, lip/o, steat/o
delivery; labor	toc/o	feeling	esthesi/o
development	troph/o	feel with	sympath/o
diaphragm	diaphragmat/o, diaphragm/o, phren/o	female	gynec/o
		femur	femor/o
digit (finger, toe)	digit/o, dactyl/o	fetus	fet/o
disease	path/o	fever	pyr/o, pyrex/o
dissolve	lys/o	few	olig/o
distant	dist/o, tele/o	fiber	fibr/o
diverticulum	diverticul/o	fibrin	fibrin/o
double	dipl/o	fibula	fibul/o, perone/o
dry	xer/o	fingernail	onycho/o, ungu/o
dull; dim	ambly/o	fingers	dactyl/o, digit/o
duodenum	duoden/o	fire	pyr/o
dura mater	dur/o	fish	ichthy/o
dust	coni/o	flow	fluor/o
ear	aur/o, auricul/o, ot/o	fluid	hydr/o
eardrum	myring/o, tympan/o	fold	plic/o

COMBINING FORMS ALPHABETIZED BY MEANING—CONT'D

MEANING	COMBINING FORM
follicle	follicul/o
foot	ped/o
foreign	xen/o
formation	plas/o, plasm/o, plast/o
fornix	fornic/o
front	anter/o
frontal	front/o, ventr/o
fundus	fund/o
fungus	myc/o
gallbladder	cholecyst/o
ganglion	gangli/o, ganglion/o
gland	aden/o
glans penis	balan/o
glassy	vitr/o
glomerulus	glomerul/o
glue	gli/o
gonad	gonad/o
grain (small)	granul/o
gray	glauc/o
groin	inguin/o
grow	phys/o
gums	gingiv/o
hair	pil/o, trich/o
hand	chir/o, man/o
hard	scler/o, kerat/o
head	capit/o, cephal/o
hearing	acous/o, audi/o
heart	cordi/o, cardi/o, coron/o
heart muscle	myocardi/o
heat	cauter/o, therm/o
heights	acr/o
hemorrhoid	hemorrhoid/o
hernia	herni/o
hidden	crypt/o
hilum	hil/o
hold back	ischem/o
horny	corne/o, kerat/o
humerus	humer/o
hump; humpback	kyph/o
hymen	hymen/o
ileum	ile/o
ilium	ili/o
inner ear	labyrinth/o
insulin	insulin/o
intestines	intestin/o
intestines (small)	enter/o
iris	ir/o, irid/o
iron	sider/o, ferr/o
ischium	ischi/o
jaw bone (lower)	mandibul/o
jaw bone (upper)	maxill/o
jejunum	jejun/o
joint	arthr/o, articul/o
juice	chym/o
ketones	keton/o
kidney	nephr/o, ren/o
knot	nod/o
knowledge	gnos/o, log/o
labia	labi/o
lacrimal duct	lacrim/o
lamina	lamin/o
larynx	laryng/o
left; left side	sinistr/o
leg	crur/o
lens	phac/o, phak/o
life; living	bi/o
life (animal)	zo/o
ligament	ligament/o, syndesm/o
light	lumin/o, phot/o
lip	cheil/o, labi/o
lipid (fat)	lip/o
liquid	humor/o
liver	hepat/o
lobe	lob/o
lower back	lumb/o
lung	pneum/o, pneumon/o, pulmon/o
lymph	lymphat/o, lymph/o
lymph gland	lymphaden/o
lymph vessel	lymphangi/o
malleolus	malleol/o
man	anthrop/o
mandible	mandibul/o
manipulation	pract/o

Continued

COMBINING FORMS ALPHABETIZED BY MEANING—CONT'D

MEANING	COMBINING FORM
mastoid process	mastoid/o
maxillary	maxill/o
measure	metr/o
meatus	meat/o
mediastinum	mediastino/o
medulla	medull/o
meninges	mening/o, meningi/o
menses	menstru/o, men/o
metacarpal	metacarp/o
metatarsal	metatars/o
middle	medi/o
midwife	obstetr/o
milk	galact/o, lact/o
mind	ment/o, psych/o, thym/o
mouth	or/o, stomat/o
movement	kinesi/o, prax/o
mucus	muc/o
muscle	muscul/o, my/o, myos/o
muscle (heart)	myocardi/o
muscle (smooth)	leiomy/o
muscle (striated)	rhabdomy/o
nail (toe, finger)	onycho/o, ungu/o
near	proxim/o
neck	cervic/o, nuch/o, trabecul/o
nerve	neur/o
nerve root	radicul/o
neutral	neutr/o
night	noct/i, nyct/o
nipple	thel/o
nipple-shaped	papill/o
nitrogen	az/o
nose	nas/o, rhin/o
nourishment	troph/o
nucleus	kary/o, nucle/o
nutrition	aliment/o
occipital	occipit/o
odor	osm/o
oil	seb/o
old age	presby/o, ger/o
opening	hiat/o, stom/o
oral cavity	or/o
orange-yellow	cirrh/o
order	tax/o
organ	viscer/o
organ; organic	organ/o
origin	gen/o
ossicle	ossicul/o
other	all/o
ovary	oophor/o, ovari/o
ovulation	ovul/o
ovum	o/o, ov/o
oxygen	ox/i, ox/o
paint	pigment/o
palate	palat/o
pancreas	pancreat/o
parathyroid gland	parathyroid/o
parietal	pariet/o
partition	sept/o
passage	por/o
patella	patell/o
pelvis	pelv/i
penis	phall/o
pericardium	pericardi/o
perineum	perine/o
peritoneum	peritone/o
phalanx	phalang/o
pharynx	pharyng/o
phosphorus	phosph/o, phosphat/o
physician	iatr/o
pimple	papul/o
pituitary gland	pituitar/o, hypophys/o
place	top/o
plaque	ather/o
platelet	thrombocyt/o
pleasure	hedon/o
pleura	pleur/o
pole	pol/o
potassium	potassi/o, kal/i
pregnancy	gravid/o
prepuce	preputi/o
pressure	press/o
prostate	prostat/o
protection	immun/o
protein	albumin/o

Combining Forms Alphabetized by Meaning—cont'd

Meaning	Combining Form
pubis; pubic bone	pub/o
pulling together	contractur/o
pupil	cor/o, core/o, pupill/o
purple	purpur/o
pus	py/o
pustule	pustul/o
pylorus	pylor/o
radius	radi/o
rectum	proct/o, rect/o
red	erythr/o
red blood cell	erythrocyt/o
renal pelvis	pyel/o
retina	retin/o
rhythm	rrhythm/o
rib	cost/o
ribose	rib/o
right; right side	dextr/o
rosy	eosin/o
sac	cyst/o, follicul/o
sacrum	sacr/o
safety	immun/o
saliva	sial/o
salivary glands	sialaden/o
same; constant	home/o
sarcoma	sarc/o
scab	eschar/o
scaly	squam/o
scanty	man/o, olig/o
scapula	scapul/o
sclera	scler/o
scrotum	scrot/o
sebum	seb/o
secrete	crin/o
section	tom/o
seed	gon/o
semen	semin/i
seminal vesicle	vesicul/o
septum	sept/o
shape	morph/o
side	later/o
sigmoid colon	sigmoid/o
sinus	sin/o, sinus/o
skin	cutane/o, derm/o, dermat/o
skull	crani/o
sleep	narc/o, somn/o
slice	tom/o
small grain	granul/o
small intestines	enter/o
smell (sense of)	osm/o
smooth	lei/o
sodium	natr/o
sound	phon/o, son/o
space between	interstit/o
speech	phas/o
spermatozoa	sperm/o, spermat/o
sphenoid	sphenoid/o
spinal column; spine	rachi/o, spin/o, myel/o
spinal nerve root	rhiz/o
spleen	splen/o
spot	macul/o
stapes	staped/o
star	astr/o
starch	amyl/o
steal	klept/o
sternum	stern/o
stiff	ankyl/o
stomach	gastr/o
stone	calcul/o, lith/o
straight	orth/o
strength	sthen/o
study of	log/o
sudoriferous gland	hidraden/o
sugar; sweet	gluc/o, glyc/o
swallow	phag/o
swayback	lord/o
sweat	hidr/o
synovial membrane	synovi/o
system	system/o
tail	caud/o
tarsal; tarsus	tars/o
tear	dacry/o
tear duct	lacrim/o
teeth	dent/i
temperature	therm/o

Continued

COMBINING FORMS ALPHABETIZED BY MEANING—CONT'D

Meaning	Combining Form
temporal bone	tempor/o
tendon	ten/o, tendin/o
tension	ton/o
testicle; testis	orch/o, orchi/o, orchid/o, test/o, testicul/o
thalamus	thalam/o
thirst	dips/o
thorax	thorac/o
three-dimensional	stere/o
throat	esophag/o, pharyng/o
thrombocyte	thrombocyt/o
thymus	thym/o
thyroid gland	thyr/o, thyroid/o
tibia	tibi/o
tissue	hist/o
toenail	onych/o
toes	dactyl/o, digit/o
tongue	gloss/o, lingu/o
tonsil	tonsill/o
tooth	odont/o
trachea	trache/o
treatment	iatr/o
tree; treelike	dendr/o
trigone	trigon/o
tumor	onc/o
turning	trop/o
ulceration	aphth/o
ulna	uln/o
umbilicus	omphal/o, umbilic/o
ureter	ureter/o
urethra	urethr/o
urinary bladder	cyst/o, vesic/o
urine; urinary system	ur/o, urin/o
uterus	hyster/o, metr/o, metri/o, uter/o
uvea	uve/o
uvula	uvul/o
vagina	colp/o, vagin/o
vagus nerve	vag/o
valve	valvul/o, valv/o
varices	varic/o
vas deferens	vas/o
vein	phleb/o, ven/o
ventral	ventr/o
ventricle	ventricul/o
venule	venul/o
vertebra	vertebr/o, spondyl/o
vessel	angi/o, vascul/o
vestibule	vestibul/o
virus	vir/o
viscera	viscer/o
vision	opt/o, optic/o
vitreous body	vitre/o
voice box	laryng/o
vomer	vomer/o
vulva	episi/o, vulv/o
walking	ambul/o
water	hydr/o
watery flow	rheumat/o
white	alb/o, albin/o, leuk/o
white blood cell	leukocyt/o
word	lex/o
wrinkle	rhytid/o
x-rays	radi/o
zygoma	zygom/o, zygomat/o

Appendix B

Combining Forms Alphabetized by Word Part

Combining Form	Meaning	Combining Form	Meaning
abdomin/o	abdomen	audi/o	hearing
acous/o	hearing	aur/o	ear
acr/o	heights; extremes	auricul/o	ear
aden/o	gland	axill/o	armpit
adenoid/o	adenoid	az/o	nitrogen
adip/o	fat	bacteri/o	bacteria
adren/o	adrenal gland	balan/o	glans penis
adrenal/o	adrenal gland	bartholin/o	Bartholin's glands
agglutin/o	clumping	bas/o	base
alb/o	white	bi/o	life; living
albin/o	white	bil/i	bile
albumin/o	protein	blast/o	embryonic; immature
aliment/o	nutrition	blephar/o	eyelid
all/o	other	bol/o	to cast
alveol/o	alveolus; small sac	bronch/o	bronchus
ambly/o	dull; dim	bronchi/o	bronchus
ambul/o	walking	bronchiol/o	bronchiole
amni/o	amnion	bucc/o	cheek
amyl/o	starch	bunion/o	bunion
an/o	anus	burs/o	bursa
angi/o	vessel	calc/o	calcium
ankyl/o	crooked; stiff	calcul/o	stone
anter/o	front	cali/o	calyx
anthrop/o	man	calic/o	calyx
antr/o	antrum	capillar/o	capillary
aort/o	aorta	capit/o	head
aphth/o	ulceration	capn/o	carbon dioxide
apic/o	apex	carcin/o	cancer of epithelial origin
append/o	appendix	cardi/o	heart
appendic/o	appendix	carp/o	carpal (wrist bone)
arteri/o	artery	cartilag/o	cartilage
arteriol/o	arteriole	caud/o	tail; lower part of body
arthr/o	joint	cauter/o	burn; heat
articul/o	joint	cec/o	cecum
astr/o	star	celi/o	abdomen
ather/o	fat; plaque	cellul/o	cell
atri/o	atrium	cephal/o	head

Continued

COMBINING FORMS ALPHABETIZED BY WORD PART—CONT'D

Combining Form	Meaning
cerebell/o	cerebellum
cerebr/o	cerebrum
cerumin/o	earwax
cervic/o	cervix; neck
cheil/o	lip
chir/o	hand
chlor/o	chloride
chol/e	bile
cholangi/o	bile vessel
cholecyst/o	gallbladder
choledoch/o	common bile duct
chondr/o	cartilage
chori/o	chorion
chorion/o	chorion
choroid/o	choroid
chrom/o	color
chromat/o	color
chym/o	juice
cirrh/o	orange-yellow
claustr/o	a closing
cleid/o	clavicle
coccyg/o	coccyx (tailbone)
cochle/o	cochlea
col/o	colon
colon/o	colon
colp/o	vagina
con/o	cone
condyl/o	condyle
coni/o	dust
conjunctiv/o	conjunctiva
contractur/o	a pulling together
cor/o	pupil
cord/o	cord
cordi/o	heart
core/o	pupil
corne/o	cornea; horny
coron/o	heart
corpor/o	body
cortic/o	cortex
cost/o	rib
crani/o	skull
crin/o	to secrete
crur/o	leg
cry/o	extreme cold
crypt/o	hidden
culd/o	cul-de-sac
cutane/o	skin
cyan/o	blue
cycl/o	cycling; ciliary body
cyst/o	urinary bladder; cyst; sac
cyt/o	cell
dacry/o	tear
dactyl/o	fingers; toes
dendr/o	tree; treelike structure
dent/i	teeth
derm/o	skin
dermat/o	skin
dextr/o	right; right side
diaphragm/o	diaphragm
diaphragmat/o	diaphragm
digit/o	digit (finger or toe)
dipl/o	double
dips/o	thirst
dist/o	distant; far
diverticul/o	diverticulum
dors/o	back of body
duoden/o	duodenum
dur/o	dura mater
electr/o	electricity
encephal/o	brain
endocardi/o	endocardium
endometri/o	endometrium
enter/o	small intestines
eosin/o	rosy; acidic
epicondyl/o	epicondyle
epididym/o	epididymis
epiglott/o	epiglottis
episi/o	vulva
epitheli/o	epithelium
erythr/o	red (blood cell)
erythrocyt/o	red blood cell
eschar/o	scab
esophag/o	esophagus; throat
esthesi/o	feeling

COMBINING FORMS ALPHABETIZED BY WORD PART—CONT'D

COMBINING FORM	MEANING
ethmoid/o	ethmoid
fasci/o	fascia
femor/o	femur
ferr/o	sider/o
fet/o	fetus
fibr/o	fiber
fibrin/o	fibrin
fibul/o	fibula
flex/o	to bend
fluor/o	to flow
follicul/o	follicle; small sac
fornic/o	fornix
front/o	frontal
fund/o	fundus
galact/o	milk
gangli/o	ganglion
ganglion/o	ganglion
gastr/o	stomach
gen/o	origin
ger/o	aging
gingiv/o	gums
glauc/o	gray; bluish green
gli/o	glue
glomerul/o	glomerulus
gloss/o	tongue
gluc/o	sweet; sugar
glyc/o	sugar
gnos/o	knowledge
gon/o	seed
gonad/o	gonad
goni/o	angle
granul/o	small grain
gravid/o	pregnancy
gynec/o	female
halit/o	breath
hedon/o	pleasure
hem/o	blood
hemat/o	blood
hemorrhoid/o	hemorrhoid
hepat/o	liver
herni/o	hernia
hiat/o	an opening
hidr/o	sweat
hidraden/o	sudoriferous gland
hil/o	hilum
hist/o	tissue
home/o	same; constant
humer/o	humerus
humor/o	liquid
hydr/o	water; fluid
hymen/o	hymen
hypophys/o	pituitary gland
hyster/o	uterus
iatr/o	treatment; physician
ichthy/o	fish
ile/o	ileum
ili/o	ilium
immun/o	safety; protection
inguin/o	groin
insulin/o	insulin
interstit/o	space between
intestin/o	intestines
ir/o	iris
irid/o	iris
ischem/o	to hold back
ischi/o	ischium
is/o	equal
jejun/o	jejunum
kal/i	potassium
kary/o	nucleus
kerat/o	hard; horny
keton/o	ketones
kinesi/o	movement
klept/o	to steal
kyph/o	hump; humpback
labi/o	labia; lip
labyrinth/o	inner ear
lacrim/o	tear duct; lacrimal duct
lact/o	milk
lamin/o	lamina
lapar/o	abdomen
laryng/o	voice box
later/o	side
lei/o	smooth

Continued

COMBINING FORMS ALPHABETIZED BY WORD PART—CONT'D

COMBINING FORM	MEANING
leiomy/o	visceral (smooth) muscle
leuk/o	white
leukocyt/o	white blood cell
lex/o	word
ligament/o	ligament
lingu/o	tongue
lip/o	lipid; fat
lith/o	stone
lob/o	lobe
log/o	study of; knowledge
lord/o	swayback
lumb/o	lower back
lumin/o	light
lymph/o	lymph
lymphaden/o	lymph gland
lymphangi/o	lymph vessel
lymphat/o	lymph
lys/o	dissolve
macul/o	spot
malleol/o	malleolus
mamm/o	breast
man/o	scanty; hand
mandibul/o	mandible (lower jaw bone)
mast/o	breast
mastoid/o	mastoid process
maxill/o	maxillary (upper jaw bone)
meat/o	meatus
medi/o	middle
mediastino/o	mediastinum
medull/o	medulla
melan/o	black; dark
men/o	menses; menstruation
mening/o	meninges
meningi/o	meninges
menstru/o	menses
ment/o	mind
metacarp/o	metacarpal
metatars/o	metatarsal
metr/o	uterus; measure
metri/o	uterus
morph/o	shape
muc/o	mucus
muscul/o	muscle
mut/a	change
my/o	muscle
myc/o	fungus
myel/o	bone marrow; spinal cord
myocardi/o	heart muscle
myos/o	muscle
myring/o	eardrum
narc/o	sleep
nas/o	nose
nat/o	birth; born
natr/o	sodium
nephr/o	kidney
neur/o	nerve
neutr/o	neutral
noct/i	night
nod/o	knot
nuch/o	neck
nucle/o	nucleus
nyct/o	night
o/o	ovum
obstetr/o	midwife
occipit/o	occipital
ocul/o	eye
odont/o	tooth
olecran/o	elbow
olig/o	scanty; few
omphal/o	umbilicus
onc/o	tumor
onych/o	nail (of toes or fingers)
oophor/o	ovary
ophthalm/o	eye
opt/o	vision; eye
optic/o	vision
or/o	mouth; oral cavity
orch/o	testicle; testis
orchi/o	testicle; testis
orchid/o	testicle; testis
organ/o	organ; organic
orth/o	straight
osm/o	sense of smell
oss/i	bone

COMBINING FORMS ALPHABETIZED BY WORD PART—CONT'D

COMBINING FORM	MEANING
osse/o	bone
ossicul/o	ossicle
oste/o	bone
ot/o	ear
ov/o	ovum; egg
ovari/o	ovary
ovi/o	egg
ovul/o	ovulation
ox/i	oxygen
ox/o	oxygen
palat/o	palate
palpebr/o	eyelid
pancreat/o	pancreas
papill/o	nipple-shaped projection
papul/o	pimple
parathyroid/o	parathyroid gland
pariet/o	parietal
patell/o	patella
path/o	disease
pector/o	chest
ped/o	child; foot
pelv/i	pelvis
pericardi/o	pericardium
perine/o	perineum
peritone/o	peritoneum
perone/o	fibula
phac/o	lens
phag/o	eat; swallow
phak/o	lens
phalang/o	phalanx
phall/o	penis
pharyng/o	pharynx (throat)
phas/o	speech
phe/o	dark
phil/o	attraction
phleb/o	vein
phon/o	sound
phor/o	to carry; to bear
phosph/o	phosphorus
phosphat/o	phosphorus
phot/o	light
phren/o	diaphragm

COMBINING FORM	MEANING
phys/o	to grow
pigment/o	paint
pil/o	hair
pituitar/o	pituitary gland
plas/o	formation
plasm/o	formation
plast/o	formation
pleur/o	pleura
plic/o	fold
pneum/o	lung; air
pneumon/o	lung
pol/o	pole; extreme
por/o	passage
poster/o	behind; back of body
potassi/o	potassium
pract/o	manipulation
prax/o	purposeful movement
preputi/o	prepuce
presby/o	old age
press/o	pressure
proct/o	rectum and anus
prostat/o	prostate
prosthes/o	addition
proxim/o	near
pseud/o	false
psych/o	mind
pub/o	pubis; pubic bone
pulmon/o	lung
pupill/o	pupil
purpur/o	purple
pustul/o	pustule
py/o	pus
pyel/o	renal pelvis
pylor/o	pylorus
pyr/o	fire; fever
pyrex/o	fever
rachi/o	spinal column
radi/o	radius; x-rays
radicul/o	nerve root
rect/o	rectum
ren/o	kidney
retin/o	retina

Continued

COMBINING FORMS ALPHABETIZED BY WORD PART—CONT'D

COMBINING FORM	MEANING
rhabdomy/o	striated muscle
rheumat/o	watery flow
rhin/o	nose
rhiz/o	spinal nerve root
rhytid/o	wrinkle
rib/o	ribose
rrhythm/o	rhythm
sacr/o	sacrum
sagitt/o	arrow
salping/o	fallopian tube
sarc/o	sarcoma; connective tissue cancer; flesh
scapul/o	scapula
scler/o	sclera; hard
scoli/o	curvature
scot/o	darkness
scrot/o	scrotum
seb/o	sebum; oil
semin/i	semen
sept/o	partition; septum
ser/o	blood serum
sial/o	saliva
sialaden/o	salivary gland
sider/o	iron
sigmoid/o	sigmoid colon
sin/o	sinus
sinistr/o	left; left side
sinus/o	sinus
som/o	body
somat/o	body
somn/o	sleep
son/o	sound
sperm/o	spermatozoon
spermat/o	spermatozoon
sphenoid/o	sphenoid
spin/o	spine; spinal column
spir/o	breathing
splen/o	spleen
spondyl/o	vertebra
squam/o	scaly
staped/o	stapes
steat/o	fat
stere/o	three-dimensional
stern/o	sternum
steth/o	chest
sthen/o	strength
stom/o	opening
stomat/o	mouth
sympath/o	to feel with
syndesm/o	ligament
synovi/o	synovial membrane
system/o	system
tars/o	tarsal; tarsus
tax/o	order; arrangement
tele/o	distant
tel/o	complete
tempor/o	temporal bone
ten/o	tendon
tendin/o	tendon
test/o	testicle; testis
testicul/o	testicle; testis
thalam/o	thalamus
thel/o	nipple
therm/o	heat; temperature
thorac/o	thorax; chest
thromb/o	clot
thrombocyt/o	thrombocyte; platelet
thym/o	thymus; mind
thyr/o	thyroid gland
thyroid/o	thyroid
tibi/o	tibia
toc/o	delivery; labor
tom/o	section; cutting; slice
ton/o	tension
tonsill/o	tonsil
top/o	place
trabecul/o	neck
trache/o	trachea
trich/o	hair
trigon/o	trigone
trop/o	turning
troph/o	nourishment; development
tympan/o	eardrum
uln/o	ulna

COMBINING FORMS ALPHABETIZED BY WORD PART—CONT'D

COMBINING FORM	MEANING
umbilic/o	umbilicus
ungu/o	nail
ur/o	urine; urinary system
ureter/o	ureter
urethr/o	urethra
urin/o	urine; urinary system
uter/o	uterus
uve/o	uvea
uvul/o	uvula
vag/o	vagus nerve
vagin/o	vagina
valv/o	valve
valvul/o	valve
varic/o	varices
vas/o	vas deferens
vascul/o	vessel
ven/o	vein
ventr/o	ventral; frontal
ventricul/o	ventricle
venul/o	venule
vertebr/o	vertebra
vesic/o	urinary bladder
vesicul/o	seminal vesicle
vestibul/o	vestibule
vir/o	virus
viscer/o	organ; viscera
vitre/o	vitreous body
vomer/o	vomer
vulv/o	vulva
xen/o	foreign
xer/o	dry
zo/o	life (animal)
zygom/o	zygoma
zygomat/o	zygoma

Appendix C

Prefixes

Prefix	Meaning
a-	no; not; without
ab-	away from
acu-	sharp
ad-	towards
amphi-	both
an-	without; not
ana-	up; apart
ante-	before; in front of
anti-	against
apo-	separate; away
auto-	self; own
bi-	two
brady-	slow
cata-	down
circum-	around
contra-	opposite; against
de-	lack of; removal
di-	through; complete; two
dia-	through; complete
dis-	apart from
dys-	bad; painful; abnormal; difficult
e-	out
ec-	out; outside; out of
echo-	sound
ecto-	outer
en-	in
end-	within
endo-	inner; within
epi-	above; on top of
eso-	inward
eu-	good; well
ex-	outside; out
exo-	outside; outward
extra-	outside; controlling
hemi-	half; partial
homo-	same
hyper-	excessive; above
hypo-	deficient; below; under
in-	in; not
infra-	below
inter-	between
intra-	within
ipsi-	same
levo-	left; left side
macro-	large
mal-	bad; poor
meso-	middle
meta-	change; beyond
micro-	small; tiny
mono-	single; one
neo-	new
non-	not
oxy-	rapid
pan-	all
par-	near; beside
para-	abnormal; near; beside
per-	through
peri-	around; surrounding
poly-	excessive; profuse; many
post-	after; behind
pre-	before
pro-	before; in front of; forward
quadri-	four
re-	back; again
retro-	backward
sub-	under; below
supra-	above
syn-	together; with
tachy-	rapid
tetra-	four
trans-	across; through
ultra-	beyond; excessive
uni-	one

Appendix D

Suffixes

Suffix	Meaning
-abrasion	scraping
-ac	pertaining to
-al	pertaining to
-algia	pain
-amnios	amnion
-an	pertaining to
-ar	pertaining to
-ary	pertaining to
-ase	enzyme
-ation	condition; process
-blast	embryonic
-cardia	heart condition
-cele	herniation; protrusion
-centesis	removal of fluid
-chalasis	relaxation; slackening
-chezia	elimination of waste; defecation
-clasis	intentional fracture; to break
-clast	breaking down; to break
-cordial	pertaining to the heart
-crine	to secrete
-cusis	hearing
-cyesis	pregnancy
-cyte	cell
-cytosis	abnormal increase of cells
-desis	binding
-dipsia	thirst
-drome	to run
-dynia	pain
-eal	pertaining to
-ectasia	dilation
-ectasis	dilation
-ectomy	removal; excision; resection
-edema	swelling
-emia	blood condition
-esis	state of
-fida	split
-flux	flow; back
-fusion	pouring; to pour
-gen	producing; produced by
-geusia	taste
-grade	to go
-gram	record; recording
-graph	instrument used to record
-graphy	process of recording
-gravida	pregnancy
-ia	condition
-iac	pertaining to
-iasis	condition
-ic	pertaining to
-ion	process
-ism	condition
-ist	one who specializes
-itic	pertaining to
-itis	inflammation
-ium	structure
-ization	process
-kine	movement
-lalia	condition of babbling
-lapse	to fall; to slide; to sag
-lepsy	seizure
-listhesis	slipping
-lithotomy	removal of a stone
-logy	study of
-lysis	separation; breakdown; destruction
-lytic	destruction; to destroy; to reduce
-malacia	softening
-mania	state of mental disorder
-megaly	enlargement
-meter	instrument to measure
-metry	process of measurement
-mission	sending
-oid	full of; resembling
-oma	tumor; mass; swelling
-opia	vision

Continued

SUFFIXES—CONT'D

SUFFIX	MEANING
-opsia	vision
-opsy	viewing
-orexia	appetite
-ose	pertaining to; sugar; full of
-osis	abnormal condition
-ous	pertaining to
-para	labor; delivery
-paresis	slight paralysis
-pathy	disease process; emotion
-penia	deficiency
-pepsia	digestion
-pexy	fixation; suspension
-phagia	condition of swallowing; eating
-philia	tendency; attraction
-phobia	fear
-phylaxis	protection
-physis	growth
-plakia	condition; plaque
-plasia	development; formation
-plasm	formation
-plasty	surgical repair
-plegia	paralysis
-pnea	breathing
-poiesis	formation
-ptosis	drooping; prolapse
-ptysis	spitting
-rrhage	bursting forth (of blood)
-rrhagia	bursting forth
-rrhaphy	suture
-rrhea	discharge; flow
-rrheic	pertaining to discharge
-rrhexis	rupture

SUFFIX	MEANING
-salpinx	fallopian tubes
-sclerosis	abnormal hardening
-scope	instrument used for visual examination
-scopic	pertaining to visual examination
-scopy	visual examination
-sis	state of
-spadia	to cut; to tear
-stalsis	contraction
-stasis	stopping; controlling
-stenosis	narrowing; stricture
-sthenia	condition of strength
-stomy	new opening
-tension	pressure
-therapy	treatment
-thorax	pleural cavity; chest
-thymia	mind
-tic	pertaining to
-tion	process of
-tocia	labor; delivery
-tome	instrument used to cut
-tomy	incision; process of cutting
-tresia	opening
-tripsy	to crush
-tripter	instrument used to crush
-trite	instrument used to crush
-trophy	development
-ule	diminutive; small
-um	structure; thing; tissue
-uria	urination; urinary condition
-us	structure; thing
-y	condition; process

Appendix E

Abbreviations

Abbreviation	Meaning
A, B, AB, O	blood types
ABR	auditory brain response
AC	air conduction
Acc	accommodation
ACTH	adrenocorticotropic hormone
AD	Alzheimer's disease; auris dextra (right ear)
ADH	antidiuretic hormone
ADHD	attention deficit hyperactivity disorder
ADLs	activities of daily living
AEB	atrial ectopic beats
AF	atrial fibrillation
AFP	alpha-fetoprotein test
AHIMA	American Health Information Management Association
AI	artificial insemination
AIDS	acquired immune deficiency syndrome
ALS	amyotrophic lateral sclerosis
AMI	acute myocardial infarction
ANA	antinuclear antibody
ANS	autonomic nervous system
AP	anteroposterior
ARF	acute renal failure
ARMD, AMD	age-related macular degeneration
AS	aortic stenosis; auris sinistra (left ear)
ASD	atrial septal defect
ASHD	arteriosclerotic heart disease
ASL	American sign language
Astigm, As, Ast	astigmatism
AU	auris uterqu (each ear)
AV	atrioventricular
BE	barium enema
BaS	barium swallow
Baso	basophils
BBB	blood-brain barrier; bundle branch block
BC	bone conduction
BD	bipolar disorder
BM	bowel movement
BMT	bone marrow transplant
BP	blood pressure
BPH	benign prostatic hyperplasia/hypertrophy
BPM	beats per minute
BSE	breast self-examination
BUN	blood urea nitrogen
bx	biopsy
c̄ gl	with glasses
C1-C7	first cervical through seventh cervical vertebrae
C1-C8	cervical nerves
Ca	calcium
CA	cancer
CA125	tumor marker for primarily ovarian cancer
CA15-3	tumor marker to monitor breast cancer
CA19-9	tumor marker for pancreatic, stomach, and bile duct cancer
CA27-29	tumor marker to check for recurrence of breast cancer
CABG	coronary artery bypass graft
CAD	coronary artery disease
CAM	complementary and alternative medicine
CAPD	continuous ambulatory peritoneal dialysis
CAT	computed axial tomography
Cath	(cardiac) catheterization
CBC	complete blood cell (count)
CC	cardiac care
CCB	calcium channel blocker(s)
CCF	congestive cardiac failure
CCS	certified coding specialist
CCS-P	certified coding specialist—physician's office
CCU	coronary care unit
CEA	carcinoembryonic antigen
CHF	congestive heart failure
CIN	cervical intraepithelial neoplasia
CK	creatine kinase
Cl	chloride
CNS	central nervous system
CO_2	carbon dioxide
COPD	chronic obstructive pulmonary disease
CP	cerebral palsy
CPAP	continuous positive airway pressure
CPK	creatine phosphokinase

Continued

Abbreviations—cont'd

Abbreviation	Meaning
CPR	cardiopulmonary resuscitation
CPT	current procedural terminology
CRF	chronic renal failure
CRT	certified respiratory therapist
CS	cesarean section
CSF	cerebrospinal fluid
CST	contraction stress test
CT	computed tomography
CT scan	computed tomography scan
CTA	clear to auscultation
CTR	certified tumor registrar
CTS	carpal tunnel syndrome
CV	cardiovascular
CVA	cerebrovascular accident
CVS	chorionic villus sampling
CWP	coal worker's pneumoconiosis
Cx	cervix
CXR	chest x-ray
D&C	dilation and curettage
D1-D12	first dorsal through twelfth dorsal vertebrae
DCB	double contrast barium enema
Decub	pressure ulcer
DEXA, DXA	dual energy x-ray absorptiometry
DI	diabetes insipidus
Diff	differential WBC count
DJD	degenerative joint disease
DM	diabetes mellitus
DOE	dyspnea on exertion
DRE	digital rectal exam
DRG	diagnosis-related group
DSA	digital subtraction angiography
DT	delirium tremens
DTR	deep tendon reflex
DUB	dysfunctional uterine bleeding
DVT	deep vein thrombosis
EBL	estimated blood loss
EBV	Epstein-Barr virus
ECC	extracorporeal circulation
ECCE	extracapsular cataract extraction
ECG, EKG	electrocardiogram
ECHO	echocardiography
ECP	emergency contraceptive pills
ECT	electroconvulsive therapy
EDD	estimated delivery date
EEG	electroencephalogram
EGD	esophagogastroduodenoscopy
EM, Em	emmetropia
EMG	electromyography
ENT	ear, nose, and throat
EOM	extraocular movements
Eosins	eosinophils
ER	emergency room
ERCP	endoscopic retrograde cholangiopancreatography
ERT	estrogen replacement therapy
ESR	erythrocyte sedimentation rate
ESRD	end-stage renal disease
ESWL	extracorporal shockwave lithotripsy
EST	exercise stress test
F	female
FB	foreign body
FBS	fasting blood sugar
FHR	fetal heart rate
FOBT	fecal occult blood test
FSH	follicle stimulating hormone
FTA-ABS	fluorescent treponemal antibody absorption test
Fx	fracture
G	grade
GAD	generalized anxiety disorder
GAF	global assessment of functioning
GB	gallbladder
Gc	gonococcus
GERD	gastroesophageal reflux disease
GI	gastrointestinal
GIFT	gamete intrafallopian transfer
GTT	glucose tolerance test
H	hypodermic
HAV	hepatitis A virus
Hb	hemoglobin
HBV	hepatitis B virus
hCG	human chorionic gonadotropin
Hct	hematocrit, packed cell volume
HD	hemodialysis
HDL	high-density lipids
HDN	hemolytic disease of the newborn
Hg	mercury
Hgb	hemoglobin
HGH	human growth hormone
HHN	hand-held nebulizer
HIV	human immunodeficiency virus
HPV	human papilloma virus
HRT	hormone replacement therapy
HSV-1	herpes simplex virus 1
HSV-2	herpes simplex virus 2; herpes genitalis
Hx	history
I&D	incision and drainage
IBS	irritable bowel syndrome
ICCE	intracapsular cataract extraction

Abbreviations—cont'd

Abbreviation	Meaning
ICD	implantable cardiac defibrillator; International Classification of Diseases
ICP	intracranial pressure
ICSI	intracytoplasmic sperm injection
ID	intradermal
IDDM	insulin-dependent diabetes mellitus (Type I diabetes)
Ig	immunoglobin
IOL	intraocular lens
IOP	intraocular pressure
IQ	intelligence quotient
IU	international unit
IUD	intrauterine device
IVF	in vitro fertilization
IVU	intravenous urogram
K	potassium
KUB	kidneys, ureters, bladder
L&A	light and accommodation
L	liter
L1-L5	first lumbar through fifth lumbar vertebrae; lumbar nerves
LA	left atrium
LAD	left anterior descending (coronary artery)
Lap	laparoscopy
LASIK	laser in situ keratomileusis
LCA	left circumflex artery, left coronary artery
LD	lactic dehydrogenase (formerly LDH)
LDH	lactate dehydrogenase
LDL	low-density lipids
LE	left eye
LH	luteinizing hormone
LLL	left lower lobe
LLQ	lower left quadrant
LMCA	left main coronary artery
LMP	last menstrual period
LP	lumbar puncture
LPN	licensed practical nurse
LRQ	lower right quadrant
LUL	left upper lobe
LV	left ventricle
Lymphs	lymphocytes
M	male
MA/OM	medical assistant/office manager
MCH	mean corpuscular hemoglobin
MCHC	mean corpuscular hemoglobin concentration
MD	muscular dystrophy
MDI	metered-dose inhaler
mets	metastases
mg	milligram
MI	myocardial infarction
MR	mental retardation; mitral regurgitation
MRI	magnetic resonance imaging
MS	multiple sclerosis; mitral stenosis; musculoskeletal
MSH	melanocyte-stimulating hormone
MUGA	multigated (radionuclide) angiogram
MV	mitral valve
MVP	mitral valve prolapse
MY	myopia
N&V	nausea and vomiting
Na	sodium
Neut	neutrophils
NGU	nongonococcal urethritis
NIDDM	non–insulin-dependent diabetes mellitus (Type II diabetes)
NK	natural killer cells
NKDA	no known drug allergy
NPO	nothing by mouth (Latin, *nil per os*)
NSAID	nonsteroidal antiinflammatory drug
NSE	neuron-specific enolase (used to detect neuroblastoma, small cell cancer)
NSR	normal sinus rhythm
NST	nonstress test
NTG	nitroglycerin
NVA	near visual acuity
O × 1	oriented to time
O × 2	oriented to time and place
O × 3	oriented to time, place, and person
O × 4	oriented to time, place, person, and objects
O_2	oxygen
OA	osteoarthritis
OAE	otoacoustic emissions
Ob	obstetrics
OCD	obsessive-compulsive disorder
OCP	oral contraceptive pill
OD	oculus dextra (right eye)
ODD	oppositional defiant disorder
OM	otitis media
Ophth	ophthalmology
OS	oculus sinistra (left eye)
OT	oxytocin
OTC	over the counter (drug)

Continued

Abbreviations—cont'd

Abbreviation	Meaning
Oto	otology
OU	oculus uterque (each eye)
P	phosphorus
PA	posteroanterior; pulmonary artery
PAC	premature atrial contractions
PAP	Papanicolaou test; prostatic acid phosphatase
PCV	packed cell volume; hematocrit
PD	Parkinson's disease
PDA	patent ductus arteriosus
PERRLA	pupils equal, round, reactive to light and accommodation
PET scan	positron emission tomography scan
PGH	pituitary growth hormone
pH	acidity/alkalinity
PHL	permanent hearing loss
PID	pelvic inflammatory disease
PK	penetrating keratoplasty (corneal transplant)
PKU	phenylketonuria
Plats	platelets; thrombocytes
PMDD	premenstrual dysphoric disorder
PMNs, polys	polymorphonucleocytes
PMS	premenstrual syndrome
PNS	peripheral nervous system
PPB	positive pressure breathing
PPD	purified protein derivative
prn	as needed (Latin, *pro re nata*)
PRK	photorefractive keratectomy
PSA	prostate-specific antigen
PSG	polysomnography
PT	prothrombin time
PTCA	percutaneous transluminal coronary angioplasty
PTH	parathyroid hormone
PTSD	posttraumatic stress disorder
PTT	partial thromboplastin time
PUD	peptic ulcer disease
PUVA	psoralen ultraviolet A
PV	pulmonary vein
PVC	premature ventricular contractions
RA	rheumatoid arthritis; right atrium
RAD	reactive airway disease
RAIU	radioactive iodine uptake
RBC	red blood cell (count)
RCA	right coronary artery
RE	right eye
RF	rheumatoid factor
RFA	radiofrequency catheter ablation
Rh	rhesus
RHIA	registered health information administrator
RHIT	registered health information technician
RIA	radioimmunoassay
RK	radial keratotomy
RLL	right lower lobe
RML	right middle lobe
ROM	range of motion
RRT	registered respiratory therapist
RUL	right upper lobe
RV	right ventricle
Rx	prescription (drug)
s̄ gl	without glasses
S1-S5	first sacral through fifth sacral vertebrae; sacral nerves
SA	sinoatrial
SAD	seasonal affective disorder
SAH	subarachnoid hemorrhage
SG	specific gravity; skin graft
SGOT	serum glutamic oxaloacetate transaminase
SNS	somatic nervous system
SOB	shortness of breath
SOM	serous otitis media
SPECT	single photon emission computed tomography
SPF	sun protection factor
SSRI	selective serotonin reuptake inhibitor
SSS	sick sinus syndrome
STD	sexually transmitted disease
STSG	split-thickness skin graft
Sx	symptoms; streptokinase
T1-T12	first thoracic through twelfth thoracic vertebrae; thoracic nerves
T_3	triiodothyronine
T_4	thyroxine
T_7	thyroid-stimulating hormone
TAH-BSO	total abdominal hysterectomy with a bilateral salpingo-oophorectomy
TB	tuberculosis
TDN	transdermal nitroglycerin
TDNTG	transdermal nitroglycerin
TEA	thromboendarterectomy
TEE	transesophageal echocardiogram
TENS	transcutaneous electrical nerve stimulation

Abbreviations—cont'd

Abbreviation	*Meaning*	*Abbreviation*	*Meaning*
TFTs	thyroid function tests	USP	United States Pharmacopeia (National Formulary)
THR	total hip replacement	UTI	urinary tract infection
TIA	transient ischemic attack	UV	ultraviolet
TKR	total knee replacement	VA	visual acuity
TMR	transmyocardial revascularization	VAD	ventricular assist device
TNM	tumor, nodes, metastases	VBAC	vaginal birth after cesarean section
TS	tricuspid stenosis	VCUG	voiding cystourethrography
TSE	testicular self-examination	VD	venereal disease
TSH	thyroid-stimulating hormone	VDRL	Venereal Disease Research Laboratory (test for syphilis)
TTS	transdermal therapeutic system	VEB	ventricular ectopic beats
TUR	transurethral resection	VF	visual field
TURP	transurethral resection of the prostate	VLDL	very low density lipids
TV	tricuspid valve	VMA	urine vanillylmandelic acid
UA	urinalysis	VP	vasopressin (also known as ADH)
UAE	uterine artery embolization	VSD	ventricular septal defect
ULQ	upper left quadrant	WAIS	Weschler Adult Intelligence Scale
Ung	ointment	WBC	white blood cell (count)
URI	upper respiratory infection	WNL	within normal limits
URQ	upper right quadrant	ZIFT	zygote intrafallopian transfer
US	ultrasound		

Answers to Exercise and Review Questions

Chapter 1 Exercises

Exercise 1

1. E 2. C 3. A 4. B
5. D

Exercise 2

1. F 2. J 3. H 4. B
5. A 6. C 7. G 8. D
9. I 10. E 11. J 12. G
13. A 14. B 15. I 16. C
17. F 18. D 19. H 20. E
21. D 22. H 23. C 24. B
25. A 26. G 27. F 28. J
29. E 30. I
31. word root, suffix
32. end, beginning
33. pronounce
34. inflammation, skin
35. A. nat, birth
    B. -al, pertaining to
    C. pre-, before
    D. pertaining to before birth
36. C 37. D 38. E 39. B
40. A
41. ps, psoriasis
42. phobia
43. xeroderma
44. eupnea
45. pneumoconiosis

Exercise 3

1. colectomy
2. odontectomy
3. ophthalmoscopy
4. arthroplasty
5. neonatology
6. gastralgia
7. osteoarthropathy
8. gastroenteritis
9. dermatitis
10. tympanoplasty
11. thrombi
12. biopsies
13. septa
14. prognoses
15. bullae
16. larynges

Exercise 4

1. A. symptom B. sign
   C. symptom D. sign
2. A. L B. I C. L D. I
3. C 4. B 5. A 6. D
7. F 8. G 9. B 10. C
11. A 12. E 13. D
14. A. arthro/tome—instrument to cut a joint
    B. electro/cardio/graph—instrument to record the electricity of the heart
    C. opthalmo/scope—instrument to visually examine the eye
    D. thermo/meter—instrument to measure heat (temperature)
    E. litho/tripter—instrument to crush stones

Exercise 5

1. H 2. I 3. F 4. A
5. D 6. E 7. J 8. G
9. C 10. B

Chapter 1 Review Questions

1. Greek, Latin
2. eponym
3. word root
4. do not
5. prefix
6. do
7. I 8. F 9. H 10. E
11. G 12. B 13. A 14. D
15. J 16. C 17. Q 18. N
19. T 20. R 21. L 22. S
23. P 24. M 25. K 26. O
27. H 28. G 29. D 30. J
31. B 32. A 33. I 34. F
35. E 36. C 37. F 38. I
39. E 40. G 41. C 42. H
43. D 44. B 45. J 46. A
47. hepatitis
48. hemigastrectomy
49. arthroscopy
50. osteotomy
51. hematology
52. cardiologist
53. neonatal
54. appendicitis
55. ophthalmoscope
56. anesthesiologist
57. pain in the eye
58. treatment of disorders of the aged
59. enlargement of the heart
60. pain of the joint
61. condition of deficient body temperature
62. instrument to visually examine a joint
63. instrument to measure temperature
64. instrument to record the electricity of the heart
65. instrument to crush stones
66. instrument to listen to the chest
67. visual examination of the inside of the body
68. instrument to visually examine the eye
69. visual examination of the ear
70. record of a joint
71. instrument to cut bone
72. pleurae
73. prognosis
74. pharynges
75. arthroscopy
76. septum
77. pre- (before)
    per- (through)
    peri- (surrounding)
78. ante- (before)
    anti- (against)
79. -ectomy (removal)
    -tomy (incision)
    -stomy (new opening)

Chapter 2 Exercises

Exercise 1

1. D 2. E 3. A 4. C
5. B

Exercise 2

1. C 2. A 3. D 4. B

Exercise 3

1. E 2. C 3. I 4. D
5. A 6. G 7. H 8. B
9. F
10. lumen
11. hilum
12. apex
13. body
14. sinuses

Exercise 4

1. E 2. K 3. H 4. J
5. C 6. B 7. A 8. D
9. I 10. F 11. G 12. L

Exercise 5

1. J 2. G 3. D 4. E
5. A 6. C 7. F 8. I
9. L 10. K 11. B 12. H
13. cardiovascular
14. inflammation, testes
15. windpipe
16. ear
17. cystoscopy

Exercise 6

1. C 2. A 3. F 4. K
5. I 6. J 7. L 8. E
9. D 10. H 11. G 12. B
13. left
14. on her back
15. sole
16. distal
17. afferent

Exercise 7

1. D 2. C 3. B 4. A
5. E
6. craniotomy
7. abdominal
8. mediastinoscopy
9. peritonitis
10. pelvic

Exercise 8

1. epigastric
2. lumbar
3. hypogastric
4. inguinal or iliac
5. hypochondriac

Exercise 9

1. transverse
2. midsagittal
3. frontal or coronal

Chapter 2 Review Questions

1. organism → systems → organs → tissues → cells
2. Homeostasis is the body's mechanism of physiologic balance to deal with internal and external change.
3. A. ribosomes
   B. mitochondria
   C. cytoplasm
   D. lysosomes
   E. nucleus
4. Muscle tissue
5. Connective tissue
6. Epithelial tissue
7. Nervous tissue
8. reproductive
9. integumentary
10. digestive
11. cardiovascular
12. urinary
13. blood, lymphatic
14. musculoskeletal
15. respiratory
16. nervous
17. endocrine
18. sensory
19. A. inferior B. supine
    C. lateral D. pronate
    E. posterior F. proximal
    G. cephalad H. superficial
    I. dorsal J. efferent
    K. contralateral
20. pronation
21. superficial
22. proximal
23. anterior
24. sinistrocardia
25. dorsal, back
26. ventral, front
27. cranial
28. spinal
29. pelvic
30. thoracic
31. mediastinum
32. pleura
33. thoracic, abdominal
34. abdominal
35. peritoneum
36. See Fig. 2-5.
37. See Fig. 2-6.
38. See Figs. 2-7 to 2-9.
39. 11:30 AM
40. arthroscopy
41. 12:30 PM
42. esophagogastroduodenoscopy
43. colonoscopy
44. fornices
45. lumina
46. apices
47. fundi
48. larynges
49. uteri
50. hila
51. nuclei
52. pleurae
53. crania
54. mitochondria
55. viscera
56. ile/o (part of small intestine); ili/o (part of hip bone)
57. my/o (muscle); myel/o (spinal cord, bone marrow)
58. cyt/o (cell); cyst/o (urinary bladder)
59. hyper- (excessive); hypo- (deficient)
60. anter/o (front); antr/o (antrum)
61. bi- (two); bi/o (life)
62. closest to the wrist
63. backwards
64. joint
65. backside

Chapter 3 Exercises

Exercise 1

1. E, J 2. C 3. I 4. G
5. H, K 6. A 7. F 8. B
9. D 10. L

Exercise 2

1. K 2. I 3. J 4. D
5. G 6. H 7. E 8. C
9. L 10. F 11. A 12. B
13. build, breakdown
14. diaphysis, epiphyses
15. periosteum, endosteum
16. depressions, processes
17. antrum

Exercise 3

See Fig. 3-3.

Exercise 4

1. zygoma
2. maxilla
3. mandible
4. lacrimal
5. vomer

Exercise 5

1. See Fig. 3-4.
2. lumbosacral

Exercise 6

1. C 2. D 3. E 4. A
5. B

Exercise 7

1. leg
2. leg
3. arm
4. shoulder girdle
5. pelvic girdle
6. pelvic girdle
7. shoulder girdle
8. leg

Exercise 8

1. D 2. G 3. F 4. E
5. B 6. A 7. H 8. C

Exercise 9

1. metatarsophalangeal
2. pubis, ilium, ischium
3. A. tibia
   B. patella
   C. femur
   D. phalanges
   E. metatarsals
   F. fibula
   G. tarsals
4. distal

Exercise 10

1. A. synarthrosis
   B. diarthrosis
   C. amphiarthrosis
2. bursae
3. bursae, joint capsules, articular cartilage

Exercise 11

1. eversion
2. supination
3. rotation
4. abduction
5. plantar flexion
6. protraction
7. flexion
8. inversion
9. adduction
10. extension
11. C 12. A 13. B

Exercise 12

1. A 2. H 3. B 4. D
5. E 6. F 7. G 8. C

Exercise 13

1. G 2. D 3. A 4. E
5. F 6. B 7. C

Exercise 14

1. A 2. D 3. F 4. G
5. I 6. E 7. B 8. H
9. C

Exercise 15

1. subluxation
2. sprain
3. strain
4. dislocation

Exercise 16

1. I 2. P 3. H 4. G
5. B 6. K 7. M 8. C
9. E 10. F 11. L 12. D
13. N 14. A 15. O 16. J
17. C 18. B 19. A

Exercise 17

1. I 2. H 3. G 4. A
5. D 6. C 7. B 8. F
9. J 10. E

Exercise 18

1. A. arthroplasty
   B. osteoclasis
   C. bunionectomy
   D. tenomyoplasty
2. H 3. C 4. G 5. A
6. B 7. J 8. F 9. I
10. E 11. D

Exercise 19

1. alendronate (Fosamax), risedronate (Actonel)
2. methotrexate, leflunomide (Arava), etanercept (Enbrel), infliximab (Remicade)
3. pain and inflammation
4. osteoarthritis

Exercise 20

1. fracture of the fifth lumbar vertebra
2. nonsteroidal antiinflammatory drugs
3. range of motion
4. CTS (carpal tunnel syndrome)
5. complementary and alternative medicine

Chapter 3 Review Questions

A. Answers will vary.

1. See Fig. 3-2.
2. A. structure within the bone
   B. structure surrounding the bone
   C. through growth (shaft of long bone)
   D. above the growth
   E. growth change
   F. embryonic bone (cells)
   G. (cells that) break down bone
   H. bone cell
3. cranium
4. ribcage
5. face
6. ribcage
7. cranium
8. face
9. spine
10. spine
11. cranium
12. cartilage (chondr/o); bursa (burs/o)
13. ad- (means towards); ab- (means away)
14. many fingers/toes
15. condition of lack of cartilage formation
16. hidden condition of spine "split" in two
17. abnormal development of muscles
18. fingers/toes joined together
19. softening of bone
20. inflammation of bone and bone marrow
21. severe muscle weakness
22. condition of slippage of vertebrae
23. abnormal condition of narrowing of spinal canal
24. simple/closed
25. comminuted
26. greenstick
27. pathologic
28. Colles'
29. subluxation
30. sprain
31. childhood
32. carpal tunnel syndrome
33. degenerative joint disease, osteoarthritis
34. rheumatoid
35. gout
36. metatarsophalangeal
37. lumbago
38. sciatica
39. kyphosis (hunchback); lordosis (swayback); scoliosis (lateral S curve of spine)
40. fibromyalgia
41. contracture
42. A. record of the spinal cord
    B. visual examination of a joint
    C. process of recording the electrical activity of a muscle
    D. process of recording a joint
43. electromyography
44. myelogram
45. arthrography
46. a DEXA scan
47. rheumatoid factor
48. A. suture of muscle
    B. surgical repair of hump (fractured vertebra)
    C. binding vertebrae together
    D. condition of stiffening
    E. removal of a lamina
    F. surgical repair of muscles and tendons
    G. surgical fracture of bone
    H. stabilization of a joint
    I. surgical puncture of a joint
    J. surgical repair of bone
49. reduction
50. open reduction
51. internal fixation
52. invasive
53. malunion
54. sequestrum
55. amputation, prosthesis
56. spondylodesis, spondylosyndesis
57. osteoporosis
58. rheumatic
59. osteoarthritis
60. pain and inflammation
61. calcium
62. fracture
63. second cervical vertebra
64. range of motion
65. degenerative joint disease, nonsteroidal antiinflammatory drugs
66. foramina
67. bursae
68. prostheses
69. phalanges
70. sulci
71. vertebrae
72. ilia
73. pelves
74. arthroscopies
75. costae

76. The process of recording the joint revealed the child's partially bent and partially broken right upper arm bone.
77. Ms. Burton-Smith was treated for inflammation of the bursa secondary to an injury with heat, rest, and nonsteroidal antiinflammatory drugs.
78. The basketball player had a surgical fracture of the bone for a bad joining of one of his hand bones.
79. The patient was sent for an ultrasonography of her heel bone to assess her abnormal condition of porosity of the bone and bone loss.
80. The patient complained of lower back pain resulting from his narrowing of the spinal canal.
81. The process of recording the electrical activity of the muscles was used to confirm the child's lack of muscle development.
82. bilateral
83. proximal
84. supine
85. transverse
86. thoracic
87. cervical
88. sacroiliac
89. myorrhaphy
90. musculoskeletal
91. ilium
92. peroneal
93. periosteum
94. calcium and phosphorus
95. acetabulum
96. radius
97. hematopoiesis
98. 150 cc
99. the front
100. kneecap
101. near the kneecap
102. incision of the joint
103. turned outward
104. instrument to cut bone
105. an overextension of a joint

Chapter 4 Exercises

Exercise 1

1. A. wastes
   B. barrier
   C. touch
   D. temperature
   E. bones, teeth

2. F 3. D 4. E 5. A
6. B 7. C

Exercise 2

1. D 2. F 3. B 4. E
5. A 6. C, G
7. sudoriferous
8. pores
9. bacteria
10. follicle
11. thermoregulation
12. cuticle
13. melanin
14. keratin
15. bed

Exercise 3

1. pruritus
2. Primary lesions are early skin lesions that have not undergone natural evolution or manipulated changes.
3. E 4. F 5. C 6. A
7. B 8. D 9. C 10. D
11. A 12. E 13. B 14. F
15. G 16. D 17. E 18. H
19. B 20. A 21. C

Exercise 4

1. eczema
2. atopic dermatitis
3. contact dermatitis
4. seborrheic dermatitis
5. paronychia
6. cellulitis
7. impetigo
8. furuncle
9. folliculitis
10. carbuncles

Exercise 5

1. D 2. C 3. F 4. B
5. E 6. A
7. pediculosis
8. herpes zoster
9. verrucae
10. HSV
11. scabies
12. dermatomycosis

Exercise 6

1. rosacea
2. psoriasis
3. hypertrichosis
4. trichotillomania
5. alopecia
6. keratinous cyst
7. acne
8. clavus
9. pressure sore or decubitus ulcer
10. milia
11. xeroderma

Exercise 7

1. hyperhidrosis
2. hypopigmentation
3. vitiligo
4. albinism
5. miliaria
6. melasma, chloasma

Exercise 8

1. D 2. A 3. B 4. E
5. C 6. F

Exercise 9

1. C 2. A 3. D 4. B
5. eschar
6. extent or percentages

Exercise 10

1. excisional
2. needle aspiration
3. incisional
4. exfoliation
5. punch
6. F 7. C 8. E 9. B
10. G 11. A 12. D

Exercise 11

1. A. skin graft from self
   B. skin graft from another human
   C. skin graft from other species
2. split thickness skin graft
3. dermatome
4. Laser therapy
5. debridement
6. cauterization
7. cryosurgery
8. curettage
9. incision and drainage
10. shaving
11. occlusive therapy
12. E 13. D 14. F 15. C
16. A 17. B 18. G

Exercise 12

1. intradermal
2. topical
3. hypodermic
4. transdermal therapeutic system
5. analgesic
6. aloe
7. acne
8. antibacterials
9. antifungal
10. aspirin, triamcinolone, hydrocortisone, fluocinonide (Lidex)
11. D 12. C 13. A 14. B
15. E 16. F 17. G

Exercise 13

1. ID
2. UV
3. SG
4. Decub
5. FB
6. OTC
7. Bx
8. Hx
9. TTS
10. Ung

Chapter 4 Review Questions

1. To cover and protect the body, help regulate body temperature, provide information through the sense of touch, eliminate waste products, and help synthesize vitamins.
2. See Fig. 4-1.
3. A. derm/o, dermat/o, cutane/o
   B. trich/o, pil/o
   C. onych/o, ungu/o
   D. hidraden/o
   E. seb/o
   F. follicul/o
4. strata
5. avascular
6. dermis, corium
7. adipose, hypodermis (subcutaneous)
8. inflammation of the skin
9. inflammation of the hair follicle
10. abnormal condition of fungus of the nails
11. tumor of a vessel
12. abnormal condition of excessive sweating
13. abnormal condition of excessive hair growth
14. abnormal condition of hardened flow of sebum
15. fat tumor
16. abnormal formation of mole
17. dry skin
18. any visible, localized abnormality of the skin
19. Primary lesions are early skin changes that have not undergone a natural evolution or change caused by manipulation. Secondary lesions have not undergone change or evolution.
20. A. pinpoint hemorrhages
    B. hemorrhage into subcutaneous tissue
    C. massive hemorrhage under the skin
    D. collection of blood trapped in tissue
    E. permanent dilation of groups of superficial capillaries and venules
21. All are lesions associated with blood vessel disruption.
22. A. vesicle
    B. crust
    C. macule
    D. cicatrix
    E. ecchymosis
    F. ulcer
    G. atrophy
23. folliculitis
24. tinea pedis
25. candidiasis or moniliasis
26. pediculosis
27. scabies
28. warts
29. herpes zoster
30. alopecia
31. ichthyosis
32. A corn is a thickened area over a bony prominence; a callus is thickening over areas of pressure or friction.
33. albinism or vitiligo
34. melasma or chloasma
35. scar tissue over a burn
36. A. epidermis—redness, hyperesthesia
    B. dermis—redness, blisters, pain
    C. subcutaneous tissue—no pain, change in skin coloration
    D. muscle and bone—bone and muscle visible, no pain
37. excisional
38. needle aspiration
39. incisional
40. exfoliation
41. punch
42. Tzanck test
43. Wood's light examination
44. tuberculosis
45. sweat
46. wound, abscess
47. viral
48. bacterial
49. fungal
50. A. instrument to cut skin
    B. surgical repair of skin
    C. incision of a scab
    D. destruction of tissue using extreme cold
    E. excision of fatty tissue
    F. excision of wrinkles
    G. surgical procedure to resurface the skin
51. A. replacement of skin with one's own skin
    B. replacement of skin with skin from a donor
    C. replacement of skin with skin from another species
52. cold, heat
53. A. slicing of thin sheets of tissue to remove a lesion
    B. removal of foreign bodies and dirt from a wound
    C. scraping material from a cavity wall for microscopic examination
54. occlusive
55. intradermal
56. topical
57. complementary and alternative medicine (CAM)
58. herbal
59. anesthetic
60. break down hardened skin
61. pediculicide
62. antipruritic
63. emollients
64. biopsy
65. split thickness skin graft
66. no known drug allergies
67. HSV
68. incision, drainage
69. decubitus ulcer, bedsore, pressure ulcer
70. transdermal therapeutic system
71. PUVA
72. Hx
73. striae
74. bullae
75. onychomycoses
76. decubiti
77. ecchymoses
78. petechiae
79. comedones
80. verrucae
81. strata
82. The patient had a wart on the bottom surface of his foot removed with extreme cold.
83. The elderly patient developed a pressure sore from lack of proper care during an extended hospital stay.
84. The patient bought a wig to cover her baldness caused by a condition of pulling out her hair.
85. Mr. Hassan complained of intense itching from hives.
86. The patient was in for an incision of a scab and a consultation for a possible replacement of skin from a human donor.
87. dorsal
88. superficial
89. word root
90. a piece of dead bone

91. A. skin tag
 B. corn
 C. birthmark
 D. hypertrichosis
 E. wart
 F. scar
 G. decubitus ulcer
92. hidr/o (sweat); hydr/o (water)
93. milia (disorder of sebaceous glands); miliaria (disorder of sudoriferous glands)
94. stria (stretch mark); strata (layers)
95. ID (intradermal); I&D (incision and drainage)
96. papill/o (papilla); papul/o (papule)
97. B
98. bulla, blisters, epidermal loss, erythema
99. the hot liquid (coffee)
100. 3 cm

Chapter 5 Exercises

Exercise 1
1. alimentary, GI
2. nutrients, cells
3. digestion
4. absorption
5. elimination
6. ingestion

7. C 8. D 9. F 10. B
11. A 12. E

Exercise 2
1. M 2. H 3. F 4. E, I
5. K, D 6. C, G 7. B 8. O
9. J 10. N 11. L 12. A
13. pharynx
14. oropharynx
15. nasopharynx
16. hypopharynx
17. esophagus
18. sphincter
19. bolus
20. parotid
21. sublingual
22. submandibular
23. lower esophageal sphincter
24. cardiac sphincter
25. gastroesophageal sphincter

Exercise 3
1. J 2. K 3. O 4. H
5. P 6. I 7. N 8. R
9. F 10. L 11. G 12. B
13. S 14. E 15. D 16. M
17. A 18. C
19. pyloric sphincter → duodenum → jejunum → ileum → ileocecal valve → cecum and appendix → ascending colon → transverse colon → descending colon → sigmoid colon → rectum → anal sphincter
20. chyme, feces
21. absorb nutrients
22. small

Exercise 4
1. G 2. D 3. A 4. C
5. B 6. E 7. F
8. A. URQ, ULQ
 B. URQ
 C. ULQ
9. adnexa
10. emulsification
11. cholecystokinin
12. bilirubin
13. cholesterol

Exercise 5
1. H 2. I 3. E 4. G
5. B 6. J 7. C 8. D
9. A 10. F 11. D 12. B
13. E 14. C 15. A

Exercise 6
1. esophageal atresia
2. cleft palate
3. Hirschsprung's disease
4. congenital megacolon
5. pyloric stenosis

Exercise 7
1. A 2. F 3. E 4. H
5. D 6. G 7. I 8. J
9. C 10. B

Exercise 8
1. F 2. D, E 3. C 4. A, H, I
5. B 6. G

Exercise 9
1. H 2. K 3. O 4. C
5. L 6. R 7. P 8. D
9. G 10. M 11. F 12. E
13. N 14. S 15. I 16. J
17. Q 18. A 19. B

Exercise 10
1. cirrhosis
2. cholelithiasis
3. cholangitis
4. choledocholithiasis
5. pancreatitis
6. hepatitis
7. cholecystitis

Exercise 11
1. A 2. B 3. F 4. C
5. D 6. E

Exercise 12
1. ultrasonography
2. barium swallow
3. cholecystography
4. CT scan
5. cholangiography
6. barium enema
7. manometry
8. stool culture
9. guaiac, hemoccult
10. biopsy
11. total bilirubin
12. gamma-glutamyl transferase
13. endoscopy
14. fluoroscopy

Exercise 13
1. B 2. E 3. A 4. F
5. H 6. N 7. J 8. M
9. G 10. L 11. D 12. I
13. K 14. C

Exercise 14
1. F 2. C 3. D 4. E
5. G 6. A 7. B

Exercise 15
1. bowel movements
2. gallbladder
3. nausea and vomiting
4. gastroesophageal reflux disease
5. irritable bowel syndrome

Chapter 5 Review Questions

1. Ingestion—taking in food. Digestion—breaking it down. Absorption—extracting nutrients. Elimination—excreting waste products of the digestive process.
2. Answers will vary.
3. See Figs. 5-1 and 5-5.
4. Tongue (lingu/o, gloss/o) → pharynx (pharyng/o) → esophagus (esophag/o) → stomach (gastr/o) → duodenum (duoden/o) → jejunum (jejun/o) → ileum (ile/o) → cecum (cec/o) → ascending colon, transverse colon, descending colon (col/o) → sigmoid colon (sigmoid/o) → rectum (rect/o) → anus (an/o)/ rectum and anus (proct/o)

5. A. mastication
   B. deglutition
   C. defecation
   D. emulsification
6. lobes
7. plicae
8. lumen
9. villi
10. -ase
11. -ose
12. bilirubin
13. cholesterol
14. chyme
15. pertaining to under the tongue
16. pertaining to the lower throat
17. pertaining to the stomach and esophagus
18. pertaining to the ileum and cecum
19. pertaining to the liver and gallbladder
20. buccal
21. gingivitis
22. cholecystitis
23. esophageal atresia
24. diverticulitis
25. hematemesis
26. inflammation of the lips
27. abnormal narrowing of the muscle between the stomach and duodenum
28. presence of stones in the common bile duct
29. pain in the anus and rectum
30. inflammation of the stomach and small intestines
31. condition of no relaxation
32. condition of white patches
33. flow/discharge of pus
34. poor/bad closure
35. bloody feces
36. difficulty swallowing
37. intussusception
38. volvulus
39. regurgitation
40. hemorrhoids
41. cirrhosis
42. dental caries
43. diarrhea
44. flatus
45. anal fissure
46. pruritus ani
47. halitosis
48. eructation
49. Hirschsprung's disease
50. herpetic stomatitis
51. dyspepsia
52. pyrosis
53. aphthous stomatitis
54. hiatal hernia
55. peptic ulcer disease
56. hemoccult test, stool guaiac
57. endoscopy
58. biopsy
59. stool culture
60. gamma-glutamyl transferase (GGT)
61. barium swallow
62. barium enema
63. cholecystography
64. tests motor function of the esophagus
65. removal of the gallbladder
66. new opening (joining) between stomach and third part of small intestine
67. new opening of the colon (large intestine)
68. removal of half the tongue
69. herniorrhaphy
70. laparotomy
71. cholelithotomy
72. gastrectomy
73. hemorrhoidectomy
74. duodenojejunostomy
75. ligation
76. lysis of adhesions
77. paracentesis
78. anastomosis
79. stoma
80. enema
81. antiemetic
82. laxative
83. cathartic
84. antibiotic
85. antidiarrheal
86. cholesterol-reducing agent
87. anorexiants
88. upper gastrointestinal, gastroesophageal reflux disease, peptic ulcer disease, hepatitis A virus, esophagogastroduodenoscopy
89. nausea and vomiting, bowel movements, gallbladder
90. gamma-glutamyl transferase, peptic ulcer disease
91. nothing by mouth
92. stomata
93. fistulae
94. endoscopies
95. esophagi
96. fundi
97. rugae
98. pharynges
99. anastomoses
100. lumina
101. villi
102. José underwent a new opening of the colon as a result of advanced ulcerative inflammation of the colon.
103. The 5-week-old patient had an incision of the pyloric sphincter to treat a case of abnormal condition of narrowing of the pyloric sphincter.
104. After reporting bloody vomit, black tarry stools, and stomach pain, the patient was found to have peptic ulcer disease.
105. The 35-year-old patient complained of upper right quadrant pain, nausea and vomiting, and fever. After inflammation of the appendix and severe short-term inflammation of the pancreas were ruled out, she was diagnosed with severe short-term inflammation of the gallbladder.
106. Blood in the feces and pain in the rectum and anus were the symptoms leading to a visual examination within the body that revealed swollen, twisted veins in the rectum.
107. LES
108. RLQ
109. smooth muscle (leiomy/o)
110. Join the terms in the order they appear using an "o" to combine the two word roots and adding an "o" in front of the suffix beginning with a consonant (gastroileostomy).
111. thoracic
112. Bx
113. surgical repair of the anus and rectum
114. condition of excessive cholesterol in the blood
115. condition of stones in the salivary glands
116. incision of the common bile duct
117. suture of the small intestine
118. A. anus
     B. up or apart
     C. no, not, without
119. A. herniation
     B. belly
120. A. mouth, opening
     B. mouth, opening
     C. organ between esophagus and small intestine
121. A. region of the abdomen
     B. stomach (an organ)
     C. belly (an area)
122. A. an intestinal obstruction
     B. third part of the small intestines
123. A. fibula
     B. lining of the abdominal cavity (peritoneum)
124. cardia of the stomach, cardiospasm, cardiomegaly
125. -ase (suffix for enzymes), -ose (suffix for carbohydrates)
126. Bovie electrocautery

127. within the trachea (windpipe)
128. below
129. back
130. tie it

Chapter 6 Exercises

Exercise 1

1. homeostasis, extracellular, proteins, urea, excreting

Exercise 2

1. C 2. F 3. D 4. A
5. E 6. G 7. B 8. L
9. J 10. H 11. M 12. I
13. K
14. nephron
15. cortex
16. glomerulus
17. Bowman's
18. afferent
19. Blood and proteins
20. renal cortex → renal medulla → renal pelvis → ureter → urinary bladder → urethra → urinary meatus

Exercise 3

1. F 2. I 3. H 4. B
5. J 6. E 7. C 8. G
9. A 10. D
11. retention
12. edema
13. abscess
14. azotemia
15. enuresis
16. diuresis
17. urgency
18. incontinence

Exercise 4

1. C 2. F 3. D 4. E
5. G 6. A 7. B
8. A. nephrolithiasis
   B. ureterolithiasis
   C. cystolithiasis
   D. urethrolithiasis

Exercise 5

1. C 2. E 3. F 4. B
5. A 6. D 7. L, K 8. I
9. D 10. G 11. J 12. C
13. H 14. A 15. F 16. B
17. K 18. E

Exercise 6

1. dehydration, blockage, strictures
2. pyelonephritis
3. diabetes or kidney damage
4. a UTI
5. UTI
6. DM or starvation
7. kidneys
8. blood, urea, and nitrogen
9. IVU
10. nephrotomography
11. VCUG
12. A. nephroscopy
    B. ureteroscopy
    C. cystoscopy
    D. urethroscopy
13. an open biopsy
14. B 15. D 16. A 17. C
18. F 19. E

Exercise 7

1. C 2. E 3. B 4. F
5. D 6. A
7. urethrolysis
8. ileal conduit
9. lithotripsy
10. dialysis procedures
11. renal transplant

Exercise 8

1. E 2. C 3. F 4. A
5. G 6. D 7. B

Exercise 9

1. diabetes mellitus, liters
2. chronic renal failure, hemodialysis
3. urinalysis specific gravity, diabetes insipidus
4. urinary tract infection
5. voiding cystourethrogram

Chapter 6 Review Questions

1. cleans the blood, regulates blood pressure, maintains homeostasis
2. urea, creatinine, uric acid
3. homeostasis
4. extra
5. voiding, urination, micturition
6. See Figs. 6-1 and 6-2.
7. See Fig. 6-3.
8. nephron, glomerulus
9. Bowman capsule
10. water, electrolytes, glucose, nitrogenous wastes
11. incontinence
12. retention
13. diuresis
14. enuresis
15. edema, hypertension
16. nephritis
17. nephropathy
18. nephrosis
19. nephroptosis
20. renal
21. abnormal narrowing of the urethra
22. surgical repair of the urethra
23. herniation of a ureter
24. inflammation of the renal pelvis
25. incision of the opening of the urethra
26. condition of stones in the kidney
27. inflammation of glomerulus of the kidney
28. pus in the urine
29. blood in the urine
30. scanty urination
31. lack of urination
32. excessive urination
33. bacteria in the urine
34. albumin in the urine
35. bacteria, appearance, blood
36. glucose
37. ketones, color, quantity
38. BUN
39. sectional radiographic exam of the kidney
40. open biopsy
41. IVU
42. A stent supports a tubular structure. A catheter is used to instill or withdraw fluid.
43. measure the specific gravity of urine
44. crush stones
45. ureterostomy
46. urethrolysis
47. transurethral procedure
48. nephrotomy
49. incision to remove stones from the kidney
50. destruction of adhesions in the urethra
51. new opening of the kidney
52. removal of kidney stone through a preexisting opening
53. incision of urinary bladder
54. catheterization
55. hemodialysis
56. transplant
57. lithotripsy
58. nephropexy
59. ileal conduit
60. stone
61. antibiotic
62. enuresis
63. diuretic
64. antidiuretic
65. ESWL
66. UTI
67. UA
68. pH
69. cyst/o
70. HD
71. Na, Cl, K
72. CAPD
73. KUB
74. VCUG

75. CRF
76. nephroses
77. urethrae
78. kidneys
79. glomeruli
80. calyces
81. nephropathies
82. calculi
83. urinalyses
84. protozoa
85. bacteria
86. A 34-year-old patient was admitted with tissue swelling and high blood pressure. Her lab work showed that she had a high blood urea nitrogen and protein in her urine.
87. The 88-year-old woman was admitted for a severe lack of water in her tissues and no production of urine.
88. Mr. Samuels was treated for his kidney stones with a procedure to crush the stones.
89. Once a urinary tract infection was ruled out, Rebecca was evaluated for ongoing bedwetting.
90. An instrument to examine the bladder was used to locate the site of a small urinary cavity containing pus.
91. superior
92. distal
93. proximal
94. lower right
95. dyspepsia
96. seven
97. compound
98. hyperhidrosis
99. verruca
100. ecchymosis
101. ilium
102. pyel/o
103. peritone/o
104. -uria
105. efferent
106. calic/o
107. a stone lodged in the tube between the left kidney and the bladder
108. normal caliber distal ureter, no strictures
109. acute exacerbation
110. yes, hydronephrosis
111. cystoscopy, retrograde pyelogram
112. atraumatically

Chapter 7 Exercises

Exercise 1

1. D 2. K 3. A 4. G
5. B 6. I 7. J 8. L
9. H 10. F 11. E 12. C
13. copulation, coitus
14. gametes
15. ejaculation
16. genitalia
17. gonads
18. spermatogenesis
19. puberty
20. conception
21. parenchymal
22. stromal

Exercise 2

1. F 2. B 3. D 4. C
5. E 6. A
7. testitis
8. benign prostatic hyperplasia
9. testicular torsion
10. varicocele
11. erectile dysfunction
12. gynecomastia
13. balanitis
14. hydrocele
15. epididymitis
16. azoospermia

Exercise 3

1. condylomata
2. chlamydia
3. syphilis
4. nongonococcal urethritis
5. gonorrhea
6. chancres
7. asymptomatic
8. human papilloma virus
9. herpes simplex virus-2

Exercise 4

1. A. DRE, PSA
   B. VDRL, FTA-ABS
   C. sperm analysis
   D. gram stain
2. digital rectal examination
3. ultrasonography

Exercise 5

1. F 2. I 3. A 4. G
5. B 6. D 7. J 8. E
9. H 10. C

Exercise 6

1. D 2. A 3. B 4. E
5. C

Exercise 7

1. BPH
2. STD
3. syphilis
4. digital rectal examination used to diagnose BPH
5. HPV
6. genitourinary

Chapter 7 Review Questions

1. Continue the human species.
2. sexual intercourse
3. release of spermatozoa and seminal fluid
4. joining of egg and sperm (fertilization)
5. See Fig. 7-1.
6. cryptorchidism
7. epididymitis
8. anorchism
9. orchitis (testitis)
10. varicocele
11. Inflammation of glans penis
12. inflammation of the urethra not caused by gonorrhea
13. condition of scant sperm
14. inflammation of the testicle
15. prostatic development of the prostate
16. hypospadias
17. phimosis
18. testicular torsion
19. BPH
20. erectile dysfunction
21. DRE, PSA
22. VDRL or FTA-ABS
23. ultrasonography
24. semen analysis (sperm count)
25. orchiopexy
26. circumcision
27. prostatectomy
28. removal of both testicles
29. excision of vas deferens
30. rejoining of vas deferens
31. castration
32. ablation
33. circumcision
34. TURP
35. sterilization
36. antibiotic
37. antiviral
38. BPH
39. antiimpotence
40. prostate
41. TPA
42. human papilloma virus
43. HSV-2

44. TURP
45. STD (VD)
46. testes
47. epididymides
48. scrota
49. penes
50. spermatozoa
51. A semen analysis revealed scanty sperm that caused the couple's inability to reproduce.
52. The patient's benign prostatic hypertrophy was diagnosed after a digital rectal examination and prostatic-specific antigen.
53. Sam's painful swelling of the testicles was diagnosed as inflammation of epididymis.
54. When the college student appeared at the clinic, he had been experiencing painful urination and a mucus and pus discharge. He was asked to bring in his girlfriend even though he said she was without symptoms.
55. The physician suggested incision to remove the foreskin from the penis to treat the patient's tightening of the foreskin.
56. unilateral
57. anastomosis
58. urinary retention
59. prone
60. vesic/o (bladder), vesicul/o (seminal vesicle)
61. cry/o (cold), crypt/o (hidden)
62. phall/o (penis), phalang/o (bone of finger or toe)
63. urethr/o (urethra), ureter/o (ureter)
64. proct/o (anus and rectum), prostat/o (prostate)
65. a protrusion of part of the stomach through the diaphragm
66. A. painful or difficult urination
    B. inability to hold urine
    C. sensation of needing to urinate
    D. frequency of urination
    E. blood in urine
67. 3
68. transurethral resection of the prostate
69. Peri- means surrounding, so they would be surrounding the prostate gland.

Chapter 8 Exercises

Exercise 1

1. C 2. D 3. A 4. E
5. B

Exercise 2

1. I 2. M 3. J 4. K
5. A 6. L 7. C 8. N
9. H 10. B 11. F 12. E
13. D 14. G

Exercise 3

1. E 2. F 3. A 4. A
5. B 6. F, G 7. C 8. D
9. F 10. A 11. B 12. H

Exercise 4

1. E 2. C 3. B 4. A
5. D 6. B, J 7. D, F 8. G
9. A, I 10. L 11. E, K 12. H
13. C

Exercise 5

1. zygote (2 weeks) → embryo (3-8 weeks) → fetus (9-38 weeks)
2. E 3. D 4. B
5. F 6. A 7. C
8. C, J, H 9. B, E 10. A, G
11. D 12. F, I 13. K

Exercise 6

1. pyosalpinx
2. adhesions
3. salpingitis
4. hematosalpinx
5. anovulation
6. ovarian cyst
7. hydrosalpinx
8. polycystic ovary syndrome

Exercise 7

1. hysteroptosis
2. leukorrhea
3. retroflexion of uterus
4. cervicitis
5. leiomyoma
6. dysplasia
7. endometriosis

Exercise 8

1. vaginal prolapse
2. vulvitis
3. vaginitis
4. vulvodynia
5. thelitis
6. mastitis
7. fibrocystic disease
8. vulvovaginitis

Exercise 9

1. amenorrhea
2. menorrhagia
3. dysmenorrhea
4. dysfunctional uterine bleeding
5. oligomenorrhea
6. premenstrual syndrome
7. menometrorrhagia
8. premenstrual dysmorphic disorder
9. polymenorrhea

Exercise 10

1. meconium
2. nuchal cord
3. placenta abruptio
4. cephalopelvic disproportion
5. ectopic pregnancy
6. abortion
7. preeclampsia
8. placenta previa
9. oligohydramnios
10. eclampsia
11. erythroblastosis fetalis

Exercise 11

1. hysterosalpingography
2. culdocentesis
3. pelvimetry
4. cervicography
5. hysteroscopy
6. colposcopy
7. mammography
8. sonohysterography
9. laparoscopy
10. culdoscopy
11. hormone levels
12. Pap smear

Exercise 12

1. human chorionic gonadotropin
2. amniocentesis
3. Apgar
4. contraction stress test
5. nonstress test
6. alpha-fetoprotein
7. congenital hypothyroidism
8. phenylketonuria
9. chorionic villus sampling

Exercise 13

1. hysteropexy
2. salpingolysis
3. bilateral oophorectomy
4. TAH-BSO
5. lumpectomy
6. pelvic exenteration
7. uterine artery embolization
8. dilation and curettage
9. colpoplasty
10. mastopexy

Exercise 14

1. tubal ligation
2. VBAC
3. episiotomy
4. vaginal delivery
5. cephalic version
6. C-section
7. sterilization

8. cerclage
9. A 10. C 11. B 12. D
13. E

Exercise 15

1. OCP
2. barrier
3. condoms
4. IUDs
5. abortifacient
6. rhythm method
7. abstinence
8. spermicides
9. ECP

Exercise 16

1. increase
2. hormone replacement therapy
3. soy proteins
4. induce
5. uterine relaxants

Exercise 17

1. H 2. D 3. F 4. B
5. G 6. E 7. C 8. A

Chapter 8 Review Questions

1. To pass on one's genetic material by producing eggs, maintaining a pregnancy, and delivering a viable neonate.
2. See Fig. 8-1.
3. ovary (oophor/o, ovari/o)
4. ovum (o/o, ov/o)
5. ovulation
6. luteinizing hormones
7. menstruation
8. menarche, menopause
9. ovarian follicles to mature and secrete estrogen, release ova
10. Estrogen and progesterone are responsible for female sex characteristics and the cyclical maintenance of the uterus for pregnancy.
11. labia (labi/o), clitoris, vaginal orifice, hymen (hymen/o), perineum (perine/o), Bartholin's glands (bartholin/o)
12. nipple (thel/o, papill/o), areola
13. lactation (lact/o, galact/o)
14. coitus, copulation
15. gestation (gravid/o, -gravida, -cyesis)
16. See Fig. 8-2.
17. human chorionic gonadotropin (hCG); prevents the corpus luteum from deteriorating
18. chorion (chorion/o), amnion (amni/o)
19. placenta
20. omphal/o, umbilic/o
21. parturition
22. A. 37 weeks
    B. premature
    C. low birth weight
23. -tocia, -para
24. oligohydraminos
25. amenorrhea
26. anovulation
27. hysteroptosis
28. leukorrhea
29. inflammation of the nipple
30. pregnancy "out of place"
31. abnormal condition of lining of uterus
32. process of turning backward
33. inflammation of the external female genitalia and the vagina
34. pus in the fallopian tube
35. meconium
36. polycystic ovary syndrome
37. abortion
38. leiomyomata (leiomyomas)
39. nuchal cord
40. preeclampsia
41. fibrocystic disease
42. menorrhagia
43. placenta placed in front of the cervical opening
44. mother's pelvis is smaller than the fetus's head
45. mammography
46. hysterosalpingography
47. culdoscopy
48. process of recording the neck of the uterus
49. instrument to visually examine the vagina
50. process of recording the uterus using ultrasound
51. detection of cervical and/or vaginal cancer
52. detection of multiple gestation and neural tube disorders of the fetus
53. used for myomectomy/polypectomy
54. detect chromosomal abnormalities
55. prediction of fetal outcome
56. fetal cardiac function
57. physical health of the newborn
58. surgical puncture to withdraw fluid from the amniotic sac for diagnostic purpose
59. If detected at birth, these conditions can be corrected. If untreated, these conditions can be detrimental or fatal.
60. bilateral oophorectomy
61. unilateral mastectomy
62. colporrhaphy
63. salpingolysis
64. episiotomy
65. pelvic exenteration
66. cerclage
67. cephalic version
68. ligation
69. dilation and curettage
70. in vitro fertilization, intracytoplasmic sperm injection (ICSI), zygote intrafallopian transfer (ZIFT)
71. estrogen and progesterone
72. tubal ligation
73. fixation of the uterus
74. destruction of adhesions in the fallopian tubes
75. incision of the vulva
76. removal of both ovaries
77. surgical repair of the vagina
78. promoting and preventing pregnancy
79. oral contraceptive pills
80. killed
81. intrauterine device
82. condom, abstinence
83. terminate a pregnancy
84. conceiving
85. to replace estrogen and progesterone to relieve symptoms of menopause
86. labor needs to be induced
87. rapid delivery
88. premenstrual syndrome
89. last menstrual period
90. 2 pregnancies, 1 delivery, 0 abortions
91. hormones
92. fetal heart rate
93. estimated date of delivery
94. intrauterine device
95. dilation and curettage
96. cervix
97. in vitro fertilization
98. papillae
99. areolae
100. ova
101. cervices
102. uteri
103. fimbriae
104. placentae
105. chorionic villi
106. Ms. Costello made an appointment to visit her gynecologist because of intense painful menstruation, dysfunctional uterine bleeding, and questions about the possibility that she might be experiencing premenstrual syndrome.
107. Anna Walker is a 37-year-old with a history of 2 pregnancies, 1 delivery, 0 abortions who is visiting her obstetrician for a surgical puncture to remove amniotic fluid for diagnostic reasons.

108. The newborn was born with an umbilical cord around his neck and was recorded as ≤2.5 kg (5 lb, 8 oz).
109. Maria Olmos presented with white discharge that was a symptom of inflammation of the cervix.
110. Ms. Robinson was treated for closure of the uterine tubes with destruction of adhesions within the fallopian tubes.
111. peri-
112. pelvic
113. bilateral
114. distal
115. greenstick
116. second
117. jejunocecostomy
118. dysuria
119. urethrolysis
120. process of measurement, uterus
121. tubes between kidneys and bladder, uterus
122. Douglas' rectouterine pouch, vagina
123. neck of uterus, vertebrae of neck
124. sprout, microorganism
125. presence of breast development in men
126. premature
127. first feces of newborn
128. fetal cord wrapped around its neck
129. neonate's cardiovascular health
130. the fetus's health due to low amount of amniotic fluid

Chapter 9 Exercises

Exercise 1

1. homeostasis
2. A. Lymphatic
   B. Immune
   C. Blood
   D. Blood
   E. Lymphatic
   F. Blood
   G. Lymphatic
   H. Blood
   I. Lymphatic

Exercise 2

1. blood cells and plasma
2. 11
3. erythrocytes, O_2 and CO_2, hemoglobin
4. millions
5. hemolysis
6. leukocytes, defend the body against disease
7. thousands
8. granulocytes, polymorphonucleocyte
9. mononuclear leukocyte, agranulocyte
10. eosinophils
11. basophils
12. neutrophils

13. C 14. D 15. B 16. A

17. liquid
18. H_2O
19. prothrombin and fibrinogen
20. thrombo, coagulation
21. prothrombin activator, thrombin, blood clot

22. G 23. L 24. W 25. Q
26. O 27. A 28. Y 29. T
30. D 31. V 32. B 33. R
34. I 35. X 36. C 37. J
38. K 39. E 40. N 41. H
42. F 43. U 44. M 45. S
46. P

Exercise 3

1. A, B, AB, O
2. antigen/antibody reaction
3. A, AB
4. universal donor, universal recipient
5. Rh

Exercise 4

1. monocytes, lymphocytes
2. They squeeze from capillaries into interstitial space.
3. right lymphatic duct, thoracic duct
4. thymus
5. spleen
6. monocytes
7. tonsils

8. D 9. A 10. I 11. F
12. E 13. C 14. H 15. G
16. B

Exercise 5

1. Nonspecific immunity is a general defense against pathogens. Specific immunity involves a recognition of a given pathogen and reaction against it.
2. Mechanical—skin, mucus. Physical—sneezing, coughing, vomiting, diarrhea. Chemical—saliva, tears, perspiration
3. phagocytosis via neutrophils and monocytes, inflammation, fever, protective proteins
4. A. viruses
   B. bacteria
   C. certain virus and cancer cells
5. bone marrow or fetal liver
6. cell-mediated
7. humoral (antibody-mediated immunity)
8. macrophages
9. agranulocyte
10. thymus
11. genetic
12. active artificial
13. passive natural
14. passive artificial
15. active natural

16. B 17. F 18. D 19. E
20. C 21. A 22. G 23. H

Exercise 6

1. I 2. J 3. C 4. E
5. F 6. A 7. G 8. H
9. D 10. B

11. sickle cell
12. autoimmune acquired hemolytic anemia
13. thalassemia
14. aplastic anemia
15. pancytopenia
16. pernicious
17. acute hemorrhagic anemia

Exercise 7

1. F 2. C 3. G 4. E
5. D 6. B 7. A

Exercise 8

1. allergy
2. autoimmune
3. immunosuppressant
4. anaphylaxis
5. mononucleosis
6. lymphopenia
7. lymphadenitis
8. hypersplenism
9. lymphocytosis
10. HIV (human immunodeficiency virus), helper T, immune

Exercise 9

1. A 2. D 3. B 4. E
5. C

Exercise 10

1. K 2. H 3. G 4. A
5. I 6. B 7. L 8. B
9. D 10. A 11. D 12. C
13. E 14. J 15. F, M

16. process of recording
17. record, vessel
18. process of recording, gland

Exercise 11

1. autologous
2. homologous
3. adenoidectomy
4. leukapheresis
5. plasmapheresis
6. splenectomy

Exercise 12

1. J 2. C 3. E 4. I
5. B 6. A 7. H 8. G
9. F 10. D

Exercise 13

1. diagnosis, Epstein-Barr virus
2. hematocrit, hemoglobin
3. acquired immunodeficiency syndrome, human immunodeficiency virus
4. estimated blood loss, cubic centimeter
5. bone marrow transplant

Chapter 9 Review Questions

1. defense
2. Answers will vary.
3. Answers will vary.
4. Blood = 45% formed elements + 55% plasma
5. erythrocyte, O_2 and CO_2 transport
6. transportation of gases and nutrients, all other body systems are involved
7. Hemoglobin is a protein-iron pigment that decomposes into hemosiderin, an iron pigment formed as a result of hemolysis.
8. granulocyte (PMN), agranulocyte (mono)
9. eosinophils, neutrophils, basophils
10. monocytes, lymphocytes
11. clot blood, platelets
12. prothrombin activator → release of Ca^+ and prothrombin → thrombin → fibrinogen → blood clot
13. water, inorganic substances, organic substances, waste products, plasma proteins
14. serum = plasma − clotting proteins
15. hematopoiesis
16. A, B, AB (universal recipient), O (universal donor)
17. antigen, agglutinogen, agglutinin
18. lymph vessel (lymphangi/o), lymph gland node (lymphaden/o), lymph (lymph/o)
19. macrophage
20. interstitial space → lymphatic capillaries → lymph nodes (glands) → right lymphatic duct or thoracic duct → venous subclavian veins → capillary
21. cytokines, lymphokines, monokines, interleukins
22. Cell-mediated immunity is a type of defense that attaches to the pathogen directly. Antibody-related immunity uses antibodies to poison the pathogen.
23. first and second, specific and nonspecific
24. Specific immunity is against one type of pathogen. Nonspecific immunity is against any pathogen.
25. dyscrasia
26. Fewer red blood cells provide less transportation for oxygen.
27. deficiency of white blood cells
28. slight increase of lymph cells
29. deficiency of iron
30. enlargement of the spleen
31. inflammation of a lymph gland
32. pancytopenia
33. leukocytosis
34. lymphadenopathy
35. lymphangitis
36. hemolytic
37. thalassemia
38. sickle cell anemia
39. hemophilia
40. mononucleosis
41. lymphedema
42. dyscrasia
43. allergy
44. anaphylaxis
45. polycythemia vera
46. diff
47. ELISA
48. hematocrit
49. Monospot
50. ESR
51. Coombs' test
52. MCH
53. PTT
54. Schilling test
55. blood cultures
56. record of lymph vessel
57. process of recording lymph gland
58. process of recording spleen
59. A. lymphangiectomy
    B. splenectomy
    C. thymectomy
    D. lymphadenectomy
60. apheresis
61. A. transfusion
    B. autotransfusion
    C. autologous transfusion
62. biopsy of lymphatic structures
63. antihistamine
64. Anticoagulants
65. Thrombolytics
66. vaccines/immunizations
67. azidothymidine (AZT)
68. cytotoxic
69. hematocrit
70. erythrocyte sedimentation rate
71. packed cell volume
72. complete blood cell count, differential WBC count
73. rhesus
74. nuclei
75. sera
76. upper left quadrant
77. lower right quadrant
78. space between the lungs
79. A. neck
    B. armpit
    C. groin
80. vomit, first
81. On physical examination, her physician observed enlargement of liver and spleen, disease of lymph glands, and massive hemorrhaging under the skin. Laboratory findings indicated deficiency of all cells. She was diagnosed with lack of formation of RBCs, and treated with red blood cells and platelet transfusions.
82. Laboratory testing revealed slight increase of white blood cells, and a lab test of blood for microorganisms was positive for staphylococci. His physician diagnosed inflammation of lymph glands.
83. Tyra Wilson worried that her weight loss, diarrhea, night sweats, and occasional fever might be symptoms of human immunodeficiency virus. After anonymous testing with a test to detect HIV types 1 and 2, she was relieved to find that she was not HIV positive.
84. Apheresis means separation of blood into components; poiesis means formation.
85. Hgb means hemoglobin; Hg means mercury.
86. Thym/o means thymus gland; thyr/o means thyroid gland.
87. Cyt/o means cell; cyst/o means bladder.
88. "pain all over his body"
89. Motrin and Darvon
90. appendix

Chapter 10 Exercises

Exercise 1

1. carry (transport)
2. heart, vessels, blood

Exercise 2

1. systemic pulmonic
2. pulmonary
3. systemic
4. CO_2

5. deoxygenated
6. away from
7. to
8. See Fig. 10-1.
9. E, G 10. F 11. B, H 12. M
13. I 14. C 15. L 16. K
17. J, D, A

Exercise 3

1. K 2. I 3. A 4. B
5. D 6. C 7. L 8. E
9. H 10. F 11. G 12. J

Exercise 4

1. Pulmonary arteries
2. tricuspid
3. mitral
4. Competent
5. ejection fraction

Exercise 5

1. diastole
2. sinus rhythm
3. SA node → AV node → bundle of His → Purkinje fibers of left and right bundle branches
4. electrocardiograph, electrocardiograph, electrocardiogram, ECG (EKG)

Exercise 6

1. nausea, ischemic pain, diaphoresis
2. DOE, SOB
3. tachycardia
4. syncope
5. thrill
6. N 7. H 8. A 9. O
10. G 11. I 12. E 13. L
14. M 15. D 16. K 17. B
18. P 19. F 20. J 21. C

Exercise 7

1. F 2. I 3. A 4. E
5. G 6. B 7. H 8. C
9. D

Exercise 8

1. C 2. D 3. B 4. A
5. left, right

Exercise 9

1. abnormal heartbeat
2. fibrillations
3. flutters
4. atrial ectopic beats
5. atrioventricular block

Exercise 10

1. heart
2. atheroma
3. angina pectoris
4. infarction
5. shortness of breath, chest pain, sense of impending doom
6. coronary artery disease
7. Infarction means tissue death; infraction means incomplete fracture.

Exercise 11

1. endocarditis
2. congestive heart failure
3. pericarditis
4. arteriosclerosis
5. atherosclerosis

Exercise 12

1. aneurysm
2. claudication
3. primary, essential
4. Secondary
5. thrombophlebitis
6. hemorrhoids
7. esophageal varices
8. peripheral artery occlusion
9. Raynaud's disease
10. varicose veins
11. D 12. G 13. F 14. B
15. A 16. E 17. C

Exercise 13

1. ECG (EKG)
2. lipid profiles
3. cardiac enzymes test
4. digital subtraction angiography
5. transesophageal echocardiography
6. radiography
7. exercise stress test
8. cardiac catheterization
9. PET scan

Exercise 14

1. atherectomy
2. CABG
3. CPR
4. hemorrhoidectomy
5. commissurotomy
6. PTCA
7. stripping, ligation, sclerotherapy
8. radiofrequency catheter ablation
9. LVAD
10. pericardiocentesis
11. L 12. I 13. O 14. P
15. K 16. T 17. C 18. D
19. E 20. N 21. R 22. J
23. S 24. A 25. M 26. F
27. Q 28. G 29. H 30. B

Exercise 15

1. C 2. A, C, D 3. A, E
4. A, D, E 5. A, D, E 6. A, E
7. B 8. F 9. G

Exercise 16

1. H 2. J 3. D 4. F
5. A 6. B 7. I 8. C
9. E 10. G

Chapter 10 Review Questions

1. Answers will vary.
2. Systemic circulation is from the heart to the cells of the body and back (excluding the lungs). Pulmonary circulation is from the heart to the lungs and back.
3. For example, if arteries are blocked, oxygen cannot be "delivered" to cells and tissue death results.
4. See Fig. 10-1.
5. by the force of the heart and the muscular structure of the arteries
6. vessels
7. the heart muscle
8. capillaries
9. away from
10. See Fig. 10-4.
11. mediastinum
12. apic/o
13. precordium
14. interatrial septum
15. endocardium
16. myocardium
17. pericardium, visceral pericardium, epicardium
18. right atrium → tricuspid valve → right ventricle → pulmonary semilunar valve → pulmonary arteries → lung capillaries → pulmonary veins → left atrium → mitral valve → left ventricle → aortic valve → aorta
19. SA node → AV node → Purkinje fibers of left and right bundle branches
20. systole
21. sphygmomanometer
22. 60-80 bpm
23. SA node
24. 120/80 to 139/84
25. stethoscope
26. ECG (EKG)
27. sinus rhythm
28. murmur
29. edema
30. shortness of breath
31. thrill

32. palpitations
33. syncope
34. pulmonary congestion
35. pallor
36. diaphoresis
37. bradycardia
38. dyspnea
39. venous distension
40. murmur
41. tachycardia
42. bruit
43. fatigue
44. cyanosis
45. holes between the bottom chambers of their hearts
46. 4
47. close
48. narrowing
49. wall defect of top chamber of the heart
50. excessive development of the ventricle
51. abnormal condition of narrowing of the aorta
52. inflammation of the valve
53. abnormal condition of blueness
54. upright breathing
55. Mitral stenosis means narrowing of the mitral valve; mitral regurgitation means backflow of blood from the left ventricle to left atrium; mitral valve prolapse means protrusion of valve leaflets back into the left atrium.
56. sinus rhythm
57. flutter
58. fibrillation
59. premature atrial contractions
60. ventricular ectopic beats
61. implantable cardiac defibrillator
62. destruction
63. sick sinus syndrome, implantable pacemaker
64. right ventricle (right bundle branch block)
65. rapid ventricular contractions
66. condition of abnormal rhythm
67. atrial contractions in abnormal rhythm
68. heart disease
69. hypoxia
70. angina
71. nitroglycerin
72. myocardial infarction
73. thrombolytic therapy
74. Both are dilated veins.
75. atherosclerosis
76. atheroma
77. atherosclerosis
78. endocarditis
79. disease of the vessels supplying blood to the heart
80. abnormal hardening of the arteries
81. tissue death of heart muscle
82. congenital
83. varicose
84. hemorrhoids
85. claudication
86. clotting and inflammation in the veins
87. high blood pressure
88. Holter monitor
89. cholesterol and triglycerides
90. myocardial infarction
91. myocardial perfusion imaging
92. echocardiography
93. size and shape
94. exercise stress test
95. Swan-Ganz catheter
96. defibrillator
97. pacemaker
98. CPR
99. MIDCAB
100. coronary artery bypass graft
101. cardiopulmonary resuscitation
102. mitral stenosis
103. left ventricular assist device
104. tying
105. radiofrequency catheter ablation
106. varicose veins
107. During MIDCAB the heart still beats during surgery; during PACAB the heart is stopped.
108. removal of fatty plaque
109. surgical repair of a coronary vessel
110. surgical puncture to remove fluid from the pericardium
111. valvuloplasty
112. commissurotomy
113. hemorrhoidectomy
114. OTC (over the counter)
115. antiadrenergics
116. anticoagulants
117. calcium channel blockers
118. ACE inhibitors
119. antiarrhythmic drugs
120. HMG-CoA reductase inhibitors
121. thrombolytics
122. antianginals (nitrates)
123. diuretics
124. clot destroyer
125. through the skin
126. against abnormal (heart) rhythms
127. transdermal nitroglycerin
128. coronary care unit, myocardial infarction
129. coronary artery disease, percutaneous transluminal coronary angioplasty
130. left carotid artery, coronary artery bypass graft
131. atrial septal defect
132. atria
133. lumina
134. apices
135. septa
136. stenoses
137. thrombi
138. Laquita Washington was born with patent ductus arteriosus that was originally detected by her doctor, who noted the presence of a continuous abnormal heart sound and fine vibrations on palpation. A left enlargement of the lower left chamber of the heart was noted on ultrasound of the heart. She was counseled as to the possibility of congestive heart failure of the disorder later in life.
139. The 72-year-old presented with advanced coronary artery disease. He had a history of cigarette smoking, high blood pressure, and blood cholesterol and triglycerides abnormalities.
140. The patient was treated with destruction of electrical pathways of the heart for his sudden, rapid contractions of the upper chambers of the heart.
141. Ms. Chong presented with breathing difficulty, pain under the breastbone, increased WBC, fever, and electrocardiography abnormalities. A diagnosis of heart inflammation was made after a chest x-ray and ultrasound of the heart.
142. A patient with varicose veins in the rectum was scheduled for a procedure to stop blood flow to an area and reroute it through nearby vessels.
143. Arteri/o means artery; atri/o means atrium; aort/o means aorta; arteriol/o means arteriole; ather/o means fatty plaque; arthr/o means joint.
144. Palpation means process of touching; palpitation means pounding of the heart.
145. Mitral regurgitation means backflow of blood to the left atrium; digestive regurgitation means backflow of the contents of the stomach.
146. Stenosis means narrowing; sclerosis means hardening.

147. Infarction means tissue death; infraction means breaking a bone.
148. apex
149. mediastinum
150. afferent, efferent
151. superior
152. inferior
153. frontal (coronal)
154. uterus
155. stenosis
156. heart muscle (cardiomy/o), skeletal muscle (rhabdomy/o), smooth muscle (leiomy/o)
157. vasectomy
158. A. difficult breathing
B. profuse sweating
C. high blood pressure
159. substernal (under the breastbone)
160. She had hypercholesterolemia.
161. echocardiogram
162. coronary artery bypass graft

Chapter 11 Exercises

Exercise 1

1. A. O_2
B. CO_2
C. pH
D. lungs
E. sound
F. olfaction

Exercise 2

1. nasal cavity, oropharynx, larynx
2. Answers will vary.
3. surfactant
4. visceral, parietal

5. T	6. N	7. S
8. V	9. O, E	10. Q
11. H	12. C	13. Z
14. AA	15. EE	16. G
17. R	18. D, L	19. U
20. B	21. X	22. F, DD
23. J, P	24. BB	25. Y
26. I	27. CC	28. W
29. K	30. M	31. A

Exercise 3

1. coughing up blood
2. nosebleed
3. hiccup
4. tachypnea
5. make sounds
6. apnea
7. pain
8. crackles
9. pleurodynia
10. wheezing
11. clubbing

12. D	13. M	14. A	15. B, L
16. G	17. K	18. I	19. C
20. E	21. F	22. H	23. J

Exercise 4

1. laryngitis
2. rhinosalpingitis
3. epiglottitis
4. coryza
5. URI
6. deviated septum
7. vocal polyps
8. Pleurisy
9. Croup
10. Atelectasis
11. Emphysema
12. Asthma
13. pulmonary abscess
14. bronchiectasis
15. pneumoconiosis
16. Cystic fibrosis
17. bradypnea
18. eupnea
19. flail chest

20. E	21. N	22. K	23. P
24. O	25. L	26. I	27. J
28. C	29. M	30. G	31. D
32. F	33. A	34. H	35. B

Exercise 5

1. Mantoux skin test
2. ABG
3. sweat test
4. lung ventilation scan
5. pulmonary angiography
6. Pulse oximetry

7. G	8. F	9. A	10. I
11. H	12. J	13. D	14. E
15. C	16. B		

Exercise 6

1. A. lobectomy
B. laryngectomy
C. tonsillectomy
D. adenoidectomy
2. A. rhinoplasty
B. septoplasty
C. bronchoplasty
3. endotracheal intubation
4. oxygen

5. K	6. O	7. B	8. C
9. L	10. M	11. J	12. D
13. I	14. A	15. N	16. E
17. G	18. H	19. F	

Exercise 7

1. C	2. E	3. D	4. A
5. B			

6. nebulizer
7. inhaler
8. ventilator

Exercise 8

1. chest x-ray, right middle lobe
2. purified protein derivative, tuberculosis
3. upper respiratory infection
4. chronic obstructive pulmonary disease, dyspnea on exertion
5. coal worker's pneumoconiosis

Chapter 11 Review Questions

1. make sounds
2. deliver O_2 to cells
3. remove CO_2 from body
4. help regulate pH of blood
5. nose (nas/o, rhin/o) → throat (pharyng/o) → voicebox (laryng/o) → windpipe (trache/o) → bronchus (bronchi/o) → bronchiole (bronchiol/o) → alveolus (alveol/o) → capillaries → blood (hem/o, hemat/o) → cells (cyt/o)
6. External respiration is the exchange of gases between the organism and the external world. Internal respiration is gas exchange within the body.
7. inhale, inspire
8. exhale, expire
9. epiglottis
10. larynx
11. See Fig. 11-1, *A*.
12. See Fig. 11-2.
13. rhinorrhea
14. epistaxis
15. fatigue
16. pyrexia
17. shortness of breath
18. Cheyne-Stokes respiration
19. cyanosis
20. wheezing
21. sputum
22. stridor
23. clubbing
24. deviated septum
25. hypoxia
26. rhonchi
27. rhinomycosis
28. multidrug-resistant TB
29. croup
30. pulmonary edema
31. pneumothorax
32. pneumonia
33. tuberculosis
34. pleurisy
35. atelectasis
36. condition of deficient oxygen
37. spitting blood
38. difficulty making sounds
39. inflammation of the voicebox

40. abnormal condition of dust in the lungs
41. pus in the pleural cavity (chest)
42. hypercapnia
43. rhinorrhea
44. tachypnea
45. bronchitis
46. rhinosalpingitis
47. auscultation and percussion
48. sputum culture
49. tuberculosis
50. mediastinoscopy
51. stethoscope
52. spirometer
53. cystic fibrosis
54. arterial blood gases (ABG)
55. how air is distributed in the lung
56. instrument to measure breathing
57. visual examination of the bronchi
58. process of recording the vessels of the lung
59. laryngoscopy
60. spirometry
61. ultrasonography
62. establish/maintain an airway
63. ventilator, cannula
64. lobectomy
65. bronchoplasty
66. tracheotomy
67. adenoidectomy
68. surgical puncture to remove fluid from the pleural cavity
69. surgical repair of the partition (between the nares)
70. excision of the tonsils
71. rhinoplasty
72. tracheostomy
73. sinusotomy
74. antitussive
75. antihistamine
76. inhaler or nebulizer
77. decongestant
78. bronchodilator/antiasthmatic
79. shortness of breath
80. left lower lobe
81. clear to auscultation
82. chest x-ray, anteroposterior
83. dyspnea on exertion
84. sinuses
85. bronchi
86. alveoli
87. pleurae
88. larynges
89. pharynges
90. Sudden, episodic difficulty with breathing, shortness of breath, and whistling sounds in the lungs were signs that Sari had asthma.
91. The patient's difficulty making sounds and inflammation of the voicebox were part of an upper respiratory infection.
92. The doctor termed the high-pitched breathing in sound heard when the baby inhaled as a high-pitched inspiratory sound, a sign of acute viral infection of early childhood.
93. The physician noted fever, difficult breathing, and chest pain before recording a working diagnosis of fluid in the pleural cavity.
94. After 3 days of severe inflammation of the throat, the patient had a lab test for microorganisms to determine the pathogen.
95. tops
96. complicated
97. psoriasis
98. micturition
99. dysphonia
100. Bronchi are tubes that bifurcate into lungs; brachi/o means arm.
101. Ox/i means oxygen; oxy- means rapid.
102. eustachian tube, fallopian tube
103. One listens, not looks, with a stethoscope.
104. slight profuse sweating, blueness around the mouth
105. through the earlobe or fingertip
106. wheezes (whistling sounds), rhonchi (rumbling sound heard when airways are blocked)
107. age
108. to measure breathing capacity
109. handheld nebulizer

Chapter 12 Exercises

Exercise 1

1. interpreting
2. endocrine
3. homeostasis

Exercise 2

1. central, peripheral (CNS, PNS)
2. transmit, to
3. efferent, from
4. somatic, autonomic

Exercise 3

1. stimulus → dendrite → cell body → axon → synapse

2. E	3. C	4. F	5. A
6. B	7. D		

Exercise 4

1. H	2. J	3. F	4. A
5. C	6. I	7. D	8. B
9. G	10. E	11. H	12. B
13. A	14. D	15. C	16. F
17. I	18. E	19. G	

20. pia mater → subarachnoid space → arachnoid membrane → subdural space → dura mater
21. 12, 31
22. Afferent
23. parasympathetic

Exercise 5

1. D	2. H	3. I	4. E
5. A	6. C	7. G	8. B
9. F	10. D	11. A	12. C
13. E	14. B		

Exercise 6

1. spina bifida
2. Huntington's chorea
3. hydrocephalus
4. Tay-Sachs
5. cerebral palsy
6. coma
7. concussion
8. cerebral contusion
9. hematoma

Exercise 7

1. Bell's palsy
2. Tourette's syndrome
3. Parkinson's disease
4. amyotrophic lateral sclerosis
5. Alzheimer's disease
6. Guillain-Barré syndrome

7. E	8. C	9. B	10. A
11. D			

Exercise 8

1. radiculitis
2. meningitis
3. sciatica
4. hemiplegia
5. transient ischemic attack
6. para

7. C	8. E	9. A	10. F
11. D	12. B	13. G	

14. thrombus, embolus, cerebral hemorrhage
15. CVA—sequelae last more than 2 hours; TIA—sequelae last less than 24 hours

Exercise 9

1. M	2. L	3. G	4. A
5. E	6. J	7. Q	8. D
9. K	10. C	11. O	12. F
13. H	14. B	15. N	16. P
17. I			

18. gait assessment rating scale

19. cerebrospinal fluid analysis
20. spinal tap
21. electroencephalogram
22. Babinski's sign
23. polysomnography
24. cerebral angiography
25. echoencephalography
26. Myelography

Exercise 10

1. P	2. F	3. H	4. J
5. Y	6. Q	7. A	8. X
9. L	10. G	11. R	12. M
13. D	14. T	15. U	16. B
17. V	18. W	19. S	20. O
21. C	22. K	23. I	24. E

25. N
26. TENS
27. CSF shunt
28. nerve block
29. vagotomy

Exercise 11

1. L	2. K	3. J	4. F
5. C	6. I	7. B	8. D
9. E	10. G	11. A	12. H

Exercise 12

1. lumbar puncture, cerebrospinal fluid
2. second cervical vertebra
3. magnetic resonance imaging, multiple sclerosis
4. polysomnography
5. activities of daily living, cerebrovascular accident

Chapter 12 Review Questions

1. The nervous system functions to sense, interpret, and act on internal and external stimuli to maintain homeostasis. Paralysis inhibits a person's ability to sense his or her environment.
2. The central nervous system consists of the brain and spinal cord. The peripheral nervous system consists of all other nerves divided into cranial and spinal nerves.
3. See Fig. 12-3 and Fig. 12-4.
4. afferent
5. meninges: dura mater → arachnoid membrane → pia mater
6. root
7. plexus
8. neurotransmitter
9. glia (neuroglia)
10. cerebrum
11. cerebellum
12. amnesia
13. insomnia
14. vasovagal attack
15. aura
16. dysarthria (dysphagia)
17. gait
18. ageusia
19. hydrocephalus
20. syncope
21. meningitis
22. Alzheimer's disease
23. Lou Gehrig's disease
24. quadriplegia
25. spina bifida
26. CVA
27. polyneuritis
28. encephalitis
29. anosmia
30. excessive sleep condition
31. seizure of sleep
32. inflammation of nerve root
33. CSF analysis
34. single photon emission computed tomography
35. CT scan
36. multiple sleep latency test, narcolepsy
37. stroke
38. process of recording the spinal cord
39. process of recording arteries of the cerebrum
40. process of recording many functions of sleep
41. activities of daily living
42. stereotactic radiosurgery
43. shunt
44. pain management
45. neurectomy
46. craniotomy
47. neurorrhaphy
48. destruction of a nerve
49. incision of a nerve root
50. stabilization of the vertebrae
51. anticonvulsant
52. stroke risk reduction drugs
53. neuroprotective agents
54. analgesics
55. antipyretic
56. cerebrovascular accident
57. electroencephalogram
58. positron emission tomography, Alzheimer's disease
59. lumbar puncture, between the third and fourth lumbar vertebrae
60. Parkinson's disease
61. gyri
62. stimuli
63. sulci
64. ganglia (ganglion)
65. thrombi
66. Mr. O'Connor had a right-sided stroke that affected the opposite side of his body. His symptoms included slight paralysis of half the body and difficulty speaking.
67. Due to a blow on the head, the patient sustained a mass of blood above the dura mater.
68. The patient reported dizziness and fainting before her arrival at the ED.
69. The baby had an abnormal opening of the spine that resulted in a protrusion of the meninges and spinal cord.
70. The neonate's abnormal accumulation of cerebrospinal fluid in the brain was treated with a tube to drain the excess cerebrospinal fluid.
71. scanty amniotic fluid
72. vesicoureteral reflex
73. transverse
74. hypothalamus
75. instrument to cut skin; skin surface area supplied by a single afferent spinal nerve; mesodermal layer
76. A. record of the spinal cord
    B. tumor of the bone marrow
    C. inflammation of bone and bone marrow
    D. herniation of the meninges and the spinal cord
    E. inflammation of the spinal cord
    F. bone marrow cell
    G. abnormal formation of spinal cord
77. Dysarthria means difficult, abnormal speech. Dysarthrosis means disorder of a joint.
78. A. bundle branch block, blood brain barrier
    B. multiple sclerosis, mitral stenosis, musculoskeletal
79. dizziness, fainting
80. blood condition of excessive cholesterol
81. benign prostatic hyperplasia with transurethral resection of the prostate
82. incoordination

Chapter 13 Exercises

Exercise 1

1. American Psychiatric Association
2. DSM
3. 10
4. spirituality
5. behavioral

Exercise 2

1. J	2. I	3. N	4. O
5. K	6. C	7. D	8. E
9. M	10. G	11. B	12. H
13. L	14. A	15. F	

16. mood
17. labile
18. projection

Exercise 3

1. severe
2. Asperger's syndrome
3. Tourette's syndrome
4. conduct disorder
5. mild
6. moderate
7. attention deficit hyperactivity disorder
8. autism
9. oppositional defiant disorder
10. Rett's disorder

Exercise 4

1. dementia
2. alcohol
3. inhalants
4. controlling substance abuse
5. schizophrenia
6. dream
7. hallucinations, delusions
8. persistent delusional
9. disorganized

Exercise 5

1. social phobia
2. claustrophobia
3. generalized anxiety disorder
4. obsessive-compulsive disorder
5. posttraumatic stress disorder
6. dissociative identity disorder
7. hypochondriacal disorder
8. bipolar disorder
9. depressive disorder
10. hypomania
11. cyclothymia
12. dysthymia
13. somnambulism
14. satyriasis
15. premature ejaculation
16. hypersomnia
17. anorexia nervosa
18. pyromania
19. paranoid
20. sadomasochism
21. kleptomania

Exercise 6

1. D	2. B	3. F	4. C
5. G	6. A	7. E	

Exercise 7

1. behavioral
2. light therapy
3. ECT
4. psychoanalysis
5. cognitive therapy

Exercise 8

1. G	2. C	3. E	4. I
5. D	6. H	7. B	8. A
9. F			

Exercise 9

1. seasonal affective disorder
2. generalized anxiety disorder
3. mental retardation, intelligence quotient, Weschler Adult Intelligence Scale
4. attention deficit hyperactivity disorder
5. posttraumatic stress disorder

Chapter 13 Review Questions

1. American Psychiatric Association, *Diagnostic and Statistical Manual of Mental Disorders*
2. Answers will vary.
3. hallucinations
4. depression
5. delusion
6. illusion
7. dementia
8. euthymia
9. akathisia
10. reduced
11. a widely changeable emotional state
12. libido
13. catatonia
14. defense mechanisms
15. hallucination
16. delirium
17. depression
18. Euphoria is an exaggerated sense of well-being; euthymia is a normal range of emotions.
19. illusion
20. dependence syndrome
21. schizophrenia
22. schizotypal disorder
23. psychotic
24. affective
25. mania, depression
26. hypersomnia, insomnia
27. sleep terrors, somnambulism
28. a mild chronic depression of mood
29. claustrophobia—fear of enclosed spaces
30. obsessive-compulsive disorder
31. posttraumatic stress disorder
32. dissociative identity disorder
33. bulimia nervosa
34. personality disorders
35. mild
36. conduct disorder
37. Tourette's syndrome
38. fear of heights
39. condition of sexual attraction to children
40. condition of well mind
41. condition of lack of pleasure
42. condition of babbling words repetitively
43. condition of inability to sit still
44. "madness" of setting fires
45. hypersomnia
46. hyperkinesis
47. euthymia
48. oneiric
49. claustrophobia
50. PET scan
51. clinical disorders, MR and personality disorders, general medical conditions, psychosocial environmental problems, global assessment of functioning
52. MMPI
53. TAT
54. intelligence
55. electroconvulsive therapy, affective disorders
56. cognitive
57. behavioral
58. substance abuse
59. seasonal affective disorder
60. anxiolytic
61. antidepressant
62. anticonvulsant
63. antipsychotic
64. nosotropic
65. stimulant
66. sedative-hypnotic
67. Food and Drug Administration
68. She is aware of who she is, the date, and where she is.
69. mental retardation
70. obsessive-compulsive disorder
71. delirium tremens alcohol
72. generalized anxiety disorder
73. The patient appeared to have a <u>diminished range of emotions</u>, <u>a depressed mood</u>, and complained of an <u>inability to sleep</u>.
74. The 15-year-old patient was admitted with a diagnosis of an <u>eating disorder in which the patient pathologically restricts his nutrition intake</u>.

75. Ariel explained that it would be difficult to go to school because she was afraid of going out to crowded places.
76. The patient's mother insisted she see a doctor regarding her sleepwalking.
77. The patient was diagnosed with an uncontrollable impulse to set fires after detectives had arrested him in connection with three intentionally set fires in his community.
78. mind, diaphragm
79. thymus gland, mind
80. condition of the mind
81. excessive movement
82. aphasia
83. tachycardia
84. esophageal varices
85. narcolepsy
86. electroencephalogram
87. depression
88. no
89. gastroesophageal reflux disorder
90. antidepressants
91. cognitive therapy

Chapter 14 Exercises

Exercise 1

1. B 2. G, E 3. A, I 4. C
5. H 6. D, F 7. K 8. J
9. orbit
10. canthi
11. palpebration
12. meibomian
13. lacrimation
14. extra-

Exercise 2

1. J 2. L 3. I, M 4. B
5. B 6. K 7. H 8. E
9. F 10. H 11. D 12. G
13. A 14. G 15. C
16. nervous
17. uvea
18. sclera
19. aqueous
20. cones
21. fovea

Exercise 3

1. D 2. I 3. F 4. B
5. A 6. E 7. G 8. J
9. C 10. H
11. emmetropia
12. esotropia
13. blepharedema
14. dacryocystitis
15. keratoconjunctivitis sicca

Exercise 4

1. J 2. I 3. F 4. G
5. C 6. H 7. B 8. A
9. E 10. D
11. keratitis
12. achromatopsia
13. nyctalopia
14. synechia
15. hemianopsia

Exercise 5

1. E 2. H 3. F 4. B
5. I 6. G 7. C 8. D
9. A 10. J 11. K

Exercise 6

1. I 2. H 3. N 4. A
5. K 6. J 7. M 8. E
9. G 10. L 11. O 12. F
13. C 14. D 15. B

Exercise 7

1. C 2. E 3. B 4. A
5. D

Exercise 8

1. myopia, left eye, with glasses
2. laser in situ keratomileusis, photorefractive keratectomy
3. visual acuity
4. age-related macular degeneration
5. in each eye
6. intraocular pressure, within normal limits
7. visual field

Exercise 9

1. J, F 2. C 3. D 4. B
5. I 6. G 7. H, K 8. E
9. A
10. auditory canal, middle ear, labyrinth
11. malleus, incus, stapes
12. cochlea
13. vestibule and semicircular canals

Exercise 10

1. A 2. H 3. K 4. G
5. F 6. I 7. B 8. D
9. C 10. E 11. J 12. L
13. sensorineural hearing loss
14. impacted cerumen
15. Ménière's disease

Exercise 11

1. E 2. D 3. F 4. A
5. B 6. C

Exercise 12

1. E 2. B 3. C 4. A
5. D

Exercise 13

1. C 2. D 3. A 4. B

Exercise 14

1. E 2. C 3. A 4. D
5. B

Chapter 14 Review Questions

1. palpebration
2. lacrimation
3. cornea
4. extraorbital
5. refraction
6. tympanic membrane
7. stapes, malleus, incus
8. cochlea
9. stapes
10. tempor/o
11. myopia
12. See Fig. 14-2.
13. hordeolum
14. epiphora
15. diabetic retinopathy
16. tinnitus
17. impacted cerumen
18. otitis externa
19. otosclerosis
20. presbycusis
21. Ménière's disease
22. macrotia
23. otalgia (otodynia)
24. otorrhea
25. xerophthalmia
26. diplopia
27. condition of unequally sized pupils
28. inflammation of the middle ear
29. abnormal hearing
30. condition of no lens
31. condition of lack of color vision
32. ophthalmic ultrasonography
33. visual acuity test
34. gonioscopy
35. Amsler grid
36. ophthalmoscopy
37. tonometry
38. Weber tuning fork test
39. tympanometry
40. speech audiometry
41. auditory brainstem response
42. blepharorrhaphy
43. LASIK
44. exenteration of the eye
45. epikeratophakia
46. intracapsular lens extraction
47. myringotomy (tympanotomy)
48. otoplasty
49. tympanostomy
50. cochlear implant
51. blepharochalasis

52. iridotomy
53. hemianopsia
54. incision of the cornea
55. surgical repair of the eyelids
56. removal of the stapes
57. lubricants
58. mydriatics
59. topical anesthetics
60. cycloplegics
61. glaucoma
62. ceruminolytic
63. otics
64. antihistamines/decongestants
65. antibacterials
66. miotics
67. Em/EM
68. OS
69. astigmatism
70. Pupil equal, round, reactive to light and accomodation
71. intraocular pressure
72. AD
73. otitis media
74. oto
75. with glasses
76. VA
77. pinnae
78. stapedes
79. mallei
80. irides
81. canthi
82. conjunctivae
83. sclerae
84. corneas
85. Maria appeared at the ED complaining of sensitivity to light, an overflow of tears, and inflammation of conjunctivae.
86. The baby appeared inconsolable when her mother brought her to the pediatrician for what was diagnosed as a middle ear infection.
87. An auto accident victim presented at the ED with unequally sized pupils, blood in the anterior chamber of the eye, and a closed ear injury after being thrown from his vehicle.
88. When the child had his first full eye exam, it was discovered that he had slight color blindness and normal vision.
89. The 80-year-old patient evaluated by one who specializes in the study of hearing loss was found to have loss of hearing common in old age.
90. The patient with condition of abnormal intraocular pressure was tested with measurement of pressure to measure her intraocular pressure.
91. medial
92. anterior
93. exophthalmos
94. Pap test, mammography
95. dyspepsia
96. leukocytosis
97. Oral means pertaining to the mouth; aural means pertaining to the ears.
98. Exotropia means eye(s) turned outward; esotropia means eye(s) turned inward.
99. sensitivity to light
100. fallopian tubes, eustachian tubes
101. Palpebrate means to blink; palpate means to examine by touch; palpitate means to pulsate rapidly.
102. Malleus is an ossicle of the ear; malleolus is a process of the tibia and fibula.
103. Diplopia means double vision; asthenopia means weakness of eye muscles; cephalgia means headache.
104. extraocular movements (EOM), each eye (OU), left eye (OS), right eye (OD)
105. nearsightedness with a malcurvature of the lens
106. Goldmann applanation tonometry
107. pertaining to near the border of the sclera and cornea

Chapter 15 Exercises

Exercise 1
1. circulatory, hormones

Exercise 2
1. hypophysis
2. hypothalamus
3. adenohypophysis
4. somatotropin
5. milk production
6. ADH, neurohypophysis
7. adrenal cortex

Exercise 3
1. metabolism, calcium
2. thyroxine
3. Calcitonin
4. parathyroid, calcium

Exercise 4
1. kidneys
2. medulla, cortex
3. steroids
4. sympathomimetic
5. electrolytes
6. secondary sex
7. cortisol
8. dopamine

Exercise 5
1. thymus
2. pancreas, glucose
3. melatonin
4. insulin and glucagon

5. S	6. G	7. L	8. C
9. A	10. W	11. R	12. F
13. X	14. E	15. I	16. J
17. B	18. O	19. K	20. N
21. P	22. D	23. M	24. V
25. T	26. H	27. Y	28. U
29. Q			

Exercise 6
1. hormones
2. medulla
3. thyroid
4. cortex
5. pituitary
6. Hypoparathyroidism
7. thyroid
8. islets of Langerhans

9. H	10. L	11. K	12. I
13. C	14. E	15. P	16. Q
17. F	18. D	19. O	20. A
21. N	22. M	23. G	24. J
25. B			

Exercise 7
1. ultrasonography
2. magnetic resonance imaging
3. A1c
4. total calcium
5. urine glucose

Exercise 8
1. adrenalectomy
2. parathyroidectomy
3. pancreatectomy
4. thyroidectomy

Exercise 9

1. C	2. A	3. D	4. B

Exercise 10

1. E	2. C	3. F	4. B
5. G	6. A	7. D	

Chapter 15 Review Questions

1. The endocrine system helps the body balance and coordinate its various functions.
2. See Fig. 15-1.

3. The hypophysis is composed of the anterior lobe (adenohypophysis) and posterior lobe (neurohypophysis). This gland secretes hormones that direct other endocrine glands.
4. Hormones can effect an action only on cells with receptor sites for those particular chemical messengers.
5. A. regulates body metabolism, amount of calcium in blood
   B. regulate calcium in bloodstream
   C. regulates blood volume and pressure, reactions to stress, secondary sex characteristics
   D. causes fight or flight response
   E. regulate blood glucose levels
   F. plays role in body's immune function
   G. affect reproductive functions
   H. thought responsible for inducing sleep
6. adrenal cortex
7. adrenal medulla
8. islets of Langerhans
9. adrenal cortex
10. thyroid
11. neurohypophysis
12. adenohypophysis
13. enlargement of the extremities
14. condition of deficient potassium in the blood
15. condition of abnormal feeling
16. condition of lacking an appetite
17. condition of excessive sodium in the blood
18. hyperglycemia
19. hypocalcemia
20. glycosuria
21. anorexia
22. hyperparathyroidism
23. glucose utilization
24. thyroid
25. diabetes mellitus
26. parathyroid function, calcium metabolism, or cancerous conditions
27. extremities, forehead, jaw, nose
28. thyroidectomy
29. adrenalectomy
30. parathyroidectomy
31. hypophysectomy
32. pancreatectomy
33. vasopressin
34. Synthroid
35. prednisone
36. insulin
37. fasting blood sugar, glucose tolerance test, diabetes mellitus (DM)
38. thyroid function tests
39. antidiuretic hormone
40. GH
41. cortices
42. thyrotoxicoses
43. After experiencing excessive urination, excessive eating, and excessive thirst, Tilda was diagnosed with diabetes mellitus.
44. Victor was treated for excess secretion of thyroid with symptoms of protrusion of eyes, rapid heartbeat, and lack of appetite.
45. Soo Lin presented with excessive body hair, easy bruising, excessive blood sugar, and deficient potassium in blood. She was subsequently diagnosed with Cushing's disease.
46. A 45-year-old patient was seen with complaints of high blood pressure, excessive calcium in the blood, kidney stones, and excessive urination.
47. A female patient is being treated with Synthroid for deficient thyroid function. Symptoms were fatigue, dry skin, slow heartbeat, and weight gain.
48. abnormal condition of dust in the lungs
49. A cesarean section is a removal of fetus through an abdominal incision. Placenta previa is a malplacement of the placenta over the cervix.
50. cranial
51. study of four. There are four heart defects present in this condition.
52. urinary tract infection, urinalysis, pus in urine
53. gland
54. adrenal gland
55. to turn
56. to nourish
57. thyroid gland
58. thymus gland
59. hormone produced by neurohypophysis
60. rapid delivery
61. excessive urination
62. polydipsia
63. A. fasting blood sugar
    B. glucose tolerance test
    C. urinalysis
64. insulin
65. Type 2

Chapter 16 Exercises

Exercise 1

1. F 2. H 3. J 4. G
5. B 6. E 7. A 8. I
9. D 10. C
11. malignant
12. carcinoma
13. sarcoma
14. myeloma
15. well
16. grading
17. staging
18. primary

Exercise 2

1. G 2. J 3. L 4. M
5. O 6. I 7. K 8. N
9. F 10. E 11. D 12. B
13. A 14. C 15. H
16. rhabdomyoma
17. basal cell carcinoma
18. benign
19. nephroma
20. malignant

Exercise 3

1. packs
2. history
3. tumor markers
4. biopsy
5. breast

Exercise 4

1. brachytherapy
2. mapping
3. sentinel
4. en bloc resection
5. margins
6. immunotherapy
7. CAM

Exercise 5

1. protocol
2. kill
3. cycle
4. antineoplastic hormones
5. alkylating agents
6. antimetabolites
7. mitotic inhibitors

Exercise 6

1. biopsy
2. grade 4
3. cancer, fecal occult blood test
4. certified tumor registrar, tumor, nodes, metastases
5. single photon emission computed tomography, metastases

Chapter 16 Review Questions

1. disruption of normal cell reproduction that triggers unregulated growth
2. Benign cancers are encapsulated, slow growing, do not metastasize, and are well differentiated. Malignant cancers are rapid growing, anaplastic, invasive, and metastasize.
3. Both mean a departure from normal formation of cells for intended cell function.
4. Staging measures the extent of disease and is important to determine the treatment.
5. Carcinoma is cancer of epithelial/endothelial tissue; sarcoma is cancer of connective tissue; lymphoma/leukemia is cancer of lymph and blood.
6. They are cancerous tumors.
7. They are tumors.
8. hypernephroma, hepatoma, thymoma, lymphoma, seminoma
9. osteosarcoma
10. rhabdomyoma
11. adenocarcinoma
12. benign tumor of cartilage
13. tumor of the nerves
14. excessive formation
15. 20
16. PAP, PSA
17. CA125
18. CEA
19. hCG
20. NSE
21. exfoliative
22. needle aspiration
23. stereotactic mammography
24. nuclear scans
25. the tumor only
26. tumor and lymph nodes
27. removal of clinically involved lymph nodes
28. first node of lymphatic drainage
29. no cancer
30. radiation with beads placed directly on cancer to destroy it
31. chemotherapy
32. defense system
33. blood
34. CAM
35. protocol
36. stimulate a patient's own immune system
37. preventing cancer cells from obtaining nutrients
38. multiplying and dividing
39. antibiotics
40. duplication
41. diagnosis, cancer, biopsy
42. breast self-examination
43. tumor, nodes, metastases
44. certified tumor registrar, metastases
45. fecal occult blood test
46. The cancer registry student had four cases to abstract: one testicular cancer, one cancer of the bone marrow, and two glandular cancers of the lung.
47. The pathologist described the cancer as appearing to have cells that retain most of their intended function.
48. The patient was diagnosed with spreading beyond control breast cancer.
49. The test for vaginal and cervical cancer revealed severe abnormal formation of the cervical cells.
50. The breast cancer patient was treated with removal of the tumor, treatment with radiation, and drug therapy.
51. long-term, part farthest from the hip, cancer of the bone
52. breast self-examination
53. abnormally formed birthmarks
54. one-sided
55. pointed area (top of the lung)
56. Sarc/o means cancer of connective tissue and flesh; sacr/o means the vertebrae between the lumbar spine and coccyx.
57. test for vaginal and cervical cancer, test for prostate cancer
58. sigmoid colon cancer
59. colonoscopy
60. sigmoid colectomy, appendectomy
61. nodes were negative for cancer

Index

C

E

F

G

M

N

O

Q

R

T

U

X

Z